# Annual Review of Biomedical Engineering

Production Editor: JENNIFER JONGSMA
Bibliographic Quality Control: MARY A. GLASS
Electronic Content Coordinator: SUZANNE K. MOSES
Subject Indexer: CHERI D. WALSH

# Annual Review of Biomedical Engineering

VOLUME 6, 2004

MARTIN L. YARMUSH, *Editor*
Center for Engineering in Medicine
Massachusetts General Hospital/Harvard Medical School, Boston

KENNETH R. DILLER, *Associate Editor*
The University of Texas at Austin

MEHMET TONER, *Associate Editor*
Center for Engineering in Medicine
Massachusetts General Hospital/Harvard Medical School, Boston

www.annualreviews.org    science@annualreviews.org    650-493-4400

ANNUAL REVIEWS
4139 El Camino Way • P.O. Box 10139 • Palo Alto, California 94303-0139

ANNUAL REVIEWS
Palo Alto, California, USA



International Standard Serial Number: 1523-9829
International Standard Book Number: 0-8243-3506-6



TYPESET BY TECHBOOKS, FAIRFAX, VA
PRINTED AND BOUND BY MALLOY INCORPORATED, ANN ARBOR, MI

Annual Review of Biomedical Engineering
Volume 6, 2004

# CONTENTS

# Related Articles

From the ***Annual Review of Biochemistry***, Volume 73 (2004)

*Nuclear Magnetic Resonance Spectroscopy of High-Molecular-Weight Proteins*, Vitali Tugarinov, Peter M. Hwang, and Lewis E. Kay

*The Molecular Mechanics of Eukaryotic Translation*, Lee D. Kapp and Jon R. Lorsch

*Mechanical Processes in Biochemistry*, Carlos Bustamante, Yann R. Chemla, Nancy R. Forde, and David Izhaky

*Analyzing Cellular Biochemistry in Terms of Molecular Networks*, Yu Xia, Haiyuan Yu, Ronald Jansen, Michael Seringhaus, Sarah Baxter, Dov Greenbaum, Hongyu Zhao, and Mark Gerstein

From the ***Annual Review of Biophysics and Biomolecular Structure***, Volume 33 (2004)

*A Function-Based Framework for Understanding Biological Systems*, Jeffrey D. Thomas, Taesik Lee, and Nam P. Suh

*Three-Dimensional Electron Microscopy at Molecular Resolution*, Sriram Subramaniam and Jacqueline L.S. Milne

*Taking X-Ray Diffraction to the Limit: Macromolecular Structures from Femtosecond X-Ray Pulses and Differentiation Microscopy of Cells with Synchrotron Radiation*, Jianwei Miao, Henry N. Chapman, Janos Kirz, David Sayre, and Keith O. Hodgson

*Rotation of $F_1$-ATPase: How an ATP-Driven Molecular Machine May Work*, Kazuhiko Kinosita, Jr., Kengo Adachi, and Hiroyasu Itoh

*Model Systems, Lipid Rafts, and Cell Membranes*, Kai Simons and Winchil L.C. Vaz

*Mass Spectral Analysis in Proteomics*, John R. Yates III

*The Thermodynamics of DNA Structural Motifs*, John SantaLucia, Jr. and Donald Hicks

From the ***Annual Review of Cell and Developmental Biology***, Volume 19 (2003)

*The Dynamic and Motile Properties of Intermediate Filaments*, Brian T. Helfand, Lynne Chang, and Robert D. Goldman

*Branching Morphogenesis of the Drosophila Tracheal System*, Amin Ghabrial, Stefan Luschnig, Mark M. Metzstein, and Mark A. Krasnow

*Adhesion-Dependent Cell Mechanosensitivity*, Alexander D. Bershadsky, Nathalie Q. Balaban, and Benjamin Geiger

From the ***Annual Review of Fluid Mechanics***, Volume 36 (2004)

*Biofluid Mechanics in Flexible Tubes*, James B. Grotberg and Oliver E. Jensen

*Engineering Flows in Small Devices: Microfluidics Toward A Lab-on-a-Chip*, H.A. Stone, A.D. Stroock, and A. Ajdari

From the ***Annual Review of Genomics and Human Genetics***, Volume 4 (2003)

*Gene Annotation: Prediction and Testing*, Jennifer L. Ashurst and John E. Collins

From the ***Annual Review of Medicine***, Volume 55 (2004)

*The Impact of the Completed Human Genome Sequence on the Development of Novel Therapeutics for Human Disease*, Christopher P. Austin

*Progress in Antisense Technology*, Stanley T. Crooke

*Serum Proteomics in Cancer Diagnosis and Management*, Kevin P. Rosenblatt, Peter Bryant-Greenwood, J. Keith Killian, Arpita Mehta, David Geho, Virginia Espina, Emanuel F. Petricoin III, and Lance A. Liotta

*Beta-Cell Replacement for Type I Diabetes*, Peter G. Stock and Jeffrey A. Bluestone

*Cochlear Implantation for the Treatment of Deafness*, Benjamin J. Copeland and Harold C. Pillsbury III

*Drug-Eluting Stents*, T. Cooper Woods and Andrew R. Marks

*New Approaches to Hemodialysis*, Andreas Pierratos

*The Impact of Minimally Invasive Surgical Techniques*, Sir Ara Darzi and Yaron Munz

*Basic Advances and New Avenues in Therapy of Spinal Cord Injury*, Bruce H. Dobkin and Leif A. Havton

From the ***Annual Review of Neuroscience***, Volume 27 (2004)

*Plasticity of the Spinal Neural Circuitry After Injury*, V. Reggie Edgerton, Niranjala J.K. Tillakaratne, Allison J. Bigbee, Ray D. de Leon, and Roland R. Roy

*Cortical Neural Prosthetics*, Andrew B. Schwartz

From the ***Annual Review of Physical Chemistry***, Volume 55 (2004)

*Single-Molecule Fluorescence Spectroscopy and Microscopy of Biomolecular Motors*, Erwin J.G. Peterman, Hernando Sosa, and W.E. Moerner

*Dynamics of Single Biomolecules in Free Solution*, Edward S. Yeung

*Biomimetic Nanoscale Reactors and Networks*, Mattias Karlsson, Max Davidson, Roger Karlsson, Anders Karlsson, Johan Bergenholtz, Zoran Konkoli, Aldo Jesorka, Tatsiana Lobovkina, Johan Hurtig, Marina Voinova, and Owe Orwar

From the ***Annual Review of Physiology***, Volume 66 (2004)

*Viral-Based Myocardial Gene Therapy Approaches to Alter Cardiac Function*, Matthew L. Williams and Walter Koch

*Live Optical Imaging of Nervous System Development*, Cristopher M. Niell and Stephen J. Smith

ANNUAL REVIEWS is a nonprofit scientific publisher established to promote the advancement of the sciences. Beginning in 1932 with the *Annual Review of Biochemistry*, the Company has pursued as its principal function the publication of high-quality, reasonably priced *Annual Review* volumes. The volumes are organized by Editors and Editorial Committees who invite qualified authors to contribute critical articles reviewing significant developments within each major discipline. The Editor-in-Chief invites those interested in serving as future Editorial Committee members to communicate directly with him. Annual Reviews is administered by a Board of Directors, whose members serve without compensation.



**Annual Reviews of**

Anthropology
Astronomy and Astrophysics
Biochemistry
Biomedical Engineering
Biophysics and Biomolecular Structure
Cell and Developmental Biology
Earth and Planetary Sciences
Ecology, Evolution, and Systematics
Entomology
Environment and Resources
Fluid Mechanics
Genetics
Genomics and Human Genetics
Immunology
Materials Research
Medicine
Microbiology
Neuroscience
Nuclear and Particle Science
Nutrition
Pharmacology and Toxicology
Physical Chemistry
Physiology
Phytopathology
Plant Biology
Political Science
Psychology
Public Health
Sociology

SPECIAL PUBLICATIONS

Excitement and Fascination of Science, Vols. 1, 2, 3, and 4

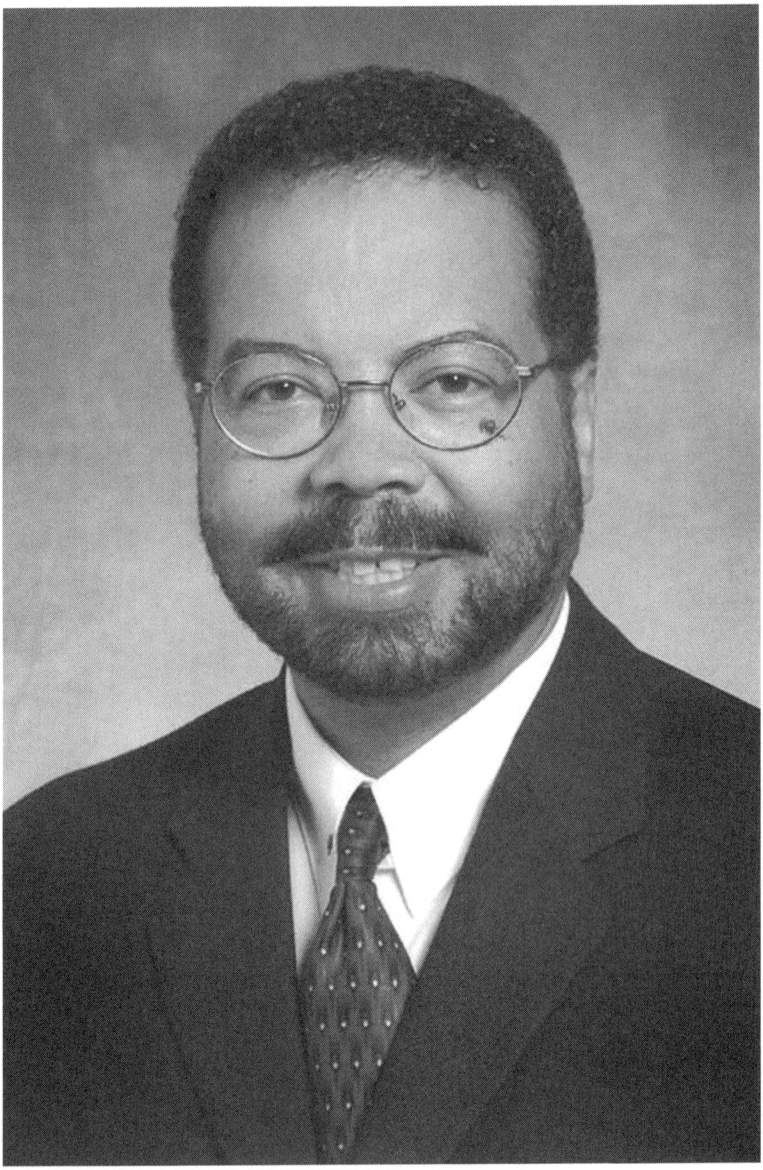

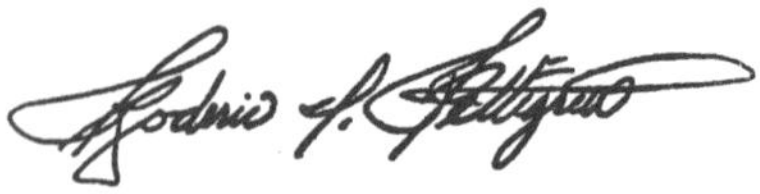

Roderic Pettigrew, M.D., Ph.D.
NIBIB Director

Annu. Rev. Biomed. Eng. 2004. 6:1–26
doi: 10.1146/annurev.bioeng.6.062403.131947

First published online as a Review in Advance on April 8, 2004

# THE NATIONAL INSTITUTE OF BIOMEDICAL IMAGING AND BIOENGINEERING

Shu Chien
*Departments of Bioengineering and Medicine, and the Whitaker Institute of Biomedical Engineering, University of California, San Diego, La Jolla, California 92093-0427; email: shuchien@ucsd.edu*

**Key Words** Academy of Radiology Research, American Institute for Medical and Biological Engineering, biomedical engineering, National Institutes of Health, research grants, training

CONTENTS

## SUMMARY

The establishment of the new National Institute of Biomedical Imaging and Bioengineering (NIBIB) has its roots in the organized activities of the biomedical imaging and bioengineering communities beginning around 1970s. The remarkable advances in biomedical engineering and imaging in the past few decades, with strong support from government agencies, especially the National Institutes of Health (NIH) and the National Science Foundation (NSF), and private foundations, particularly the Whitaker Foundation, have led to important contributions to the enhancement of health and the development of new methods for diagnosis, treatment, and prevention of disease. A series of actions in Congress and the presidential signing of Public Law 106–580 led to the establishment of the NIBIB, whose mission is improving health by the promotion of fundamental discoveries, design, and development and the translation and assessment of technological capabilities in biomedical imaging and bioengineering, in coordination with the relevant programs of other agencies and institutes and centers (ICs) of the NIH. The emphasis of the NIBIB is to foster biomedical imaging and bioengineering activities that cut across institutional boundaries and to complement such programs in other NIH ICs. Currently, the NIBIB funds approximately 15% of all NIH grants related to biomedical imaging and bioengineering. Following its formal establishment in April 2001, the NIBIB has made significant progress. Dr. Roderic I. Pettigrew took office as Director in September 2002, and the National Advisory Council for Biomedical Imaging and Bioengineering was formed and held its first meeting in January 2003. The NIH consulted extensively with the extramural community in establishing the NIBIB; Dr. Pettigrew and Dr. Donna Dean, first as Acting Director and later Deputy Director, spoke at more than 70 professional meetings and visited more than 40 academic institutions. The appropriation of a new budget starting in fiscal year (FY) 2002, together with the transfer of grant funds from other ICs, have built up the NIBIB's grant portfolio, which includes grants for R01, the Bioengineering Research Partnership (BRP), small business innovation research (SBIR) and small business technology transfer (STTR) grants, as well as training grants. The FY2003 budget of the NIBIB was nearly 2.5 times that of FY2002, but the proposed FY2004 budget shows only a slight increase over FY2003. The NIH Center for Scientific Review (CSR) is reorganizing integrated review groups (IRGs) and study sections, with a significant emphasis on the review of grants for biomedical imaging and bioengineering. NIH Director Dr. Elias Zerhouni has formulated a new roadmap for the NIH that focuses on new pathways of discovery, research teams for the future, and the re-engineering of the clinical research enterprise. The NIBIB is initiating a series of new activities to realize the vision of the NIH roadmap. The timely establishment of the new institute, with appropriate support for its growth and development, will play a major role in fostering the advancement of biomedical engineering and imaging to improve the health and well-being of people.

# HISTORY OF DEVELOPMENT OF THE NATIONAL INSTITUTE OF BIOMEDICAL IMAGING AND BIOENGINEERING

The establishment of the National Institute of Biomedical Imaging and Bioengineering (NIBIB) in April 2001 was a major event at the National Institutes of Health (NIH) and for the biomedical imaging and bioengineering communities. A summary of the history of these developments is given below. The reader is also referred to an earlier article by Hendee et al. (1).

## Developments in the Biomedical Imaging Community Prior to 1996

In the mid-1970s, the Conjoint Committee on Diagnostic Radiology was formed under the leadership of Drs. Herbert Abrams and Russell Morgan, with sponsorship by the American College of Radiology, the Association of University Radiologists, and the Society of Chairmen of Academic Radiology Departments, to represent the diagnostic imaging community's interests to Congress, the NIH, and other federal agencies. The committee, led by its first two Chairs, Drs. James Youker and Charles Putman, played significant roles in several developments of imaging research at the NIH. The primary focus of NIH-wide imaging research (cancer and noncancer) was transferred from the National Institutes of General Medical Sciences (NIGMS) to the National Cancer Institute (NCI) in 1978, and the intramural Laboratory of Diagnostic Radiology Research (LDRR) was established in 1992. The NIH-sponsored Conference on Developing a Long-Term Plan for Imaging Research was held in 1994, and NIH research funding in this field has increased steadily since (2).

In 1995, the Academy of Radiology Research (ARR) was created as an alliance of 19 (currently 25) scientific and professional societies, with the primary goal of establishing a new institute for imaging research at the NIH. In 1995–1996, the NCI expanded its Diagnostic Imaging Research Branch into a Diagnostic Imaging Program [later renamed the Biomedical Imaging Program (BIP) and, more recently, the Cancer Imaging Program (CIP)], with Dr. Daniel Sullivan as the first Director. Although the success of the CIP demonstrated the potential of imaging research, its limitation to cancer reinforced the imaging community's view that the NIH needed a new institute, with a broad range of applications for all ICs, to support basic research in imaging science (3, 4).

## Developments in the Biomedical Engineering Community Prior to 1996

In 1967–1968, NIH Director James Shannon requested the National Academy of Engineering to conduct a study on how to apply engineering to the pursuit of NIH activities. This led to the formation of the Committee on Interplay of

Engineering with Biology and Medicine, which was chaired by Dr. John Truxell followed by Dr. Robert Marshall, with Dr. Gilbert Devey as Executive Secretary. The establishment of an Institute of Biomedical Engineering was considered, but the final recommendation was to first set up subcontracts with universities to form prototype biomedical engineering departments. In the 1970s, the biomedical engineering research community formed the Alliance for Engineering in Medicine and Biology (AEMB) to organize annual scientific conferences for biomedical engineering and to foster the discipline in the NIH and other federal agencies. In 1991, the American Institute for Medical and Biological Engineering (AIMBE) was formed under the leadership of Dr. Robert Nerem and other key members of the AEMB as a federation of 15 scientific societies[1] to represent the community on public policy issues. AIMBE is also an honorary society that elects outstanding medical and biological engineering investigators and leaders in academia, industry, and other sectors as Fellows. The strong support by the Whitaker Foundation and the AIMBE constituency (including industrial support and generous donations by its Fellows, led by Dr. Jen-Shih Lee), together with excellent leadership and collaboration, have made possible its continued growth and development.

AIMBE works to enhance the visibility and impact of biomedical engineering in and beyond the NIH, and supports the efforts of biomedical engineers to heighten Congress' awareness of the need for increased support for research in the field. In concert with these efforts, Senator David F. Durenberger (R-MN) inserted language into the NIH Revitalization Act of 1993 (PL 103–43) to direct the Department of Health and Human Services to report on the state of bioengineering research at the NIH. In response to this call from Congress, the NIH prepared a report entitled *Support for Bioengineering Research* (5), for which Dr. John Watson of the National Heart, Lung, and Blood Institute (NHLBI) played a critical role. The NIH also formed the External Consultants Committee, chaired by Dr. Robert Nerem. The committee's report (6), submitted in 1995, made five specific recommendations, including the establishment of a central focus at the highest level in the NIH for basic bioengineering research, with resources for support of extramural research in collaboration with the NIH ICs. Concurrent with these developments, biomedical engineering was making great strides in merging biology, medicine, and engineering to foster tissue engineering, nanoscience and nanotechnology,

[1]The 15 founding societies of AIMBE are the American Association of Physicists in Medicine; American College of Clinical Engineering; American Institute of Chemical Engineers: Food, Pharmaceutical, and Bioengineering Division; American Medical Informatics Association; American Society of Agricultural Engineers; American Society for Artificial Internal Organs; American Society of Biomechanics; American Society of Mechanical Engineers: Bioengineering Division; Biomedical Engineering Society; IEEE Engineering in Medicine and Biology Society; Institute of Biological Engineering; Orthopaedic Research Society; Rehabilitation Engineering and Assistive Technology Society of North America; Society for Biomaterials; and SPIE: The International Society for Optical Engineering. They were later joined by the Controlled Release Society, the International Society for Magnetic Resonance in Medicine, and the Surfaces in Biomaterials Foundation.

functional genomics, smart biomaterials, biosensors, molecular imaging, and their applications for the prevention, diagnosis, and treatment of disease (see, e.g., 7, 8). The strong and timely support for biomedical research and training by the Whitaker Foundation has played a pivotal role in the advancement of biomedical engineering as a discipline.

## Developments in Biomedical Imaging and Bioengineering Between 1996 and 1999/2000

The fields of bioengineering and biomedical imaging continued to advance at rapid rates to become frontier areas of biomedical research, making possible earlier detection, improved diagnosis, and more effective treatments for a variety of diseases and, hence, improvements in health care. The remarkable advances in bioengineering and biomedical imaging and the potential of these disciplines to contribute in a profound way to fulfill the mission of the NIH have been presented by Hendee et al. (1) and are not repeated here.

Both ARR and AIMBE grew significantly and began to cooperate in achieving the common goal of enhancing biomedical imaging and bioengineering activities at the NIH and other federal agencies. ARR is currently comprised of 25 societies with a combined membership of over 45,000 radiologists and scientists in the field of biomedical imaging. AIMBE currently has 18 member societies comprised of more than 35,000 engineers, scientists, and clinicians; 83 academic programs in the field; over 700 Fellows; and an industrial council of manufacturers and industries.

Through the efforts of Senator William H. Frist (R-TN), Congress responded to the report on *Support for Bioengineering Research* by including an amendment to the reauthorization legislation for the NIH, which led the Secretary of Health and Human Services (HHS) Donna Shalala to prepare a report to Congress outlining specific plans and time frames for implementing the report's recommendations. The legislation passed in the Senate but was not acted upon by the House. In September 1996, at the urging of the ARR's Dr. Douglas Maynard, Representative Richard M. Burr (R-NC) introduced legislation (HR 4196) to establish the National Institute of Biomedical Imaging at the NIH at the end of the Congressional session, but it did not advance. The bill was reintroduced in the House in 1997 (HR 1715), and a companion bill (SR 990) was introduced in the Senate by Senator Lauch Faircloth (R-NC). These bills also failed to advance. In 1997, Senator Frist introduced SR 1030 to create an NIH Center for Bioengineering Research. Because the proposed center would not have funding authority and would have been located within one existing institute, i.e., the NHLBI, the bill did not receive the broad support of the biomedical engineering community and it did not pass out of committee.

At the NIH, the efforts of NIH Deputy Director for Extramural Research Dr. Wendy Baldwin, Dr. John Watson, and others led to increasing recognition of the role of biomedical engineering as an important discipline in health science and health care. In February 1997, NIH Director Dr. Harold Varmus established the

Bioengineering Consortium (BEACON), with the mission of coordinating bioengineering activities within the NIH and between the NIH and other relevant federal agencies. BECON, which was chaired by Dr. Wendy Baldwin and comprised of senior representatives from each of the NIH ICs, together with representatives from other federal agencies, holds monthly meetings to discuss common interests, problems, and strategies. The first BECON Symposium on Bioengineering, organized by Dr. Dov Jaron of the National Center of Research Resources and Dr. John Watson of the NHLBI, was held in February 1998. As a result of the recommendations of the BECON, NIH developed several major new grant programs, e.g., the Bioengineering Research Partnerships (BRPs) and bioengineering research grants (BRGs). The BRPs, by bringing together investigators from bioengineering, physical sciences, computational fields, and medicine, have contributed greatly to the advancement of interdisciplinary research on bioengineering problems. Dr. Varmus stated in his 1998 plenary lecture at the American Association of the Advancement of Science (9), "We are also fostering new efforts in materials science, bioengineering, instrumentation development, and informatics. In short, biology is not only for biologists." Annual BECON meetings have since been held on specific topics in biomedical imaging and engineering (symposia on biomedical imaging in 1999, nanoscience and nanotechnology in 2000, reparative medicine in 2001, sensors in biological research and medicine in 2002, and catalyzing team science in 2003). The rapid advances in bioengineering, its increasing recognition by the NIH and Congress, and the varied views of how to foster its growth at the NIH are summarized by Agnew (10).

At its annual meeting in March 1999, following considerable discussions, the AIMBE adopted the following resolution: "AIMBE should represent its constituent societies and its Fellows as a unified voice seeking to enhance the identity and support of biomedical engineering at the National Institutes of Health through pursuit of the following objectives: (a) Establishment of a free-standing Center or Institute of Biomedical Engineering with a director with authority equal to that of directors of other NIH centers and institutes. (b) Designation of grant-making authority to the Center or Institute for funds allocated in support of basic science, engineering and mathematics underlying biomedical engineering. (c) Funding the Center or Institute entirely through new appropriations without transfer of funds from existing centers and institutes."

Thus, the biomedical engineering and imaging communities converged on the opinion that the proper support of these rapidly evolving fields required an institute dedicated to these disciplines.

Concurrent with the move to establish a new institute, the biomedical engineering and imaging communities also had concerns that the NIH review process was focused on hypothesis-driven research and rendered it nearly impossible to obtain funding support for research aimed at the design and development of innovative technologies, which are indispensable for the advancement of hypothesis-driven research. In 1999–2000, the NIH took several steps to address these concerns and began to foster design-directed research and technology development.

Dr. Ellie Ehrenfeld, then Director of the NIH Center for Scientific Review (CSR), formed an adhoc working group, chaired by Dr. Lee Huntsman (with Linda Engel as Executive Secretary), to recommend ways to make the NIH peer-review process more receptive to the nonhypothesis-driven research that is essential for advancing basic and clinical research (11). As stated in the current version of the PHS 398 grant application instructions (12), "List the broad long-term objectives and what the specific research proposed in this application is intended to accomplish, e.g., to test a stated hypothesis, create a novel design, solve a specific problem, or develop new technology," as opposed to only "to test a stated hypothesis," as was specified in the previous version.

The CSR also formed an ad hoc Boundary Panel, chaired by Dr. Bruce Alberts of the National Academy of Sciences, to restructure the NIH peer-review organization into integrated review groups more responsive to the array of research applications received by the NIH (13). In May 2000, using the BECON as a model, the NIH established the Biomedical Information Science and Technology Initiatives Consortium (BISTI), which was aimed at making optimal use of computer science and technology to address problems in biology and medicine.

Although the NIH had been active in fostering biomedical engineering and biomedical imaging during the 1990s, it did not plan to add any new institutes (14). The initial action was to establish the Office of Bioengineering, Bioimaging, and Biocomputing (OB3) in the Office of the NIH Director in response to a Congressional directive in the FY2000 NIH Appropriations Act. OB3 would assume the responsibility of BECON and also work with those ICs in areas of bioimaging and biocomputing, with the goal of coordinating the activities of the various NIH institutes in developing collaborative initiatives and budget in these fields. A search committee, chaired by Dr. Baldwin, was formed to find a scientist with stature in these fields to serve as the OB3 Director, who would report directly to the NIH Director. However, OB3 would not have grant-making authority and its budget would be kept small, in the $2 million range, mainly for holding the Annual BECON Symposia and for supporting the necessary staff to carry out the coordinating functions. Furthermore, the plan was to terminate the OB3 after ten years; the reasoning was that either it would have succeeded in accomplishing its mission or need to be replaced by some other structure. Although the OB3 was a positive move toward fostering research in bioengineering and bioimaging, the scientific community generally felt that it would fall short of supporting the full potential for these rapidly developing disciplines and that it lacked permanence. As the keynote speaker at the AIMBE Annual Meeting on March 3, 2000, Dr. Baldwin spoke on the NIH plan for biomedical engineering, including the OB3. On March 5, after thorough discussions, the AIMBE Board decided to support the OB3 initiative, but expressed the view that their resolution adopted a year ago was the preferred action.

The evolution of the events during the period of 1996–2000 made it clear to the biomedical imaging and bioengineering communities that it was necessary for them to work together in order to achieve the goal of infrastructure reorganization

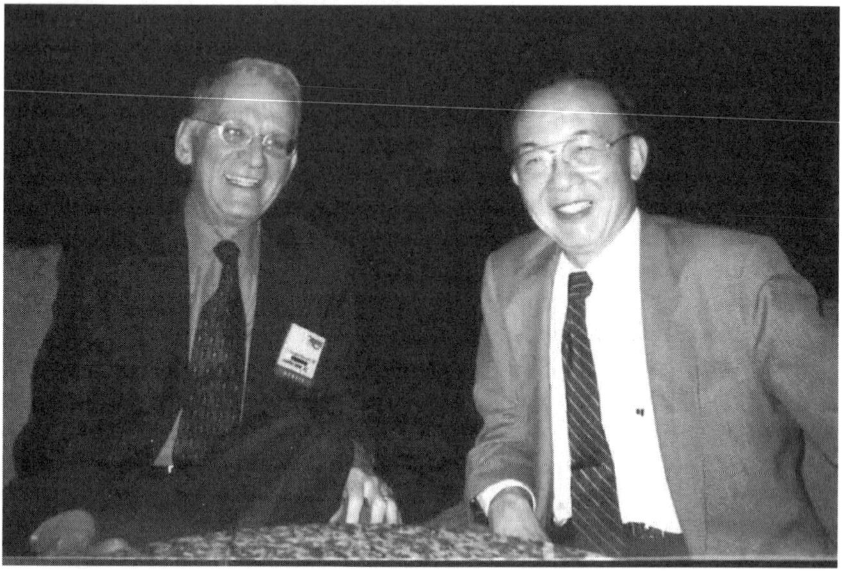

**Figure 1** ARR President Douglas Maynard and Shu Chien, May 2000, American Roentgen Ray Society Meeting, Washington, D.C.

at the NIH and to increase the recognition and enhance the activities of these fields. ARR President Douglas Maynard and I met several times to discuss the ways in which ARR and AIBME could collaborate toward our common goal (Figure 1). The establishment of the NIBIB was made possible following the joining of forces of the two communities.

## Legislative and Executive Actions to Establish NIBIB in 1999/2000

The remarkable advances in biomedical imaging and bioengineering, the great potential of these disciplines to fulfill the mission of the NIH, and the combined efforts of the two advocacy communities set the stage for a series of extraordinary events, which culminated in the establishment of the NIBIB.

As a result of the AIMBE/ARR coalition, Representative Burr modified his 1996 bill and introduced HR 1795 with Representative Anna Eshoo (D-CA) in 1999, calling for the establishment of a National Institute of Biomedical Imaging and Engineering at the NIH. This bill noted that biomedical engineering and imaging require an identity and research home at the NIH that is independent of the existing structure to ensure the development and transfer of new techniques and technologies that are critical to improving health care for the twenty-first century. Shortly thereafter, majority leader Trent Lott (R-MS) introduced a companion bill (SR1110) in the Senate for the establishment of a National Institute of

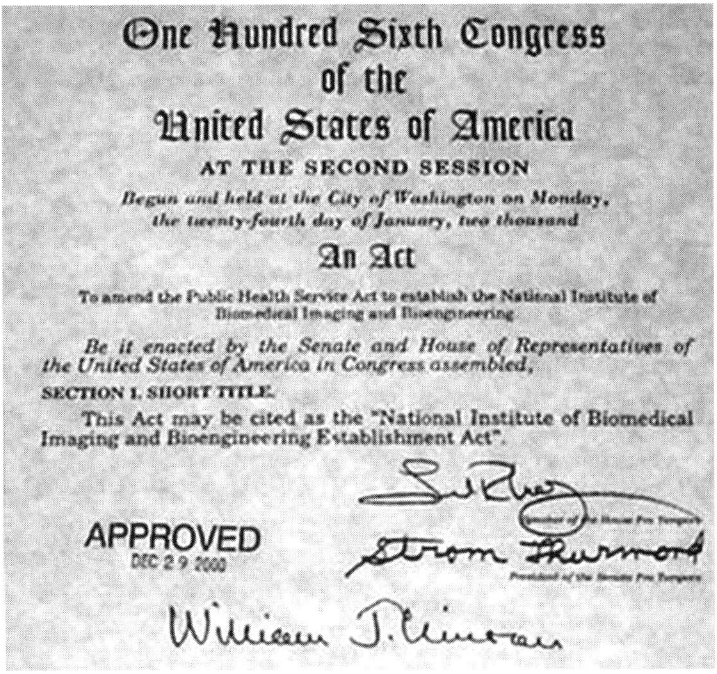

One Hundred Sixth Congress
of the
United States of America
AT THE SECOND SESSION
*Begun and held at the City of Washington on Monday,
the twenty-fourth day of January, two thousand*

An Act

To amend the Public Health Service Act to establish the National Institute of Biomedical Imaging and Bioengineering

*Be it enacted by the Senate and House of Representatives of the United States of America in Congress assembled,*

SECTION 1. SHORT TITLE.

This Act may be cited as the "National Institute of Biomedical Imaging and Bioengineering Establishment Act".

APPROVED
DEC 2 9 2000

**Figure 2** The National Institute of Biomedical Imaging and Bioengineering Establishment Act (Public Law 106–580), signed by President Clinton on December 29, 2000.

Bioengineering and Biomedical Imaging. Introduction of these bills was accompanied by an intense grassroots campaign in the biomedical imaging and bioengineering communities to generate legislative support for their passage. After some debates, the House of Representatives voted to pass HR 1795 on September 27, 2000. The Senate passed the same bill without debate on the last evening (December 15, 2000) of the second session of the 106th congressional session.

On December 29, 2000, then President William J. Clinton signed into law the National Institute of Biomedical Imaging and Bioengineering Establishment Act (Public Law 106–580) (Figure 2). This was the last law signed by President Clinton.

## Cooperation of Extramural Communities with the NIH in the Establishment of the NIBIB

In the processes leading to the establishment of the NIBIB and during the initial years of its operation, the NIH made extraordinary efforts to involve the extramural scientific communities. During the formative years of the NIBIB, the NIH leadership consulted extensively with the relevant scientific communities, especially the two federated organizations in biomedical engineering and biomedical imaging, i.e., AIMBE and ARR, respectively. Because I was AIMBE President in 1999–2000 and directly involved in these developments, some of the descriptions in this section are written from a personal perspective.

As mentioned above, AIMBE was working with the biomedical imaging community, especially ARR, to facilitate the passage and signing of the bill (HR 1795). Until the final signing of the bill into law, however, it had been uncertain whether the new Institute would become a reality; if President Clinton had not signed it by December 31, 2000, it would have been a pocket veto, which would make all the efforts for naught and everything would have to start from ground zero in the next Congressional sessions.

As the situation unfolded in December 2000, I realized that if the new institute were to become a reality, the major question would be how bioengineering and bioimaging activities at the NIH, especially their funding, would be distributed between the new institute and the existing ones. Most of the members of the bioengineering community felt that, although it would be beneficial to the field to have increased support through the new institute, we should keep most of the current support in the existing institutes.

By the very nature of the interdisciplinary approach in bioengineering research and training, it is critical to have the activities linked to the various institutes focusing on specific diseases and organs. Therefore, I drafted a letter in late December for submission to *Science* (15) to express AIMBE's support of the new institute and the opinion that the transfer of resources from existing NIH institutes to the new institute, as legislatively required, should be done with prudence. That is, our aim was to continue the activities related to bioengineering and bioimaging in the existing institutes, which are very valuable to the growth of these fields. The letter recommended that the new institute focus on fostering activities that cut across institutional boundaries, including fundamental and applied research and training in these fields, and that it should strengthen and complement (not subtract from or substitute for) research programs in the other NIH ICs.

Immediately after the Presidential signing of Public Law 106–580, Dr. Ruth Kirschstein (Figure 3), Acting Director of the NIH, asked me, the AIMBE President, to go to Bethesda to discuss the establishment of the new institute. On January 2, 2001, I met with Dr. Kirschstein and five other high-level NIH administrators, including Dr. Wendy Baldwin and Dr. Donna Dean, who would head the new NIBIB in its transition phase. Dr. Kirschstein told me that the NIH would form an internal working group to draft a mission statement and would welcome the formation of an external advisory group to provide inputs from the extramural scientific community. She and Dr. Dean wanted to work closely with the extramural community for the success of this new institute. We went through various scenarios of how the new institute might function, and the NIH leadership supported what I had drafted in the letter to *Science*.

The draft letter received valuable inputs and was unanimously approved by the AIMBE Board, and ARR President Doug Maynard accepted the invitation to cosign the letter, with approval by the ARR Board. On January 4, 2001, an

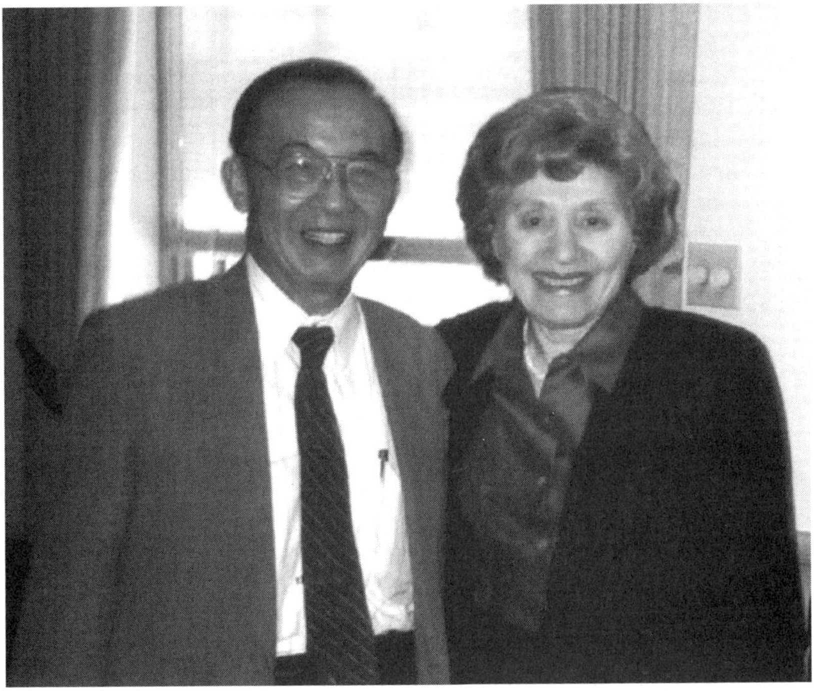

**Figure 3** Shu Chien and NIH Acting Director Ruth Kirschstein, January 2001, NIH Director's Office, Bethesda, MD.

AIMBE/ARR Joint Committee was established to provide extramural advice on the new institute as requested by the NIH. The members from AIMBE were Drs. William Hendee, John Linehan, Peer Portner, Buddy Ratner, and Shu Chien. The members appointed by ARR were Drs. Maynard, Stanley Baum, Reed Dunnick, Bruce Hillman, and Elias Zerhouni, the current NIH Director. Dr. Baum and I cochaired this joint committee. AIMBE and AAR Executive Directors Kevin O'Connor and Edward Nagy were ex officio members.

On January 8, 2001, Drs. Kirschstein and Dean held a teleconference call with representatives of AIMBE and ARR to discuss the developments of the new institute. Dr. Kirschstein established an internal task force chaired by Dr. Steven Hyman, Director of the National Institute of Mental Health, with four other institute directors: Dr. Stephen Katz (National Institute of Arthritis, Musculoskeletal and Skin Diseases), Dr. Richard Klausner (NCI), Dr. Claude Lenfant (NHLBI), and Dr. Lawrence Tabak (National Institute of Dental and Craniofacial Research).

In January 2001, the AIMBE-ARR Joint Committee proposed the mission statement and goals for the NIBIB, which were sent to Drs. Kirschstein and Dean on January 30. In February 2001, the joint committee representatives met on several occasions with Dr. Dean and Dr. Hyman, who said that the NIH internal task force used the letter to *Science* (15), among other documents, as content for the mission statement for the NIBIB. The statement was quite congruent with that drafted by the joint committee. The joint committee stressed the importance of a significant budget base and pointed out the importance of R01 funding, together with other funding mechanisms, and training support, as well as the need for an intramural program in the NIH on biomedical imaging and bioengineering.

The NIH internal task force formed a working group composed of program officials from several ICs with experience on relevant research areas to work with the task force to review their existing research grant portfolio for the identification of grants that are appropriate for transfer to the NIBIB. The amount transferred was $67 million (see FY2002, below).

On March 1, 2001, Dr. Kirschstein gave the keynote address at the AIMBE Tenth Anniversary Meeting on "Partnerships for the New Millennium," in which she outlined the plans for the new NIBIB and invited the medical and biological communities to provide input. Her address was followed by active and constructive discussions. On March 2, AIMBE held a forum on "NIH and Bioengineering." At the forum, Dr. Dean gave a speech on the current developments and future directions of NIBIB and served with Drs. Baum (ARR) and Linehan (AIMBE) as panelists in an open forum, where I served as the moderator. The discussions were very fruitful, with active participation by the audience, on issues related to the operation of NIBIB, e.g., grant funding mechanisms, areas of emphasis, transfer of grants from other institutes, etc.

On March 19, 2001, representatives of ARR and AIMBE met with Drs. Kirschstein and Dean at the NIH. Dr. Kirschstein was pleased with the publication of the letter in *Science* on March 2, 2001 (15). The NIH had just sent the plans and timelines for establishing the NIBIB to Secretary Tommy Thompson, Department of HHS, for approval. Dr. Kirschstein encouraged the bioimaging and bioengineering communities to submit nominations for members of the NIBIB Director Search Committee and candidates to be considered as NIBIB Director, as well as members of the Advisory Council. Dr. Kirschstein stated that the new Institute would start with an appropriate budget that would be ramped up over a five-year period, as in the case of the National Human Genome Research Institute, and that the NIBIB would foster training as well as research in bioimaging and bioengineering.

On April 20, 2001, Secretary Thompson approved the NIBIB Establishment Plan, which described the initial infrastructure, organization, budget requirements, and mission of the NIBIB.

On April 26, 2001, Dr. Donna Dean was designated as Acting Director of the NIBIB (Figure 4). She initiated the internal implementation steps: recruiting scientific and administrative staff, organizing program areas, establishing referral guidelines for grant applications, finalizing transfer of funded grants into the NIBIB, establishing a Web site (http://www.nibib.nih.gov), setting up NIBIB's central offices in the NIH's building 31, and extending outreach and communications to the potential research constituencies. On April 29, 2001, Dr. Dean spoke about

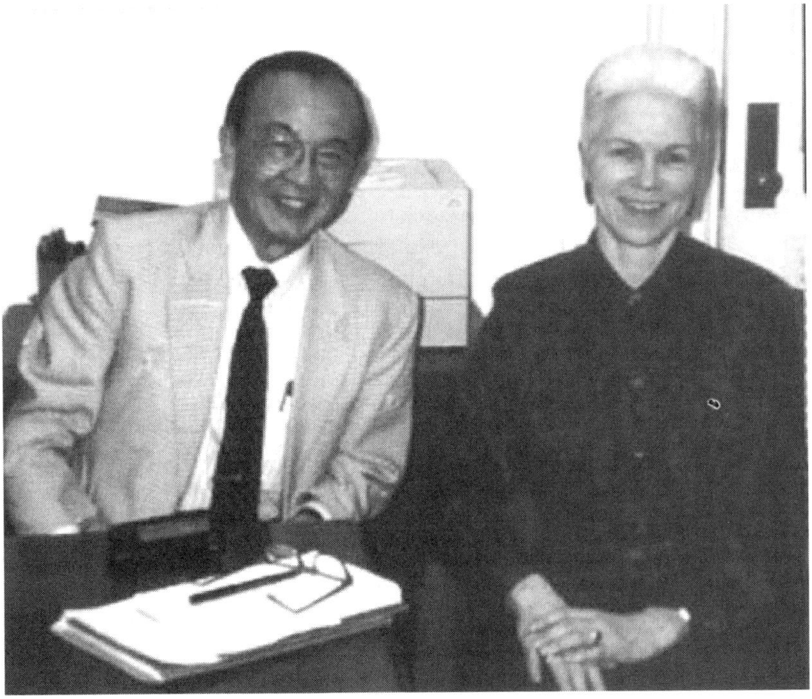

**Figure 4** Shu Chien and NIBIB Acting Director (2001–2002) Donna Dean, May 2001, NIBIB Acting Director's Office, Bethesda, MD.

the NIBIB at the American Roentgen Ray society annual meeting in Seattle and met with the Board members of ARR and AIMBE.

## MISSION STATEMENT OF THE NIBIB

The mission statement of the NIBIB was first developed by the NIH task force and was made public on March 5, 2001:

> "The mission of the National Institute of Biomedical Imaging and Bioengineering is to improve health by promoting fundamental discoveries, design and development, and translation and assessment of technological capabilities in biomedical imaging and bioengineering, enabled by relevant areas of information science, physics, chemistry, mathematics, materials science, and computer sciences. The Institute plans, conducts, fosters, and supports an integrated and coordinated program of research and research training that can be applied to a broad spectrum of biological processes, disorders and diseases and across organ systems. The Institute coordinates with the biomedical

imaging and bioengineering programs of other agencies and NIH Institutes to support imaging and engineering research with potential medical applications and facilitates the transfer of such technologies to medical applications." (An abbreviated version is shown on the home page of http://www.nibib.nih.gov)

In support of its mission, the institute will perform the following:

- Support research and research training through existing NIH funding mechanisms, and take the lead in exploring novel approaches for funding technology development and interdisciplinary research
- Form partnerships with NIH ICs to translate fundamental discoveries into research and applications for specific diseases, disorders, or biological processes
- Coordinate with other government agencies to translate fundamental or cross-cutting discoveries and developments in imaging, engineering, and related areas of information science and technology assessment into biomedical applications
- Encourage and support the development of relevant standards and guidelines that will enable widespread adaptability for biomedical imaging, bioengineering, and related information science and technology and computation, by taking a leadership and coordinating role for the NIH.

The principles outlined above form the basis of the congressional budget justifications for the NIBIB.

## NIBIB DIRECTOR AND ADVISORY COUNCIL

At the end of August 2001, the NIH advertised the position of the Director of the NIBIB in many scientific and professional publications, as well as on a number of Web sites. A search committee was formed, which was cochaired by Drs. Lawrence Tabak and Stephen Katz of the NIH, with seven members from the biomedical imaging and bioengineering communities and four other members from the NIH. The cochairs solicited qualified applicants from over 20 relevant professional organizations. The requirements included having a doctoral degree, senior-level research expertise and knowledge in relevant areas, outstanding scientific competence respected nationally and internationally, demonstrated leadership of an interdisciplinary research program, a track record of resolution of operational problems, and experience in management of financial and human resources.

Many excellent candidates were nominated and applied for the position. The search committee selected the seven most qualified candidates for interviews, and three finalists were presented to the NIH. Following further interviews with the NIH leadership, Dr. Roderic I. Pettigrew (Figure 5), who had superb expertise in biomedical imaging and bioengineering and outstanding leadership ability, was selected and appointed as the first permanent Director of the NIBIB in May 2002.

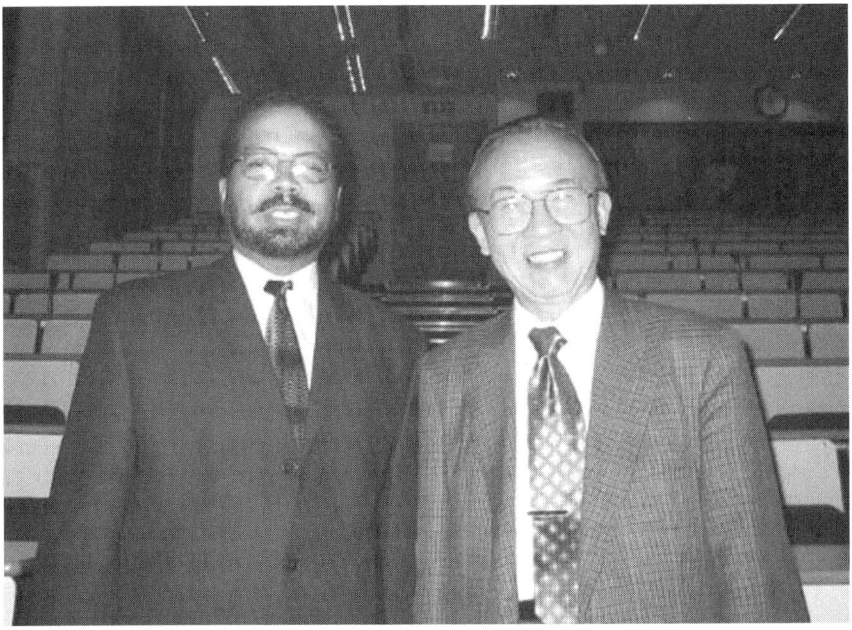

**Figure 5** NIBIB Director Roderic Pettigrew and Shu Chien, July 2002, Medical Imaging Meeting at Imperial College, London.

Dr. Pettigrew received his Ph.D. degree in applied radiation physics from the Massachusetts Institute of Technology and his M.D. from the University of Miami School of Medicine. He did his internship and residency in internal medicine at Emory University and completed his residency in nuclear medicine at the University of California, San Diego. Prior to assumption of the NIBIB Directorship in September 2002, he was Professor of Radiology, Medicine (Cardiology), and Bioengineering at Emory University School of Medicine in Atlanta, and Director of the Emory Center for MR Research.

Dr. Dean was appointed as Deputy Director of NIBIB, a position she held until November 2003. In December 2003, Dr. Belinda Seto (Figure 6), previously serving as Acting Deputy Director for Extramural Research at the NIH, was appointed as the NIBIB Deputy Director.

The National Advisory Council for Biomedical Imaging and Bioengineering (NACBIB) was established by HHS Secretary Tommy Thompson under the Public Health Service Act to advise, assist, consult with, and make recommendations to the Secretary and the NIBIB Director on matters related to the activities carried out by and through the Institute and the policies related to these activities. The advisory council has 12 scientific members composed of scientists, engineers, physicians, and other health professionals. Of these, six represent disciplines in biomedical engineering and imaging; the other six represent other disciplines and

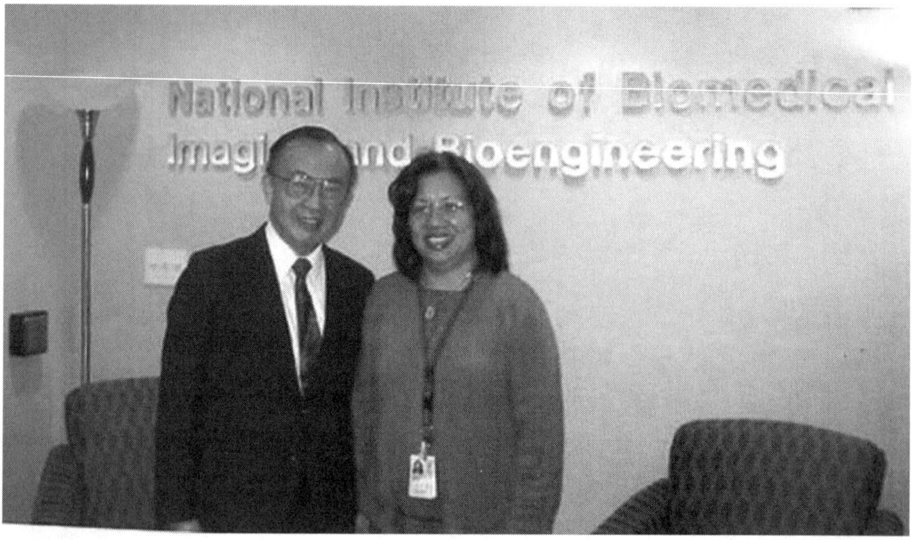

**Figure 6** Shu Chien and NIBIB Deputy Director Belinda Seto, February 2004, NIBIB Office, Bethesda, MD.

are knowledgeable about the applications of biomedical engineering and imaging in medicine. Ex officio members of the advisory council include the Director of the Centers for Disease Control and Prevention, the Director of the NSF, and the Director of the National Institute of Standards and Technology (or their designees). The advisory council held its first meeting on January 16–17, 2003, and meets three times a year. The roster of the advisory council and the minutes of past meetings can be found at http://www.nibib.nih.gov/about/NACBIB/NACBIB.htm.

Under the excellent leadership of Dr. Pettigrew, assisted by Dr. Dean and other very capable staff members, the NIBIB has made remarkable advances in less than three years. The leaders of various programs and divisions in the NIBIB, together with its organizational chart, are provided in Figure 7.

Drs. Pettigrew and Dean made unprecedented efforts to communicate with extramural communities, reaching out for input and providing information on developments at the NIBIB. In 2002 and 2003, they spoke at more than 70 scientific and professional society meetings and visited more than 40 academic institutions. These interactions between the NIBIB leadership and the biomedical imaging and bioengineering communities have been very valuable in the development of the NIBIB in concert with the opportunities and challenges of the frontiers of these disciplines.

To enhance the participation of bioengineering leaders in the NIBIB policy matters, Dr. Pettigrew appointed Dr. Robert M. Nerem of the Georgia Institute of Technology and Emory University as a part-time senior advisor for bioengineering in January 2003. The other senior advisor is Dr. Richard Swaja.

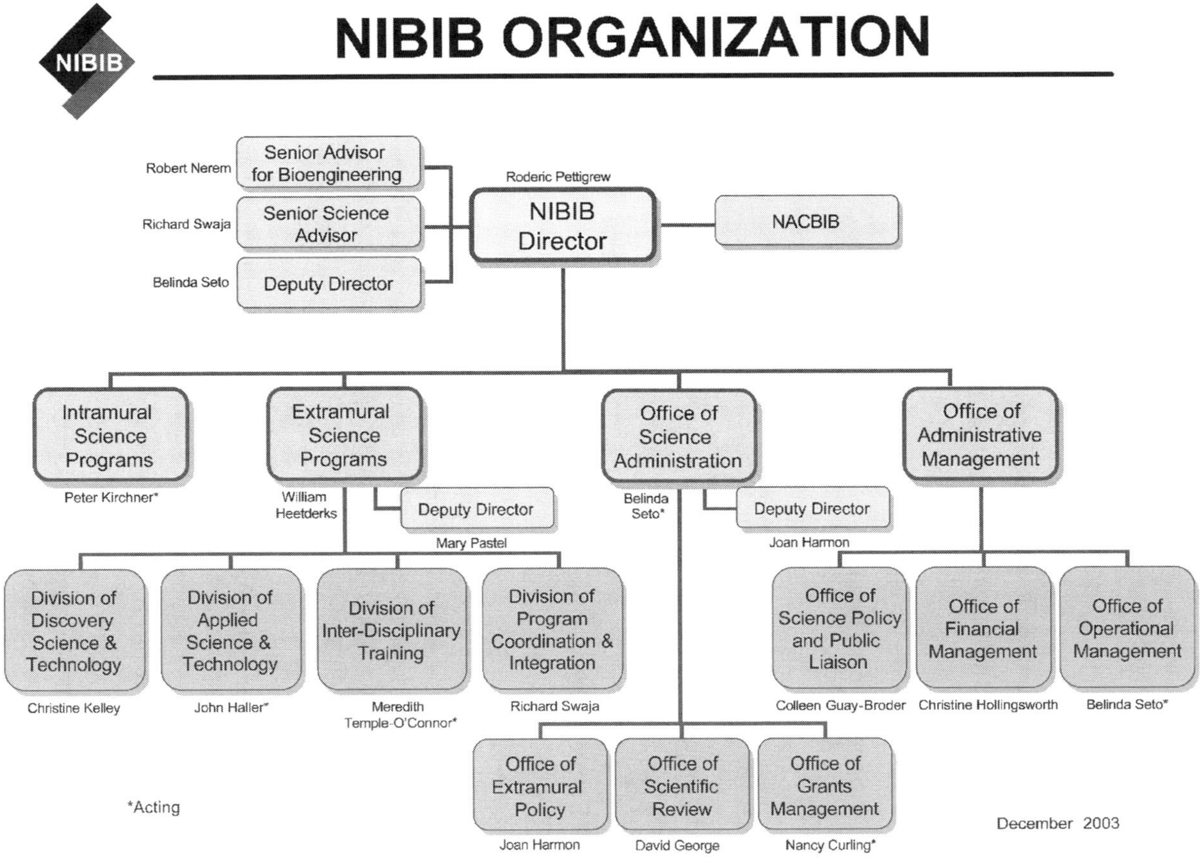


**Figure 7** NIBIB organizational chart.

# NIBIB ACTIVITIES

## NIBIB Symposia and Workshops

The NIBIB has organized, sponsored, or cosponsored many symposia and workshops. The most recent ones held between August 2002 and August 2003 are given below:

- NIBIB Workshop on Biomedical Imaging and Bioengineering Training
- NIH/NSF Workshop on Image-Guided Interventions
- BMIS Medical Implant Information, Performance, and Policies Workshop
- Third Inter-Institute Workshop on Diagnostic Optical Imaging
- NIBIB Workshop on Future Research Directions
- Symposium on Defining the State of the Art in Biomedical Imaging: Research for the Future
- Symposium on Imaging the Pancreatic Beta Cell
- BECON 2003 Symposium: Catalyzing Team Science [the sixth in a series of annual BECON meetings (see Developments in the Biomedical Engineering Community Prior to 1996)]
- Symposium on Modeling of Complex Biological Systems

## NIBIB Requests for Applications in 2002

The NIBIB held several workshops (see previous section) to identify the highest priority research focus areas that are appropriate in relation to its mission and national priorities, as well as promising emerging technologies or high-impact projects. The research focus areas thus identified led to the issuance in early 2003 of ten requests for applications (RFA) on development of advanced biomaterials, development of novel drug and gene delivery systems and devices, image-guided interventions, improvements in imaging methods and technologies, research opportunities in tissue engineering, low-cost medical imaging devices, telehealth technologies development, research and development of systems and methods for cellular and molecular imaging, systems and methods for small animal imaging, and operation of sensors in vivo.

## NIBIB Grant Portfolio Areas in 2003 and Initiatives for FY2004

Analysis of the NIBIB research grants portfolio in 2003 using program class codes has identified the following subject areas: biosensors; biomaterials; biomechanics; bioinformatics; computational biology; drug and gene delivery; image-guided therapies; medical devices/implants; magnetic resonance imaging and spectroscopy; nanotechnology; nuclear medicine; optical imaging; platform technology; rehabilitation engineering; surgical tools and techniques; tissue engineering; ultrasonics; and X ray, electron microscopy, and ion beam.

The NIBIB has been working on identifying concept areas for exploration in FY2004. Examples of these research areas include the following:

- Data integration
- Quantum projects
- Tissue engineering
- Multiscale modeling
- Computer-assisted image-guided surgery
- Microimaging of pancreatic islets
- Chemistry of imaging agents and molecular probes
- Brain computer interface
- Translational research in nanotechnology-based diagnoses and therapy

Currently, the NIH is operating under a continuing resolution, as indicated below, and an approved budget is needed for the initiation of new projects.

## NIBIB BUDGET

The legislation establishing the NIBIB was not passed until the end of 2000, thus precluding the NIBIB's inclusion in the FY2001 NIH budget, which had been developed almost a year earlier. However, the NIH FY2001 appropriation contained $1.975 million originally designated for the OB3 within the Office of the NIH Director, and this amount was used to support the administrative activities necessary to create the new institute.

The FY2002 operating budget totaled $111.7 million, which included $67 million in grants and funds that were transferred from other ICs of the NIH (see above). The majority of the funds over and above the transfer, approximately $40 million, were used to support the NIBIB's mission, which included research grants and contracts, training grants, and operations (Table 1).

The transfer of funds from the existing ICs to the NIBIB was not an easy process. It is often difficult to clearly differentiate grants that are crosscutting versus those that are organ/disease-specific. As a result of the cooperative efforts between NIH leadership and the scientific community in a working group examining the grant

**TABLE 1** NIBIB operating budget figures for fiscal years 2002 and 2003 (million $)

| | Training | RMS[a] | Contracts | Other res. | Centers | RPG[b] | Total |
|---|---|---|---|---|---|---|---|
| FY2002 | 0.2 | 11.7 | 1.3 | 2.9 | 1.3 | 94.3 | 111.7 |
| FY2003 | 2.8 | 13.8 | 7.3 | 4.5 | 23.6 | 226.2 | 278.2 |

[a]RMS: Research management and support funds.

[b]RPG: Research project grants including BRP and SBIR/STTR. SBIR funds were $0.89 million in 2002 and $10.9 million in 2003.

portfolios, a solution was attained with the transfer of an additional $150 million from the various NIH ICs to the NIBIB. The extramural members of the working group were Drs. Don P. Giddens, Peer M. Portner, and Matthew Tirrell from AIMBE and Drs. Stanley Baum, Reed Dunnick, and Etta Pisano from ARR. The intramural members were Drs. Robert Balaban, Suzanne Fisher, and King C.P. Li, with staff support from Dr. Mary Pastel and Ms. Stacy Wallick. Kevin O'Connor (AIMBE), Edward C. Nagy (AAR), and Dr. Dean were ex officio members.

The FY2003 budget appropriation was passed in February 2003. The total operating budget was increased to $278.2 million, which included the $150 million in grants and funds transferred from other ICs. The approximately $128.2 million over and above the transfer was used to carry out the NIBIB's mission, including a significant increase in its funding of research and training, especially research project grants and center grants. In FY2003, the NIBIB funded 38 BRP grants with $30 million, which constitute approximately 30% of all BRPs in the NIH (130 grants with an annual budget of $106 million). For all biomedical imaging– and bioengineering–related NIH grants, approximately 15% were supported by the NIBIB and the remainder by other ICs.

The budget appropriation for FY2004 is yet to be passed. The president's budget and the House mark both have $282 million for the NIBIB, whereas the Senate mark is slightly higher at $289 million. The FY2004 president's budget provides only a 1.4% increase over FY2003.

## REVIEW OF BIOMEDICAL IMAGING AND BIOENGINEERING GRANTS

As mentioned above (see Developments in the Biomedical Engineering Community Prior to 1996, above), the CSR has implemented its reorganization of the peer review system at the NIH (13). The reorganization of the review system involves (*a*) the establishment of IRGs, each with approximately six to eight study sections, to replace the initial review groups and (*b*) the realignment of study sections. The CSR is proceeding with implementation plans for the IRGs that were approved in January and May 2003. Descriptions of the IRGs and their study sections can be found on the CSR's IRG description page located at http://www.csr.nih.gov/review/irgdesc.htm. Lists of the scientific review administrators (SRAs) and provisional membership rosters are available on the CSR study section roster index page at http://www.csr.nih.gov/Committees/rosterindex.asp. Investigators are encouraged to read these Web pages to identify the IRG and study section most suited for the review of their applications. With each grant application, the principal investigator may submit a cover letter to suggest an IRG or study section, as well as the areas of science and engineering needed for appropriate peer review.

As a result of the reorganization of the review system, two new IRGs related to biomedical imaging and bioengineering, namely, Bioengineering Sciences and

Technologies (BST) and Surgical Sciences, Biomedical Imaging, and Bioengineering (SBIB), have been formed in place of the previous Surgery, Radiology, and Bioengineering (SRB) IRG. These two new IRGs are described below. The study sections in these IRGs review the applications for research project grants (R01, R21, R15, etc.) and SBIR and STTR grants.

## Bioengineering Sciences and Technologies IRG

The BST IRG reviews grant applications that focus on fundamental aspects of bioengineering and technology development in the following areas: gene and drug delivery systems, imaging principles for molecules and cells, modeling of biological systems, bioinformatics and computer science, statistics and data management, instrumentation, chips and microarrays, biosensors, and biomaterials. Although biological context is important in bioengineering, a central premise in organizing this IRG is the need for effective review of bioengineering and technology development in early stages before specific practical uses are proven. The current BST IRG includes the following study sections:

- Gene and Drug Delivery Systems (GDD)
- Microscopic Imaging (MI)
- Modeling and Analysis of Biological Systems (MABS)
- Biodata Management and Analysis (BDMA)
- Instrumentation and Systems Development (ISD)
- Biomaterials and Biointerfaces (BMBI)

## Surgical Sciences, Biomedical Imaging, and Bioengineering IRG

The SBIB IRG reviews applications for research grants that address topics in a variety of areas at the interface between a physical science or engineering and biomedical or clinical research. Major areas include the following: (*a*) Development of molecular probes and contrast agents; development of molecular imaging techniques; and basic, applied, and preclinical aspects of the design and development of medical imaging systems (including hardware, software, and mathematical methods of image analysis) for studying organs or whole animals (including humans). (*b*) Application of computational sciences to knowledge and information in biological and clinical medicine, healthcare, and their integration. (*c*) Development of biomedical sensing and measurement instrumentation; diagnostic instrumentation creating knowledge to enhance organ system function and recovery; innovative biologics, materials, processes, implants, devices; and informatics approaches to prevent, diagnose, and treat disease. (*d*) Surgery and anesthesiology, host response to sepsis and injury, surgical and microsurgical therapies, surgical critical care and emergency medicine, treatment of trauma; multi-organ responses to surgery.

The following scientific review groups are included within this IRG:

- Biomedical Imaging Technology (BMIT)
- Medical Imaging (MEDI)
- Biomedical Computing and Health Informatics (BCHI)
- Bioengineering, Technology, and Surgical Sciences (BTSS)
- Surgery, Anesthesiology, and Trauma (SAT)
- Small Business Biomedical Imaging (SBMI)
- Small Business Bioengineering, Surgical Sciences, and Technology (SBTS)
- Small Business Biomedical Sensing, Measurement, and Instrumentation (SSMI)
- Small Business Bioelectromagnetics Special Emphasis Panel

Deliberations are under way on the development of recommendations for other IRGs that may share interests in areas of research with these IRGs. Tentative proposals on shared-interest guidelines are being developed for each of the study sections, pending further input from the remaining study section design teams, the scientific community, the CSR Advisory Committee to the Director, and the CSR.

For the most part, all grant applications are reviewed by the CSR; however, training grant applications, program project grants, and applications in response to RFAs are mainly reviewed by the institutes. The review administrators receive the applications, set up the reviews, and compile the summary statements. The program administrators give guidance to the applicants before submission and after review. In September 2003, the NIBIB Special Emphasis Panel was established, which enables the institute's Office of Review to hold special review meetings. The first review meetings in November 2003 encompassed reviews of applications of institutional training grants and research career-development awards.

## NIBIB PARTICIPATION IN NIH ROADMAP ACTIVITIES

Following his appointment as the Director of the NIH in May 2002, Dr. Elias Zerhouni initiated the creation of a new research vision for the NIH that focused the attention of the biomedical research community on three main themes: new pathways of discovery, research teams for the future, and the re-engineering of the clinical research enterprise (the Web site for the NIH roadmap is located at http://nihroadmap.nih.gov). This roadmap strategy was developed after extensive discussions involving the directors of NIH's 27 ICs. The three main themes include the following nine implementation groups:

- New Pathways to Discovery
  - Building Blocks, Pathways, and Networks Implementation Group
  - Molecular Libraries and Imaging Implementation Group
  - Structural Biology Implementation Group

  - Bioinformatics and Computational Biology Implementation Group
  - Nanomedicine Implementation Group
- Research Teams of the Future
  - Interdisciplinary Research Implementation Group
  - High-Risk Research Implementation Group
  - Public-Private Partnerships Implementation Group
- Re-Engineering the Clinical Research Enterprise
  - Clinical Research Implementation Group

The aim of these roadmap activities is to improve health by providing researchers with tools and capabilities to make innovative, novel, and multidisciplinary discoveries in science, engineering, and technology, and to ensure that these basic research discoveries are translated quickly into new approaches for diagnosis, treatment, and prevention of disease. Because the broad mission of the NIBIB is to improve health by leading the development and application of emerging and breakthrough biomedical technologies based in the physical and engineering sciences, there is a direct tie between the NIBIB's mission and the roadmap initiatives. The NIBIB is designated as a participant in all the roadmap initiatives.

Under New Pathways to Discovery, a key focus at the NIBIB is individualized molecular medicine. Technologies will be developed to evaluate specific diseases and their presentation in individual patients, with the goal of enabling physicians to obtain personalized profiles of molecular and genetic disease markers. Using this information, treatments can be tailored to each patient.

The goals of the initiatives under the Building Blocks, Pathways, and Networks Implementation Group include developing a network of research centers to create new tools to describe the dynamics of protein interactions, developing novel technologies to study cellular metabolites, establishing standards for proteomics and metabolomics, and assessing critical reagents for proteomics.

For the initiatives on Molecular Libraries and Imaging, an emphasis will be placed on the development of high-resolution probes for cellular imaging. The goals are to support multidisciplinary teams for the development of new technologies that enable higher-sensitivity biological imaging in living cells; to encourage and facilitate novel, high-risk strategies to create fundamentally new probes with enhanced spectral characteristics; to improve detection schemes by a factor of 10–100; and to develop probes that can be used to routinely achieve single-molecule sensitivity for imaging dynamic processes in living cells.

The NIBIB will participate in the initiative of the Bioinformatics and Computational Biology Implementation Group through the activities of the trans-NIH BISTI. The goals of this initiative include providing key building blocks for the national biomedical computing environment, the formation of single or multisite consortia, and the establishment of National Centers for Biomedical Computing.

For the initiative on Nanomedicine, the NIBIB focuses on nanoscience and nanotechnology. The goals are to obtain quantitative measurements on biological molecular system components and their interactions, and to combine these measurements using mathematical and analytical tools for the fundamental understanding of biological circuits/processes and their precise interactions, with the aim of effecting desired changes in human health.

Under Research Teams of the Future and Re-Engineering the Clinical Research Enterprise, the NIBIB focuses on the implementation of interdisciplinary research. The goals are to supplement existing programs to promote research training experiences and to create new initiatives for the (*a*) promotion of curriculum development and short course development and (*b*) revitalization of clinical research scientist training for M.D.s and Ph.D.s.

## CONCLUSIONS AND PERSPECTIVES

The establishment of the NIBIB is a timely event that allows the NIH to capitalize on the remarkable advances in these fields to realize its mission to improve the health and well-being of our citizens. The establishment of the Institute was the result of the outstanding accomplishments of the scientists and engineers in the fields; the sustained and coordinated efforts of the relevant communities; the timely and generous support by the Whitaker Foundation; and the increasing recognition of the importance of these disciplines by the NIH, the public, and Congress.

The extraordinary cooperation between the NIH and the extramural communities has played a significant role in the establishment of NIBIB. The visionary leadership at the NIH and the NIBIB has led to its significant growth and development in a short period of time. The NIBIB now funds 800 grants in biomedical imaging and bioengineering. In addition to this active extramural program, we look forward to the establishment of an intramural program in these important frontier areas.

Because of the suddenness of its formation, however, the NIBIB started with a relatively limited budget. The budget for FY2003 did show a healthy increase over that of FY2002, but the proposed FY2004 budget does not provide much of an increase. For this new institute to further enhance its activities and to fully implement its mission, it is necessary to have a progressive increase in funding with a relatively steep slope for several years before attaining a quasi-steady state. The extramural community and the individual investigators need to reflect this need to our congressional and administrative leaders, emphasizing the vital importance of biomedical engineering and imaging in contributing to the infrastructure essential to advances in biomedical sciences and critical to the improvement of health care. By fostering biomedical imaging and biomedical engineering, the NIBIB will synergize with the other ICs at the NIH to elucidate the mechanisms underlying health at all levels of biological hierarchy; the diagnosis, treatment, and prevention of diseases; and the training of future generations of biomedical engineers and biomedical imagers. NIBIB is still in its beginning phase. To accomplish these important missions, it is essential that it grow to become at least a medium-sized institute among the NIH ICs and to have a high-quality intramural program.

We are indeed at a very exciting time. The NIBIB, if provided an adequate budget, will be able to seize the unprecedented opportunity presented by the rapid advancements of biomedical engineering and imaging and meet the grand challenge of taking the research frontiers of these disciplines to new heights, with the ultimate goal of enhancing the health and well-being of people in the United States and throughout the world.

## ACKNOWLEDGMENTS

The author wishes to express his gratitude to the valuable advice, comments, and provision of information by officials in NIBIB and other components of the NIH, especially Drs. Roderic Pettigrew, Donna Dean, Wendy Baldwin, Robert Nerem, Elliot Postow, Donald Schneider, Richard Swaja, John Watson, Cheryl Fee, Christine Kelley, and Peter Moy. I would like to thank many friends and colleagues in biomedical imaging (Dr. Douglas Maynard and Edward Nagy) and bioengineering (Dr. William Hendee, Dr. Jack Linehan, Patricia Horner, and Kevin O'Connor) for their valuable input and critiques. I am grateful to all the friends and colleagues with whom I have had the pleasure and privilege to work with toward the common goal of establishing the NIBIB for enhancing the health and well-being of people.



## LITERATURE CITED

1. Hendee WR, Chien S, Maynard CD, Dean DJ. 2002. The National Institute of Biomedical Imaging and Bioengineering: history, status and potential impact. *Ann. Biomed. Eng.* 30:2–10; Radiology 222:12–18
2. Putman CE, Frank JA. 1993. Enhancement of diagnostic radiologic research and education. *Invest. Radiol.* 28(Suppl. 2):552–56
3. Holman BL, Nagy EC. 1998. Why we need a National Institute of Biomedical Imaging. *Acad. Radiol.* 5:211–14
4. Academy of Radiology Research. 1998. Imaging Research and the Federal Government: A White Paper. Washington, DC, September
5. National Institutes of Health Report on Support for Bioengineering Research. 1994. National Institutes of Health, Bethesda, MD, http://www.becon1.nih.gov/nihreport.htm
6. Nerem RM, Taylor KD, Arnold F, Chien S, Katona PG, et al. 1995. Support for Bioengineering Research, Department of Health and Human Services, Public Health Service, National Institutes of Health, http://www.becon1.nih.gov/externalreport.htm
7. Bronzino JD. 2000. *The Biomedical Engineering Handbook*. Boca Raton, FL: CRC Press
8. Griffith LG, Grodzinsky AJ. 2001. Advances in biomedical engineering. *JAMA* 285:556–61

9. Varmus H. 1998. *New directions in biology and medicine*. AAAS Plenary Lecture, http://www.nih.gov/about/director/021398.htm
10. Agnew B. 1998. Multidisciplinary research. Biology by design: from software to skin. *Science* 280:1516–18
11. Huntsman LL, Chien S, Davis RW, Griffith LG, Hendee WR, et al. 1999. Expanding opportunities. *NIH Work. Group Rep.*, Rev. Bioeng. Technol. Instrum. Dev. Res. Natl. Inst. Health, Bethesda Md. http://www.drg.nih.gov/bioopp1/select.htm
12. U.S. Department of Health and Human Services. *Public Health Service Grant Application (PHS 398 Instructions) Rev. 05/2001* (ftp://ftp.grants.nih.gov/forms/phs398.pdf)
13. Alberts BM, Ayala FJ, Botstein D, Frank E, Holmes EW, et al. 2000. Recommendations for change at the NIH's Center for Scientific Review. *Phase 1 Rep.*, Panel Sci. Bound. Rev, Natl. Inst. Health, Bethesda, Md. http://www.csr.nih.gov/bioopp/select.htm
14. Varmus H. 2001. Proliferation of National Institutes of Health. *Science* 291:1903–5
15. Chien S, Maynard CD. 2001. Newest member of the NIH family. *Science* 291:1701–2

Annu. Rev. Biomed. Eng. 2004. 6:27–40
doi: 10.1146/annurev.bioeng.6.012204.115707

First published online as a Review in Advance on February 18, 2004

# TISSUE ENGINEERING APPLICATIONS OF THERAPEUTIC CLONING

Anthony Atala and Chester J. Koh
*Wake Forest Institute for Regenerative Medicine, Wake Forest University School of Medicine, Winston Salem, North Carolina 27157; email: aatala@wfubmc.edu*

**Key Words** kidney, muscle, regenerative medicine, embryonic stem cells, tissue-specific stem cells, tissue transplantation, organ transplantation

■ **Abstract** Few treatment options are available for patients suffering from diseased and injured organs because of a severe shortage of donor organs available for transplantation. Therapeutic cloning, where the nucleus from a donor cell is transferred into an enucleated oocyte in order to extract pluripotent embryonic stem cells, offers a potentially limitless source of cells for replacement therapy. Scientists in the field of tissue engineering apply the principles of cell transplantation, material science, and engineering to construct biological substitutes that will restore and maintain normal function in diseased and injured tissues. The present chapter reviews recent advances that have occurred in therapeutic cloning and tissue engineering and describes applications of these new technologies that may offer novel therapies for patients with end-stage organ failure.

CONTENTS



## INTRODUCTION

Cloning techniques are already widely utilized in the modern world, where gardeners perform plant cuttings and commercial companies propagate desirable plant strains and animal breeds (1). However, since the birth of Dolly as the first animal cloned from an adult somatic cell in 1997, tremendous further interest in cloning has arisen, and cloning has been envisioned as having utility in medical applications as well.

Regenerative medicine has the potential to benefit from advances in cloning technology. The field of regenerative medicine seeks to relieve the suffering of patients from the consequences of disease and injury by restoring the form and function of their damaged tissue and organs. Many disorders, such as congenital anomalies, cancer, trauma, infection, inflammation, iatrogenic injuries, and other conditions, can lead to organ damage or loss and to the eventual need for reconstruction. In the United States, approximately one person in five reaching 65 years of age will receive temporary or permanent organ-replacement therapy during his or her remaining life span (2). In addition, using the kidney as an example, over 2 million patients are projected to suffer from end-stage renal disease by 2010, and the aggregate health care costs for treating these patients has been estimated to be over $1 trillion dollars (3).

The majority of current reconstructive techniques rely on donor tissue for replacement; however, a shortage of donor tissue may limit these types of reconstruction, and usually significant morbidity is associated with the harvest procedure. Furthermore, the functional aspects of the damaged organ are rarely replaced by these reconstructive procedures, and they may even lead to complications because of the inherently different functional parameters of reconstructed tissue. Other potential sources of tissue include homologous tissues from cadavers, heterologous tissues from animal sources (bovine), and artificial materials (silicone, polyurethane, Teflon). Artificial devices made from these alternative sources were noted to be biocompatible and could provide structural replacement; however, the functional component of the original tissue was usually not recovered. Although caution and disease prevention may never completely eradicate the incidence of disease and injury, regenerative medicine physicians and researchers hope to relieve the suffering of their patients from these unfortunate entities, and if possible, to repair or restore the damaged tissue with the hope of regenerating essentially normal body parts.

Organ transplantation was one of the first methods to restore form and function in modern medicine. In 1955, Murray performed the first successful organ transplant (kidney), and in the early 1960s, he performed the first allogeneic kidney transplantation from a genetically dissimilar donor into an unrelated recipient (4). As one of the first procedures to overcome the immunologic barrier, this revolutionary procedure marked the modern era in which transplantation could be used as means of therapy for diseased and injured organs. Since then, advances in immunosuppressive medications, in the matching of similar donors to recipients, and in the treatment of rejections have resulted in thousands of patients each year undergoing successful transplantation of donor organs. In 2001, over 23,000 patients received a transplanted organ in the United States (5).

However, despite the advances in transplantation over the past 50 years, a severe shortage of donor organs limits the availability of this treatment, such that in 2001,

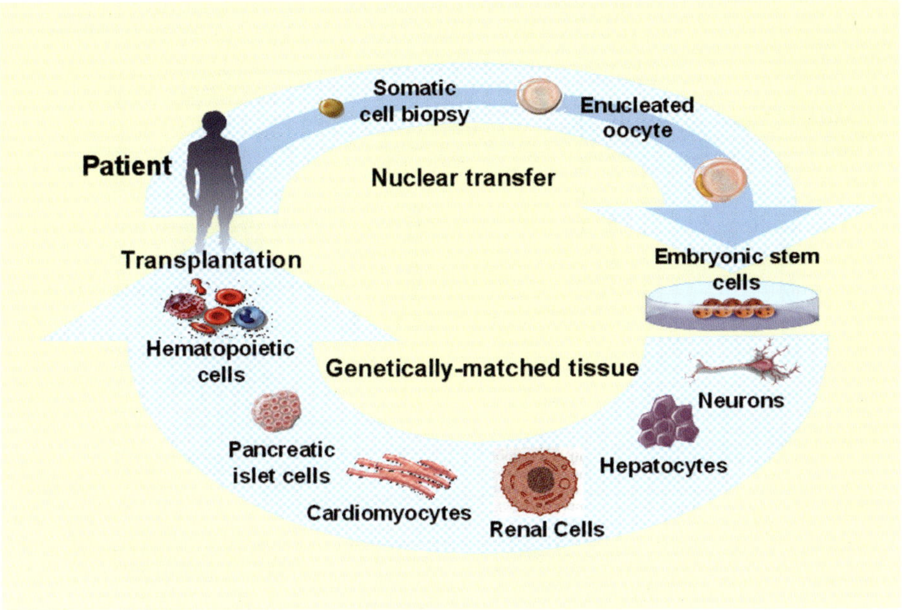


**Figure 1** Strategy for therapeutic cloning and tissue engineering.

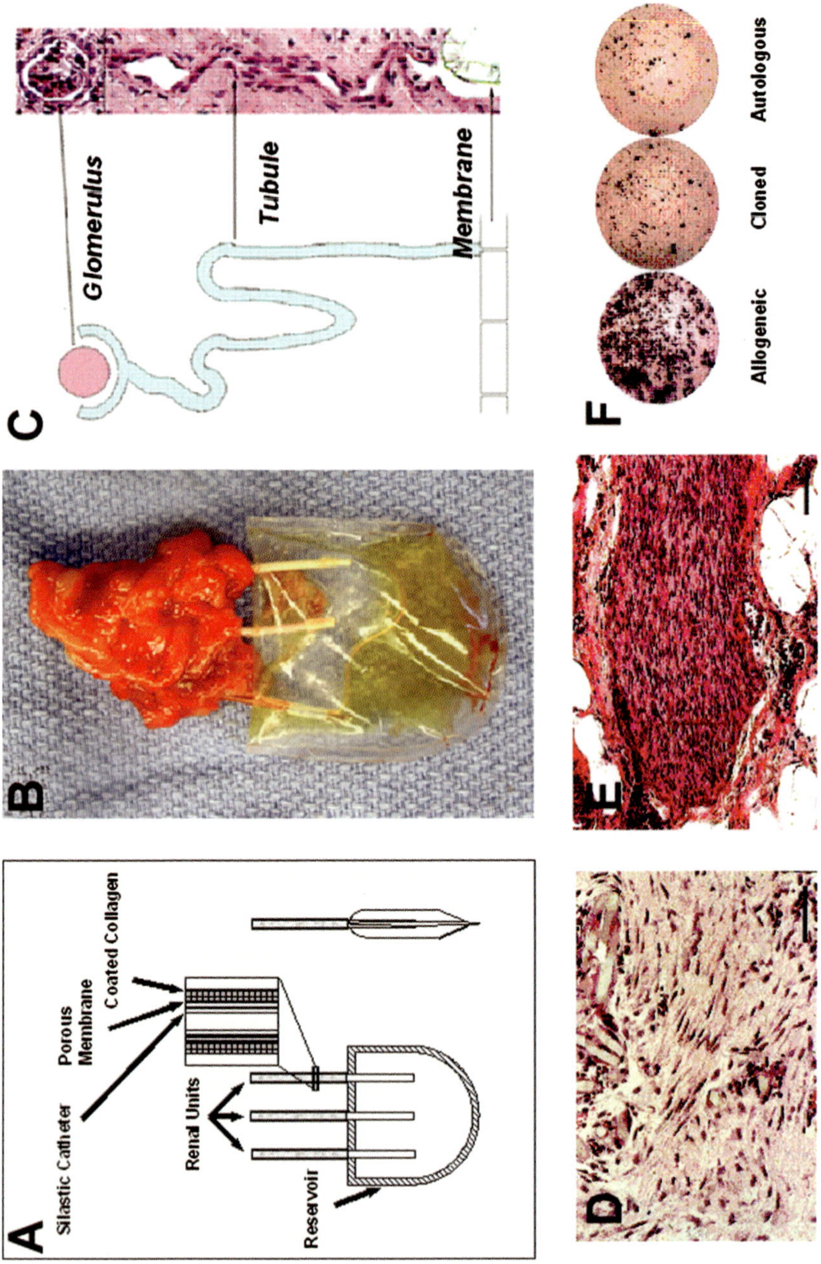


See legend on next page

**Figure 2** Applications of therapeutic cloning and tissue engineering. (*A*) Illustration of the tissue-engineered renal unit. (*B*) Renal unit seeded with cloned cells, three months after implantation, showing the accumulation of urine-like fluid. (*C*) There was a clear unidirectional continuity between the mature glomeruli, their tubules, and the polycarbonate membrane. (*D*) Retrieved cloned cardiac muscle tissue shows a well-organized cellular orientation six weeks after implantation. (*E*) Retrieved cloned skeletal muscle tissue show spatially oriented muscle fibers 12 weeks after implantation. (*F*) Elispot analyses of the frequencies of T cells that secrete IFN-gamma after primary and secondary stimulation with allogeneic renal cells, cloned renal cells, or nuclear donor fibroblasts.

nearly 80,000 patients were awaiting a donor organ and over 6000 patients were reported to have died while awaiting an organ transplant (5). This has spawned the search for alternate therapies, such as therapeutic cloning, that can be used in regenerative medicine applications.

## DEFINITION OF THERAPEUTIC CLONING

Nuclear cloning, which has also been called nuclear transplantation and nuclear transfer, involves the introduction of a nucleus from a donor cell into an enucleated oocyte to generate an embryo with a genetic makeup identical to that of the donor.

Although there has been tremendous interest in the field of nuclear cloning since the birth of Dolly in 1997, the first successful nuclear transfer was reported over 50 years ago by Briggs & King (6). Cloned frogs, which were the first vertebrates derived from nuclear transfer, were subsequently reported by Gurdon in 1962 (7), but the nuclei were derived from nonadult sources. In the past six years, tremendous advances in nuclear cloning technology have been reported, indicating the relative immaturity of the field. Dolly was not the first cloned mammal to be produced from adult cells; in fact, live lambs were produced in 1996 using nuclear transfer and differentiated epithelial cells derived from embryonic discs (8). The significance of Dolly was that she was the first mammal to be derived from an adult somatic cell using nuclear transfer (9). Since then, animals from several species have been grown using nuclear transfer technology, including cattle (10), goats (11, 12), mice (13), and pigs (14–17).

Two types of nuclear cloning, reproductive cloning and therapeutic cloning, have been described, and a better understanding of the differences between the two types may help to alleviate some of the controversy that surrounds these revolutionary technologies (18, 19). Banned in most countries for human applications, reproductive cloning is used to generate an embryo that has the identical genetic material as its cell source. This embryo can then be implanted into the uterus of a female to give rise to an infant that is a clone of the donor. Conversely, therapeutic cloning is used to generate early stage embryos that are explanted in culture to produce embryonic stem cell lines whose genetic material is identical to that of its source. These autologous stem cells have the potential to become almost any type of cell in the adult body and thus would be useful in tissue and organ replacement applications (20). Some useful applications would be in the treatment of diseases, such as end-stage kidney disease, neurodegenerative diseases, and diabetes, for which there is limited availability of immunocompatible tissue transplants.

Therefore, therapeutic cloning, which has also been called somatic cell nuclear transfer, provides an alternative source of transplantable cells that theoretically may be limitless. Figure 1 (see color insert) shows the strategy of combining therapeutic cloning with tissue engineering to develop tissues and organs. According to data from the Centers for Disease Control, it has been estimated that approximately 3000 Americans die every day of diseases that could have been treated with embryonic stem cell–derived tissues (21). With current allogeneic tissue transplantation protocols, rejection is a frequent complication because of immunologic incompatibility, and immunosuppressive drugs are usually administered to treat and hopefully prevent host-versus-graft disease (20). The use of transplantable tissue and organs derived from therapeutic cloning may lead to the avoidance of immune responses that typically are associated with transplantation of nonautologous tissues. As a result, with therapeutic cloning, the variety of serious and potentially life-threatening complications associated with immunosuppressive treatments may be avoided (22).

## STEM CELLS AND THERAPEUTIC CLONING

Most current strategies for tissue/organ replacement therapy depend upon a sample of autologous cells from the diseased organ of the host. However, for many patients with extensive end-stage organ failure, a tissue biopsy may not yield enough normal cells for expansion and eventual transplantation. In these situations, embryonic stem cells are envisioned as an alternative source of cells from which the desired tissue can be derived. Combining the techniques learned in tissue engineering over the past few decades with this potentially endless source of versatile cells could lead to novel sources of replacement organs.

Embryonic stem cells exhibit two remarkable properties: the ability to proliferate in an undifferentiated but pluripotent state (self-renew) and the ability to differentiate into many specialized cell types (23). They can be isolated by immunosurgery from the inner cell mass of the embryo during the blastocyst stage (5 days postfertilization) and are usually grown on feeder layers consisting of mouse embryonic fibroblasts or human feeder cells (24). More recent reports have shown that these cells can be grown without the use of a feeder layer (25), thus avoiding the exposure of these human cells to mouse viruses and proteins. These cells have demonstrated longevity in culture by maintaining their undifferentiated state for at least 80 passages when grown using current published protocols (26, 27).

Human embryonic stem cells have been shown to differentiate into cells from all three embryonic germ layers in vitro. Skin and neurons have been formed, indicating ectodermal differentiation (28–31). Blood, cardiac cells, cartilage, endothelial cells, and muscle have been formed, indicating mesodermal differentiation (32–34). And pancreatic cells have been formed, indicating endodermal differentiation (35). In addition, as further evidence of their pluripotency, embryonic stem cells can form embryoid bodies, which are cell aggregations that contain all three embryonic germ layers, while in culture and can form teratomas in vivo (36).

However, the harvesting of human embryonic stem cells requires the destruction of human embryos, which has raised significant ethical and political concerns in the United States. On August 9, 2001, in a compromise between stem cell research advocates and critics, the federal government ordered that only previously generated human embryonic stem cell lines could be approved for federal research funding; over 70 different cell lines met this criterion at that time. However, as stated in National Institutes of Health (NIH) testimony before Congress in April 2003, only 11 stem cell lines are currently available, which has had deleterious effects on the progress of stem cell research in the United States (37). In addition, most of the approved cell lines were grown in the presence of mouse cells (feeder cells), which can supply many needed growth factors, but which also expose the human cells to potential contamination from mouse viruses or proteins. This may render the current cell lines unsuitable for human therapeutic purposes.

These barriers to progress in embryonic stem cell research have spawned the search for alternate sources of embryonic stem cells. Therapeutic cloning may be a potentially viable source of embryonic stem cells that avoids the ethical and political controversies described above.

## FURTHER IMPROVEMENTS IN SOMATIC CELL NUCLEAR TRANSFER TECHNOLOGY

Although promising, somatic cell nuclear transfer technology has certain limitations that require further improvements before therapeutic cloning can be applied widely in replacement therapy.

Currently, the efficiency of the overall cloning process is low. The majority of embryos derived from animal cloning do not survive after implantation (38–40). In practical terms, multiple nuclear transfers must be performed in order to produce one live offspring for animal cloning applications. The potential for cloned embryos to grow into live offspring is between 0.5% to 18% for sheep, bovine, pigs, and mice (41). However, greater success (80%) has been reported in cattle (42), which may be in part due to the availability of advanced bovine supporting technologies, such as in vitro embryo production and embryo transfer, which have been developed for this species for agricultural purposes. To improve cloning efficiencies, further improvements are required in the multiple complex steps of nuclear transfer, such as enucleation and reconstruction, activation of oocytes, and cell cycle synchronization between donor cells and recipient oocytes (43), which will more readily produce viable sources of cells.

Furthermore, common abnormalities have been found in newborn clones if they survive to birth, including enlarged size with an enlarged placenta (large-offspring syndrome) (44); respiratory distress and defects of the kidney, liver, heart, and brain (45); obesity (46); and premature death (47). These may be related to the epigenetics of the cloned cells, which involve the reversible modifications of the DNA or chromatin, whereas the original DNA (genetic) sequences remain intact. Faulty epigenetic reprogramming in clones, where the DNA methylation patterns, histone modifications, and the overall chromatin structure of the somatic nuclei are not being reprogrammed to an embryonic pattern of expression, may explain the above abnormalities (20). Reactivation of key embryonic genes at the blastocyst stage is usually not present in embryos cloned from somatic cells, whereas embryos cloned from embryos consistently express early embryonic genes (48, 49). Proper epigenetic reprogramming to an embryonic state may help to improve the cloning efficiency and reduce the incidence of abnormal cloned cells.

## TISSUE ENGINEERING PRINCIPLES

After an adequate amount of cells are expanded from a cloned source, tissue engineering will be required to produce transplantable tissue or organs. The field of tissue engineering has emerged over the past 40 years to address the shortcomings of previous replacement therapies. Scientists in this relatively new field aim to combine the principles of cell transplantation, material science, and engineering to construct biological substitutes that will restore and maintain normal function in diseased and injured tissues. Over the past two decades, scientists have attempted to engineer tissue replacements for virtually every tissue and body part of the human body.

Tissue engineering strategies generally fall into two categories: acellular matrices, where matrices are used alone and depend on the body's natural ability to regenerate new tissue, and matrices with cells. Acellular tissue matrices are usually prepared by removing cellular components from tissues via mechanical and chemical manipulation to produce collagen-rich matrices (50–53). These matrices tend to slowly degrade on implantation and are generally replaced by the extracellular matrix (ECM) proteins that are secreted by the ingrowing cells.

When cells are used for tissue engineering, a small piece of donor tissue or cloned tissue is dissociated into individual cells. These cells are either implanted directly into the host or are expanded in culture, attached to a support matrix, and then reimplanted into the host after expansion. The source of donor tissue can be heterologous (such as bovine), allogeneic (same species, different individual), or autologous. Ideally, both structural and functional tissue replacement will occur with minimal complications. The most preferred cells to use are autologous cells, where a biopsy of tissue is obtained from the host, the cells are dissociated and expanded in culture, and the expanded cells are implanted into the same host (53–70). The use of autologous cells or cloned cells avoids rejection and, thus, the deleterious side effects of immunosuppressive medications can be avoided.

One of the initial factors that inhibited progress in cell-based tissue engineering in the past was the difficulty of growing the cells in culture in quantities sufficient for transplantation. Although cells could be grown in a laboratory setting for in vitro studies, there was an inherent difficulty in expanding them into large enough quantities in the laboratory, such that tissue formation could occur in vivo after transplantation. This was thought to be due to a natural senescence that was difficult to overcome. However, over the past two decades, protocols have been developed in many laboratories that allow for sufficient expansion in vitro that produce adequate numbers of cells for tissue formation. As an example, urothelial cells can now be harvested and expanded without the use of any enzymes or serum (59, 71–73).

With urothelial cells, a single specimen of cells that initially covers a surface area of 1 $cm^2$ can be expanded into enough cells that covers a surface area of 4202 $m^2$ (the equivalent area of one football field) within 8 weeks (59). This serves as an example that a small sample of autologous cells can be collected from a human patient, expanded in culture, and then returned to the same patient in sufficient quantities for reconstructive purposes.

For transplantation, the expanded cells are seeded onto a scaffold synthesized with the appropriate biomaterial. In tissue engineering, biomaterials replicate the biologic and mechanical function of native ECM found in tissues in the body by serving as an artificial ECM. As a result, biomaterials provide a three-dimensional space for the cells to form into new tissues with appropriate structure and function and also can allow for the delivery of cells and appropriate bioactive factors (e.g., cell adhesion peptides, growth factors) to desired sites in the body (74). As the majority of mammalian cell types are anchorage dependent and will die if no cell-adhesion substrate is available, biomaterials provide a cell-adhesion substrate that can deliver cells to specific sites in the body with high loading efficiency. Biomaterials can also provide mechanical support against in vivo forces such that the predefined three-dimensional structure is maintained during tissue development. Furthermore, bioactive signals, such as cell-adhesion peptides and growth factors, can be loaded along with cells to help regulate cellular function.

The ideal biomaterial should be biocompatible in that it is biodegradable and bioresorbable to support the replacement of normal tissue without inflammation. Incompatible materials are destined for an inflammatory or foreign-body response that eventually leads to rejection and/or necrosis. In addition, the degradation products, if produced, should be removed from the body via metabolic pathways at an adequate rate that keeps the concentration of these degradation products in the tissues at a tolerable level (75). Furthermore, the biomaterial should provide an environment in which appropriate regulation of cell behavior (e.g., adhesion, proliferation, migration, differentiation) can occur such that functional tissue can form. Cell behavior in the newly formed tissue has been shown to be regulated by multiple interactions of the cells with their microenvironment, including interactions with cell-adhesion ligands (76) and with soluble growth factors (77). In addition, biomaterials provide temporary mechanical support that allows the tissue to grow in three dimensions while the cells undergo spatial tissue reorganization. The properly chosen biomaterial should allow the engineered tissue to maintain sufficient mechanical integrity to support itself in early development, whereas in late development, the properly chosen biomaterial should have begun degradation such that it does not hinder further tissue growth (74).

## APPLICATIONS OF THERAPEUTIC CLONING

We applied the principles of both tissue engineering and therapeutic cloning in an effort to produce genetically identical renal, cardiac, and skeletal muscle tissue in a large animal model, the cow (*Bos taurus*) (78). Unfertilized bovine donor oocytes were retrieved from abbatoir-derived ovaries, and the nuclear material from these eggs was removed by mechanical enucleation 18–22 h after maturation. Complete enucleation of the metaphase plate was confirmed with *bis* Benzimide dye under fluorescence microscopy. Bovine skin fibroblasts from adult Holstein steers were obtained by ear notch, and single donor cells were isolated and microinjected into the perivitelline space of the enucleated oocytes (nuclear transfer). Neoembryogenesis with fusion of the cell-oocyte complexes was initiated by applying a single electrical pulse of 2.4k V/cm for 15 $\mu$s. The resulting blastocysts were implanted into progestrin-synchronized recipients to allow for further in vivo growth.

After 12 weeks, cloned renal and muscle cells were harvested, expanded in vitro, then seeded onto biodegradable scaffolds. The constructs, which consist of the cells and the scaffolds, were then implanted into the subcutaneous space of the same steer from which the cells were cloned to allow for tissue growth.

## Muscle

Cloned bovine cardiac and skeletal muscle cells seeded on polyglycolic acid scaffolds were retrieved 6 weeks after transplantation. Histologic examination of the cloned muscle constructs revealed well-organized cellular orientation with spindle-shaped nuclei (Figures 2*D*,*E*, see color insert), and immunohistochemical analysis identified muscle fibers within the implanted constructs. In addition, semiquantitative RT-PCR and Western blot analysis confirmed the expression of muscle-specific mRNA and proteins. Furthermore, histologic examination revealed extensive vascularization within the implants, which is essential for the survival and future growth of the cloned tissue.

The control implants that were seeded with allogeneic cells were noted to have a lack of muscle bundle formation, and histology revealed an abundance of inflammatory cells, fibrosis, and necrotic debris consistent with acute rejection. Using immunocytochemical analyses and CD4- and CD8-specific antibodies, the control implants were noted to have an approximately twofold increase in CD4+ and CD8+ T cells as compared to the cloned implants. Furthermore, Western blot analyses indicated a significant increase in the expression intensities of both CD4 and CD8 in the control implants when compared with that in the cloned implants.

## Kidney

The kidney is a complex organ with multiple cell types and a complex functional anatomy that renders it one of the most difficult to reconstruct (54, 79). Previous efforts in tissue engineering of the kidney have been directed toward the development of extracorporeal renal support systems made of biological and synthetic components (80–86), and ex vivo renal replacement devices are known to be life-sustaining. However, there would be obvious benefits for patients with end-stage kidney disease if these devices could be implanted long term without the need for an extracorporeal perfusion circuit or immunosuppressive drugs.

For the production of cloned kidney tissue, renal cells were isolated and expanded in vitro. The presence of renal-specific proteins, such as synaptopodin (produced by podocytes), aquaporin-1 (produced by proximal tubules and the descending limb of the loop of Henle), aquaporin-2 (produced by the ascending loop of Henle), Tamm-Horsfall protein (produced by the ascending loop of Henle), and Factor VII (produced by endothelial cells), was confirmed by immunohistochemistry on in vitro samples. In addition, the renal cells were noted to produce two important kidney proteins, erythropoietin and 1,25-dihydroxyvitamin $D_3$.

After the renal cells were characterized and expanded, the cloned cells were seeded on scaffolds consisting of three collagen-coated cylindrical polycarbonate membranes (Figure 2*A*). The ends of the three membranes of each scaffold were connected to catheters that terminated into a collecting reservoir. This created a renal neo-organ with a mechanism for collecting the excreted urinary fluid. These scaffolds with the collecting devices were transplanted subcutaneously into the same steer from which the genetic material originated and retrieved 12 weeks after implantation.

Upon retrieval, a straw-yellow fluid was seen in the reservoirs of the cloned cells (Figure 2*B*). Chemical analysis noted the presence of urea nitrogen and creatinine in the fluid at levels that approached physiologically normal levels. In addition, after analysis of the electrolyte levels, specific gravity, and glucose concentrations of the collected fluid, the implanted renal cells were noted to possess filtration, reabsorption, and secretory capabilities.

Histological examination of the retrieved implants revealed extensive vascularization and self-organization of the cells into glomeruli- and tubule-like structures. The glomeruli-like structures were noted to have a variety of cell types with abundant red blood cells, whereas the tubule-like structures were lined with cuboidal epithelial cells with large, spherical, and pale-stained nuclei. A clear continuity between the glomeruli, the tubules, and the polycarbonate membrane was noted that allowed the passage of urine into the collecting reservoir (Figure 2*C*). Immunohistochemical analysis with renal-specific antibodies revealed the presence of renal proteins corresponding to tubular (AQP1), collecting tubule (AQP2), and glomerular (synaptopodin) segments within the cloned constructs. RT-PCR analysis confirmed the transcription of the corresponding renal-specific RNA in the cloned specimens, and Western blot analysis confirmed the presence of elevated renal-specific protein levels.

## Mitochondrial DNA (mtDNA) Analysis

Because previous studies have shown that bovine clones harbor the oocyte mitochondrial DNA (87–89), the donor egg's mitochondrial DNA was thought to be a potential source of immunologic incompatibility. Differences in mtDNA-encoded proteins expressed by cloned cells could stimulate a T cell response specific for mtDNA-encoded minor histocompatibility antigens when the cloned cells are implanted back into thc original nuclear donor (90). We used nucleotide sequencing of the mtDNA genomes of the clone and fibroblast nuclear donor to identify potential antigens in the muscle constructs. Only two amino acid substitutions were noted to distinguish the clone and the nuclear donor, and as a result, a maximum of two minor histocompatibility antigens could be defined. Given the lack of knowledge regarding peptide-binding motifs for bovine major histocompatability complex (MHC) class I molecules, there is no reliable method to predict the impact of these amino acid substitutions on bovine histocompatibility.

Oocyte-derived mtDNA was also thought to be a potential source of immunologic incompatibility in the cloned renal cells. Maternally transmitted minor histocompatibility antigens in mice have been shown to stimulate both skin allograft rejection in vivo and cytotoxic T lymphocytes expansion in vitro (90) that could prevent the use of these cloned constructs in patients with chronic rejection of MHC-matched human renal transplants (91, 92). We tested for a possible T cell response to the cloned renal devices using delayed-type hypersensitivity testing in vivo and Elispot analysis of interferon-gamma secreting T cells in vitro. Both analyses revealed that the cloned renal cells showed no evidence of a T cell response, suggesting that rejection will not necessarily occur in the presence of oocyte-derived mitochondrial DNA (Figure 2*F*). This finding may represent a step forward in overcoming the histocompatibility problem of stem cell therapy (79).

These studies demonstrated that cells derived from nuclear transfer can be successfully harvested, expanded in culture, and transplanted in vivo with the use of biodegradable scaffolds on which the single suspended cells can organize into tissue structures that are genetically identical to that of the host. These studies were the first demonstration of the use of therapeutic cloning for regeneration of tissues in vivo.

Eventually, physicians may be able to take a single skin cell from a patient and generate any type of tissue for replacement therapy. The advantage of this system, as opposed to current transplantation techniques, is that the transplanted tissue would be genetically identical to that of the recipient and thus would be fully immunocompatible. Conceivably, each patient could have a ready-made supply of autologous tissue stored for their own use should the need arise in the future.



## LITERATURE CITED

1. Gurdon JB, Colman A. 1999. The future of cloning. *Nature* 402:743–46
2. Lysaght MJ, O'Loughlin JA. 2000. Demographic scope and economic magnitude of contemporary organ replacement therapies. *ASAIO J.* 46:515–21
3. Lysaght MJ. 2002. Maintenance dialysis population dynamics: current trends and long-term implications. *J. Am. Soc. Nephrol.* 13:S37–40
4. Murray JE, Merrill JP, Harrison JH. 1955. Renal homotransplantation in identical twins. *Surg. Forum* 6:432–36
5. UNOS. 2002. 2002 OPTN/SRTR Annual Report. www.optn.org
6. Briggs R, King TJ. 1952. Transplantation of living nuclei from blastula cells into enucleated frogs' eggs. *Proc. Natl. Acad. Sci. USA* 38:455–63
7. Gurdon JB. 1962. Adult frogs derived from the nuclei of single somatic cells. *Dev. Biol.* 4:256–73

8. Campbell KH, McWhir J, Ritchie WA, Wilmut I. 1996. Sheep cloned by nuclear transfer from a cultured cell line. *Nature* 380:64–66
9. Wilmut I, Schnieke AE, McWhir J, Kind AJ, Campbell KH. 1997. Viable offspring derived from fetal and adult mammalian cells. *Nature* 385:810–13. Erratum. 1997. *Nature* 386(6621):200
10. Cibelli JB, Stice SL, Golueke PJ, Kane JJ, Jerry J, et al. 1998. Cloned transgenic calves produced from nonquiescent fetal fibroblasts. *Science* 280:1256–58
11. Baguisi A, Behboodi E, Melican DT, Pollock JS, Destrempes MM, et al. 1999. Production of goats by somatic cell nuclear transfer. *Nat. Biotechnol.* 17:456–61
12. Keefer CL, Keyston R, Lazaris A, Bhatia B, Begin I, et al. 2002. Production of cloned goats after nuclear transfer using adult somatic cells. *Biol. Reprod.* 66:199–203
13. Wakayama T, Perry AC, Zuccotti M, Johnson KR, Yanagimachi R. 1998. Full-term development of mice from enucleated oocytes injected with cumulus cell nuclei. *Nature* 394:369–74
14. Betthauser J, Forsberg E, Augenstein M, Childs L, Eilertsen K, et al. 2000. Production of cloned pigs from in vitro systems. *Nat. Biotechnol.* 18:1055–59
15. Polejaeva IA, Chen SH, Vaught TD, Page RL, Mullins J, et al. 2000. Cloned pigs produced by nuclear transfer from adult somatic cells. *Nature* 407:86–90
16. Onishi A, Iwamoto M, Akita T, Mikawa S, Takeda K, et al. 2000. Pig cloning by microinjection of fetal fibroblast nuclei. *Science* 289:1188–90
17. De Sousa PA, Dobrinsky JR, Zhu J, Archibald AL, Ainslie A, et al. 2002. Somatic cell nuclear transfer in the pig: control of pronuclear formation and integration with improved methods for activation and maintenance of pregnancy. *Biol. Reprod.* 66:642–50
18. Colman A, Kind A. 2000. Therapeutic cloning: concepts and practicalities. *Trends Biotechnol.* 18:192–96
19. Vogelstein B, Alberts B, Shine K. 2002. Genetics. Please don't call it cloning! *Science* 295:1237
20. Hochedlinger K, Jaenisch R. 2003. Nuclear transplantation, embryonic stem cells, and the potential for cell therapy. *N. Engl. J. Med.* 349:275–86
21. Lanza RP, Cibelli JB, West MD, Dorff E, Tauer C, Green RM. 2001. The ethical reasons for stem cell research. *Science.* 292:1299
22. Lanza RP, Cibelli JB, West MD. 1999. Prospects for the use of nuclear transfer in human transplantation. *Nat. Biotechnol.* 17:1171–74
23. Brivanlou AH, Gage FH, Jaenisch R, Jessell T, Melton D, Rossant J. 2003. Stem cells. Setting standards for human embryonic stem cells. *Science* 300:913–16
24. Richards M, Fong CY, Chan WK, Wong PC, Bongso A. 2002. Human feeders support prolonged undifferentiated growth of human inner cell masses and embryonic stem cells. *Nat. Biotechnol.* 20:933–36
25. Amit M, Margulets V, Segev H, Shariki K, Laevsky I, et al. 2003. Human feeder layers for human embryonic stem cells. *Biol. Reprod.* 68:2150–56
26. Reubinoff BE, Pera MF, Fong CY, Trounson A, Bongso A. 2000. Embryonic stem cell lines from human blastocysts: somatic differentiation in vitro. *Nat. Biotechnol.* 18:399–404. Erratum. 2000. *Nat. Biotechnol.* 18(5):559
27. Thomson JA, Itskovitz-Eldor J, Shapiro SS, Waknitz MA, Swiergiel JJ, et al. 1998. Embryonic stem cell lines derived from human blastocysts. *Science* 282:1145–47. Erratum. 1998. *Science* 282(5395):1827
28. Reubinoff BE, Itsykson P, Turetsky T, Pera MF, Reinhartz E, et al. 2001. Neural progenitors from human embryonic stem cells. *Nat. Biotechnol.* 19:1134–40
29. Schuldiner M, Eiges R, Eden A, Yanuka O, Itskovitz-Eldor J, et al. 2001. Induced neuronal differentiation of human embryonic stem cells. *Brain Res.* 913:201–5

30. Schuldiner M, Yanuka O, Itskovitz-Eldor J, Melton DA, Benvenisty N. 2000. Effects of eight growth factors on the differentiation of cells derived from human embryonic stem cells. *Proc. Natl. Acad. Sci. USA* 97:11307–12
31. Zhang SC, Wernig M, Duncan ID, Brustle O, Thomson JA. 2001. In vitro differentiation of transplantable neural precursors from human embryonic stem cells. *Nat. Biotechnol.* 19:1129–33
32. Kaufman DS, Hanson ET, Lewis RL, Auerbach R, Thomson JA. 2001. Hematopoietic colony-forming cells derived from human embryonic stem cells. *Proc. Natl. Acad. Sci. USA* 98:10716–21
33. Kehat I, Kenyagin-Karsenti D, Snir M, Segev H, Amit M, et al. 2001. Human embryonic stem cells can differentiate into myocytes with structural and functional properties of cardiomyocytes. *J. Clin. Invest.* 108:407–14
34. Levenberg S, Golub JS, Amit M, Itskovitz-Eldor J, Langer R. 2002. Endothelial cells derived from human embryonic stem cells. *Proc. Natl. Acad. Sci. USA* 99:4391–96
35. Assady S, Maor G, Amit M, Itskovitz-Eldor J, Skorecki KL, Tzukerman M. 2001. Insulin production by human embryonic stem cells. *Diabetes* 50:1691–97
36. Itskovitz-Eldor J, Schuldiner M, Karsenti D, Eden A, Yanuka O, et al. 2000. Differentiation of human embryonic stem cells into embryoid bodies compromising the three embryonic germ layers. *Mol. Med.* 6:88–95
37. Kennedy D. 2003. Stem cells: still here, still waiting. *Science* 300: 865
38. Solter D. 2000. Mammalian cloning: advances and limitations. *Nat. Rev. Genet.* 1:199–207
39. Rideout WM 3rd, Eggan K, Jaenisch R. 2001. Nuclear cloning and epigenetic reprogramming of the genome. *Science* 293:1093–98
40. Hochedlinger K, Jaenisch R. 2002. Nuclear transplantation: lessons from frogs and mice. *Curr. Opin. Cell Biol.* 14:741–48
41. Tsunoda Y, Kato Y. 2002. Recent progress and problems in animal cloning. *Differentiation* 69:158–61
42. Kato Y, Tani T, Sotomaru Y, Kurokawa K, Kato J, et al. 1998. Eight calves cloned from somatic cells of a single adult. *Science* 282:2095–98
43. Dinnyes A, De Sousa P, King T, Wilmut I. 2002. Somatic cell nuclear transfer: recent progress and challenges. *Cloning Stem Cells* 4:81–90
44. Young LE, Sinclair KD, Wilmut I. 1998. Large offspring syndrome in cattle and sheep. *Rev. Reprod.* 3:155–63
45. Cibelli JB, Campbell KH, Seidel GE, West MD, Lanza RP. 2002. The health profile of cloned animals. *Nat. Biotechnol.* 20:13–14
46. Tamashiro KL, Wakayama T, Akutsu H, Yamazaki Y, Lachey JL, et al. 2002. Cloned mice have an obese phenotype not transmitted to their offspring. *Nat. Med.* 8:262–67
47. Ogonuki N, Inoue K, Yamamoto Y, Noguchi Y, Tanemura K, et al. 2002. Early death of mice cloned from somatic cells. *Nat. Genet.* 30:253–54
48. Bortvin A, Eggan K, Skaletsky H, Akutsu H, Berry DL, et al. 2003. Incomplete reactivation of Oct4-related genes in mouse embryos cloned from somatic nuclei. *Development* 130:1673–80
49. Boiani M, Eckardt S, Scholer HR, McLaughlin KJ. 2002. Oct4 distribution and level in mouse clones: consequences for pluripotency. *Genes Dev.* 16:1209–19
50. Chen F, Yoo JJ, Atala A. 1999. Acellular collagen matrix as a possible "off the shelf" biomaterial for urethral repair. *Urology* 54:407–10
51. Dahms SE, Piechota HJ, Dahiya R, Lue TF, Tanagho EA. 1998. Composition and biomechanical properties of the bladder acellular matrix graft: comparative analysis in rat, pig and human. *Brit. J. Urol.* 82:411–19
52. Piechota HJ, Dahms SE, Nunes LS, Dahiya R, Lue TF, Tanagho EA. 1998. In vitro

functional properties of the rat bladder regenerated by the bladder acellular matrix graft. *J. Urol.* 159:1717–24
53. Yoo JJ, Meng J, Oberpenning F, Atala A. 1998. Bladder augmentation using allogenic bladder submucosa seeded with cells. *Urology* 51:221–25
54. Amiel GE, Atala A. 1999. Current and future modalities for functional renal replacement. *Urol. Clin. North Am.* 26:235–46, xi
55. Atala A. 1999. Future perspectives in reconstructive surgery using tissue engineering. *Urol. Clin. North Am.* 26:157–65, ix–x
56. Atala A, Freeman MR, Vacanti JP, Shepard J, Retik AB. 1993. Implantation in vivo and retrieval of artificial structures consisting of rabbit and human urothelium and human bladder muscle. *J. Urol.* 150:608–12
57. Atala A, Guzman L, Retik AB. 1999. A novel inert collagen matrix for hypospadias repair. *J. Urol.* 162:1148–51
58. Atala A, Kim W, Paige KT, Vacanti CA, Retik AB. 1994. Endoscopic treatment of vesicoureteral reflux with a chondrocyte-alginate suspension. *J. Urol.* 152:641–43; discuss. 4
59. Cilento BG, Freeman MR, Schneck FX, Retik AB, Atala A. 1994. Phenotypic and cytogenetic characterization of human bladder urothelia expanded in vitro. *J. Urol.* 152:665–70
60. Fauza DO, Fishman SJ, Mehegan K, Atala A. 1998. Videofetoscopically assisted fetal tissue engineering: bladder augmentation. *J. Pediatr. Surg.* 33:7–12
61. Fauza DO, Fishman SJ, Mehegan K, Atala A. 1998. Videofetoscopically assisted fetal tissue engineering: skin replacement. *J. Pediatr. Surg.* 33:357–61
62. Godbey WT, Atala A. 2002. In vitro systems for tissue engineering. *Ann. N.Y. Acad. Sci.* 961:10–26
63. Kershen RT, Atala A. 1999. New advances in injectable therapies for the treatment of incontinence and vesicoureteral reflux. *Urol. Clin. North Am.* 26:81–94, viii
64. Oberpenning F, Meng J, Yoo JJ, Atala A. 1999. De novo reconstitution of a functional mammalian urinary bladder by tissue engineering. *Nat. Biotechnol.* 17:149–55
65. Park HJ, Yoo JJ, Kershen RT, Moreland R, Atala A. 1999. Reconstitution of human corporal smooth muscle and endothelial cells in vivo. *J. Urol.* 162:1106–9
66. Yoo JJ, Atala A. 1997. A novel gene delivery system using urothelial tissue engineered neo-organs. *J. Urol.* 158:1066–70
67. Yoo JJ, Lee I, Atala A. 1998. Cartilage rods as a potential material for penile reconstruction. *J. Urol.* 160:1164–68; discuss. 78
68. Atala A, Lanza RP. 2001. Preface. In *Methods of Tissue Engineering*, ed. A Atala, RP Lanza. San Diego, CA: Academic
69. Atala A, Mooney D. 1997. Preface. In *Tissue Engineering*, ed. A Atala. Boston: Birkhauser Press
70. Machluf M, Atala A. 1998. Emerging concepts for tissue and organ transplantation. *Graft* 1:31
71. Liebert M, Hubbel A, Chung M, Wedemeyer G, Lomax MI, et al. 1997. Expression of mal is associated with urothelial differentiation in vitro: identification by differential display reverse-transcriptase polymerase chain reaction. *Differentiation* 61:177–85
72. Puthenveettil JA, Burger MS, Reznikoff CA. 1999. Replicative senescence in human uroepithelial cells. *Adv. Exp. Med. Biol.* 462:83–91
73. Scriven SD, Booth C, Thomas DF, Trejdosiewicz LK, Southgate J. 1997. Reconstitution of human urothelium from monolayer cultures. *J. Urol.* 158:1147–52
74. Kim BS, Mooney DJ. 1998. Development of biocompatible synthetic extracellular matrices for tissue engineering. *Trends Biotechnol.* 16:224–30
75. Bergsma JE, Rozema FR, Bos RR, Boering G, de Bruijn WC, Pennings AJ. 1995. In vivo degradation and biocompatibility study of in vitro pre-degraded as-polymerized polyactide particles. *Biomaterials* 16:267–74

76. Hynes RO. 1992. Integrins: versatility, modulation, and signaling in cell adhesion. *Cell* 69:11–25
77. Deuel TF. 1997. Growth factors. In *Principles of Tissue Engineering*, ed. RP Lanza, R Langer, WL Chick, pp. 133–49. New York: Academic
78. Lanza RP, Chung HY, Yoo JJ, Wettstein PJ, Blackwell C, et al. 2002. Generation of histocompatible tissues using nuclear transplantation. *Nat. Biotechnol.* 20:689–96
79. Auchincloss H, Bonventre JV. 2002. Transplanting cloned cells into therapeutic promise. *Nat. Biotechnol.* 20:665–66
80. Aebischer P, Ip TK, Panol G, Galletti PM. 1987. The bioartificial kidney: progress towards an ultrafiltration device with renal epithelial cells processing. *Life Support Syst.* 5:159–68
81. Amiel GE, Yoo JJ, Atala A. 2000. Renal therapy using tissue-engineered constructs and gene delivery. *World J. Urol.* 18:71–79
82. Humes HD, Buffington DA, MacKay SM, Funke AJ, Weitzel WF. 1999. Replacement of renal function in uremic animals with a tissue-engineered kidney. *Nat. Biotechnol.* 17:451–55
83. Ip TK, Aebischer P, Galletti PM. 1988. Cellular control of membrane permeability. Implications for a bioartificial renal tubule. *ASAIO Trans.* 34:351–55
84. Joki T, Machluf M, Atala A, Zhu J, Seyfried NT, et al. 2001. Continuous release of endostatin from microencapsulated engineered cells for tumor therapy. *Nat. Biotechnol.* 19:35–39
85. Lanza RP, Hayes JL, Chick WL. 1996. Encapsulated cell technology. *Nat. Biotechnol.* 14:1107–11
86. MacKay SM, Funke AJ, Buffington DA, Humes HD. 1998. Tissue engineering of a bioartificial renal tubule. *ASAIO J.* 44:179–83
87. Evans MJ, Gurer C, Loike JD, Wilmut I, Schnieke AE, Schon EA. 1999. Mitochondrial DNA genotypes in nuclear transfer-derived cloned sheep. *Nat. Genet.* 23:90–93
88. Hiendleder S, Schmutz SM, Erhardt G, Green RD, Plante Y. 1999. Transmitochondrial differences and varying levels of heteroplasmy in nuclear transfer cloned cattle. *Mol. Reprod. Dev.* 54:24–31
89. Steinborn R, Schinogl P, Zakhartchenko V, Achmann R, Schernthaner W, et al. 2000. Mitochondrial DNA heteroplasmy in cloned cattle produced by fetal and adult cell cloning. *Nat. Genet.* 25:255–57
90. Fischer Lindahl K, Hermel E, Loveland BE, Wang CR. 1991. Maternally transmitted antigen of mice: a model transplantation antigen. *Annu. Rev. Immunol.* 9:351–72
91. Hadley GA, Linders B, Mohanakumar T. 1992. Immunogenicity of MHC class I alloantigens expressed on parenchymal cells in the human kidney. *Transplantation* 54:537–42
92. Yard BA, Kooymans-Couthino M, Reterink T, van den Elsen P, Paape ME, et al. 1993. Analysis of T cell lines from rejecting renal allografts. *Kidney Int. Suppl.* 39:S133–38

Annu. Rev. Biomed. Eng. 2004. 6:41–75
doi: 10.1146/annurev.bioeng.6.040803.140027

First published online as a Review in Advance on March 24, 2004

# BIOMATERIALS: Where We Have Been and Where We Are Going

Buddy D. Ratner[1,2] and Stephanie J. Bryant[1]
*[1]Department of Bioengineering and [2]Department of Chemical Engineering, University of Washington, Seattle, Washington 98195; email: ratner@uweb.engr.washington.edu*

**Key Words** surface-modified biomaterials, synthetic polymers, biomimetic materials, self-assembling peptides, patterned biomaterials

■ **Abstract** Since its inception just over a half century ago, the field of biomaterials has seen a consistent growth with a steady introduction of new ideas and productive branches. This review describes where we have been, the state of the art today, and where we might be in 10 or 20 years. Herein, we highlight some of the latest advancements in biomaterials that aim to control biological responses and ultimately heal. This new generation of biomaterials includes surface modification of materials to overcome nonspecific protein adsorption in vivo, precision immobilization of signaling groups on surfaces, development of synthetic materials with controlled properties for drug and cell carriers, biologically inspired materials that mimic natural processes, and design of sophisticated three-dimensional (3-D) architectures to produce well-defined patterns for diagnostics, e.g., biological microelectromechanical systems (bioMEMs), and tissue engineering.

CONTENTS



## INTRODUCTION

A commonly used definition of biomaterial is "a nonviable material used in a medical device, intended to interact with biological systems" (1). If the words "used in a medical device" are removed, this definition becomes more inclusive to the wide range of applications where we interface synthetic materials and modified natural materials with biology. Table 1 lists some of these applications, both medical and nonmedical. Biomaterials and medical devices have evolved over the last 50 or so years to a $100 billion endeavor. The subject of biomaterials resides at a multidimensional interface between chemistry, chemical engineering, materials science, mechanics, surface science, bioengineering, biology, and medicine, with considerable input from ethicists, government-regulated standards organizations, and entrepreneurs. The field has seen consistent growth since its inception and a steady introduction of new ideas and productive branches. Some examples of these outgrowths from biomaterials that have evolved into identifiable

**TABLE 1** Uses for biomaterials (almost A to Z)

| Medical uses | Non-medical uses |
|---|---|
| Artery graft | Arrays for DNA and diagnostics |
| Breast implant | Bioremediation materials |
| Cochlear implant | Biosensors |
| Ear drainage tube | Bioseparations, chromatography |
| Dental implant | Biofouling-resistant materials |
| Feeding tube | Biomimetics for new materials |
| Glaucoma drainage tube | Cell culture |
| Hydrocephalous shunt | Controlled release for agriculture |
| Intraocular lens | Electrophoresis materials |
| Joints (hip, knee, shoulder) | Fuel cells (biomass) |
| Keratoprosthesis | MEMS |
| Left ventricular assist device (LVAD) | Muscles (artificial) and actuators |
| Mechanical heart valve | Nanofabrication |
| Nerve guidance tube | NEMS |
| Ophthalmic drug delivery device | Neural computing/biocomputer |
| Pacemaker | Smart clothing for biowarfare |
| Renal dialyzer | Yeast array chip |
| Stent | |
| Tissue adhesive | |
| Urinary catheter | |
| Valve, heart | |
| Wound dressing | |
| X-ray guide | |
| Zirconium knee joint | |

fields of their own include controlled release, diagnostic arrays, and tissue engineering.

The numerous facets of the field of biomaterials make a comprehensive review article impossible. However, in general terms, we can review where we have been, the state of the art today, and where we might be in 10 or 20 years.

## TRADITIONAL BIOMATERIALS

Although medical implant materials have been used for at least 2000 years (some historians trace sutures back 32,000 years), most early medical implants were doomed to failure because important concepts relating to infection, materials, and the biological reaction to materials were not yet established. The modern era of medical implants might be traced back to an observation made by British ophthalmologist Harold Ridley in the late 1940s. While examining Spitfire fighter pilots who had shards of canopy plastic unintentionally implanted in their eyes from enemy machine gun fire, he noted that these shards seemed to heal without ongoing reaction. He concluded that the canopy plastic, poly(methyl methacrylate), might be appropriate for fashioning implant lenses for replacing cataractous natural lenses. His first implantation of such a lens was in 1949. His observation and innovation led to the development of modern intraocular lenses (IOLs) that are now being implanted in over 10 million human eyes each year and have revolutionized treatment for those with cataracts. At about the same time that Harold Ridley was innovating IOLs, Charnley was developing the hip implant, Vorhees invented the vascular graft, Kolff was revolutionizing kidney dialysis, and Hufnagel invented the ball and cage heart valve. These pioneers, in an era before principles for medical materials were established, proved feasibility, saved lives, and evolved the foundations that we build on today. By the late 1960s engineers, chemists, and biologists, in collaboration with physicians, were formalizing design principles and synthetic strategies for biomaterials. In particular, the idea that the release of toxic leachables from biomaterials will adversely affect healing was formalized—this toxicology idea is implicit in today's definition of biocompatibility. As developments took place in biology and materials science, biomaterials researchers were quick to incorporate these new ideas into biomaterials. Molecular biology concepts are now opening new frontiers for biomaterials design—a path to biomaterials that will work with the normal physiology and seamlessly integrate into the human body.

The appreciation of the host response (healing) of implanted materials helps us understand the performance of today's biomaterials and also aids us in envisioning how we might improve the body's response to biomaterials in the future. The following section reviews our understanding of the reaction of a living organism to an implanted synthetic material.

## Host Response to Biomaterials

When a tissue is injured, the normal healing response is initiated through a series of complex events that include acute inflammation, the formation of granulation tissue, and eventual scar formation. The immediate response is to flood the injured area with blood. Fibrinogen within the blood is cleaved into fibrin to form a blood clot that promotes platelet adhesion and aggregation. Cytokines and growth factors are released to recruit white blood cells, mainly neutrophils. Monocytes are then called to the wound site where they differentiate into macrophages. The macrophages are responsible for cleaning up the wound site, which may contain foreign material, bacteria, and dead cells, and also for recruiting cells such as fibroblasts and endothelial cells, which convert the fibrin clot into a highly vascularized granulation tissue. The formation of blood vessels is essential to the healing wound. The granulation tissue is subsequently replaced by an extracellular matrix (ECM) deposited primarily by fibroblasts. The degree of ECM remodeling depends on the extent and location of the injury. In some cases, complete restoration of the tissue architecture is possible; however, in most cases the granulation tissue is remodeled into scar tissue.

A biomaterial implanted into the body, however, induces a different response, termed the foreign body reaction. This response is illustrated in Figure 1. The biological response to materials has been reviewed in detail by Anderson (2). In brief, a biomaterial elicits nonspecific protein adsorption immediately upon implantation. Many different proteins adsorb to the surface in a range of conformations from native to denatured. Non-specific protein adsorption, however, never occurs in the normal physiological process of wound healing. Thus, nonspecific protein adsorption may be an instigator in the foreign body reaction. A number of different cells, such as monocytes, leukocytes, and platelets (cells that are key players in normal wound healing), adhere to these biomaterial surfaces and as a result may lead to upregulation of cytokines and subsequent proinflammatory processes. In addition, the implant is significantly larger than the adhered macrophages, preventing them from phagocytosing the foreign body. Chronic inflammation at the biomaterial interface ensues, and the frustrated macrophages fuse together to form multinucleated foreign body giant cells that often persist for the lifetime of the implant (3). The end stage of the foreign body reaction involves the walling off of the device by an avascular, collagenous fibrous tissue that is typically 50–200 $\mu$m thick.

## The Performance of Contemporary Biomaterial Implants

Although many medical devices are implanted in humans each year that save lives and improve the quality of life, there is substantial room for improvement of medical devices. In particular, the fibrous capsule that forms around implants can lead to complications. Capsular contracture of breast implants, insulating barriers around electrodes, scarring of heart valve sewing rings, and tough, fibrous layers

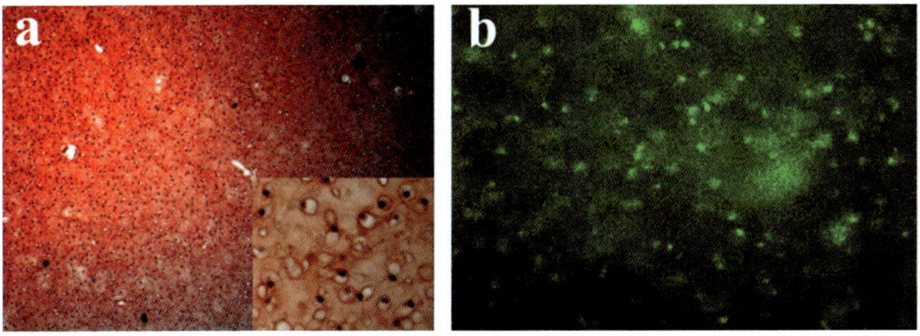


**Figure 4** Photopolymerized hydrogels for tissue scaffolds for cartilage tissue engineering. The degradation behavior of hydrogels fabricated from poly(ethylene glycol) and poly(vinyl alcohol) were tailored to match neotissue growth by encapsulated chondrocytes. The panel in (*a*) illustrates glycosaminoglycans, a primary component of proteoglycans, produced by chondrocytes after 6 weeks in vitro (complete degradation of the gel has occurred). Original magnification is 40× and 200× (*inset*). In (*b*), chondrocytes express green fluorescent protein (GFP) after 15 days in vitro when coencapsulated with lipofectamine-complexed DNA encoded for GFP in degradable PEG gels. Images courtesy of Kristi S. Anseth.

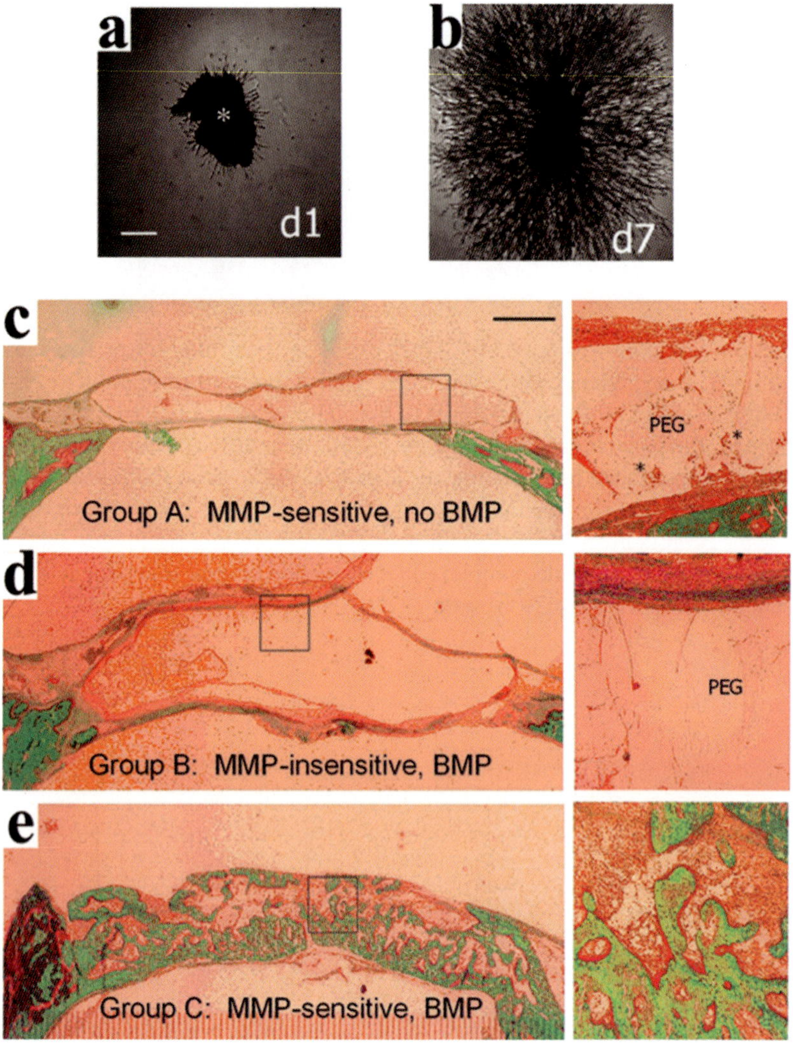


**Figure 9** Three-dimensional migration of human foreskin fibroblasts from a fibrin cluster of cells (*labeled* *) into an RGD-adhesive and MMP-sensitive PEG hydrogel at (*a*) day 1 and (*b*) day 7. PEG hydrogels containing RGD-adhesive peptides were placed in a rat calvaria critical-sized defect to monitor bone healing in response to (*c*) MMP-sensitive crosslinks, (*d*) bone morphogenic protein (BMP), or (*e*) both. Reproduced with permission from (107).

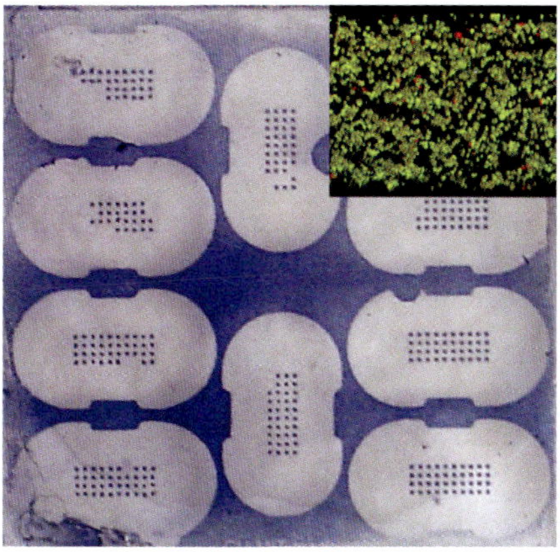

**Figure 12** A device based on living radical polymerizations containing a microarray of cells encapsulated in 3-D PEG hydrogels; (*inset*) a cross-section of cells within the hydrogel where live cells fluoresce green and dead cells fluoresce red. Image courtesy of Kristi S. Anseth.

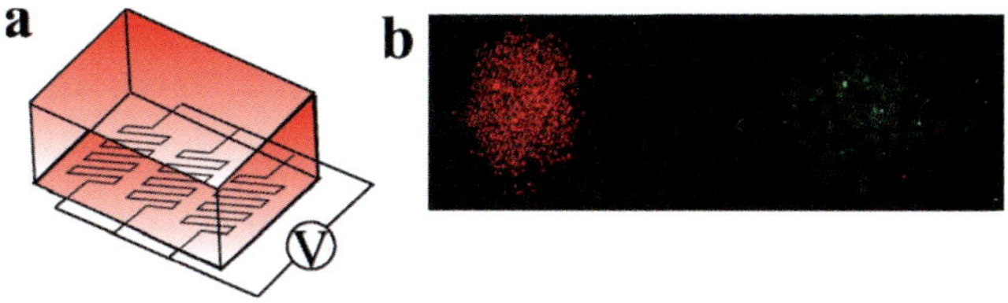


**Figure 13** (*a*) A schematic of the 3-element heater array device fabricated on plasma deposited pNIPAAm treated glass. Each of the heaters can be independently controlled and switched on demand to create a hydrophobic, cell-adhesive surface. (*b*) When the heaters were turned on separately, local adhesion of bovine aortic endothelial cells with different fluorescent tags were possible (a *red tag* was used for cells adhered to the region around the left heater and a *green tag* for cells adhered to the region around the right heater).

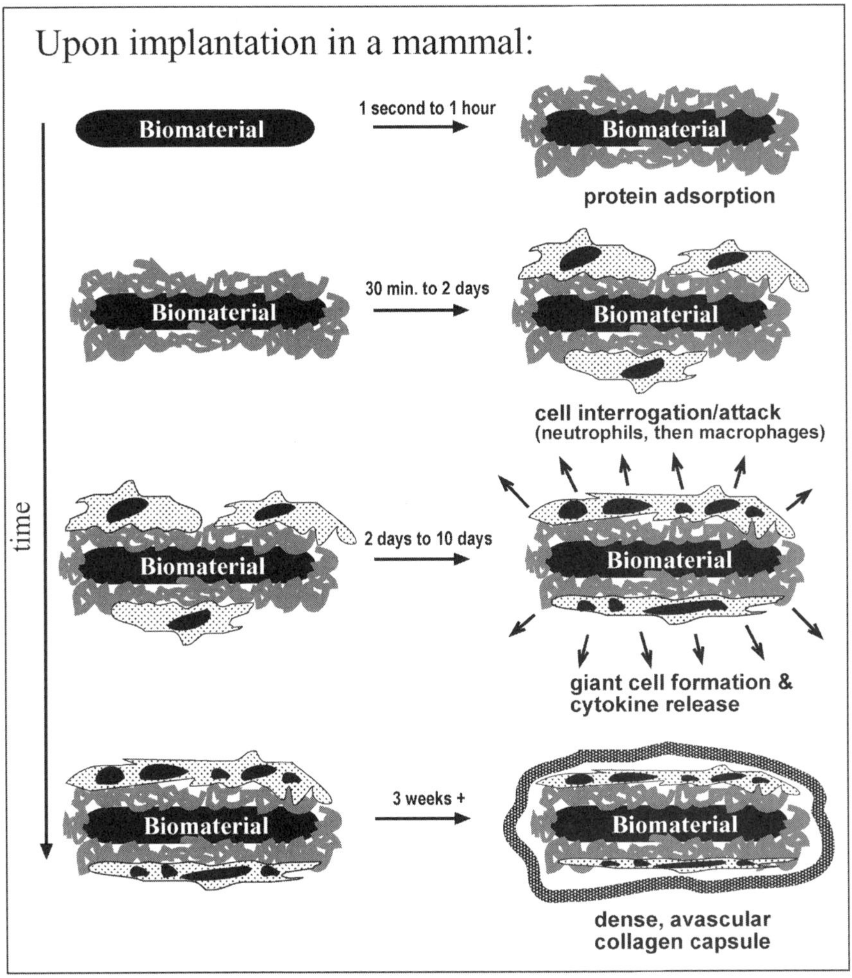


**Figure 1** The foreign body reaction as illustrated here is the normal reaction by higher organisms to an implanted synthetic material.

surrounding vascular grafts are examples of this poor healing. Furthermore, posterior capsular opacification seen in IOLs, the poor luminal healing of porous vascular grafts, and inflammation seen with some contact lenses may be manifestations of the interfacial encapsulation reaction observed for implanted materials.

In general, today's biomaterials do not control the biological response induced by them. The biological response is stochastic and unplanned. Clearly, an engineering approach that controls the interfacial response with precision is a strategy worth considering. The next generation of biomaterials may realize this vision.

# A NEW GENERATION OF BIOMATERIALS

The next generation of biomaterials will be based upon knowledge of the biology of wound healing and inflammation and will control bioreaction responses with precision. One approach to achieve such healing biomaterials is to modify surfaces of existing devices to minimize the foreign body reaction and to promote normal wound healing. This approach is elaborated on shortly. For longer-term solutions, however, researchers must turn to biology to develop ways to help the body mend itself and regenerate new tissue that can last for the patient's lifetime. The only way to replace function to damaged tissue is with similar tissue that contains the appropriate tissue architecture of cells and ECM. A number of different approaches are being investigated including drug and cell delivery. In both cases, a carrier is required to deliver the drug to a particular site successfully and, in the case of cells, to provide a 3-D structure that facilitates tissue growth. Many different types of biomaterials have been investigated for both drug and cell carriers. In tissue engineering, a combination of drugs, cells, and a suitable carrier with tailored macroscopic properties, a well-tuned degradation profile, and specific biological cues may be necessary to promote normal tissue growth.

This section highlights the next generation of biomaterials, which include surface modification of biomaterials to overcome nonspecific protein adsorption in vivo, precision immobilization of signaling groups on surfaces, the development of synthetic materials with controlled and tailored properties for drug and cell carriers, biologically inspired materials that mimic natural processes, and finally the design of sophisticated 3-D architectures to produce well-defined patterns for developing bioMEM devices and tissue-engineering scaffolds. Because of the fast growth of this field, this section aims to highlight several exciting new research areas. We present some of the most recent developments in the different subfields of biomaterials and provide references to recent reviews for more in-depth discussions. This section aims to demonstrate the powerful impact that biomaterials will have on the future of medicine.

## Surface-Modified Biomaterials

The surface chemistry and topography of a biomaterial are important parameters that influence protein adsorption, cell interaction, and the host response. For example, surface chemistry has been shown to alter monocyte adhesion in vitro (4). However, in vivo the foreign body reaction seems independent of simple surface chemistry. For instance, materials that are polymeric, ceramic, or metallic based and that exhibit different surface properties, from hydrophilic to hydrophobic or hard to soft, all elicit the same response in vivo (5–7). This observation has been attributed to nonspecific protein adsorption. In contrast, all of nature's processes employ specific molecular (i.e., protein and saccharide) interactions. Where organisms seem insensitive to relatively simple surface chemistries, the complex surfaces associated with biological recognition are effective in controlling biological responses. Thus, to address this issue, efforts have focused on modifying surfaces to control protein interaction and to decorate the surface appropriately with signaling molecules. Specifically, a considerable amount of research has explored surfaces that are resistant to protein adsorption, termed nonfouling surfaces, and more recently surfaces that control protein adsorption.

NONFOULING SURFACES Poly(ethylene glycol) (PEG), also known as poly (ethylene oxide) (PEO), has been most widely studied for its protein and cell resistance. There have been many approaches to attaching PEG to materials and rendering them nonfouling, such as through covalent immobilization, adsorption, or interpenetration. A recent novel approach takes advantage of the highly adhesive nature of mussel adhesive protein (8). Specifically, PEG was covalently attached to the mussel adhesive protein to form a copolymer that exhibited a nonfouling segment and a sticky segment. The sticky segment adhered well to gold and titanium surfaces presenting the PEG chains at the new interface. These modified surfaces were found to resist cell adhesion for up to 2 weeks in vitro (8).

Although PEG is effective in preventing nonspecific protein adsorption, its nonfouling character is dependent on surface chain density and can be damaged by oxidants. As an alternative, Lopez et al. (9) have investigated PEG-like surfaces prepared by radio frequency plasma deposition of tetraethyleneglycol dimethylether (tetraglyme), which forms a highly nonfouling crosslinked structure. In plasma-deposited tetraglyme, there are no chains longer than 3 tetraethyleneglycol units, demonstrating that the conformation of PEG is not the controlling variable in its nonfouling ability. These surfaces exhibit little protein adsorption with levels as low as 2 ng/cm$^2$ (9). These surfaces have also been shown to significantly reduce blood platelet (10) and monocyte (11, 12) adhesion in vitro.

A recent study investigated the in vivo response of untreated fluorinated ethylene propylene copolymer (FEP) and FEP treated with plasma-polymerized tetraglyme when implanted subcutaneously in the backs of mice (13). After 4 weeks, a fibrous capsule had formed around all the implants. The capsule thickness was similar regardless of treatment. Interestingly, macrophage adhesion was significantly higher in the tetraglyme-treated samples compared with the untreated samples. This study further confirms the differences between in vitro and in vivo responses. It was hypothesized that the tetraglyme surface binds very little protein in vivo, as seen in vitro, but that the conformation, not quantity, of the adsorbed protein may promote the foreign body response. For example, tetraglyme may prevent a protein from fully spreading, and therefore more active sites (i.e., cell adhesion sites) become available. Alternatively, degradation of the tetraglyme surface, and subsequent loss of the nonfouling character, may occur under in vivo conditions.

There are many nonfouling surfaces in addition to PEG. The most commonly studied are phospholipid surfaces (14) and saccharide surfaces (15). A number of novel classes of nonfouling surfaces have recently been reported (16). Theoretical and experimental studies on the nature of the nonfouling phenomenon are expanding our understanding of the important parameters driving protein adsorption (17,

18). In general, a number of different chemistries minimize protein adsorption and, consequently, cell adhesion in vitro. However, the in vivo response is quite different. To develop a long-term nonfouling surface for implanted devices will require better ex vivo model systems that can capture the complex processes of the in vivo environment.

SURFACE SPECIFICITY Cell adhesion to adsorbed proteins is mediated through integrin and other receptors located within the cell membrane. Upon adhering to the protein film, a cascade of intracellular signaling events is triggered. Therefore, controlling protein adsorption on the surface of biomaterials may be critical to controlling and directing cell responses to biomaterials. Several approaches have been examined, from incorporating short oligopeptides that exhibit specific binding domains to incorporating whole proteins on the surface of the biomaterial.

Several short oligopeptide sequences that make up the receptor-binding domains within large proteins have been elucidated. A number of different short amino acid sequences have been identified that mediate cell-specific adhesion and function, and these have been recently reviewed (19). The most widely investigated cell-adhesive oligopeptide is arginine-glycine-aspartic acid (or RGD), which is found in a number of different extracellular matrix proteins, such as fibronectin (20), laminin (21), collagen (22), and vitronectin (23). Short oligopeptides are relatively inexpensive, are easy to synthesize, and offer greater flexibility for surface modification compared with the bulky and labile intact proteins. As a result, RGD has been applied to a number of different surfaces to direct cell adhesion and render them bioactive. When a surface was modified with a combination of nonfouling PEG (99%) and RGD (1%), protein adsorption was minimal (2 $ng/cm^2$), but a sufficient number of RGD sites was present to promote fibroblast cell adhesion (24). Furthermore, the structure and the conformation of these oligopeptides are important in modulating cell adhesion. For example, immobilization of a cyclic RGD peptide resulted in increased human bone marrow stromal cell adhesion compared with linear RGD peptides (25). Recently, an oligopeptide containing the integrin $\alpha_2\beta_1$ binding domain found in collagen type I was synthesized in such a way that it adopted a triple-helical conformation similar to the native collagen structure that is necessary for integrin binding (26). When the mimetic peptide was immobilized on the surface, cell adhesion was similar compared with collagen type I, but interestingly when the peptide was passively adsorbed on the surface, where a range of orientations can exist, including disruption of the tertiary structure, cell adhesion decreased.

In many cases, incorporation of the entire protein is desired to promote multiple integrin-mediated responses (where often the exact roles are not yet understood). However, nonspecific binding of a protein to a surface may render it nonfunctional owing to changes in orientation or conformation, i.e., the active sites may be hidden or the protein may become denatured. Surface chemistry influences the conformation of adsorbed fibronectin (27). Self-assembled monolayers of alkanethiols with different terminal endgroups (e.g., $CH_3$, OH, COOH, and $NH_2$) on gold provide a well-controlled method to explore such surface chemistry effects. It was found

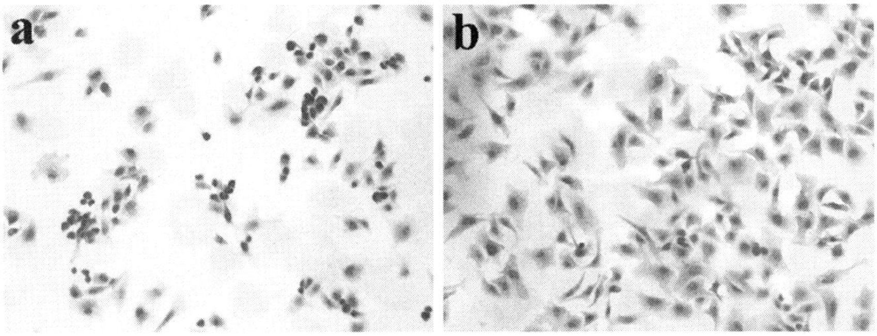


**Figure 2** Bovine aortic endothelial cells cultured for 1.5 h on poly(2-hydroxyethyl methacrylate) surfaces (*a*) immobilized with osteopontin or (*b*) immobilized with collagen then incubated with osteopontin to allow the natural binding of osteopontin to collagen.

that fibronectin adsorbed onto gold surfaces exhibiting the OH headgroup chemistry increased cell adhesion compared with fibronectin adsorbed onto to COOH and $NH_2$ and even more so to $CH_3$. Integrin binding to fibronectin by cells using these receptors also depended on the surface chemistry, but the dependence varied for each integrin studied, suggesting that the orientation of the fibronectin is altered by surface chemistry (27). Osteopontin is one protein of particular interest because of its potential role in mediating wound healing (28). We have successfully immobilized osteopontin on poly (2-hydroxyethyl methacrylate) (pHEMA) surfaces to promote endothelial cell adhesion (29) (Figure 2*a*). However, when collagen type I was first immobilized on the pHEMA surface, followed by the addition of osteopontin that was allowed to affinity bind to the immobilized collagen, endothelial cell adhesion increased significantly compared with cell adhesion to immobilized osteopontin, as shown in Figure 2*b* (29). By allowing osteopontin to adopt a more native conformation by binding to collagen type I, protein function may be preserved.

SURFACE MICROARCHITECTURE The microarchitecture of the implant, particularly at the surface, is an important parameter that influences the host response. Nonporous implants result in densely packed, well-organized fibrous capsules, whereas certain porous implants lead to a less dense, more open and disorganized fibrous capsule (30, 31). The latter loose collagenous capsule exhibits increased vascularization leading to enhanced diffusion of small molecules across the fibrous capsule to the implant (32). Porous membranes, with pores between 5 and 15 $\mu$m, resulted in significantly increased vascularization adjacent to the implant and within the fibrous capsule compared with smooth surfaces, regardless of chemistry (31). In an effort to develop porous materials that can be used to enhance the vascularity of implants, pHEMA hydrogels with well-defined and controlled pore sizes have been synthesized by a sphere-template technique that allows

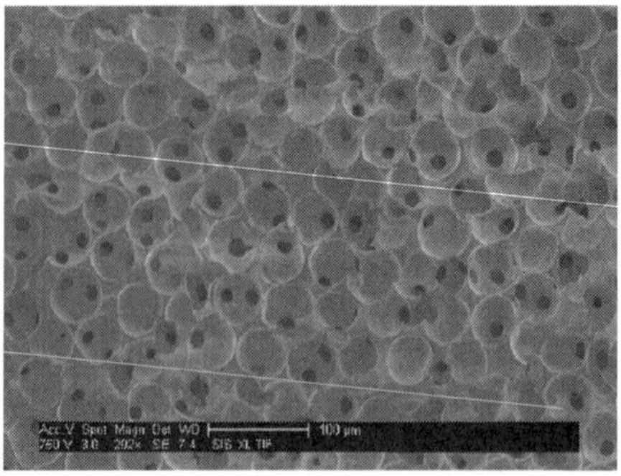


**Figure 3** A scanning electron microscopy image of a porous poly(2-hydroxyethyl methacrylate) hydrogel prepared by a sphere templating method with well-defined monodisperse pore sizes. Bar = 100 $\mu$m.

monodisperse and uniformly shaped pores (33). An example of these porous pHEMA hydrogels is shown in Figure 3. By tightly controlling pore size and shape, we may better understand this apparent influence of implant microarchitecture on the host response. Preliminary results from our group show a strong vascularization effect of these porous materials (34).

The diameter of polymer fibers influences capsule thickness (35–37). Fibers with diameters greater than 5 $\mu$m induced the classic foreign body response, whereas fiber diameters between 1 and 5 $\mu$m exhibited little or no capsule (35). Fiber chemistry, not surface charge, appeared to have an effect on fibrous capsule thickness, although not as dramatic as fiber diameter (36, 37). Furthermore, blood vessel density surrounding the fibers was unaffected by fiber density for fiber diameters between 1 and 15.9 $\mu$m (36).

## The Synthesis of New Biomaterials

Because of the growing interest and need for new biomaterials, a great deal of research has been devoted to synthesizing new materials from a range of natural and synthetic chemistries and 3-D macrostructures to offer materials with a wide range of properties and/or controlled responses that can be used for many different applications. The list of new materials developed specifically for biological applications is far too long to describe here. We have chosen to focus on two types of synthetic biomaterials: (*a*) hydrogels, which are attractive owing to their high water content and tissue-like properties, and (*b*) smart materials, which can rapidly respond to changes in the in vivo environment.

HYDROGELS Hydrogels are crosslinked polymer networks that are insoluble but swellable in aqueous medium. These materials offer an environment that resembles the highly hydrated state of natural tissues, making them excellent candidates for tissue engineering and drug delivery. Several types of crosslinking mechanisms have been investigated to develop hydrogels for tissue scaffolds and drug delivery devices. These mechanisms include ionic (e.g., alginate), physical (e.g., pluronics and peptide self-assembling gels described in the section on Self-Assembled Biomaterials, below), chemical (e.g., fibrin glue and multivinyl methacrylate and acrylate derivatives), and hydrogen bonding (e.g., a new class of hydrogels described below). Several synthetic and natural hydrogels have been recently reviewed (38–40).

Hydrogels that are chemically crosslinked via a radical-initiated chain polymerization of multivinyl monomers or macromers have gained considerable interest because of their chemical versatility and ease of fabrication. The polymerization reaction of methacrylate- or acrylate [(meth)acrylate]-modified macromers can be initiated using photoinitiators or redox initiators under physiological pH and temperature enabling in situ formation. Photoinitiators offer spatial and temporal control over the polymerization process allowing for fabrication of complex 3-D shapes, whereas redox initiators (e.g., ammonium persulfate and vitamin A) are typically milder and potentially less toxic. Both synthetic (e.g., poly(ethylene glycol)-co-poly(lactic acid) (PEG-*co*-PLA) (41), poly(vinyl alcohol) (PVA) (42), PVA-g-PLA (43) and natural polymers (e.g., hyaluronic acid (44, 45) and chondroitin sulfate (46)) have been modified with meth(acrylates) to form crosslinkable macromers that form hydrogels with a range of different chemistries. Alternatives to meth(acrylates) include novel hydrogels based on poly(propylene fumarate-co-ethylene glycol) developed by Mikos and coworkers (47). The propylene fumarate repeat unit contains a polymerizable vinyl group and a hydrolytically degradable ester group, whereas ethylene glycol segments increase the hydrophilicity of the gels; together these facets make this copolymer an attractive candidate for tissue engineering (48, 49). In general, crosslinked hydrogels afford tight control over the final gel chemistry, macroscopic properties, and degradation. Simple changes in the processing conditions (e.g., macromer concentration, macromer molecular weight) can lead to a range of gel properties (42, 50), whereas simply mixing different macromers in solution prior to polymerization can lead to networks that contain both synthetic and natural components (46). Gel degradation is easily tailored by varying the length and/or chemistry of the hydrolytic labile group, such as, for example, poly(lactic acid) (PLA) versus $\varepsilon$-caprolactone (41), by incorporating enzyme cleavable peptide sequences within the crosslinker (51), or by employing natural polymers such as those mentioned above, which are also sensitive to enzymatic degradation (45).

Photopolymerized hydrogels have been used more recently to successfully encapsulate pancreatic islets (52), smooth muscle cells (53), osteoblasts (54), chondrocytes (55–57), and growth factors (53, 58) while maintaining cell viability and protein activity. In a recent study, osteoconductive growth factors delivered from photopolymerized PEG hydrogels were found to enhance osteoblast mineralization (58). Degradable hydrogels based on PEG and PVA have been tuned to degrade at a rate that parallels the production of ECM by photoencapsulated chondrocytes. This led to the development of a cartilaginous tissue throughout the hydrogel scaffold

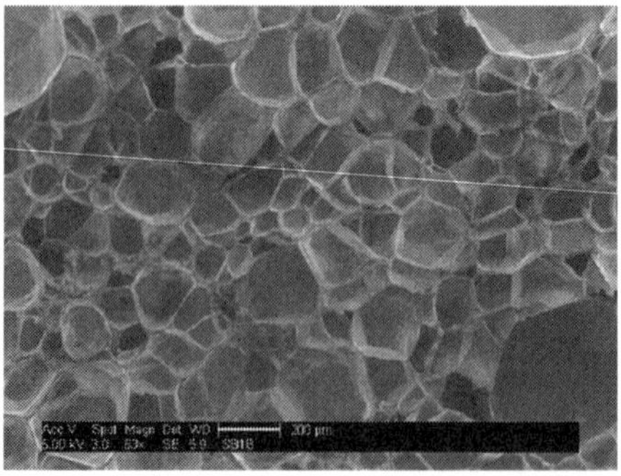

**Figure 5** A scanning electron microscopy image of a hydrogel foam prepared by solid colloidal gas aphrons of a PVA and arginine. Bar = 200 $\mu$m.

as illustrated by the uniformly distributed glycosaminoglycans in Figure 4*a* (see color insert) (59). Furthermore, DNA encoding for the green fluorescent protein (GFP) was co-encapsulated with chondrocytes in degradable photocrosslinked PEG hydrogels as a method for in situ gene delivery (60). Figure 4*b* demonstrates successful in situ transfection of chondrocytes within the hydrogel.

A new class of hydrogels has been recently discovered by Nair et al. (61) that involves a unique interaction between PVA and amino acids. Initial results based on nuclear magnetic resonance (NMR) and infrared spectrometry suggest that hydrogen bonding is responsible for gel formation (62). We have combined these unique hydrogels with a new approach to fabricate tissue scaffolds using solid colloidal gas aphrons (CGAs) (63). CGAs or microfoams contain uniform air bubbles that produce pores from 50–500 $\mu$m in size, suitable for tissue scaffolds. An example of a PVA and arginine amino acid hydrogel scaffold prepared from CGAs is shown in Figure 5. This new class of hydrogels offers several advantages over conventional gels, including the use of nontoxic aqueous solvent, Food and Drug Administration (FDA) approved components, and short preparation times.

SMART BIOMATERIALS Materials that can respond to changes in their surrounding environment are attractive because these changes, particularly in vivo, can be exploited to control parameters such as drug release, cell adhesiveness, mechanical properties, or permeability. Several approaches have been examined for stimulants such as pH (64, 65), temperature (66, 67), and light (68, 69).

The body employs changes in pH to facilitate a range of different processes. For example, along the gastrointestinal track, food is broken down into nutritive substances in the stomach under acidic pH ~2 and subsequently absorbed in the small intestine (pH ~ 7). Drug delivery by oral administration is attractive to many patients who require routine, periodic delivery of drugs. However, for the drug to remain effective, it must survive the acidic pH of the stomach. Researchers have developed pH-sensitive materials that take advantage of pH changes in the gastrointestinal tract and carry drugs through the stomach for successful delivery in the small intestine. pH responsive hydrogels prepared from poly(methacrylic acid) grafted with poly(ethylene glycol) (PMAA-g-PEG) have been widely explored. These materials undergo changes in swelling in response to pH. For example, the gel shrinks (trapping the drug cargo) at low pH $\sim 2$ owing to the formation of interpolymer complexes, whereas at physiological pH $\sim 7$ the gel can swell 3–25 times depending on its composition (releasing its cargo in the desired compartment) (65). In vitro, these gels have low cytotoxicity (70) and have been shown to improve protein transport across epithelial cell monolayers (71). As a practical demonstration of this strategy, insulin loaded PMAA-g-PEG gels were delivered orally to diabetic mice. Their glucose levels decreased significantly, suggesting that these materials can protect protein function under acidic environments and in the presence of digestive enzymes (72).

Another natural process that employs a drop in pH is intracellular waste disposal. This process involves trafficking of molecules to the lysosome for degradation. Many molecules are taken up by the cells through receptor-mediated endocytosis, where they are entrapped in endosomes and brought to the lysosome for destruction as depicted in Figure 6. Both endosomes and lysosomes exist at pH values between 5.0 and 6.5, whereas the cytoplasm is at a pH of 7.4. The delivery of therapeutics, e.g., DNA, RNA, and proteins, into a cell requires that the drug get into the cell without being trafficked to the lysosome and degraded. To escape the degradative process, a number of researchers have examined ways to take

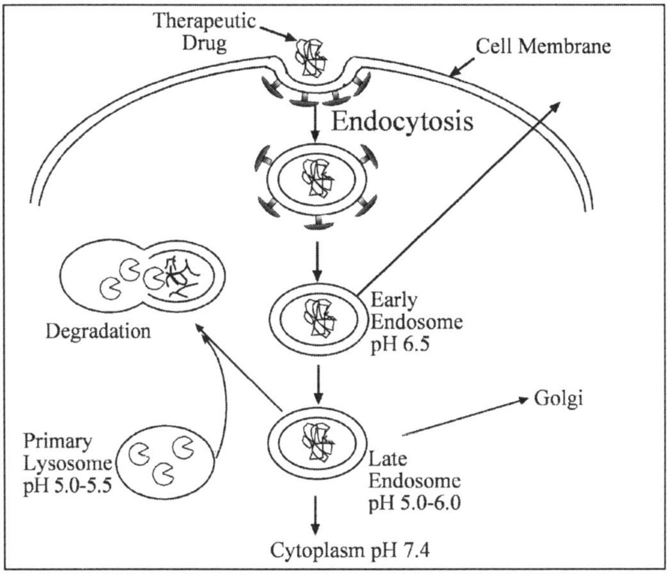


**Figure 6** A schematic of receptor-mediated endocytosis and the potential intracellular trafficking routes of therapeutics.

advantage of the pH gradient between the endosome and the cytosol. A new class of polymers has been developed that targets disrupting the endosomal membrane (64). These polymers have several unique features: (*a*) a membrane-disruptive backbone (composed of dimethylaminoethyl methacrylate, butyl methacrylate, and a styrene derivative); (*b*) PEG oligomers, which act as stabilizers at neutral pH, are grafted to the membrane-disruptive backbone via an acid degradable linkage that enables the release of the stabilizer under acidic environments; and (*c*) multiple specificities conjugated to the PEG stabilizer for drug attachment and delivery allowing, for example, hexalysine to bind oligonucleotides and lactose to target the ASGP receptor on hepatocytes (73). This new class of polymers conjugated to a therapeutic drug forms a stable drug-polymer complex at physiological pH. This complex can enter the cells via receptor-mediated endocytosis. Once in the endosome, the acid-degradable acetal linkers are hydrolyzed, releasing both the stabilizing PEG chains and the drug from the core membrane-disruptive polymer. As a result, the membrane-disruptive polymer is free to disrupt the endosomal membrane and release the drug into the cytoplasm. When these novel encrypted polymers were tested with fluorescein isothiocyanate (FITC) conjugated to PEG, cytoplasmic delivery to hepatocytes was observed by fluorescences. With a smaller oligonucleotide as a model drug, delivery to the nucleus was possible (73).

A healthy human body maintains a constant temperature of 37°C, and many researchers have designed materials that can respond to changes in temperature from room temperature to body temperature. Polymers that phase separate because of a change in temperature are often driven by solution conformational changes of the hydrophobic and the hydrophilic moieties. Thermally responsive biopolymers have been recently reviewed (66). Here, we briefly describe several temperature-responsive polymers, with details deferred to the more focused reviews. The usefulness of thermally responsive biopolymers is primarily based on their demonstration of a polymer lower critical solution temperature (LCST). Two polymers that have been extensively investigated are poly(N-isopropylacrylamide) (pNIPAAm) and elastin-like peptide (ELP) (see reviews 67, 74). For example, pNIPAAm has an LCST at 32°C (75), whereas the LCST of ELP can be controlled by varying the length of the ELP molecule and/or its amino acid composition to obtain transition temperatures ranging from 30°C to greater than 90°C (76). The ELPs have been used in tissue-engineering applications for chondrocyte encapsulation (77) and as a drug carrier for cancer therapy (74). pNIPAAm and its derivatives have been used for a number of different applications, including drug delivery (78), biological microelectromechanical systems (bioMEMs) (79), and tissue engineering (80). A unique technique, termed cell sheet engineering, has arisen from this thermally responsive polymer. At 37°C, pNIPAAm becomes hydrophobic, promoting protein adsorption and, subsequently, cell adhesion. By lowering the temperature below 32°C, cells cultured on pNIPAAm surfaces can be lifted off of the surface. This change from hydrophobic to hydrophilic character over this transition results in the release of proteins and, thus, adherent cells from the surface. This technique maintains intact cell-cell connections and their associated extracellular matrix. Several approaches have been examined, including layering cell sheets to reconstruct a homogenous tissue (81, 82) and layering several sheets made from various types of cells to reconstruct multicellular tissues (83, 84). The detachment of the cell sheet was accelerated when small amounts of PEG were grafted to the surface with pNIPAAm (85).

Thermally responsive biopolymers can also be useful in controlling enzyme activity. Polymer-enzyme conjugates have been constructed in which the polymer has been conjugated to the enzyme near the site of enzymatic activity. At temperatures above the LCST, the polymer conjugated to the enzyme assumes a collapsed state, blocking the active site and preventing substrate interaction with the enzyme; however, at temperatures below its LCST, the polymer is expanded, allowing substrate-enzyme interaction. This phenomenon has been demonstrated by conjugating a short protein sequence derived from the active region of the enzyme endoglucanase, which hydrolyzes amorphous cellulose, to the responsive copolymer *N,N*-dimethylacrylamide-*co*-*N*-4-phenylazo-phenylacrylamide (69). Interestingly, this copolymer is both thermo- and photo-sensitive. Upon exposing to UV or visible light, the LCST shifts, giving additional control over enzyme activity. Furthermore, this strategy can be adapted to other enzymes by changing polymer size and the conjugation site.

Alternatives to environmental changes have also been investigated that are stimulated by a more specific response. In 1985, Kost et al. (86) published a paper on a new hydrogel that swelled in response to glucose. The crosslinked pHEMA was copolymerized with a monomer containing pendant amine groups. The hydrogel system contained entrapped glucose oxidase. In the presence of glucose, the enzyme produced gluconic acid, which lowered the pH, protonated the amines, and induced the gel to swell. More recently, a unique approach to glucose sensing also based on swellable gels was developed by Asher and coworkers (87). Specifically, the sensor employed an anionic hydrogel fabricated from crosslinked polyacrylamide with tethered boronic acids (4-amino-3-fluoro-phenylboronic acid, which are known to bind glucose reversibly) and stabilized by PEG (87). Within the hydrogel was an embedded crystalline colloidal array (CCA) that diffracts light. In this unique system, shown in Figure 7*a*, changes in glucose concentration result in anionic gel swelling (high glucose concentration) or deswelling (low glucose concentration). Changes in the gel volume cause a change in the CCA structure and hence a change in the diffraction wavelength. This unique combination of elements allows the sensor to work effectively at physiological pH and salt concentrations. The diffraction wavelengths are given in Figure 7*b* as a function of glucose concentration. Such materials could be useful in providing an easy visual recognition of glucose levels by sensing tear glucose levels.

## Biologically Inspired Materials

In an effort to design materials that will perform their intended functions in the presence of cells and/or in vivo, we as engineers and scientists can look to biology

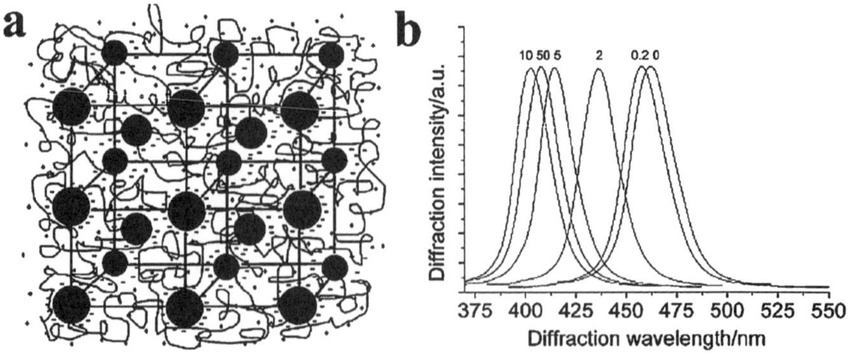


**Figure 7** (*a*) A schematic of a glucose sensor fabricated from a polymerized crystalline colloidal array (CCA) embedded in an ionic hydrogel containing a molecular recognition element for glucose. (*b*) Under physiological pH, changes in glucose concentration affect gel swelling and subsequently affect the lattice structure of the CCA, causing a shift in the diffraction wavelength. Glucose concentration (mM) is shown above the diffraction peaks. Reproduced with permission from (87).

and take advantage of biological processes that have evolved over thousands of years. In this section, we present some of the most current advances in biomaterials that have emerged by mimicking properties or processes that occur in the body.

SELF-ASSEMBLED BIOMATERIALS One of the many fascinating aspects of biology is the self-organization of molecules into hierarchal structures that perform a specific task. This self-organization or self-assembly is based on the formation of weak noncovalent bonds, typically hydrogen, ionic, or van der Waals bonds or hydrophobic interactions (88). For example, amphiphilic molecules have hydrophobic and hydrophilic segments that self-assemble into distinct structures, such as micelles, vesicles, and tubules that are nanometers in length. When dispersed in an aqueous solvent, the hydrophobic segments in the amphiphilic molecules agglomerate, driving out water and, as a result, producing a well-ordered structure that can be useful in a number of different biomedical applications. A naturally occurring amphiphilic molecule is a phospholipid, which largely composes the cell membrane. Alternatively, a polymer (or oligomer) of amino acids can be synthesized to contain a number of different regions (hydrophobic, hydrophilic, charged, etc.) that under certain conditions will self-assemble into a macroscopic hydrogel (89). In general, the final three dimensional structure of the self-assembled material is dependent on the molecule's length and composition (90–93). Thus, by systematically synthesizing a molecule, a desired 3-D structure can be produced. These self-assembled biomaterials are promising new materials that can be engineered for applications in nanotechnology and in tissue engineering for drug and cell carriers. These materials may be particularly beneficial because the engineered peptides will take on a 3-D shape that may be recognized by the in vivo environment, more so than a conventionally synthesized material, and furthermore will breakdown into amino acids that the body is well equipped to deal with.

There have been significant investigations into the primary sequence of engineered peptides to better understand the composition-structure relationships responsible for self-assembly. With such an understanding, biomaterials can be tailored to achieve desired structures and functions. For example, chemistry affects the packing of hydrophobic tails in peptide amphiphiles that results in a variety of 3-D structures. In one study, changes to the hydrophobic tail length and amino acid composition (where cysteine residues were replaced with alanine to prevent crosslinking of cysteine thiols) did not alter a molecule's ability to self-assemble into nanofibers, but did change the morphology of the nanofibers (93). Changes in the amino acid sequence can lead to morphological changes in self-assembled nanofibers by introducing kinks (94) or even branches (95) into otherwise linear nanofibers.

In many cases, an external stimulus [e.g., pH (89), temperature (92), or salt concentration (91)] is necessary to activate (or terminate) the self-assembly process. The amino acid sequence can influence the point at which self-assembly occurs for a given external condition. Oligopeptides with amino acid repeat units in the configuration of hydrophobic-negatively charged–hydrophobic-positively charged can self-assemble in the presence of salt solutions (91). For example, increasing the hydrophobicity of the oligopeptide results in a decrease in the critical salt concentration required to induce self-assembly (91). In addition, the critical salt concentration was affected by the overall length of the oligopeptide (91). Tuning the primary peptide sequence to develop biomaterials that self-assemble in situ under physiological conditions has also been investigated. For example, manipulating the amino acid sequence to give the oligopeptide a net positive charge at neutral pH and low salt concentration prevented self-assembly, but when the salt concentration was increased to physiological levels, the molecules self-assembled into a hydrogel. Alternatively, certain oligopeptides self-assemble in the presence of divalent calcium at physiological pH (93).

The design of tissue-engineering constructs requires scaffolds with appropriate mechanical stability and biological cues, e.g., adhesive proteins. It was found that the overall length (but not hydrophobicity) of the oligopeptide (the hydrophobic-negatively charged–hydrophobic-positively charged configuration described above) significantly influenced the shear modulus of the self-assembled biomaterial (96). Oligopeptides containing an elastin-like repeat unit can be crosslinked after self-assembly using bifunctional N-hydroxysuccinimidyl ester, which results in crosslinking between two available amine groups, to further control the mechanical properties of these materials (97). As a result, the tensile modulus was varied an order of magnitude by simply adjusting the amount of crosslinker added to the gel (97). Self-assembled molecules with sequence Ac-QQKFQFQFEQQ-Am can be further modified after gelation by tethering bioactive molecules using transglutaminase as a catalyst to connect a peptide ligand, e.g., RGD, to the self-assembled protein via a glutamine and/or lysine residue in the presence of calcium (98).

A unique advantage of developing biomaterials from self-assembled oligopeptides is the ability to incorporate biological cues within the material by simply integrating sequences directly into the peptide backbone. Two peptide amphiphiles were designed to exhibit a hydrophobic alkyl tail and a hydrophilic head group containing a biologically recognized amino acid sequence of RGD or YIGSR (tyrosine-isoleucine-glycine-serine-arginine) derived from fibrinogen (20) and laminin (99), respectively (100). Their chemical structures are shown in Figure 8*a*. At neutral pH, molecule 1 has a net negative charge whereas molecule 2 has a net positive charge. Upon combining, the two molecules self-assemble, and nanofibers spontaneously form at neutral pH (Figure 8*b*).

The nanostructure of these self-assembled peptides offers a unique matrix structure containing fibers that are three orders of magnitude smaller than typical fiber scaffolds used in tissue-engineering applications [e.g., poly(lactic-co-glycolic acid) (PLGA) fibers typically range from 10–100 $\mu$m in diameter]. Self-assembled

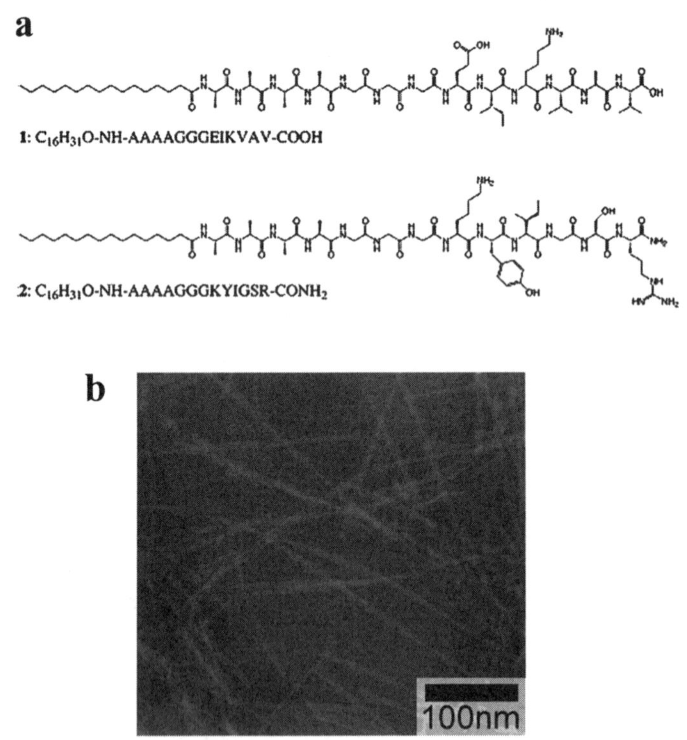


**Figure 8** Chemical structures of peptide-amphiphiles (*a*) that self-assemble into nanofibers (*b*) at neutral pH. Reproduced with permission from (100).

peptides have been shown to support cell adhesion for a number of different cell types (cell lines and primary cells) (101), as well as to support neurite outgrowth by PC12 cells and primary neurons (102). In another study, 3T6 Swiss albino mouse embryo fibroblasts were seeded onto a self-assembled layer containing a hydrophobic moiety comprised of cholesterol and a PLA segment (103). A greater number of cells were present on the self-assembled layers compared with a PLA control surface. Interestingly, the adhered cells on the self-assembled layer were found to take up the cholesterol segment, suggesting a potential mechanism for delivering a hydrophobic molecule to cells.

Self-assembled peptide hydrogels have only recently been explored as cell carriers for tissue engineering. The first study examined encapsulating chondrocytes in a peptide gel (with sequence AcN-KLDLKLDLKLDL-$CNH_2$) (104). Accumulation of glycosaminoglycans and the presence of type II collagen (the two main components of cartilage) were observed in gels cultured up to 28 days. Furthermore, the equilibrium modulus and dynamic stiffness increased nearly 100-fold from 0 to 28 days, indicative of tissue development. In a separate study, an oligopeptide with the amino acid sequence Ac-RADARADARADARADA-$CONH_2$ (RAD), which self-assembles into a 3-D peptide gel with interwoven fibers on the order of 10–20 nm (102), was used as a tissue-engineering scaffold (105). Specifically, liver progenitor cells were encapsulated in the peptide gel (105). The encapsulated cells stopped proliferating and expressed the liver developmental marker (C/EBP$\alpha$) as well as other hepatocyte markers such as albumin and cytochromes P450 (CYP1A1 and CYP1A2), all indicative of differentiated liver cells. Furthermore, when two different peptide sequences (n-AEAEAKAKAEAEAKAK-c and RAD described above) were injected and formed in situ within the leg muscle of rats, no inflammation or immune response was detected (102).

BIOMIMETIC BIOMATERIALS Direct mimicry of biological processes represents an important strategy in modern biomaterials. Hydroxyapatite is the natural mineral in bone. There is now a huge amount of literature describing the use of hydroxyapatite and other forms of calcium phosphate coupled with synthetic and other natural biomaterials to induce bone formation. Nacre, the aragonite-rich lining of many seashells, also induces rapid bone formation. Nacre contains about 5% protein that serves as a "mortar" to bind together a brick-like mineral structure. A biomimetic approach to creating synthetic nacre-like structures has been published (106).

Normal tissues have a complex 3-D architecture important for the mechanics and functionality of the biological organism. Biomimetically, we might emulate such structures with synthetic biomaterials. Synthetic materials offer the ability to generate many different kinds of 3-D structures with precise control over the final macroscopic properties and degradation profiles by varying the chemistry and processing techniques. However, synthetic materials provide little control over cell behavior and tissue response in vivo. Thus, to generate a biomaterial for a specific cell type and/or tissue, efforts have focused on adding biological cues to synthetic materials in an attempt to mimic the native tissue while simultaneously maintaining control over the material properties.

The primary focus of the biomimetic approach of emulating the extracellular matrix and tissue architectures has been to incorporate short oligopeptides into synthetic materials to create bioactive materials. The most studied sequence is RGD. Other sequences have also been discovered that mediate cell adhesion, cell-specific adhesion, neurite extension, and degradation, to name few—these ideas have been reviewed elsewhere (19). A recent study examined cell migration into a synthetically derived hydrogel matrix based on PEG (107). The PEG hydrogel was fabricated to contain a matrix metalloproteinase (MMP)–sensitive amino acid sequence as the crosslink and RGD-tethered ligands throughout the bulk of the hydrogel. Interestingly, fibroblast invasion (Figures 9*a*,*b*, see color insert) into the gel was mediated by the presence of both the protease-sensitive crosslinks and cell-adhesive moieties. When either was lacking, cell invasion was not observed. This hydrogel was also placed in a rat calvarial critical-sized defect to examine bone ingrowth. Intramembranous bone formation was observed throughout the defect area when the MMP-sensitive gel was used in conjunction with human recombinant bone morphogenic protein-2 (Figures 9*c*–*e*). The ability of cells to infiltrate a matrix loaded with a growth factor was essential for bone ingrowth. This study demonstrates the importance of developing biomaterials that express multiple bioactive elements. Such a combination of elements is likely necessary for regeneration of new tissues.

ACELLULAR TISSUES Naturally derived tissues are attractive materials for cell seeding and tissue-engineering applications because they are comprised of an extracellular matrix in native conformation and composition. The tissue is decellularized and cell debris removed to reduce host immune response. The resulting material retains many of the natural tissue's mechanical and biological properties. An acellular tissue commonly used in humans today to replace damaged malfunctioning heart valves is a glutaraldehyde-fixed porcine heart valve. Glutaraldehyde crosslinking increases the life span of the implant by minimizing enzymatic degradation; however, it significantly alters the mechanics of the implant (108). In tissue-repair or tissue-engineering applications, a resorbable tissue is desired. Acellular porcine small intestinal submucosa (SIS) has been studied extensively as a naturally derived, resorbable material (109). Submucosa has been used as a xenogeneic scaffold for tissue repair in both animal studies and human clinical trials. Interestingly, upon implantation in the bladder, SIS exhibits no inflammation, has good vascularization, and lacks the foreign body reaction typically observed for biomaterials. Submucosa enables tissue ingrowth and has been used in a number of different applications as a graft to promote tissue repair. In many cases, SIS is rapidly remodeled by host tissue and 90% degraded within 4 weeks (110). Submucosa has been approved by the FDA for use in humans for skin repair, soft-tissue support, and rotator-cuff repair. The success of SIS has been attributed to its ECM proteins and glycosaminoglycans, cytokines, and growth factors that are retained within the matrix, for example vascular endothelial growth factor (111), transforming growth factor $\beta_1$ (TGF$\beta_1$), and basic fibroblast growth factor (112). Endogenous TGF$\beta_1$ in the SIS has been implicated in the immunosuppressiveness of helper T (Th) cells (113). When compared with type I collagen and PLGA subcutaneous implants, a marked increase in recruited marrow-derived cells was observed for the SIS implants (114). This study further demonstrates the importance of scaffold chemistry (and structure) and the presence of growth factors that, combined, are important for tissue growth.

## Patterned Biomaterials

The ability to pattern biomaterials has enabled researchers to create cost-effective diagnostic tools by miniaturizing and combining laboratory procedures onto a single device. Patterning can also assist us in better understanding many biological processes by mimicking in vivo structures. In this section, we present some recent advances in bioMEMs technology and tissue-engineering scaffold developments that exploit patterned biomaterials.

BIOMEMS BioMEMs are technologies that can offer micrometer- and even nanometer-scaled devices designed specifically for biological applications. These miniaturized, engineered biosystems have many benefits in biology; in particular, experiments can be performed at the scale of a single cell. Furthermore, these devices reduce cost by shortening reaction times and minimizing reagent volumes. These biological devices have led to the idea of a total microanalysis system, or lab-on-a-chip technology, in which multiple analyses can be performed in series and/or in parallel on one device (115). Such a system has the potential to revolutionize medicine in both diagnostics and in basic research. Before a total microanalysis system can be fully developed, many specific fabrication and biointeraction challenges must be addressed. The promise these systems hold for advancing medicine has stimulated a huge bioMEMs research endeavor. Because bioMEMs is one of the fastest growing areas that rely on biomaterials, we present some of the latest findings in bioMEMs technology. In particular, we discuss material processing using soft lithography and new techniques in photolithography, as well as devices that take advantage of smart polymers. We direct the reader to a number of recently published reviews on bioMEMs for a more complete discussion (116–124).

SOFT LITHOGRAPHY Soft lithography has emerged in recent years as a popular microfabrication technique that is inexpensive, facile, and bio-friendly (118). Soft lithography begins with a patterned elastomeric material, typically poly(dimethylsiloxane) (PDMS), that is fabricated using standard photolithography procedures and can generate patterns as small as 30 nm, as illustrated in Figure 10 (125). There are several merits of soft lithography: (*a*) Multiple PDMS stamps can be made from one mask; (*b*) the PDMS stamps are often reusable (minimizing clean room time); (*c*) the elastomeric and hydrophobic properties help establish and

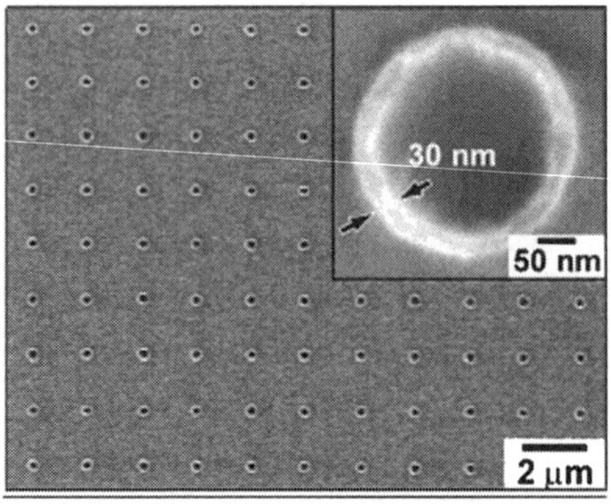


**Figure 10** Scanning electron micrograph of 30 nm features fabricated from composite PDMS masks and phase-shifting photolithography. Reproduced with permission from (125).

maintain good contact with rough surfaces; (*d*) PDMS is transparent, allowing visualization through the stamp; (*e*) the surface chemistry of the PDMS is easily modified; and finally, (*f*) PDMS is a nontoxic material through which oxygen and carbon dioxide can permeate.

A multitude of uses has emerged because of the versatility of these PDMS stamps. Figure 11 illustrates several recent applications of these materials. Microcontact printing of proteins has enabled the facile transfer of proteins to surfaces either directly or indirectly using microcontact-printed alkanethiols with defined geometries (126–129) (Figure 11*a*). By spatially controlling protein adsorption on a surface, researchers have been able to better understand cell processes (130, 131). For example, Chen et al. (130) found that focal adhesions, which mediate cell adhesion to ECM, do not depend on the total amount of ECM but rather on cell spreading. Gray-scale photolithography (132) used PDMS stamps to provide a means to generate structures of varying heights in one easy step (133, 134). One example is shown in Figure 11*b* (134) where the channels were filled with a solution containing a gradient of UV-absorbing dye. Upon irradiation with UV light (made possible by the PDMS transparency), the underlying photoresist was exposed to a gradient of light intensities, resulting in structures of different heights. The last example, illustrated in Figure 11*c* and experimentally demonstrated in Figure 11*d*, shows that these materials can be used to examine subcellular processes (135). Because flow in microchannels is laminar, a bioactive molecule can be introduced into one of the inlets, resulting in localized flow through the channel. Thus, microchannels provide a means to expose only a portion of a cell to a particular molecule. Figure 11*d* demonstrates the effects of treating a part of a single bovine capillary endothelial cell with trypsin, an enzyme that digests the underlying ECM proteins. The sequential micrographs demonstrate that only the part of the cell exposed to trypsin detached from the surface, and when trypsin was replaced with medium containing serum, cell reattachment occurred.

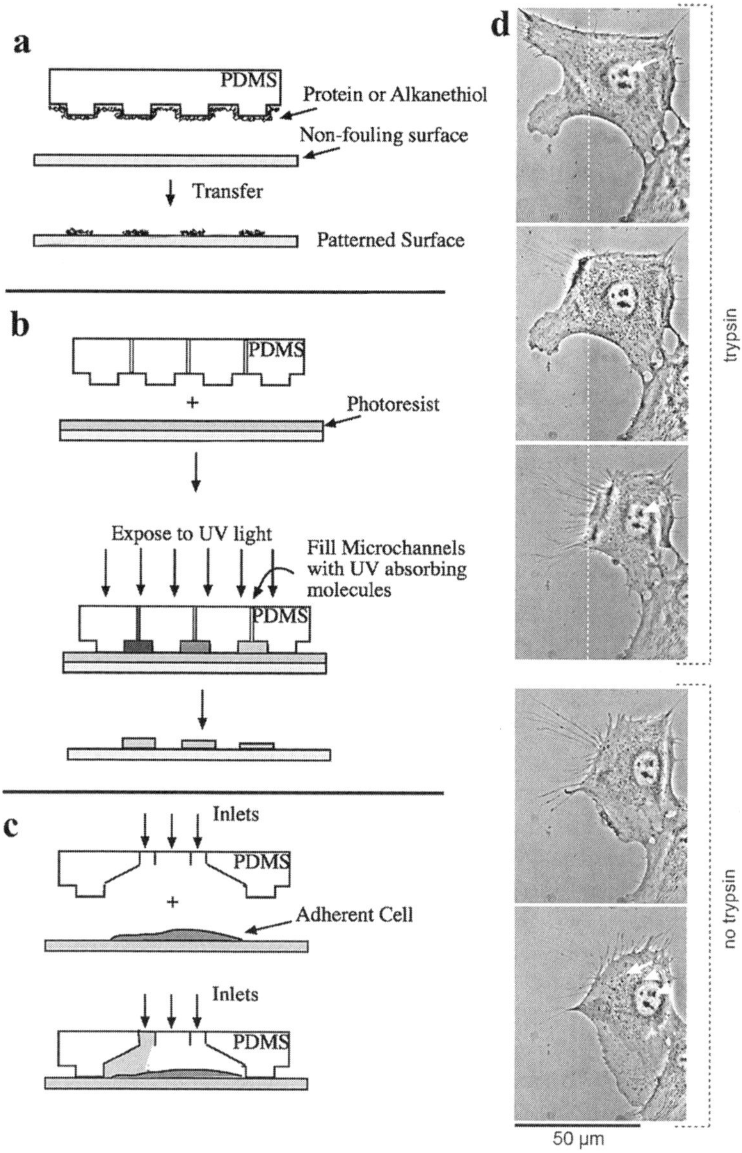


**Figure 11** Schematics illustrating several applications of PDMS stamps: (*a*) Microcontact printing allows transfer of materials, including biologically active molecules, e.g., proteins, to a surface in a well-defined pattern; (*b*) gray scale photolithography provides a facile method with which to pattern structures of varying heights; and (*c*) partial cell treatment uses laminar flow within microfluidic channels to treat part of a cell to a particular molecule. Panel (*d*) illustrates the partial treatment of a bovine capillary endothelial cell with trypsin, an enzyme that digests the underlying extracellular matrix proteins, causing cell detachment. Panel (*d*) reproduced with permission from (135).

PHOTOLITHOGRAPHY When precision on the micron scale is desired (typical in biological applications), simple photopolymerization reactions can be used to minimize the lengthy preparatory procedures involved in designing a mold for soft lithography. An ultra-rapid prototyping method for designing channels in a microfluidic device uses a solution of photoreactive monomers, a photoinitiator, and a photomask. A device with channels as small as 25 $\mu$m can be easily prepared in a matter of minutes (136).

In an effort to design a versatile and simple patterning method, living radical polymerization (LRP) has been investigated for designing microfluidic devices. In LRP, a photoiniferter [a derivative of dithiocarbamate that acts as an initiator, transfer agent, and terminator in radical polymerizations (137)] is bound to a surface from which a polymer chain can be grafted. The grafting can be controlled by using a photomask in which grafting occurs only where UV light is transmitted (138, 139). Furthermore, LRP enables 3-D micropatterning up to 1 mm. For example, the microfluidics group at the University of Colorado has demonstrated the ability to form bioMEM devices that have cells entrapped in 3-D PEG hydrogels that have been grafted to the surface using LRP technology (140, 141). This device, shown in Figure 12 (see color insert), enables cell culture without the need for individual wells and has potential for use in high-throughput screening to develop and/or optimize tissue-engineering scaffolds and culture conditions in 3-D matrices.

SMART POLYMERS The future of bioMEMs technology relies on the development of inexpensive devices that respond to either external or internal stimuli. Several approaches have been investigated. For example, coating a surface with a thermoresponsive polymer such as pNIPAAm allows control over the surface chemistry by simple changes in temperature, as described in detail above. Cheng et al. (79) has fabricated a device with microheater arrays that allows the surface chemistry of a small region to be reversibly switched on demand. The results shown in Figure 13 (see color insert) demonstrate that cell adhesion can be localized to a certain region by simply turning on one of the microheater array elements through an external power supply. Such a technology allows for attaching several different types of cells in a given device. Huber et al. (142) demonstrated that the initial adsorption of proteins on heated pNIPAAm surfaces is driven by kinetics and is a function of the size of the protein. Thus, by controlling adsorption times, protein separation was possible. In another study, genetically engineered, temperature-sensitive, elastin-like polypeptides were used to selectively recover a protein, ELP fusion peptide, directly from a cell lysate (143). The ELP polypeptides can selectively bind ELP fusion peptide above the LCST of the polypeptide (allowing separation of the protein of interest), whereas below the LCST the protein can be recovered for downstream processing, thus minimizing the lengthy purification steps.

BioMEMs that respond to internal stimuli are attractive because the device can be portable, allowing analysis to be performed offsite and potentially by the patient him/herself. Many of these advances have examined responsive polymers that act as valves. For example, Zhao et al. (144) modified channels within a microfluidic device, using simple photolithography techniques, to pattern surfaces with different free energies to serve as pressure-sensitive valves. In another study, LRP was used to generate pH-sensitive microchannels that could be opened and closed by simple changes in the pH (139). Strategies that use environmentally responsive polymers as pumps to induce flow through the microchannels are also a subject of intense interest.

TISSUE ENGINEERING Tissue engineering requires a 3-D matrix that will not only guide tissue formation into the desired shape but also provide adequate transport of nutrients and growth factors to promote tissue growth. In an effort to develop complex scaffolds that better match natural tissue structure, several approaches have been investigated to three dimensionally pattern materials. For example, an indirect solid free-form (SSF) fabrication (145) has been developed that combines direct SSF [that uses computational design to generate an exact external shape and macroporous architecture with minimum features of 100 $\mu$m (146)] with standard techniques to generate porous tissue-engineering scaffolds (e.g., salt leaching). For example, PLA scaffolds were fabricated that exhibited a 3-D structure similar to that of human trabecular bone with macropores (500–800 $\mu$m) to micropores (50–100 $\mu$m) (145).

Efforts have also been explored to develop 3-D scaffolds that contain multiple cell types wherein their spatial arrangement is controlled through 3-D patterning. Tan et al. (147) used channels from a PDMS stamp as a 3-D template for encapsulating human umbilical vein endothelial cells in a collagen type I matrix. A second cell type, human lung fibroblasts, was then selectively patterned onto the collagen-cell matrices. Alternative and simpler methods have used photopolymerization reactions to generate patterned 3-D hydrogel scaffolds. In one such study, fluorescently labeled HepG2 cells were photoencapsulated in PEG hydrogels during patterning to generate multiple layers of cells in defined geometries (148).

## THE FUTURE OF BIOMATERIALS

There are trends in biomaterials, many of them highlighted in this review, that suggest the future of biomaterials. Medical implants and in vitro systems are addressed separately.

Implanted medical devices are essential to modern medical practice, and they save lives or improve the quality of life for millions. However, they still heal like foreign objects—they are encapsulated and walled off. With the major investment by medical-device companies in development, manufacture, marketing, surgeon acceptance, and regulatory approval, it is unlikely that medical devices as we know them will change substantially in the next ten years. However, by surface modification of existing medical devices, we might expect to see devices that heal in a physiologically normal fashion (a vascularized reconstruction of the anatomy). Such a normal healing will improve the performance of many devices that are now hampered by poor healing (e.g., the problems associated with the foreign body capsule). For example, with integrative healing characteristics coupled with advances in materials and robotics, implanted limbs may not only replace the functionality of lost limbs but also provide some functionality even superior to that possible in flesh and blood limbs.

Another area of research that will lead to improvements in the performance of implants is a reduction in the propensity toward infection. This may be accomplished through antibacterial surface treatments, nonfouling surfaces, and antibiotic controlled release strategies. Also, general advances in controlled drug release will permit the development of devices with both device and drug functionality. The potential of this approach is now being realized with drug eluting cardiovascular stents that inhibit restenosis. Finally, advanced smart materials may be used for tissue, organ, and system replacement. A polymeric artificial muscle or an insulin-releasing system that intrinsically responds to blood glucose are examples of possible in vivo systems that use smart materials concepts and also may substantially advance the treatment of diseases or organ/tissue replacement.

Two technologies, tissue engineering and regenerative medicine, both in development now, will ultimately revolutionize medical implants. Tissue engineering will allow replacement of many tissues and organs with living, functional replacements. Tissue-engineering advances will rest upon advances in biodegradable polymers, rapid prototyping, drug delivery, cell culture, stem cell methodologies, angiogenesis, and biomimetic strategies for recreating extracellular, matrix-like biomimetics. Also, advances in cell culture, gene delivery, cell and tissue storage, sterilization, and surgery will be needed to fully realize the potential of tissue engineering. Regenerative medicine, permitting in vivo regeneration of whole organs and tissues, will ultimately replace tissue engineering. Technologies important to making regenerative medicine a reality include advances in biology, gene delivery, and controlled release.

With respect to in vitro systems, regulatory issues are not so constraining, and we can expect to see substantial advances in devices both for diagnostics and therapeutics. Smart materials, nonfouling surfaces, and MEMS concepts will enter into these devices. A chip array with complementary DNA to 100 different bacteria can rapidly recognize the origin of a bacterial infection. An array device with the whole human genome on it will permit infants to be diagnosed at birth with problems likely to crop up later in life. Preventative medicine, buttressed by this foreknowledge of conditions that probably will develop later, can greatly improve the quality of life. Possibly, a MEMS device containing a living culture of cells from a person's body might be used to synthesize on demand specific pharmaceuticals tuned to the physiology of the individual. The possibilities are almost limitless for developments using smart systems and micro- and nanofabrication. These in vitro systems of the future will be grounded in an advanced understanding of the way biological systems interact with synthetic surfaces. Careful ethical deliberation will also enter into these new technologies that have the potential to alter the expectations for humans.

## CONCLUSIONS

Biomaterials is a field with just over a half century of innovation and development. The success of biomaterials is seen in the importance to modern medical therapies, the economic potential of the market, and the steady growth of the field over more than 50 years. Tissue engineering will change the face of biomaterials, but tissue engineering still makes use of biomaterials. Regenerative medicine will reduce the need for synthetic materials in the body. Still many applications will require synthetics, and we can envision the need for biomaterials well through this century.

### ACKNOWLEDGMENTS

The authors are grateful for financial support from the NSF-Engineering Research Center program, UWEB (grant EEC-95,29161), the NIH through a research grant (R24HL64387) and an NRSA fellowship (1 F32 HL 74,6199-01) to S.J.B. We are also grateful for the helpful comments and thorough review from Dr. Kip D. Hauch and Elizabeth E. Donaldson. We also thank Kristi S. Anseth for the images in Figures 4 and 12.

**The *Annual Review of Biomedical Engineering* is online at http://bioeng.annualreviews.org**

### LITERATURE CITED

1. Williams DF. 1987. *Definitions in Biomaterials. Progress in Biomedical Engineering, 4*. Amsterdam: Elsevier. 72 pp.
2. Anderson JM. 2001. Biological responses to materials. *Annu. Rev. Mater. Res.* 31: 81–110
3. Salthouse TN. 1984. Some aspects of macrophage behavior at the implant interface. *J. Biomed. Mater. Res.* 18:395–401
4. Collier TO, Anderson JM. 2002. Protein and surface effects on monocyte and macrophage adhesion, maturation, and survival. *J. Biomed. Mater. Res.* 60:487–96
5. Behling CA, Spector M. 1986. Quantitative characterization of cells at the interface of long-term implants of selected polymers. *J. Biomed. Mater. Res.* 20:653–66
6. Johansson CB, Albrektsson T, Ericson LE, Thomsen P. 1992. A quantitative comparison of the cell response to commercially pure titanium and Ti-6Al-4V implants in the abdominal wall of rats. *J. Mater. Sci. Mater. Med.* 3:126–36
7. Piglowski J, Gancarz I, Staniszewska-Kus J, Paluch D, Szymonowicz M, Konieczny A. 1994. Influence of plasma modification on biological properties of poly(ethyleneterephthalate). *Biomaterials* 15:909–20
8. Dalsin JL, Hu BH, Lee BP, Messersmith PB. 2003. Mussel adhesive protein mimetic polymers for the preparation of nonfouling surfaces. *J. Am. Chem. Soc.* 125:4253–58
9. Lopez GP, Ratner BD, Tidwell CD, Haycox CL, Rapoza RJ, Horbett TA. 1992. Glow discharge plasma deposition of tetraethylene glycol dimethyl ether for fouling-resistant biomaterial surfaces. *J. Biomed. Mater. Res.* 26:415–39
10. Tsai WB, Grunkemeier JM, McFarland CD, Horbett TA. 2002. Platelet adhesion

to polystyrene-based surfaces preadsorbed with plasmas selectively depleted in fibrinogen, fibronectin, vitronectin, or von Willebrand's factor. *J. Biomed. Mater. Res.* 60:348–59
11. Shen MC, Horbett TA. 2001. The effects of surface chemistry and adsorbed proteins on monocyte/macrophage adhesion to chemically modified polystyrene surfaces. *J. Biomed. Mater. Res.* 57:336–45
12. Shen MC, Pan YV, Wagner MS, Hauch KD, Castner DG, et al. 2001. Inhibition of monocyte adhesion and fibrinogen adsorption on glow discharge plasma deposited tetraethylene glycol dimethyl ether. *J. Biomater. Sci. Polym. Ed.* 12:961–78
13. Shen MC, Martinson L, Wagner MS, Castner DG, Ratner BD, Horbett TA. 2002. Peo-like plasma polymerized tetraglyme surface interactions with leukocytes and proteins: in vitro and in vivo studies. *J. Biomater. Sci. Polym. Ed.* 13:367–90
14. Ishihara K, Ziats NP, Tierney BP, Nakabayashi N, Anderson JM. 1991. Protein adsorption from human plasma is reduced on phospholipid polymers. *J. Biomed. Mater. Res.* 25:1397–407
15. Holland NB, Qiu Y, Ruegsegger M, Marchant RE. 1998. Biomimetic engineering of non-adhesive glycocalyx-like surfaces using oligosaccharide surfactant polymers. *Nature* 392:799–801
16. Chapman RG, Ostuni E, Takayama S, Homlin E, Yan L, Whitesides GM. 2000. Surveying for surfaces that resist the adsorption of proteins. *J. Am. Chem. Soc.* 122:8303–4
17. Harder P, Grunze M, Dahint R, Whitesides GM, Laibinis PE. 1998. Molecular conformation in oligo(ethylene glycol)-terminated self-assembled monolayers on gold and silver surfaces determines their ability to resist protein adsorption. *J. Phys. Chem. B* 102:426–36
18. Pertsin AJ, Grunze M, Garbuzova IA. 1998. Low-energy configurations of methoxy triethylene glycol terminated alkanethiol self-assembled monolayers and their relevance to protein adsorption. *J. Phys. Chem. B* 102:4918–26
19. Shin H, Jo S, Mikos AG. 2003. Biomimetic materials for tissue engineering. *Biomaterials* 24:4353–64
20. Pierschbacher MD, Ruoslahti E. 1984. Cell attachment activity of fibronectin can be duplicated by small synthetic fragments of the molecule. *Nature* 309:30–33
21. Aumailley M, Gerl M, Sonnenberg A, Deutzmann R, Timpl R. 1990. Identification of the Arg-Gly-Asp sequence in laminin A chain as a latent cell-binding site being exposed in fragment P1. *FEBS Lett.* 262:82–86
22. Staatz WD, Fok KF, Zutter MM, Adams SP, Rodriguez BA, Santoro SA. 1991. Identification of a tetrapeptide recognition sequence for the $a_2b_1$ integrin in collagen. *J. Biol. Chem.* 266:7363–67
23. Smith JW, Cheresh DA. 1988. The Arg-Gly-Asp binding domain of the vitronectin receptor. Photoaffinity cross-linking implicates amino acid residues 61–203 of the beta subunit. *J. Biol. Chem.* 263:18726–31
24. VandeVondele S, Voros J, Hubbell JA. 2003. RGD-grafted poly-L-lysine-graft-(polyethylene glycol) copolymers block non-specific protein adsorption while promoting cell adhesion. *Biotechnol. Bioeng.* 82:784–90
25. Verrier S, Pallu S, Bareille R, Jonczyk A, Meyer J, et al. 2002. Function of linear and cyclic RGD-containing peptides in osteoprogenitor cells adhesion process. *Biomaterials* 23:585–96
26. Reyes CD, Garcia AJ. 2003. Engineering integrin-specific surfaces with a triple-helical collagen-mimetic. *J. Biomed. Mater. Res.* 65A:511–23
27. Keselowsky BG, Collard DM, Garcia AJ. 2003. Surface chemistry modulates fibronectin conformation and directs integrin binding and specificity to control

cell adhesion. *J. Biomed. Mater. Res.* 66A:247–59
28. Giachelli CM, Steitz S. 2000. Osteopontin: a versatile regulator of inflammation and biomineralization. *Matrix Biol.* 19:615–22
29. Martin SM, Schwartz JL, Giachelli CM, Ratner BD. 2003. Investigation of immobilized type-1 collagen as an affinity coating to bind osteopontin to poly(2-hydroxyethyl methacrylate). *Polym. Preprints* 44:177–78
30. Sharkawy AA, Klitzman B, Truskey GA, Reichert WM. 1998. Engineering the tissue which encapsulates subcutaneous implants. II. Plasma-tissue exchange properties. *J. Biomed. Mater. Res.* 40:586–97
31. Brauker JH, Carr-Brendel VE, Martinson LA, Crudele J, Johnston WD, Johnson RC. 1995. Neovascularization of synthetic membranes directed by membrane microarchitecture. *J. Biomed. Mater. Res.* 29:1514–24
32. Sharkawy AA, Klitzman B, Truskey GA, Reichert WM. 1998. Engineering the tissue which encapsulates subcutaneous implants. III. Effective tissue response times. *J. Biomed. Mater. Res.* 40:598–605
33. Marshall A, Ratner BD. 2002. Sphere templated porous hydrogels for tissue engineering. *Trans. Am. Chem. Soc. Symp. Polym. Med. Biol., Sonoma, CA*
34. Marshall A, Barker T, Sage EH, Hauch KD, Ratner BD. 2004. *Pore size controls angiogenesis in subcutaneously implanted porous matrices*. World Biomater. Congr., 7th, Sydney, Australia
35. Sanders JE, Stiles CE, Hayes CL. 2000. Tissue response to single-polymer fibers of varying diameters: evaluation of fibrous encapsulation and macrophage density. *J. Biomed. Mater. Res.* 52:231–37
36. Sanders JE, Cassisi DV, Neumann T, Golledge SL, Zachariah SG, et al. 2002. Relative influence of polymer fiber diameter and surface charge on fibrous capsule thickness and vessel density for single-fiber implants. *J. Biomed. Mater. Res.* 65A:462–67
37. Sanders JE, Bale SD, Neumann T. 2002. Tissue response to microfibers of different polymers: polyester, polyethylene, polylactic acid, and polyurethane. *J. Biomed. Mater. Res.* 62:222–27
38. Lee KY, Mooney DJ. 2001. Hydrogels for tissue engineering. *Chem. Rev.* 101:1869–79
39. Drury JL, Mooney DJ. 2003. Hydrogels for tissue engineering: scaffold design variables and applications. *Biomaterials* 24:4337–51
40. Hoffman AS. 2001. Hydrogels for biomedical applications. *Ann. NY Acad. Sci.* 944:62–73
41. Sawhney AS, Pathak CP, Hubbell JA. 1993. Bioerodible hydrogels based on photopolymerized poly(ethylene glycol)-co-poly(alpha-hydroxy acid) diacrylate macromers. *Macromolecules* 26:581–87
42. Martens P, Anseth KS. 2000. Characterization of hydrogels formed from acrylate modified poly(vinyl alcohol) macromers. *Polymer* 41:7715–22
43. Nuttelman CR, Henry SM, Anseth KS. 2002. Synthesis and characterization of photocrosslinkable, degradable poly(vinyl alcohol)-based tissue engineering scaffolds. *Biomaterials* 23:3617–26
44. Leach JB, Bivens KA, Patrick CW, Schmidt CE. 2003. Photocrosslinked hyaluronic acid hydrogels: natural, biodegradable tissue engineering scaffolds. *Biotechnol. Bioeng.* 82:578–89
45. Park YD, Tirelli N, Hubbell JA. 2003. Photopolymerized hyaluronic acid-based hydrogels and interpenetrating networks. *Biomaterials* 24:893–900
46. Luo N, Bryant S, Anseth K. 2001. *Photopolymerizable PVA and chondroitin sulfate hydrogels for cartilage tissue engineering*. Annu. Meet. Trans. Soc. Biomater., 27th, p. 327, St. Paul, MN
47. Peter SJ, Suggs LJ, Yaszemski MJ, Engel PS, Mikos AG. 1999. Synthesis of

poly(propylene fumarate) by acylation of propylene glycol in the presence of a proton scavenger. *J. Biomater. Sci. Polym. Ed.* 10:363–73
48. Behravesh E, Mikos AG. 2003. Three-dimensional culture of differentiating marrow stromal osteoblasts in biomimetic poly(propylene fumarate-co-ethylene glycol)-based macroporous hydrogels. *J. Biomed. Mater. Res. A* 66A:698–706
49. Shin H, Ruhe PQ, Mikos AG, Jansen JA. 2003. In vivo bone and soft tissue response to injectable, biodegradable oligo(poly(ethylene glycol) fumarate) hydrogels. *Biomaterials* 24:3201–11
50. Metters AT, Anseth KS, Bowman CN. 2000. Fundamental studies of a novel, biodegradable PEG-b-PLA hydrogel. *Polymer* 41:3993–4004
51. West JL, Hubbell JA. 1999. Polymeric biomaterials with degradation sites for proteases involved in cell migration. *Macromolecules* 32:241–44
52. Cruise GM, Hegre OD, Lamberti FV, Hager SR, Hill R, et al. 1999. In vitro and in vivo performance of porcine islets encapsulated in interfacially photopolymerized poly(ethylene glycol) diacrylate membranes. *Cell Transplant.* 8:293–306
53. Mann BK, Schmedlen RH, West JL. 2001. Tethered-TGF-$\beta$ increases extracellular matrix production of vascular smooth muscle cells. *Biomaterials* 22:439–44
54. Burdick JA, Anseth KS. 2002. Photoencapsulation of osteoblasts in injectable RGD-modified PEG hydrogels for bone tissue engineering. *Biomaterials* 23:4315–23
55. Elisseeff J, Anseth K, Sims D, McIntosh W, Randolph M, Langer R. 1999. Transdermal photopolymerization for minimally invasive implantation. *Proc. Natl. Acad. Sci. USA* 96:3104–7
56. Bryant SJ, Anseth KS. 2001. Hydrogel properties influence ECM production by chondrocyte photoencapsulated in poly(ethylene glycol) hydrogels. *J. Biomed. Mater. Res.* 59:63–72
57. Bryant SJ, Anseth KS. 2003. Controlling the spatial distribution of ECM components in degradable PEG hydrogels for tissue engineering cartilage. *J. Biomed. Mater. Res.* 64A:70–79
58. Burdick JA, Mason MN, Hinman AD, Thorne K, Anseth KS. 2002. Delivery of osteoinductive growth factors from degradable PEG hydrogels influences osteoblast differentiation and mineralization. *J. Control. Release* 83:53–63
59. Martens PJ, Bryant SJ, Anseth KS. 2003. Tailoring the degradation of hydrogels formed from multivinyl poly-(ethylene glycol) and poly(vinyl alcohol) macromers for cartilage tissue engineering. *Biomacromolecules* 4:283–92
60. Quick DJ, Anseth KS. 2003. Gene delivery in tissue engineering: a photopolymer platform to co-encapsulate cells and plasmid DNA. *Pharmaceut. Res.* 20(11):1730–37
61. Nair P, Ratner BD, Vogel V, Nerem RN. 2002. *Porous scaffolds containing amino acid networks as matrixes for tissue engineering.* Annu. Meet. Trans. Soc. Biomater., 28th, p. 654, Tampa, FL
62. Boeckl MS, Perry J, Leber ER, Nair P, Ratner BD. 2003. Development and characterization of poly(vinyl alcohol)-amino acid hydrogels for the use as biomaterials. *Polym. Preprints* 44:677–78
63. Donaldson EE, Boeckl MS, Hauch KD, Zhang M, Ratner BD. 2003. *Solid, polymeric microfoams for use as novel tissue engineering scaffolds.* Soc. Biomater. Annu. Meet. Trans., 29th, p. 638, Reno, NV
64. Murthy N, Campbell J, Fausto N, Hoffman AS, Stayton PS. 2003. Bioinspired pH-responsive polymers for the intracellular delivery of biomolecular drugs. *Bioconjugate Chem.* 14:412–19
65. Kim B, La Flamme K, Peppas NA. 2003. Dynamic swelling behavior of pH-sensitive anionic hydrogels used for protein delivery. *J. Appl. Polym. Sci.* 89: 1606–13

66. Jeong B, Kim SW, Bae YH. 2002. Thermosensitive sol-gel reversible hydrogels. *Adv. Drug Deliver. Rev.* 54:37–51
67. Chilkoti A, Dreher MR, Meyer DE. 2002. Design of thermally responsive, recombinant polypeptide carriers for targeted drug delivery. *Adv. Drug Deliver. Rev.* 54:1093–111
68. Shimoboji T, Larenas E, Fowler T, Kulkarni S, Hoffman AS, Stayton PS. 2002. Photoresponsive polymer-enzyme switches. *Proc. Natl. Acad. Sci. USA* 99: 16592–96
69. Shimoboji T, Larenas E, Fowler T, Hoffman AS, Stayton PS. 2003. Temperature-induced switching of enzyme activity with smart polymer-enzyme conjugates. *Bioconjugate Chem.* 14:517–25
70. Torres-Lugo M, Garcia M, Record R, Peppas NA. 2002. Physicochemical behavior and cytotoxic effects of p(methacrylic acid-g-ethylene glycol) nanospheres for oral delivery of proteins. *J. Control. Release* 80:197–205
71. Torres-Lugo M, Garcia M, Record R, Peppas NA. 2002. pH-sensitive hydrogels as gastrointestinal tract absorption enhancers: transport mechanisms of salmon calcitonin and other model molecules using the Caco-2 cell model. *Biotechnol. Progr.* 18:612–16
72. Lowman AM, Morishita M, Kajita M, Nagai T, Peppas NA. 1999. Oral delivery of insulin using pH-responsive complexation gels. *J. Pharm. Sci.* 88:933–37
73. Murthy N, Campbell J, Fausto N, Hoffman AS, Stayton PS. 2003. Design and synthesis of pH-responsive polymeric carriers that target uptake and enhance the intracellular delivery of oligonucleotides. *J. Control. Release* 89:365–74
74. Dreher MR, Raucher D, Balu N, Colvin OM, Ludemann SM, Chilkoti A. 2003. Evaluation of an elastin-like polypeptide-doxorubicin conjugate for cancer therapy. *J. Control. Release* 91:31–43
75. Heskins M, Guillet JE. 1968. Solution properties of poly(n-isopropylacrylamide). *J. Macromol. Sci. Chem.* A2:1441–55
76. Meyer DE, Chilkoti A. 2002. Genetically encoded synthesis of protein-based polymers with precisely specified molecular weight and sequence by recursive directional ligation: examples from the elastin-like polypeptide system. *Biomacromolecules* 3:357–67
77. Betre H, Setton LA, Meyer DE, Chilkoti A. 2002. Characterization of a genetically engineered elastin-like polypeptide for cartilaginous tissue repair. *Biomacromolecules* 3:910–16
78. Sershen S, West J. 2002. Implantable, polymeric systems for modulated drug delivery. *Adv. Drug Deliver. Rev.* 54:1225–35
79. Cheng X, Wang Y, Hanein Y, Bohringer KF, Ratner BD. 2004. Novel cell patterning using microheater controlled thermoresponsive plasma films. *J. Biomed. Mater. Res.* In press
80. Stile RA, Burghardt WR, Healy KE. 1999. Synthesis and characterization of injectable poly(n-isopropylacrylamide)-based hydrogels that support tissue formation in vitro. *Macromolecules* 32:7370–79
81. Shimizu T, Yamato M, Isoi Y, Akutsu T, Setomaru T et al. 2002. Fabrication of pulsatile cardiac tissue grafts using a novel 3-dimensional cell sheet manipulation technique and temperature-responsive cell culture surfaces. *Circ. Res.* 90:E40–E48
82. Shimizu T, Yamato M, Akutsu T, Shibata T, Isoi Y, et al. 2002. Electrically communicating three-dimensional cardiac tissue mimic fabricated by layered cultured cardiomyocyte sheets. *J. Biomed. Mater. Res.* 60:110–17
83. Harimoto M, Yamato M, Hirose M, Takahashi C, Isoi Y, et al. 2002. Novel approach for achieving double-layered cell sheets co-culture: overlaying endothelial cell sheets onto monolayer hepatocytes utilizing temperature-responsive culture dishes. *J. Biomed. Mater. Res.* 62:464–70

84. Nandkumar MA, Yamato M, Kushida A, Konno C, Hirose M, et al. 2002. Two-dimensional cell sheet manipulation of heterotypically co-cultured lung cells utilizing temperature-responsive culture dishes results in long-term maintenance of differentiated epithelial cell functions. *Biomaterials* 23:1121–30
85. Kwon OH, Kikuchi A, Yamato M, Okano T. 2003. Accelerated cell sheet recovery by co-grafting of PEG with PIPAAm onto porous cell culture membranes. *Biomaterials* 24:1223–32
86. Kost J, Horbett TA, Ratner BD, Singh M. 1985. Glucose-sensitive membranes containing glucose oxidase: activity, swelling and permeability studies. *J. Biomed. Mater. Res.* 19:1117–33
87. Alexeev VL, Sharma AC, Goponenko AV, Das S, Lednev IK, et al. 2003. High ionic strength glucose-sensing photonic crystal. *Anal. Chem.* 75:2316–23
88. Zhang SG. 2002. Emerging biological materials through molecular self-assembly. *Biotechnol. Adv.* 20:321–39
89. Petka WA, Harden JL, McGrath KP, Wirtz D, Tirrell DA. 1998. Reversible hydrogels from self-assembling artificial proteins. *Science* 281:389–92
90. Caplan MR, Lauffenburger DA. 2002. Nature's complex copolymers: engineering design of oligopeptide materials. *Ind. Eng. Chem. Res.* 41:403–12
91. Caplan MR, Schwartzfarb EM, Zhang SG, Kamm RD, Lauffenburger DA. 2002. Control of self-assembling oligopeptide matrix formation through systematic variation of amino acid sequence. *Biomaterials* 23:219–27
92. Wright ER, McMillan RA, Cooper A, Apkarian RP, Conticello VP. 2002. Thermoplastic elastomer hydrogels via self-assembly of an elastin-mimetic triblock polypeptide. *Adv. Funct. Mater.* 12:149–54
93. Hartgerink JD, Beniash E, Stupp SI. 2002. Peptide-amphiphile nanofibers: a versatile scaffold for the preparation of self-assembling materials. *Proc. Natl. Acad. Sci. USA* 99:5133–38
94. Ryadnov MG, Woolfson DN. 2003. Engineering the morphology of a self-assembling protein fibre. *Nat. Mater.* 2: 329–32
95. Ryadnov MG, Woolfson DN. 2003. Introducing branches into a self-assembling peptide fiber. *Angew. Chem. Int. Ed.* 42: 3021–23
96. Caplan MR, Schwartzfarb EM, Zhang SG, Kamm RD, Lauffenburger DA. 2002. Effects of systematic variation of amino acid sequence on the mechanical properties of a self-assembling, oligopeptide biomaterial. *J. Biomater. Sci. Polym. Ed.* 13:225–36
97. Di Zio K, Tirrell DA. 2003. Mechanical properties of artificial protein matrices engineered for control of cell and tissue behavior. *Macromolecules* 36:1553–58
98. Collier JH, Messersmith PB. 2003. Enzymatic modification of self-assembled peptide structures with tissue transglutaminase. *Bioconjugate Chem.* 14:748–55
99. Graf J, Iwamoto Y, Sasaki M, Martin GR, Kleinman HK, et al. 1987. Identification of the major epithelial-cell attachment site (YIGSR) in the B1-chain of laminin. *J. Invest. Dermatol.* 88:491–91
100. Niece KL, Hartgerink JD, Donners J, Stupp SI. 2003. Self-assembly combining two bioactive peptide-amphiphile molecules into nanofibers by electrostatic attraction. *J. Am. Chem. Soc.* 125:7146–47
101. Zhang SG, Holmes TC, Dipersio CM, Hynes RO, Su X, Rich A. 1995. Self-complementary oligopeptide matrices support mammalian-cell attachment. *Biomaterials* 16:1385–93
102. Holmes TC, de Lacalle S, Su X, Liu GS, Rich A, Zhang SG. 2000. Extensive neurite outgrowth and active synapse formation on self-assembling peptide scaffolds. *Proc. Natl. Acad. Sci. USA* 97:6728–33
103. Hwang JJ, Iyer SN, Li LS, Claussen R, Harrington DA, Stupp SI. 2002.

Self-assembling biomaterials: liquid crystal phases of cholesteryl oligo(l-lactic acid) and their interactions with cells. *Proc. Natl. Acad. Sci. USA* 99:9662–67

104. Kisiday J, Jin M, Kurz B, Hung H, Semino C, et al. 2002. Self-assembling peptide hydrogel fosters chondrocyte extracellular matrix production and cell division: implications for cartilage tissue repair. *Proc. Natl. Acad. Sci. USA* 99:9996–10001
105. Semino CE, Merok JR, Crane GG, Panagiotakos G, Zhang SG. 2003. Functional differentiation of hepatocyte-like spheroid structures from putative liver progenitor cells in three-dimensional peptide scaffolds. *Differentiation* 71:262–70
106. Ni M, Ratner BD. 2003. Nacre surface transformation to hydroxyapatite in a phosphate buffer solution. *Biomaterials* 24:4323–31
107. Lutolf MR, Weber FE, Schmoekel HG, Schense JC, Kohler T, et al. 2003. Repair of bone defects using synthetic mimetics of collagenous extracellular matrices. *Nat. Biotechnol.* 21:513–18
108. Trowbridge EA, Lawford PV, Crofts CE, Roberts KM. 1988. Pericardial heterografts—why do these valves fail. *J. Thorac. Cardiovasc. Surg.* 95:577–85
109. Badylak SF. 1993. Small intestinal submucosa (SIS): a biomaterial conducive to smart tissue remodeling. In *Tissue Engineering: Current Perspectives*, ed. E Bell, pp. 179–89. Cambridge, MA: Burkhauser
110. Record RD, Hillegonds D, Simmons C, Tullius R, Rickey FA, et al. 2001. In vivo degradation of $^{14}$C-labeled small intestinal submucosa (SIS) when used for urinary bladder repair. *Biomaterials* 22:2653–59
111. Hodde JP, Record RD, Liang HA, Badylak SF. 2001. Vascular endothelial growth factor in porcine-derived extracellular matrix. *Endothelium* 8:11–24
112. Voytik-Harbin SL, Brightman AO, Kraine MR, Wainer B, Badylak SF. 1997. Identification of extractable growth factors from small intestinal submucosa. *J. Cell. Biochem.* 67:478–91
113. Palmer EM, Beilfuss BA, Nagai T, Semnani RT, Badylak SF, van Seventer GA. 2002. Human helper T cell activation and differentiation is suppressed by procine small intestinal submucosa. *Tissue Eng.* 8:893–900
114. Badylak SF, Park K, Peppas N, McCabe G, Yoder M. 2001. Marrow-derived cells populate scaffolds composed of xenogeneic extracellular matrix. *Exp. Hematol.* 29:1310–18
115. Figeys D, Pinto D. 2000. Lab-on-a-chip: a revolution in biological and medical sciences. *Anal. Chem.* 72:330A–35A
116. Xia YN, Whitesides GM. 1998. Soft lithography. *Annu. Rev. Mater. Res.* 28:153–84
117. Folch A, Toner M. 2000. Microengineering of cellular interactions. *Annu. Rev. Biomed. Eng.* 2:227–56
118. Whitesides GM, Ostuni E, Takayama S, Jiang XY, Ingber DE. 2001. Soft lithography in biology and biochemistry. *Annu. Rev. Biomed. Eng.* 3:335–73
119. Beebe DJ, Mensing GA, Walker GM. 2002. Physics and applications of microfluidics in biology. *Annu. Rev. Biomed. Eng.* 4:261–86
120. Brehmer M, Conrad L, Funk L. 2003. New developments in soft lithography. *J. Disper. Sci. Technol.* 24:291–304
121. Weigl BH, Bardell RL, Cabrera CR. 2003. Lab-on-a-chip for drug development. *Adv. Drug Deliver. Rev.* 55:349–77
122. Kovacs GTA. 2003. Electronic sensors with living cellular components. *Proc. IEEE* 91:915–29
123. Selvaganapathy PR, Carlen ET, Mastrangelo CH. 2003. Recent progress in microfluidic devices for nucleic acid and antibody assays. *Proc. IEEE* 91:954–75
124. Andersson H, van den Berg A. 2003. Microfluidic devices for cellomics: a review. *Sens. Actuators B-Chem.* 92:315–25

125. Odom TW, Thalladi VR, Love JC, Whitesides GM. 2002. Generation of 30–50 nm structures using easily fabricated, composite PDMS masks. *J. Am. Chem. Soc.* 124:12112–13
126. Bernard A, Delamarche E, Schmid H, Michel B, Bosshard HR, Biebuyck H. 1998. Printing patterns of proteins. *Langmuir* 14:2225–29
127. James CD, Davis RC, Kam L, Craighead HG, Isaacson M, et al. 1998. Patterned protein layers on solid substrates by thin stamp microcontact printing. *Langmuir* 14:741–44
128. Singhvi R, Kumar A, Lopez GP, Stephanopoulos GN, Wang DI, et al. 1994. Engineering cell shape and function. *Science* 264:696–98
129. Chen CS, Mrksich M, Huang S, Whitesides GM, Ingber DE. 1997. Geometric control of cell life and death. *Science* 276:1425–28
130. Chen CS, Alonso JL, Ostuni E, Whitesides GM, Ingber DE. 2003. Cell shape provides global control of focal adhesion assembly. *Biochem. Biophys. Res. Commun.* 307:355–61
131. Brock A, Chang E, Ho CC, LeDuc P, Jiang XY, et al. 2003. Geometric determinants of directional cell motility revealed using microcontact printing. *Langmuir* 19:1611–17
132. Kley EB. 1997. Continuous profile writing by electron and optical lithography. *Microelectron. Eng.* 34:261–98
133. Wu HK, Odom TW, Whitesides GM. 2002. Reduction photolithography using microlens arrays: applications in gray scale photolithography. *Anal. Chem.* 74:3267–73
134. Chen CC, Hirdes D, Folch A. 2003. Gray-scale photolithography using microfluidic photomasks. *Proc. Natl. Acad. Sci. USA* 100:1499–504
135. Takayama S, Ostuni E, LeDuc P, Naruse K, Ingber DE, Whitesides GM. 2003. Selective chemical treatment of cellular microdomains using multiple laminar streams. *Chem. Biol.* 10:123–30
136. Khoury C, Mensing GA, Beebe DJ. 2002. Ultra rapid prototyping of microfluidic systems using liquid phase photopolymerization. *Lab Chip* 2:50–55
137. Otsu T, Yoshida M. 1982. Role of initiator-transfer agent-terminator (iniferter) in radical polymerizations—polymer design by organic disulfides as iniferters. *Makromol. Chem. Rapid* 3:127–32
138. Nakayama Y, Matsuda T. 1996. Surface macromolecular architectural designs using photo-graft copolymerization based on photochemistry of benzyl n,n-diethyldithiocarbamate. *Macromolecules* 29:8622–30
139. Luo N, Metters AT, Hutchison JB, Bowman CN, Anseth KS. 2003. A methacrylated photoiniferter as a chemical basis for microlithography: micropatterning based on photografting polymerization. *Macromolecules* 36:6739–45
140. Haraldsson KT, Sebra RP, Luo N, Hutchison JB, Anseth KS, Bowman CN. 2002. *3D-microfluidic devices using LRPP.* Annu. Meet. Arch.—Am. Inst. Chem. Eng., Indianapolis IN, Nov. 3–8, pp. 157–60
141. Sebra RP, Hutchison JB, Haraldsson KT, Anseth KS, Bowman CN. 2003. Living radical photopolymerizations to modify surfaces in microfluidic devices for biological applications. *Polym. Preprints* 44: 833–34
142. Huber DL, Manginell RP, Samara MA, Kim BI, Bunker BC. 2003. Programmed adsorption and release of proteins in a microfluidic device. *Science* 301:352–54
143. Nath N, Chilkoti A. 2003. Fabrication of a reversible protein array directly from cell lysate using a stimuli-responsive polypeptide. *Anal. Chem.* 75:709–15
144. Zhao B, Moore JS, Beebe DJ. 2003. Pressure-sensitive microfluidic gates fabricated by patterning surface free energies inside microchannels. *Langmuir* 19:1873–79

145. Taboas JM, Maddox RD, Krebsbach PH, Hollister SJ. 2003. Indirect solid free form fabrication of local and global porous, biomimetic and composite 3D polymer-ceramic scaffolds. *Biomaterials* 24:181–94
146. Hutmacher DW. 2000. Scaffolds in tissue engineering bond and cartilage. *Biomaterials* 21:2529–43
147. Tan W, Desai TA. 2003. Microfluidic patterning of cells in extracellular matrix biopolymers: effects of channel size, cell type, and matrix composition on pattern integrity. *Tissue Eng.* 9:255–67
148. Liu VA, Bhatia SN. 2002. Three-dimensional photopatterning of hydrogels containing living cells. *Biomed. Microdevices* 4:257–66

Annu. Rev. Biomed. Eng. 2004. 6:77–107
doi: 10.1146/annurev.bioeng.6.040803.140250

First published online as a Review in Advance on March 24, 2004

# TISSUE GROWTH AND REMODELING

Stephen C. Cowin
*The New York Center for Biomedical Engineering and the Departments of Biomedical and Mechanical Engineering, School of Engineering, City College and Graduate School, The City University of New York, New York 10031; email: scowin@earthlink.net*

**Key Words** simulation, modeling, morphogenesis, development, adaptation

■ **Abstract** The growth and remodeling of a tissue depends on certain features in the history of its mechanical environment as well as its genetic makeup. The mechanical environment influences the tissue's developing morphology, the process of simply increasing the size of existing morphological structures, and the formation of the proteins of which the tissue is constructed. The relationships between genetic information, various epigenetic mechanisms and tissue development are discussed. The developmental growth and remodeling of most structural tissues are enhanced by the use of those tissues and retarded by their disuse. The mechanical or mathematical modeling of tissue growth and development using cellular automata models and continuum mechanical models is reviewed.

CONTENTS



1523-9829/04/0815-0077$14.00

# INTRODUCTION

A tissue is a composite material whose constituents, and therefore structure, are continually changing owing to the growth and response of the tissue to its physical and chemical environment. A tissue's physiochemical environment includes the environment it is experiencing and the recent history of that environment. A tissue is a collection of cells and extracellular matrices (ECMs) that perform specialized functions. The ECM consists of fibers (e.g., the proteins collagen and elastin) and a ground substance (e.g., proteoglycans). Animal tissues are classified into four main groups: connective, epithelial, muscle, and nerve. The main tissue examples considered in this review are connective tissues. Connective tissue connects the body organs and tissues; it holds organs in place and provides the structure that gives the body shape. Compared with other types of tissue, connective tissue has relatively few cells and much extracellular substance. Connective tissues include cartilage, tendons, ligaments, the matrix of bone, and the adipose (fatty) tissues, as well as skin, blood, and lymph.

Growth is the process of gradual increase in the net volume of a tissue, but it may also include some resorption. There is evidence that growth in length of an organism is proportional to the cube root of growth in volume (1). A distinction is made between appositional growth and interstitial growth; that is, the difference between growth on the surface and growth within a volume of tissue. Appositional growth occurs, for example, when a tree adds another layer to the outside of its trunk, and interstitial growth occurs within the cavities or spaces in the tissues of animals or plants. Hard tissues, bone and teeth, grow by apposition and soft tissues grow interstitially. This review focuses on the influence of the recent history of mechanical loading on growth rate; although, growth rate may also be slowed or accelerated by hormones, vitamins, bioelectrical factors, surgical intervention, imbalances between deposition and resorption, and other factors.

In addition to, and apart from, growth, mature tissues may remodel their ECM to adapt its structure to the mechanical loading environment it is and has been experiencing. As an illustration of the adaptation of tissues to a changed mechanical load environment, consider the data on the response to microgravity. Almost 1000 mature humans have accumulated almost 70 person-years of space flight. The direct and indirect effects of microgravity are numerous. The removal of gravity means that the limbs no longer have weight and muscles are no longer required to maintain posture. The stretch sensors in the musculoskeletal system then receive a signal different from the one they receive on Earth. They no longer have to maintain the normal musculoskeletal structure of the body against gravity and the system begins to diminish its capacity. Bone mass is lost from key parts of the skeleton at the rate of approximately 1% per month, and some muscles atrophy rapidly. The vestibular system in the inner ear, the system that allows us to control our balance and equilibrium, automatically compensates for gravity, and some adaptation of this system is necessary when there is microgravity. A researcher studying the effect of microgravity on the vestibular system has indicated that we are not able to predict whether, after a yearlong trip from Earth, an astronaut would be able to stand up on Mars (2). Much of the body is fluid, and therefore the body, designed for life on Earth, experiences a fluid shift to the head and away from the feet in microgravity. The fluid shift initiates a number of interacting renal, hormonal, and mechanical effects that regulate fluid and electrolyte levels (3). The kidney filtration rate, for example, is increased by 20%, and the skull may actually gain bone rather than lose it because of the increased fluid pressure within the skull owing to the caudal shift of fluids in microgravity.

Morphogenesis refers to the processes that are responsible for producing the complex shapes of adults from the simple ball of cells that derives from division of the fertilized egg. Morphogenetic events include pattern and template formation in tissue development. Morphogenetic processes interact with the growth and remodeling processes and often all three process types occur simultaneously.

The subject of this review is the simulation and mathematical modeling of tissue growth and remodeling. These subjects are viewed from the perspective of how they are, or could be, mathematically modeled. In 1885, Wilhelm Roux stated the need for mechanical modeling in the study of tissue development in his statement of objective (4) for his new journal, the *Archiv für Entwickelungsmechanik der Organismen*, a journal that is still published. His statement of objective was contained in an introductory essay entitled "The Problems, Methods, and Scope of Developmental Mechanics" (4). Readers not familiar with Roux could see many of the same ideas in the first (1917) edition of D'Arcy Thompson's *On Growth and Form* (5), and almost all writers in this area indicate the influence of D'Arcy Thompson as a starting point. In spite of this perceptive start a century ago, innovative mechanics is only beginning to be applied to the study of tissue development. The biologist Albert Harris (6) wrote, "Systems of interacting forces and stimuli don't have to be very complicated before the unaided human intuition can no longer predict accurately what the net result should be. At this point computer simulations, or other mathematical models, become necessary. Without the aid of mechanicians, and others skilled in simulation and modeling, developmental biology will remain a prisoner of our inadequate and conflicting physical intuitions and metaphors." In 1990, the geneticist Jonathan Bard wrote "I . . . assert that the process of tissue formation is in many ways the cellular equivalent of molecular self-assembly and that the appropriate language in which to analyze morphogenesis is that of the differential equation . . ." (7).

In the next section, the relationship between genetic information and tissue development is discussed. Various epigenetic mechanisms for tissue patterning that have been suggested are also described below. After a short section on the supramolecular assembly of tissues, the mechanical or mathematical modeling of tissue growth and development occupies the remainder of the review. A section on modeling considerations is followed by four sections on continuum models: kinematic models of growth; bone remodeling; soft tissue growth and remodeling; and heart and joint growth, remodeling, and morphogenesis. The final section concerns cellular automata models for cell sorting.

Anthropologists and forensic experts study bone because, owing to its mineralized character, it lasts many lifetimes and furnishes a readable record, whereas it is more difficult to discern structure in soft tissue and the soft tissue disappears relatively quickly, seldom leaving a record to be studied. The development of mechanical models for growth and remodeling of bone have preceded those for soft tissue because bone models are also easier to construct because bone deformations under load are small and because they grow by apposition rather than interstitially. It is for these reasons that there are so many examples associated with bone tissue in this chapter and not the fact that the author has studied bone tissue more than the other tissues.

## GENETIC INFORMATION AND THE DEVELOPMENT OF BIOLOGICAL TISSUE

Biological tissues form distinctive and repeated patterns found throughout the animal kingdom. The relationship of genetic information to biological structure, and to the proteins that form the structure, is indirect and not yet fully understood. The three viewpoints are (7) the genetic view, the epigenetic view, and the middle view. In the (strong) genetic view, tissue structure is predetermined by precise information stored in the genome interpreted by cells as specific instructions. Tissue structure is directly determined by DNA-coded information laid down in the egg. In the epigenetic view, tissue structure develops by a process of interaction of cells with their environment. Tissue structure arises from changes in the properties of the cells and the then existing tissue structure. In the middle view, both genetic and epigenetic contribute, and the extent to which both contribute depends on the animal or the tissue under consideration (4). The answer most preferred is the middle route, as recommended by Daedalus to Icarus. The combination of genetic and epigenetic contributions also applies to the making of proteins. The folding of a protein is created by the interactions of the polypeptide chain within itself, and in the development of a tissue, there are also interactions of the developing tissue with the tissue's external environment that contribute to the determination of the resulting structure (8).

Separation of the influence of genetics and epigenetics was apparently achieved for a specific period in the development phase of a tissue in an animal experiment (9). In this experiment, the cartilaginous primordia or anlage (template) of the femur in a developing mouse was transplanted into the mouse's spleen, a site where the usual mechanical loading of the femur was absent. Cartilaginous primordia are the result of genetic information and epigenetic developmental processes. After development, the bone was compared with that developed in the mouse hind limb under normal physiological loading. It is assumed that neither genetic information nor its usual mechanical loading is delivered to the developing femur for the period that it is in the spleen. The influence of genes and the influence of the combination of normal mechanical loading and the genes can be discerned by comparing these two mouse femora, as illustrated in Figure 1 (see color insert). The morphologically normal mouse femur was developed within a normal functional loading environment (Figure 1*a*). The morphology of a mouse femur deprived of its normal mechanical loading was produced by having the bone develop from its cartilage anlage, without normal mechanical loading, in the spleen (Figure 1*b*). Although the bone developed as a recognizable femur, it lacked the refinements associated with the normal functional bone. The major features induced by normal mechanical loading were the organization of the internal trabecular structure, the width of the medullary cavity and thickness of the cortical wall, the wasting of the femoral neck, and the curvature of the femoral diaphysis (10).

A basic method of approach in science and engineering is reductionism. The philosophy of this approach is to decompose the object of study into its constituent parts, analyze each part separately, and then reconstruct the object and predict its response to stimuli from a knowledge of response of the constituent parts to stimuli. The partial separation of the influence of the primordial template contained in the cartilage anlage and epigenetics in the animal experiment described in the previous paragraph is an illustration of the reductionist idea that the development of a biological structure can be separated into the effect of the primordial template and the effect of the history of mechanical loading on the biological structure. The idea underlying the primordial template is that in the absence of mechanical loading, the form of a skeletal element will revert to a form determined by the information in the primordial template. As noted above, the information contained in the primordial template comes from both genetic and epigenetic sources. The experiment described in the paragraph above provides insight into the nature of the primordial template for the mouse femur. The reductionist hypothesis is that any decrease in the functional loading of a bone induces remodeling changes that reduce the bony mass and allow the form of the bone to revert to its primordial template. Studies of the development of cultured chick limb in vitro have shown that some of the prominences on specific bones developed in culture and some did not. This indicates that some bony features required functional loading for development, whereas others were part of the primordial template. There is a caveat associated with the use of the concept of a primordial template because this reductionist idea does not easily allow for the interaction of genetic and epigenetic influences that occur during development. Some development genes are only activated at the stage of development where they are to be effective and

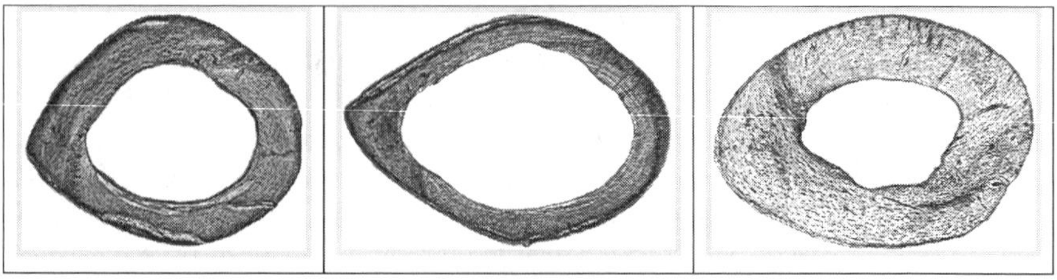

**Figure 2** Images of femoral cross-sections at the mid diaphysis of three strains of 16-week-old female mice. The names of the inbred strains are (*left*) A/J, (*center*) C57BL/6J (Black 6), and (*right*) C3H/HeJ (C3H). From Tommasini et al. (12).

are inactive at other stages. In mathematical terms, the separation of genetic and epigenetic effects can be nonlinear rather than linear and therefore not open to reductionism.

The information contained in the primordial template may be different for different strains of a species. Mice from different inbred strains have noticeable structural differences in their bones (11, 12). The cross-sections of femurs at the mid diaphysis and the vertebrae of three inbred strains of 16-week-old female mice are shown in Figures 2 and 3, respectively. The age of peak bone mass is 16 weeks in these animals. The names of the inbred strains in the two figures are (left) A/J, (center) C57BL/6J (Black 6), and (right) C3H/HeJ (C3H). The A/J strain have slender femurs, small cortical area, small polar moment of inertia, high ash content, low whole-bone stiffness, low maximum strength, and are brittle. The B6 femurs have small cortical area, large polar moment of inertia, low ash content, low whole-bone stiffness, low maximum strength, and are ductile. The C3H femurs

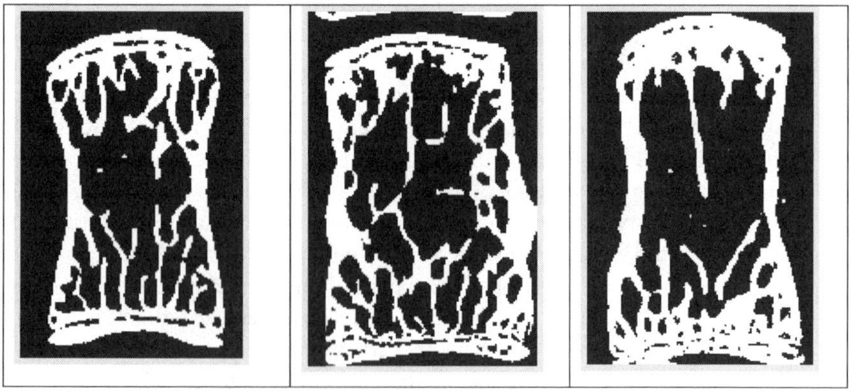

**Figure 3** Images of vertebral cross-sections of three strains of 16-week-old female mice. The names of the inbred strains are (*left*) A/J, (*center*) C57BL/6J (Black 6), and (*right*) C3H/HeJ (C3H). From Tommasini et al. (12).

have large cortical area, large polar moment of inertia, intermediate ash content, high whole-bone stiffness, high max load, and moderate brittleness. The A/J vertebrae have small cross-sectional area, small cortical area, intermediate bone mineral content, low stiffness, moderate brittleness, and low strength. The B6 vertebrae have large cross-sectional area, small cortical area, low bone mineral content, low stiffness, are ductile, and have high strength. The C3H vertebrae have large cross-sectional area, large cortical area, high bone mineral content, high stiffness, high brittleness, and high strength. All three strains have similar vertebral solid volume fraction of bone matrix. Thus, the primordial template for a species is not unique. If one views the development of a skeleton or a biological structure as the solution to a mathematical problem, one concludes that the solution is not unique, as well as being development-path dependent.

Fortunately, with the present rate of decoding the human genetic information, a great deal more will be understood in a decade. Certain basic features of the full organism are recorded in the primordial template, but during embryonic development and during early growth the structure of the organism is modified or molded by epigenetic factors. For example, the skin forming the soles of the feet is already thickened in the human fetus, but our common experience shows that walking barefoot or wearing poorly fitting footwear will contribute to the thickness and distribution of this tissue on the foot bottom.

In the following section, the various proposals for epigenetic mechanisms that may contribute to the patterning of tissue development are considered.

## EPIGENETIC MECHANISMS FOR TISSUE PATTERNING

The most important epigenetic mechanisms that are considered determinants of individual development are (*a*) interactions of cell metabolism with the physicochemical environment within and external to the organism, (*b*) interactions of tissue masses with the physical environment, and (*c*) interactions among tissues themselves, according to a temporally evolving set of rules (8). Different epigenetic processes have prevailed at different stages of morphological evolution, and the forms and characters assumed by metazoan organisms (i.e., the broad class of multicellular animals having cells differentiated into tissues and organs and usually a digestive cavity and nervous system) originated in large part by the action of such processes.

### Epigenetic Mechanisms Associated with the Interactions of Cell Metabolism with the Physicochemical Environment

Alan Turing, famous for his 1936 creation of the prototype plan for digital computers and for his effort in deciphering the German Enigma cipher during World War II, is also renowned for the chemical reaction mechanism hypothesis. In his 1952 paper entitled "The Chemical Basis of Morphogenesis," he hypothesized

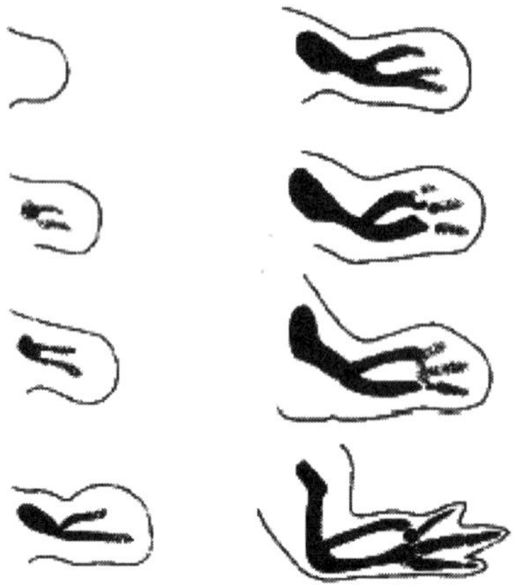

**Figure 4** Development of the chick limb bud between four and seven days of incubation. The solid black regions represent definitive cartilage; striped areas represent early cartilage. From Newman & Frisch (15).

that the diffusing patterns of reacting chemicals can form steady-state heterogeneous spatial patterns, and this phenomenon could be a biological mechanism of pattern formation (13). Turing introduced the term morphogen to describe the particular chemical substance that was the signal for structural change or development. The development and application of the Turing system to biological and mathematical problems is summarized in the book by Murray (14). One particularly graphic use of the Turing system described by Murray is his application of the reaction-diffusion equations to mammalian coat patterns. A Turing-related diffusion model to explain the development of skeletal pattern in the embryonic chick limb bud was presented by Newman & Frisch (15). The pattern of development of the chick limb bud between four and seven days of incubation is shown in Figure 4. The solid black regions represent definitive cartilage; striped areas represent early cartilage. The predicted pattern of limb development using the diffusion model of Newman & Frisch (15) for the morphogen is shown in Figure 5. The solid black regions in this figure represent cartilage or precartilage condensation; the striped regions represent the distribution of the morphogen preceding chondrogenesis.

There is another set of models in which diffusion-like equations are combined with equations describing mechanical activity. The model of mesenchymal morphogenesis gives an example where an active stress exerted by cells is taken into account. The mesenchyme is part of the embryonic mesoderm, consisting of loosely packed, unspecialized cells set in a gelatinous ground substance consisting of proteoglycans, from which connective tissue, bone, cartilage, and the circulatory and lymphatic systems develop. The condensation of cartilaginous skeletal rudiments in the developing vertebrate limb was also modeled in Oster et al. (16) with equations similar to those in Newman & Frisch (15), but with a model that incorporated

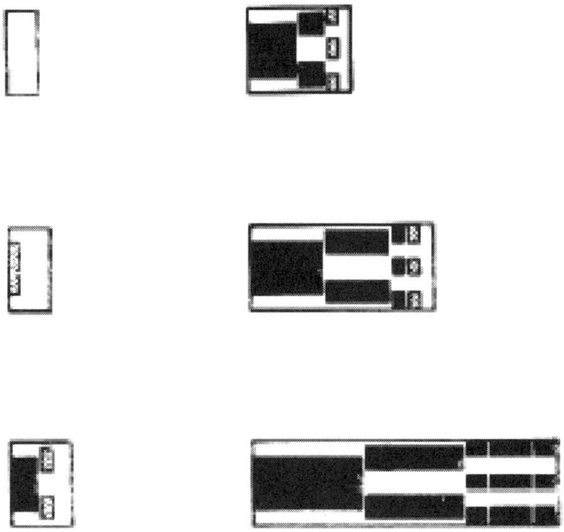

**Figure 5** The predicted pattern of limb development using the Newman & Frisch (15) diffusion model. The solid black regions represent cartilage or pre-cartilage condensation; striped regions represent the distribution of the morphogen preceding chrondrogenesis. Elongation of the domain is based on empirical measurements; it represents growth superposed on the diffusion in the domain. From Newman & Frisch (15).

the cumulative effects of cell-generated forces (17) in place of the purely chemical diffusive mechanism used in Newman & Frisch (15).

A second mechanism for the morphogenetic event of pattern formation in tissue development is that cells somehow sense the tissue in which they reside and make use of this positional information to trigger further steps in development. This concept is credited to developmental biologist Lewis Wolpert, who suggests that there is both a weak statement of the positional information mechanism and a strong statement (18, 19). In the weak statement of the concept, the operational mechanism of positional information is not specified. In this case, a cell does something just by being in a certain tissue at a certain stage of its development; the cell knows where it is. In the strong statement of the positional information concept, Wolpert suggests that the cell knows where it is because it can sense the concentration of some chemical or, to use Turing's term, morphogen. There is a gradient of the morphogen and the cell knows from the concentration of the morphogen that it measures where it is located along the gradient.

The idea underlying the differential adhesion hypothesis (20, 21) is that combinations of different cell types behave as immiscible liquids because of surface tension, but with the cell-to-cell adhesion forces playing the role of molecule-molecule attraction forces. Two fluids are said to be immiscible if they do not mix

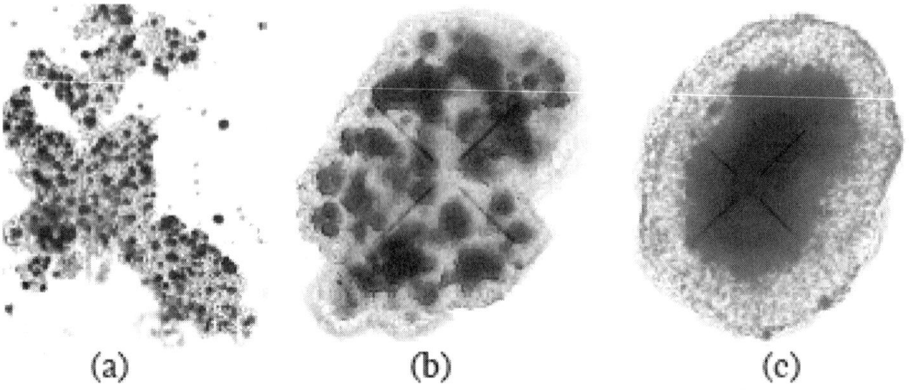


**Figure 6** Experimental images from chicken embryo cells in culture: light cells are neural retinal cells and dark cells are pigmented retinal cells. An initial random mixture of light and dark cells (*a*) forms dark clusters after approximately 10 h (*b*), and eventually sorts to produce a dark cell core surrounded by light cells after approximately 72 h. From Alber et al. (23).

and miscible if they do mix. The most well-known examples of immiscible fluids are oil and water. In immiscible liquids, a liquid with a higher surface tension will form droplets enclosed by drops of another liquid with lower surface tension. In combinations of different cell types, cells with higher surface tension will band more tightly together, forcing the cells with a lower surface tension to the outside. The last statement is the differential adhesion hypothesis. This sorting is illustrated schematically in Figure 8*A*, (see color insert), as discussed below; Figure 6 shows experimental images from the sorting of chicken embryo cells in culture (22, 23). In Figure 6 the light cells are neural retinal cells and dark cells are pigmented retinal cells. The initial situation, shown in the first panel, is a random mixture of light and dark cells. The second panel shows the dark clusters formed in 10 h, and the third panel shows the dark cell core surrounded by a light cell shell at 72 h. It has been experimentally demonstrated (24) that the mean size of the interconnected cellular domains, like those in panel (*b*) of Figure 6, increase linearly in time, consistent with the analogy between combinations of different cell types and immiscible fluids.

A mechanism other than surface tension–induced relative adhesiveness has been suggested to be consistent with the analogy between combinations of different cell types and immiscible fluids. Harris (25) suggested that the observations that support the surface tension–induced relative adhesiveness mechanism are equally consistent with an explanation based on the cell's own contractility of its cytoskeletal structure. The idea is that the contraction of the surface layer of a cell induced by the contraction of the underlying cytoskeleton simulates surface tension because surface tension is due to the mutual attraction of subunits in a surface layer.

## Epigenetic Mechanisms Associated with Interactions of Tissue Masses with the Tissue's Physical Environment

Wolff's law is generally considered as a statement on the epigenetic effect of mechanical loading on a tissue, generally to the effect that, over time, the mechanical load applied to a living tissue influences the structure of the tissue. The sensors of this mechanical load applied to the tissue are thought to be the tissue cells, e.g., the endothelial cells in blood vessels, the chondrocytes in articular cartilage, and the osteocytes in bone. This weak or loose statement of Wolff's law represents the common usage of the term Wolff's law today, although Wolff only concerned himself with bone tissue (26, 27). Wolff's precise claim was that his law was a rigorous mathematical statement, namely that the pattern of trabecular architecture of cancellous bone coincided with stress trajectories in the bone. This strong form of Wolff's law is not valid, as many students of the subject over the past century have concluded (28). The concept of functional adaptation to mechanical loading of a tissue (Wolff's law) is more legitimately credited to Roux (29).

## Epigenetic Mechanisms Associated with Interactions Among Tissues Themselves

Mechanical instability, or buckling, is another mechanism that might classify as a positional information mechanism of the weak type. Examples of mechanical instability are numerous and include column and plate buckling. Realistic models for some biological pattern-forming processes are the deflections associated with column and plate buckling when the beam or plate is on an elastic foundation under axial compression (such as a column with lateral support from springs). The supporting springs are considered to be so close together that they can be treated as continuous elastic support. As the compressive axial load acting on this beam is increased, it will deflect from its straight-line shape into the shape of $(N + 1)$ half-sine waves, where $N = 0, 1, 2, 3$, etc., and where N depends on the value of the compressive load. This is just one example of a mechanical instability, or buckling, situation that might be used by developing organisms to generate patterns for their structure. This particular example gives rise to a one-dimensional pattern, whereas plates compressed in two directions will give rise to a great variety of two-dimensional patterns. A fascinating buckling plate pattern formation hypothesis for the patterns associated with leaf and petal formation, phyllotaxis, has been developed in Green (30, 31). A buckling pattern formation hypothesis for spiral phyllotaxis was developed in Green (30, 31). The apical meristem, or growth tip, of a plant was modeled as a circular undulating shell on an elastic foundation subjected to several types of compressive stress systems owing to turgor and/or growth. The compressive stress systems included one in the tangent plane of the circular undulating shell and one pushing the circular undulating shell from below, on the plant tissue side of the growth tip. The existence of compressive stresses at the appropriate shifting active region between two circles on the undulating surface of the shell representing the meristem surface is demonstrated in Dumais & Steele (32) using meristem experiments and numerical calculations of the stresses in the shell (tissue). The results of the numerically calculated stresses in the shell (tissue) produced a buckling pattern characterized by the same pattern as the spiral phyllotaxis (Figure 7, see color insert). Figure 7 appeared on the July 1999 cover of the *American Journal of Botany*, the month before the article by Green (30) appeared. Half of this illustration is the spiral of the calculated buckling pattern (right) and the other half is the spiral phyllotaxis of a flower with the same pattern (left). The viewer of this illustration observes a great deal of similarity between the flower structure and the calculated buckling pattern. The buckling pattern of a circular undulating shell on an elastic foundation is not the only model for the pattern displayed by the spiral phyllotaxis; there are a number of other models, including reaction-diffusion models.

The proponents of buckling mechanisms suggest that these mechanisms are favored over Turing's morphogen approach for a number of reasons. First, mechanical instabilities can directly create physical structures in one step, in contrast to the two or more steps required with morphogens if positional information first had to be specified by morphogen gradients and then implemented in physical form. Second, physical forces act at much longer ranges (and more quickly) than diffusing chemicals. A difficulty with the morphogen approach is the identification of morphogens and the fact that quite different morphogen systems can produce the same pattern. Some argue that the mechanical activities of cells can accomplish the morphogenetic functions usually attributed to the diffusion and reactions of chemical morphogens. Systems of cells may also accomplish this by exerting traction forces by which they can propel themselves and rearrange extracellular materials, in particular the fibrous protein collagen. Because the compression and alignment created by these cellular forces can, in turn, affect cell behavior, several kinds of positive feedback cycles arise, and these cycles are capable of spontaneously generating regular geometric patterns of cells and matrix.

## Illustrative Cartoons of Epigenetic Mechanisms of Tissue Morphogenesis

The biological mechanisms described above are illustrated in this subsection by Figures 8 and 9 (see color inserts). These figures are described and discussed here; the material in this subsection is adapted from the figure captions of the illustrations in their source (8).

Figure 8 illustrates generic processes that occur in tissue morphogenesis. Figure 8*A* is a schematic representation of the behavior of intermixed cells and corresponding tissue fragments in the case where the two cell populations are differentially adhesive. The cell mixture segregates its more adhesive cells by establishing more stable bonds with one another than with cells of the less-adhesive population; this is consistent with the differential adhesive hypothesis discussed above. Random motion leads to the formation of cohesive islands of these cells, which will ultimately coalesce into a separate tissue phase, or compartment. This process is illustrated with chicken embryo cells in culture in Figure 6. The equilibrium configuration of the cell mixture is identical to that formed by fusion and spreading of fragments of tissue consisting of the same differentially adhesive cell populations. Figure 8*B* is a step-by-step illustration of the formation of a lumen or internal cavity by differential adhesion in an epithelioid tissue consisting of polarized cells. In the original state (top), the cells are uniformly adhesive and make contacts around their entire peripheries. Upon expression of an antiadhesive protein (green) in a polarized fashion in a random subpopulation of cells (center), and during random movement of the cells throughout the mass, bonds between adhesive surfaces are energetically favored over those between adhesive and nonadhesive surfaces, resulting in lumen formation (bottom). This step-by-step illustration is in the form of the graphic representation of a cellular automata calculation (see Continuum Models for Heart and Joint Growth, Remodeling, and Morphogenesis). Figure 8*C* is a schematic cross-sectional view of the five main types of gastrulation, which is an embryonic developmental process in which a gastrula is formed from a blastula. The blastula is a hollow sphere formed by cells, and gastrulation folds a portion of the spherical surface into the center of the sphere. In each case illustrated in the figure, a new population of cells differentiates from a solid or hollow embryo and assumes a position that would be attained by a similarly situated differentially adhesive population. Figure 8*D* is a schematic representation of two modes of tissue segmentation that can arise when the tissue's cells contain a biochemical circuit that generates a chemical oscillation or molecular clock, and the oscillating species directly or indirectly regulates the strength or specificity of cell adhesivity. In the mechanism shown on the left, the periodic change in cell adhesivity occurs in a growth zone in which the cell cycle has a different period from the regulatory oscillator; as a result, bands of tissue are sequentially generated with alternating cohesive properties. In the mechanism shown on the right, one or more of the biochemical species can diffuse, leading to a set of standing waves of concentration of the regulatory molecule by a reaction-diffusion mechanism. This leads to the simultaneous formation of bands of tissue with alternating cohesive properties.

Figure 9 illustrates the epigenetic mechanisms of tissue morphogenesis and organogenesis. Figure 9*A* is a schematic representation of major modes of epithelial morphogenesis resulting from extrinsic alteration of cell parameters. In (*a*), a pattern formation mechanism (e.g., a reaction-diffusion system) is activated in a flat epithelial sheet (green), possibly mediated by a subjacent mesenchymal layer (brown), and marks a subset of cells to undergo alteration of one or more "potential functions" (e.g., adhesive strength, cytoskeletal tension). In (*b*)–(*e*), resulting epithelial morphologies are indicated. A placode (*b*), a region of thickened ectoderm in the embryo from which a nerve ganglion or a sense organ will develop, will form if the lateral regions of the epithelial cells become more adhesive than the apical and basal regions. An evagination (*b*), such as a developing intestinal villus, or an invagination (*d*), such as a developing hair or feather, will form if the change in cell potential gives rise to a locally concentrated couple that destabilizes the flat configuration. Progressive cycles of patterning and invagination will give rise to a branched tubular structure (*e*), such as salivary gland morphogenesis. Figure 9*B* is a schematic representation of mesenchymal condensation, as occurs during skeletal morphogenesis and many other developmental processes. Such condensations can be initiated by local patches of elevated production of ECM molecules and consolidated by cell-cell adhesion. Figure 9*C* is an illustration of the morphogenesis of connective tissue elements, such as cartilage rods and nodules. This morphogenesis occurs through the regulation of the pattern of mesenchymal condensation formation. An example of this regulation of the pattern is the diffusion model of limb development shown in Figure 5 to predict the development of the chick limb bud shown in Figure 4. One way that this can occur is by the interplay of a positively autoregulatory diffusible activator of ECM production, such as transforming growth factor-beta (TGF-beta) (red arrows), with a diffusible inhibitor of its activity (violet arrows). In the absence of the inhibitor (top), resulting cartilage forms as an amorphous mass; in its presence, the patterns of well-spaced nodules and rods may form as centers of activation and become surrounded by domains of inhibition. Figure 9*D* is an illustration of the origin of the fibular crest in a subclass (including crocodiles, alligators, and dinosaurs) of reptilian hindlimbs by mechanical regulation of mesenchymal morphogenesis. Progressive evolutionary reduction of the fibula increases the mechanical load on the connective tissue between the tibia (yellow) and the fibula (brown), exerted by the pulling action of the iliofibularis muscle (red). A stress-dependent cartilage (gray-blue) forms in response and becomes later incorporated into the ossifying tibia to form a prominent crest (stippled), a homologue shared by theropod dinosaurs and carinate birds. This tight fixation of the proximal fibula permits its further distal reduction in avian limbs.

## SUPRAMOLECULAR ASSEMBLY

The question of how a tissue evolves from its primordial template to a mature, functioning tissue has not been fully answered. Exactly what is both known and conjectured about the mechanisms used to form one tissue, the tendon, from collagen molecules in vivo is described in Silver et al. (33). It is clear from the fact that animals generally mature in repeatable fashion that a tendon must grow in length so as to maintain its connection to both bone and muscle during the maturation process. It must also grow in cross-sectional area so that it can transmit increasingly greater forces between muscle and bone during the maturation process. The production of the collagen molecule by the cell is now well understood, and the structure of the collagen molecule has been deduced. The structural hierarchy of the collagen fibrils and the tendon is also well understood. An excellent summary of both in vivo and in vitro supramolecular assembly of the tendon is recorded in Silver et al. (33).

## MODELING CONSIDERATIONS

Models to describe tissue growth and remodeling may be classified as phenomenological or mechanistic. The phenomenological models attempt to simulate cause and effect (e.g., changed mechanical loading leading to changed tissue architecture) without a consideration of the intermediary mechanical and biological mechanisms involved. Phenomenological models allow for conveniently testing the consequences of different hypotheses of tissue growth and adaptation. This approach is often useful for eliminating some assumptions that do not match experimental or clinical results and observations (e.g., only compressive static loading leads to a particular tissue formation) or stimulate further investigations (e.g., strain rates and spatial gradients may regulate adaptation). The theory of adaptive elasticity for bone, reviewed and critiqued below in Continuum Models for Bone Remodeling, is a phenomenological model. The basic concepts underlying phenomenological models for soft tissue growth and adaptation are described below in Continuum Models for Soft Tissue Growth and Remodeling.

Mechanistic models, on the other hand, start instead with parameters (e.g., cell activities and microenvironment) that are linked to portions of the biological processes involved in tissue maintenance, turnover, and repair. These models, currently less developed than some of the phenomenological models because they are more complex, may lead to successfully linking mechanical and biological causes and effects. These models offer the promise of not only extending the descriptive and predictive capabilities of phenomenological models, but may offer insights into manipulation of the tissue response and development of pharmacological therapeutic agents. A mechanistic model for bone adaptation is described by Cowin (34). A mechanistic model that relates the effect of mechanical load applied to a whole bone, to the bone fluid flow around the cells buried in the bone, and, most significantly, to the bone adaptation process has been presented in a series of papers over the past decade by Cowin, Weinbaum, and associates (35–44). Mechanistic bone models are not reviewed here; instead, these models are reviewed by Cowin in References 34 and 45.

In the creation of phenomenological mathematical models for tissue growth and remodeling, the modeler must select a parameter to represent the effect of the mechanical loading on the development and remodeling of the tissue. In a mechanistic model, such a parameter would arise from biophysical considerations. Do biological tissues sense stress, strain, strain rate, or some other parameter of the mechanical loading? This is equivalent to asking if a tissue has baroreceptors (stress receptors), stretch receptors (strain receptors), or another type of receptor. One answer to the question is that tissues sense strain, stretch, strain rate, or stretch rate but not stress (46). The reason that tissues sense strain or strain rate and not stress is that strain is a primary, directly measurable, physical quantity, whereas stress is not. Stress is an abstract concept, a creation of man that can be measured only indirectly. Baroreceptors are described as "a spray-type nerve ending lying in the walls of arteries that are stimulated when stretched" (compare, e.g., 47). Clearly, baroreceptors sense stretch. From this perspective, the terminology baroreceptor is a misnomer; they are stretch receptors.

Strain is excluded as a possible growth stimulus for soft tissue (48) because of the difficulty in defining a reference configuration for its measurement in a growing material. The question is one of gauge length. If the gauge length is changing owing to the addition of new tissue, how can one measure strain? Several studies have considered this question of the appropriate stimulus (49, 50) and some have developed models in which the growth of soft tissue is dependent upon applied stress (48, 51–54). The substantial and important structure of these studies is independent of the fact that it is assumed that the growth of soft tissue is dependent upon applied stress; the alternative structure necessary to convert the stimulus from applied stress to loading rate of deformation or loading strain is easily constructed. The exact stimulus for growth is presently unknown (in bone there is strong evidence to suggest that it is strain rate). However, the argument sometimes presented is that strain requires a reference configuration and stress does not. There is a concern that the reference configuration for strain will change in time owing to tissue growth and remodeling. If this is a problem, can it be addressed in another way?

First, is the changing reference configuration really the problem? It is possible that the gauge length used for the sensing of strain does not change as the tissue grows, as noted by Cowin (55). For example, the cell may sense the strain and not change its length on the remodeling timescale t. Numerous cell culture studies have shown that the key connective tissue building cells begin to respond to strains above approximately 0.5%, with various signals that indicate the cells are aware that they are being excited. Generally, cells in tissues at different stages of growth are the same size. Some cells do not change their length on the timescale t as the tissue grows; cells can, however, stiffen or relax their cytoskeleton on a timescale that is greater than the loading timescale $\tau$ and less than the remodeling timescale t. The tissue either adds or subtracts cells or ECM to achieve the volume change; in most tissues the (sensor) cell size is unchanged. One cell does not likely determine the response of a tissue; it is more likely that the response of the tissue is determined by averaging the response of numerous cells by intercellular communication. Thus, one possibility is that the gauge length used for the sensing of strain does not change as the tissue grows. However, this observation does not entirely solve the problem because it leaves open the question of how to construct a model with such an invariant microstructural gauge length.

Second, if changing gauge length is a problem, can it be addressed in another way? Appropriate measures of the rate of deformation or strain on which the growth stretch may depend may be constructed if the two timescales in living tissue mechanics are recognized. These timescales differ by many orders of magnitude (55). Let $T_r$ denote the time that biological processes take to complete significant growth (or remodeling) associated with a mechanical loading, and let $T_L$ denote the characteristic period of mechanical loading. Rough estimates of $T_r$ and $T_L$ are two weeks and one second, respectively; thus, $T_L/T_r$ is a small number, of the order $10^{-6}$. To keep these timescales separate, let $\tau$ denote time on the loading timescale and t denote time on the remodeling timescale. Measures of tissue strain may be constructed using two facts: tissue is strained on the timescale $\tau$ and the gauge length changes on the timescale t, which is a million times longer.

The loading rate of deformation of an object is an instantaneous kinematic measure independent of reference configuration or gauge length, and thus does not have the disadvantage that might exclude strain as a growth stimulus. The rate

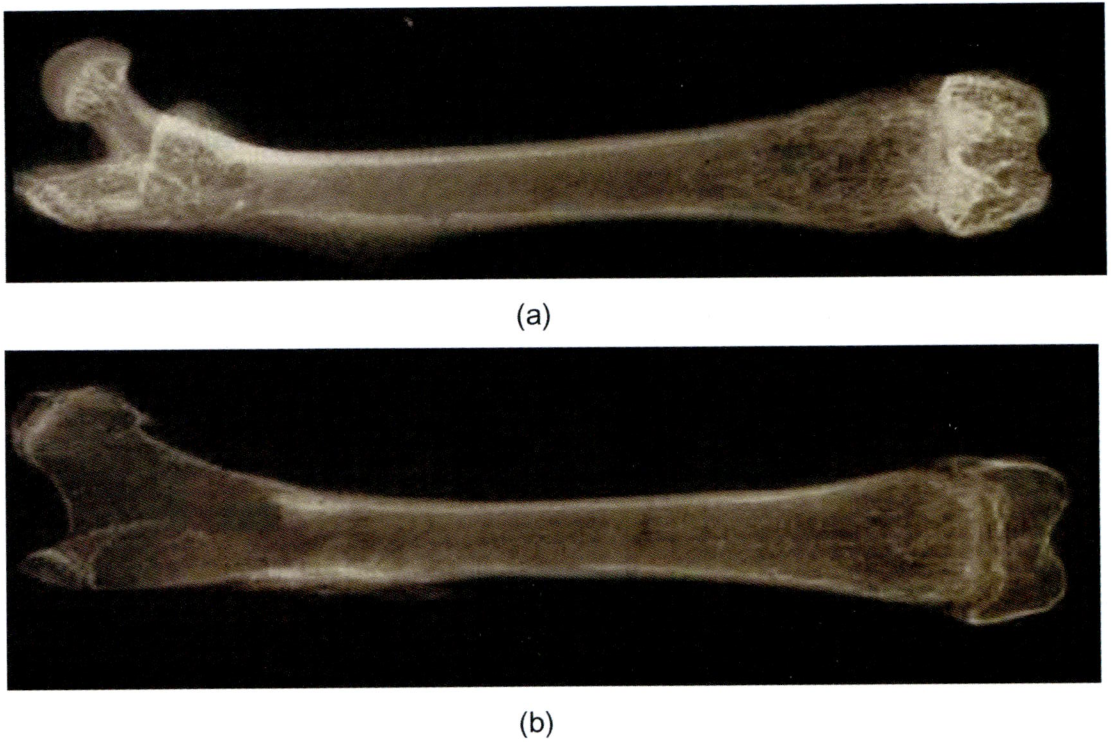


**Figure 1** Two mouse femora illustrate the effects of genetics and the effects of normal mechanical loading and genetics. (*a*) Normal morphology of a mouse femur developed within a normal functional loading environment. (*b*) Morphology of a mouse femur deprived of its normal mechanical loading. This femur was produced by transplanting the primordial template to the spleen and allowing it to develop there. The experiment thus provides insight into the nature of the primordial template for the mouse femur. From Chalmers & Ray (9).

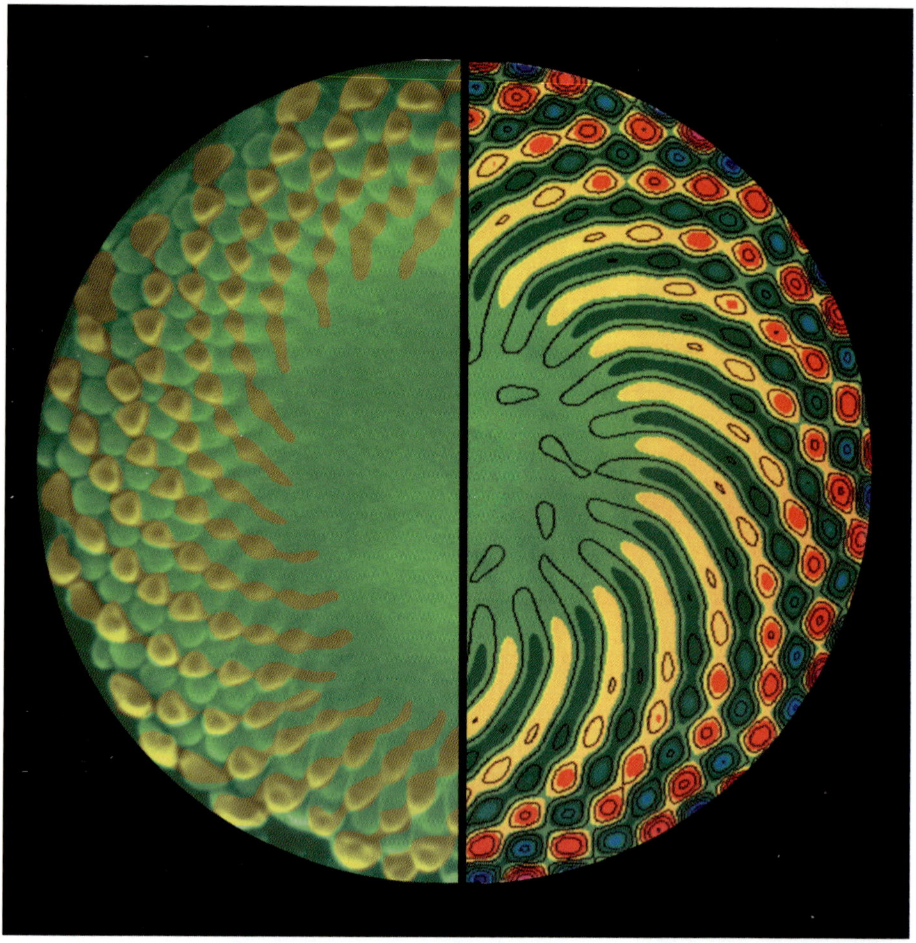

**Figure 7** Scanning electron micrograph of a young sunflower capitulum (*left*) and simulation of the same structure based on mechanical buckling of a thin circular plate (*right*). One family of spirals is highlighted in yellow. This illustration was composed by Jacques Dumais (Biological Sciences, Stanford) based on a micrograph he obtained and a computer buckling simulation of the sunflower capitulum using a thin circular plate model by Steven C. Rennich (Aeronautics and Astronautics, Stanford University). [A version of this figure appeared on the cover of the July 1999 issue of the *American Journal of Botany* (30)].

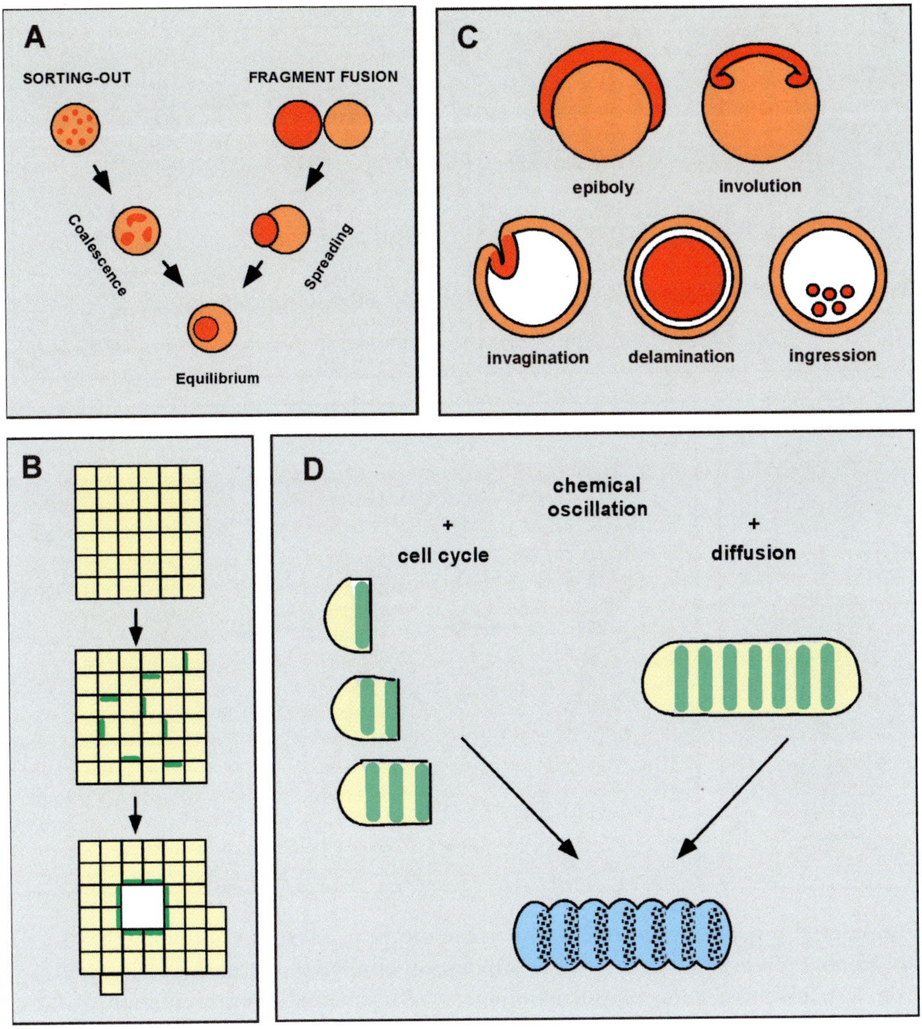


**Figure 8** Generic processes in tissue morphogenesis. (*A*) Schematic representation of the behavior of intermixed cells and corresponding tissue fragments where the two cell populations are differentially adhesive. (*B*) Schematic view of formation of a lumen or internal cavity by differential adhesion in an epithelioid tissue consisting of polarized cells. (*C*) Schematic cross-sectional views of the five main types of gastrulation. (*D*) Schematic representation of two modes of tissue segmentation. See the text for a more detailed description. From Newman & Müller (8).

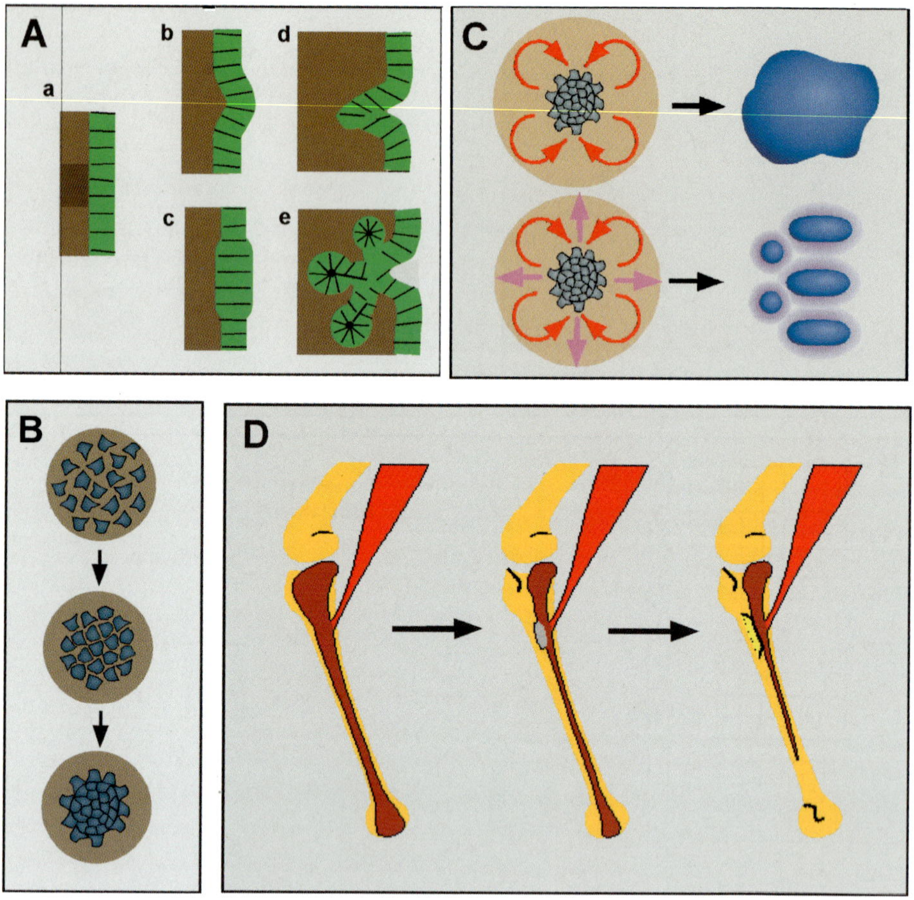


**Figure 9** Epigenetic mechanisms of tissue morphogenesis and organogenesis. (*A*) Schematic representation of major modes of epithelial morphogenesis resulting from extrinsic alteration of cell parameters. (*B*) Schematic representation of mesenchymal condensation. (*C*) Morphogenesis of connective tissue elements, such as cartilage rods and nodules. (*D*) Origin of the fibular crest in archosauran hindlimbs by mechanical regulation of mesenchymal morphogenesis. See the text for a more detailed description. From Newman & Müller (8).

of deformation is suggested as a remodeling stimulus for endothelial and bone cells in the sense that the shear stress owing to fluid motion over these epithelial cells is a stimulus for their activity and shear stress is proportional to the rate of deformation of a fluid. It is unknown how much of the rate of deformation is actually transferred to the epithelial cells. The cell layer is compliant and the undulations of the cell contour are observed in laminar shear flows in which the cells are attached to a supporting plate. Adaptive remodeling of the vasculature has been observed so as to maintain nearly constant endothelial fluid shear stress (rate of deformation to the cell) throughout the entire arterial side of the circulation (56). Cowin (55) presents explicit forms of appropriate or plausible measures of loading rate of deformation or loading strain of the growth stretch rate, see also Luo et al. (57). The recognition of the two timescales in the growth process, the loading timescale and the growth (or remodeling) timescale, which differ by many orders of magnitude, permit the consideration of strain and rate of deformation as growth stimuli in finite growth models of soft tissues.

## CONTINUUM KINEMATIC MODELS OF GROWTH

The growth and development of hard and soft tissues are kinematically different. The growth of hard tissues is appositional; that is, the growth is by deposition and resorption at a surface. The growth of soft tissues is interstitial volumetric growth. Thus, an increase in a hard tissue occurs by adding material onto an existing surface, whereas soft tissues grow by adding material internally. The kinematics of growth of an organism was a primary interest of D'Arcy Thompson, and the subject is well illustrated in his famous book (5). The classical ideas of growth kinematics were recast in the mathematics of contemporary continuum mechanics in Skalak et al. (58). This included continuum kinematics models for volumetrically and surface-distributed growth by deposition or resorption; the growth of horns and spiral shells (a favorite of D'Arcy Thompson); allometric growth; and the initial idea for a kinematic model in which simultaneously occurring growth and deformation are considered as a sequence of two mappings, one representing stress-free growth and the other representing the deformations of the tissue owing to forces acting on the tissue. This last topic is discussed below in Continuum Models for Heart and Joint Growth, Remodeling, and Morphogenesis. However, the other topics on the modeling of the kinematics of growth of an organism are not reviewed here; instead, the reader is referred to the review of Skalak et al. (58), with its refinements (59, 60).

## CONTINUUM MODELS FOR BONE REMODELING

The first continuum model for bone adaptation to mechanical loading was the (phenomenological) theory of adaptive elasticity (61–63). The objective of these studies was to formulate a model for the understanding and prediction of the strain-controlled remodeling properties of normal living bone. The strain-adapting properties of living bone are represented by a strain-controlled chemical reaction that transfers mass, momentum, entropy, and energy to and from the porous elastic solid. The addition of mass to the porous solid modifies its porosity. Bone adaptation to environmental strain is a collective phrase for the continual processes of growth, reinforcement, and resorption that occur in living bone. The resulting theory describes an elastic material that adapts its structure to applied loading, hence the term adaptive elasticity. There were major successes in the 1976 theory of adaptive elasticity; however, there are things that should be done differently if the theory is to be renovated. The largest success was the development of a thermodynamic open-system model of tissue adaptation. This model has been followed, or assumed as a starting point, by most subsequent models of tissue adaptation [a survey of these models appears in Hart (64)]. The model assumed that the load-adapting properties of living bone can be modeled by a chemically reacting porous medium in which the rate of reaction is strain controlled. The porous medium has two components: a porous elastic solid representing the matrix structure of bone, including the bone cells, and a perfusant bath that represents the extracellular fluid and the blood plasma, which flow through the matrix structure. A schematic diagram of this model is shown in Figure 10. The reality that living bone is always within its host organism is modeled by placing the porous structure representing bone in a bath of the perfusant representing body fluids. The perfusant bath is assumed to be an isothermal heat reservoir, an assumption that appears to be easily justified by common knowledge concerning living organisms. The mechanical load is applied directly to the porous structure across the walls of the perfusant bath as illustrated in Figure 10. The system consisting of the porous structure and its perfusant bath is considered to be closed

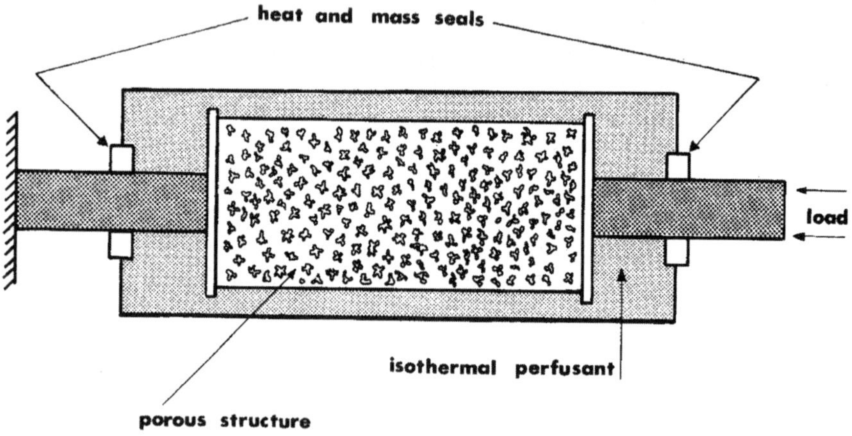


**Figure 10** A schematic diagram of the conceptual model for bone adaptation to mechanical loading. From Cowin (61).

with respect to mass, heat energy, and entropy transfer, but open with respect to momentum transfer from loading. The system consisting of only the porous structure without its entrained perfusant is open with respect to momentum transfer as well as mass, energy, and entropy transfer. The bone matrix is considered to be the control system because the mechanical properties of the bone matrix alone determine the mechanical properties of the bone. Balance and constitutive equations were developed only for the bone matrix. The perfusant delivers the tissue-building constituents to the bone matrix but it does not contribute to the mechanical properties of the bone matrix. Thus, the perfusant plays a prominent role in the transfer of mass, momentum, energy, and entropy to the bone matrix. The rate at which mass, momentum, energy, and entropy transfer occurred was assumed to depend on the local strain and the other independent variables. One of the strongest assumptions made was the assumption that the internal energy of the mass added to the porous tissue was equal to the internal energy of the porous tissue at the site where the mass is added. In retrospect, this assumption is easily justified by recalling how bone tissue is deposited and if the bone adaptation is viewed on two timescales as discussed in Some Modeling Considerations, above. New bone deposition begins with a deposit of osteoid onto an existing bone surface. The osteoid is of much lower modulus than the existing bone. Over a time period of a month, the osteoid becomes mineralized and its modulus increases approximately linearly with the mineralization. Because the mechanical loading timescale is much shorter than the adaptation timescale, the osteoid/bone undergoes many million cycles of mechanical loading in the course of the adaptation tissue deposition time period. It follows that the internal energy can be gradually increased with the mineralization in the tissue deposition time period so that, when viewed from the long-term adaptation timescale, it will be equivalent to having the new mass deposited at the same internal energy as the existing mass in the porous bone structure. Other features common to most of the later models [these models are described by Hart (64)] of internal adaptation include the formulation of the theory in terms of a constitutive relation for the mass supply term introduced by the open system formulation of the mass balance equation; the porosity of the medium could be increased or decreased. The increased or decreased porosity is then assumed to influence the elastic constants through their constitutive dependence on porosity.

Reformulating the theory of adaptive elasticity requires a few changes. A major change is the introduction of the two timescales discussed in Modeling Considerations, above. The reformulated theory of adaptive elasticity should allow the mass supply and the free energy to depend on the remodeling time and the history of deformation; thus, functions of deformation gradients in the original theory should be replaced by functionals of the history of reference solid volume fraction and deformation gradients. Such strain history–dependent relationships are familiar from nonlinear viscoelasticity. The reformulated theory would then consist of the usual equations for an elastic object and equations that change on the long timescale, slowly adding or subtracting mass and free energy and, thereby, changing the elastic constants. The theory of adaptive elasticity's stimulus for remodeling requires perhaps the most revision. The model points to time-averaged strain and strain-energy as the first measures of stimulus. The experimental literature suggests, however, that it must be a stimulus that involves the rate of strain or the rate of loading. A moderate periodic strain applied to living bone is more effective in causing remodeling than a static strain of the same magnitude. A constant load applied with fixed springs to isolated living bone caused the bone to resorb as if there were no load placed on it (65). The living bone showed no effect from the constant, non-time varying loading. Further evidence that the effective stimulus was strain rate is provided in O'Connor et al. (66) and Rubin & Lanyon (67). The mechanistic models (see Modeling Considerations, above) that relate the effect of mechanical load–driven bone fluid flow around the cells buried in bone to the bone adaptation process strongly suggest strain rate as a strong mechanical stimulus (34, 36).

Cowin (68) recently reviewed and critiques the theory of adaptive elasticity. Hart (64) recently reviewed this model and other phenomenological models for cortical and cancellous bone adaptation.

# CONTINUUM MODELS FOR SOFT TISSUE GROWTH AND REMODELING

## The Separability Hypothesis

The final section of the Skalak et al. paper on the analytical description of growth (59), discussed above in Continuum Kinematic Models of Growth, describes a kinematic model in which simultaneously occurring growth and deformation are considered as a sequence of two mappings, one representing stress-free growth and the other representing the deformations of the tissue owing to forces acting on the tissue. This may be the first statement of the separability hypothesis: simultaneously occurring growth and deformation may be decomposed into a growth deformation and an elastic deformation associated with the instantaneous loading. The validity of this hypothesis is easy to imagine in a thought experiment involving a whole bone without residual stress. By measuring the size of the bone in a fixed, unstressed, situation periodically over a significant growth period, the measurement represents the growth of the bone. The hypothesis is not valid if there is an inelastic deformation of the bone, as there would be in an Ilizarov lengthening procedure.

The hypothesis was extended (48) to a general three-dimensional theory of mechanically modulated volumetric growth for soft incompressible biological tissues. Rodriguez et al. (48) rendered the mapping composition idea described in Skalak et al. (58) as a composition of deformation gradient mappings. The overall growth deformation is represented by a mapping, denoted by $\mathbf{F}_{eg}$, of the initial configuration of the object $B(t_0)$ into the instantaneous configuration $B'(t_1)$. The decomposition of the mapping suggested by Rodriguez et al. (48) is represented by

$$\mathbf{F}_{eg} = \mathbf{F}_e\mathbf{G}, \tag{1}$$

where **G** is a symmetric tensor representing the growth deformation gradient and $\mathbf{F}_e$ represents an elastic deformation necessary to maintain overall compatibility of the mapping $\mathbf{F}_{eg}$. The representation (Equation 1) follows from the fact that any deformation gradient can be decomposed into a product of deformation gradients as long as there is a definition of one of the decomposition elements that provides a method to calculate the other decomposition element. That is the case because of our ability to measure growth (69). The symmetry of **G** follows from the fact that any deformation gradient may be decomposed into the product of an orthogonal tensor representing the rigid object rotation and a symmetric positive tensor representing the shape-changing deformation. When growth is measured, any effect of rigid object rotation is easily removed; hence, **G** is necessarily symmetric as pointed out by Skalak et al. (58). The mapping decomposition (Equation 1) is illustrated in Figure 11. Note that there is no mechanical loading applied to any of the objects in Figure 11, but it is possible for the final configuration $B'(t_1)$ to have residual stresses owing to incompatibilities induced by growth. It is interesting to compare Figure 11 with the two photos of mouse femora shown in Figure 1. It is reasonable to associate the normal morphology of a mouse femur developed within a normal functional loading environment (Figure 1*a*) with the final configuration $B'(t_1)$

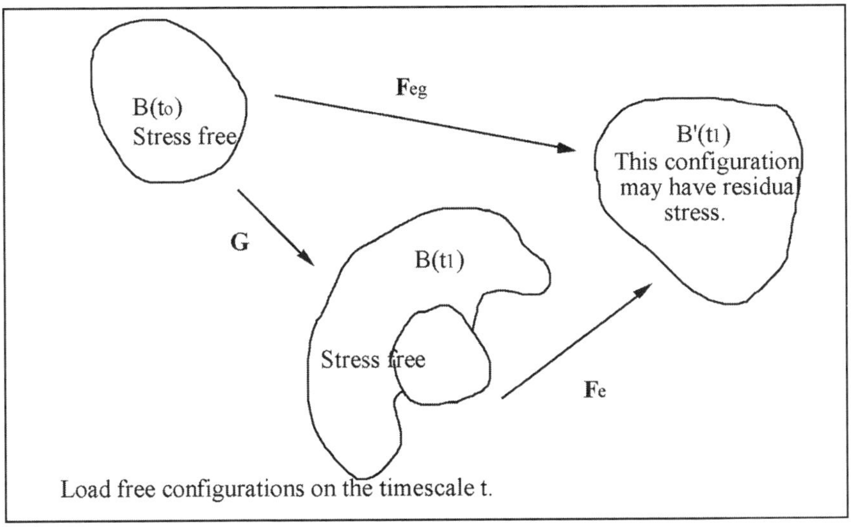


**Figure 11** An illustration of the relationship between the various (unloaded) configurations considered and the deformation gradients that represent mappings between these configurations. This diagram is conceptually identical with figure 1 of Rodriguez et al. (48). Adapted from Cowin (55).

in Figure 11, and the mouse femur deprived of its normal mechanical loading (Figure 1*b*) with the configuration $B(t_l)$ in Figure 11, the configuration resulting from growth without loading.

This decomposition (Equation 1) is analogous to the decomposition of the deformation gradient, which has been used in plasticity theory to separate finite elastic and plastic deformations since the 1960s (70–73), and in the literature on polymeric swelling to separate elastic and swelling deformations since the 1940s (M. Boyce, private communication, 2003). Each biological situation in which the assumption (Equation 1) might be applied must be carefully scrutinized to evaluate the justification of the separation of the growth and deformation effects. The separability hypothesis is an example of the reductionism problem discussed above in Genetic Information and the Development of a Biological Tissue. When the growth tensor **G** is known because the growth is well mapped, there should be no difficulty; for example, the development and loading of the mouse femur suggested by the photos in Figure 1. However, if there is any morphological development event occurring that cannot be represented by the growth tensor **G**, the decomposition (Equation 1) is not possible. This restriction is due to the definition of growth; if we were able to describe morphological events mathematically, the growth tensor could be replaced by a growth and morphogenesis tensor and the predictive capacity of the model would increase.

Models of tissue growth in the cardiovascular system employing these ideas have been described by Taber and coworkers (52–54) and Rodriguez et al. (75, 76).

## The Loading Timescale and the Growth Timescale

The recognition of two timescales in the growth process, the loading timescale and the growth (or remodeling) timescale, which differ by many orders of magnitude, permits the consideration of strain and rate of deformation as growth stimuli in finite growth models of soft tissues, as noted above in Modeling Considerations. Explicit forms of appropriate or plausible measures of loading rate of deformation or loading strain on which the growth stretch rate may depend may be constructed using the two timescales, the loading timescale $\tau$ and the remodeling timescale t. An extension of the representation in Figure 11 to include these two timescales and two loaded configurations is shown in Figure 12; Figure 11 is repeated in the box outlined with dotted lines in Figure 12. The growth tensor **G** is now a function of t, thus $\mathbf{G} = \mathbf{G}(t)$. The deformation gradient associated with the loaded configuration from the unloaded, but not necessarily stress-free, configuration is denoted by $\mathbf{F}_L(\tau, t)$. The tissue is mechanically strained on the loading timescale $\tau$, and therefore the deformation gradient of loading $\mathbf{F}_L$ is considered to be dependent on both timescales. If the residual elastic deformation $\mathbf{F}_e$ is significant and thought to be a growth stimulus, then rather than employing the loading deformation $\mathbf{F}_L$ as the basis for the independent constitutive variable in the growth stimulus, the basis could be provided by the composition $\mathbf{F}_{eL}$, $\mathbf{F}_{eL} = \mathbf{F}_e\mathbf{F}_L$, of the residual elastic deformation $\mathbf{F}_e$ and the loading deformation $\mathbf{F}_L$. This would make the growth

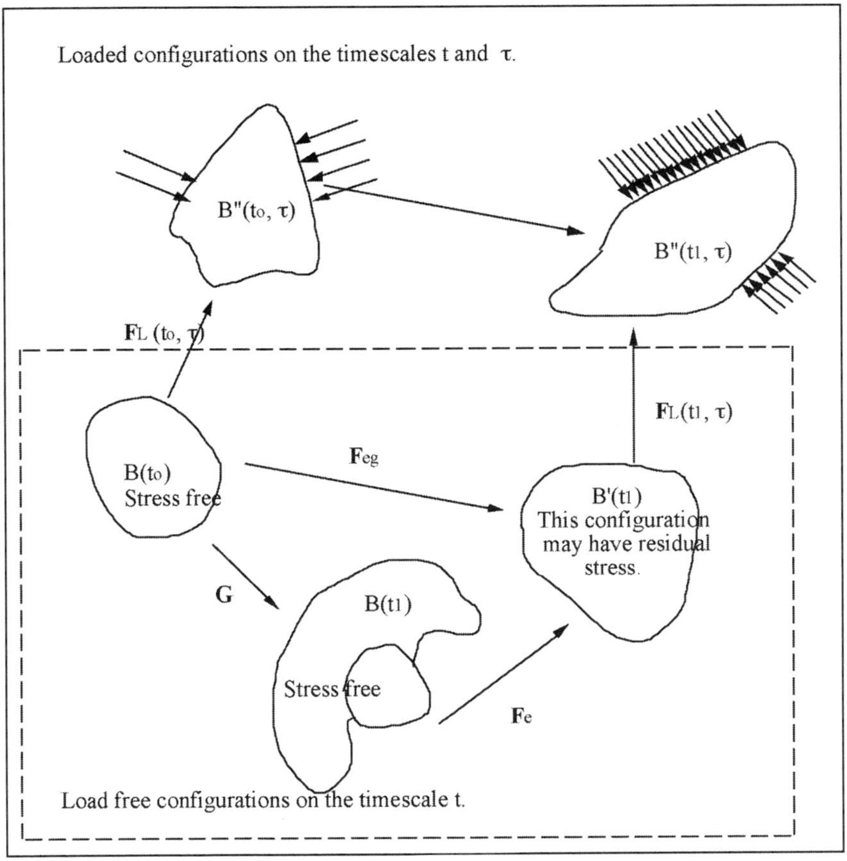


**Figure 12** An illustration of the relationship between the various configurations considered. There are two broad classes of configurations, loaded and unloaded. The unloaded configurations are within the portion of the diagram outlined with the dotted lines. This portion of the diagram is identical with Figure 11 above. The loaded configurations are above and outside of the dotted lines. The deformation gradient associated with the deformation to the loaded configuration from the unloaded (but not necessarily stress-free) configuration is denoted by $F_L(\tau, t)$. It is shown at times $t_0$ and $t_1$. Adapted from Cowin (55).

stimulus dependent on the loading and the residual strain:

$$\mathbf{F} = \mathbf{F}_{eg}\mathbf{F}_{\mathrm{L}} = \mathbf{F}_e(\tau, \mathrm{t}) \cdot \mathbf{G}(\mathrm{t}) \cdot \mathbf{F}_{\mathrm{L}}(\tau, \mathrm{t}). \tag{2}$$

## Residual Stresses

The presence of residual stress in biological tissues has been widely reported in the past two decades. Residual stresses in the arteries were demonstrated by performing experiments on unloaded arterial rings dissected from blood vessels (77–80). Two transverse cuts of an artery yield an unloaded arterial ring. If that arterial ring is cut so that it is no longer an approximately circular ring, but instead a sector of a circular ring, the unloaded sector of the arterial ring opens and displays an opening angle, indicating that when it was a complete ring it had internal stresses. If one keeps cutting the sector of the circular ring into smaller pieces, each cut produces a new opening angle, indicating the presence of internal stresses in each progressively smaller piece. The presence of residual stress has been established in a number of other tissues, including veins (81), ventricular myocardium (82, 83), and the trachea (84). The residual stress in biological organs is thought to be a consequence of nonuniform growth, resorption, and remodeling (58, 85, 86). Residual stresses in the heart and arteries are thought to minimize the peak stresses experienced by these tissues in vivo (79, 87, 88), and thus improve their mechanical function. The inclusion of the residual stress in the stress constitutive equations used to describe these soft tissues has been the focus of Hoger and coworkers (89–91).

### General Continuum Models of Growth

A general constitutive theory of the stress-modulated growth of soft tissues was developed by Lubarda & Hoger (92). The work provides an explicit representation of **G** for various material symmetries, and an incremental formulation for stress-modulated growth process. A theory of material growth (mass creation and resorption) is presented in Epstein & Maugin (93). In this study, growth is viewed as a local rearrangement of material inhomogeneities. The question of growth in continuum growth models is examined from a rigorous mathematical approach in DiCarlo & Quiligotti (73).

## CONTINUUM MODELS FOR HEART AND JOINT GROWTH, REMODELING, AND MORPHOGENESIS

Modeling the development of an organ or an organism is an objective that is presently experiencing a pioneering exploration. Such models will necessarily involve the processes of growth, remodeling, and morphogenesis. Two examples are briefly described here: the modeling of the embryonic chicken heart (49, 94–96) and a model for articular joint morphogenesis (97, 98).

The heart is the first functioning organ in the embryo, and it continues to function without interruption, although its morphology changes dramatically during development. Development consists of a coordinated, dynamic interaction between genetic and environmental factors that regulate the primary developmental processes of volume change (growth), tissue property change (remodeling), and shape change (morphogenesis). Taber & Perucchio (94) give a mathematical model for the embryonic heart development in the chicken as it transforms from a single tube into a four-chambered pump.

Heegaard and coworkers (97, 98) described a mathematical model for joint morphogenesis that contained the hypothesis that the stress distribution created in a functional joint will modulate the growth of the primordial template and lead to the development of congruent articular surfaces. In a computational model, the morphogenesis of a human finger joint (proximal interphalangeal joint) was simulated for the period between days 55 and 70 of fetal life. The biological growth rate was assumed to be proportional to the chondrocyte density in the growing tissue. Cyclic hydrostatic stress caused by joint motion was assumed to modulate the baseline biological growth, with compression slowing it and tension accelerating it. The model prediction was that the articular surfaces became more congruent, and the primordial template exhibited an asymmetric sagittal profile similar to that observed in adult phalangeal bones.

## CELLULAR AUTOMATA TYPE IMMISCIBLE FLUID MODELS FOR CELL SORTING

The models considered thus far in this review are calculus-based continuum models. In a large and extensively illustrated book, Wolfram (99) argues that the computational capabilities now available permit investigators to change their methods of calculation from calculus-based to computational algorithm–based. Thus, equations are replaced by the simple step-by-step procedures of computer programs. In these algorithms, time and space are no longer considered as continuous, but as digital steps. The continuum is replaced by a grid or lattice. The algorithms for the accomplishment of this objective are called cellular automata.

On first encounter with cellular automata, they appear similar to a chess or checker board because they involve arrays of squares (see Figure 8*B*). The rules for any system, including chess or checkers, "can be viewed as corresponding to a program, so its behavior can be viewed as corresponding to a computation" (99, p. 165).

Recall from Epigenetic Mechanisms Associated with the Interactions of Cell Metabolism with the Physiochemical Environment, above, that immiscible fluids are of interest in the mechanical modeling of biological tissue development because cell sorting is analogous to the separation of phases in the immiscible fluids. Lattice models of immiscible fluids are effective calculational tools. Recall also the differential adhesion hypothesis described in Epigenetic Mechanisms Associated with the Interactions of Cell Metabolism with the Physiochemical Environment, above, the hypothesis that combinations of different cell types behave as immiscible liquids (for example, oil and water) because of surface tension, but with the cell-to-cell adhesion forces playing the role of molecule-molecule attraction forces. In immiscible liquids, a liquid with a higher surface tension will form droplets enclosed by another liquid with lower surface tension. In combinations of different cell types, cells with higher surface tension will band more tightly together, forcing the cells with a lower surface tension to the outside, also known

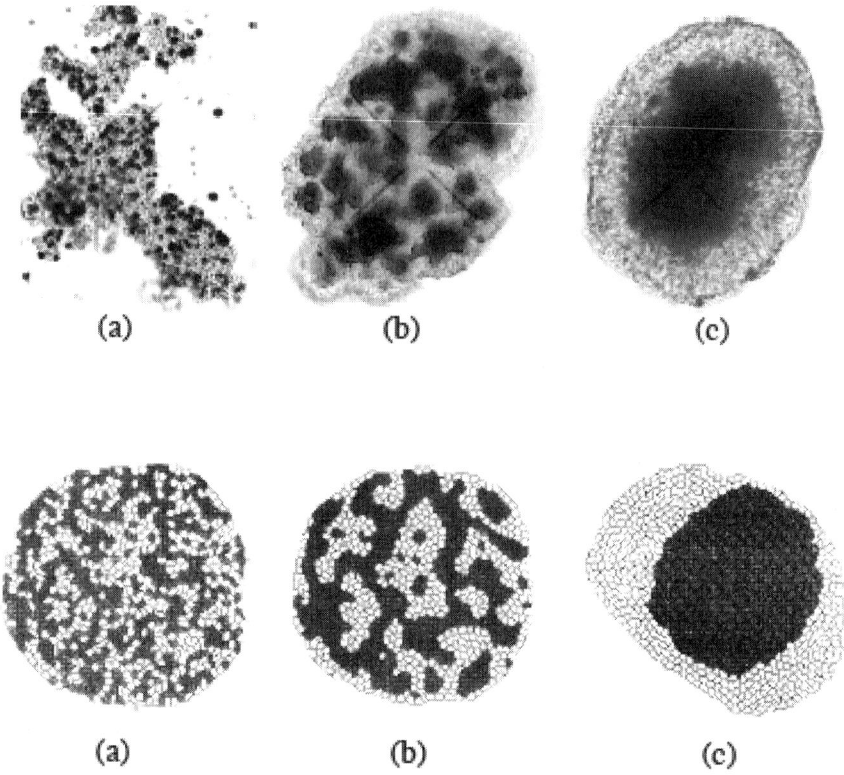


**Figure 13** The top panel repeats Figure 6 and represents experimental images from chicken embryo cells in culture: Light cells are neural retinal cells and dark cells are pigmented retinal cells. An initial random mixture of (*a*) light and dark cells forms (*b*) dark clusters after approximately 10 h, and eventually sorts to produce (*c*) a dark cell core surrounded by light cells after approximately 72 h. The bottom panels show the corresponding images from a simulation with three cell types: light cells, dark cells, and medium. From Alber et al. (23).

as the differential adhesion hypothesis. This sorting was illustrated in Figures 6 and 8*A*; Figure 6 is repeated as the top set of three panels in Figure 13. These three panels show the experimental images from chicken embryo cells in culture. The light cells are neural retinal cells and dark cells are pigmented retinal cells. The initial situation, shown in the first of the three panels, is a random mixture of light and dark cells. The second panel shows the dark clusters formed in 10 h, and the third panel shows the dark cell core surrounded by a light cell shell at 72 h. The bottom set of three panels in Figure 13 shows the corresponding images from an immiscible lattice gas simulation with three cell types: light cells, dark cells, and medium (22, 23).

There appears to be a great deal of potential for modeling the mechanics of biological tissue development using cellular automata.

## ACKNOWLEDGMENTS

A number of people were consulted and helpful in the preparation of this work. They include Anne Hoger at UCSD, Jacques Dumais in Biology at Stanford, Allen Goodship of the Royal Veterinary College and Institute of Orthopaedics in London, Karl Jepsen and Steven Tommasini in Orthopedics at the Mount Sinai School of Medicine in New York, and Stuart Newman in Cell Biology and Anatomy at the New York Medical College at Valhalla. The Whitaker Foundation, the NIH, the NSF, and the PSC-CUNY Research Award Program of the City University of New York supported this work.



## LITERATURE CITED

1. Gilbert SF. 2000. *Developmental Biology*. Sunderland, MA: Sinaur. 6th ed.
2. Young LR. 1993. Guest editorial: space and the vestibular system: what has been learned? *J.Vestib. Res.* 3:203–6
3. White RJ. 1998. Weightlessness and the human body. *Sci. Am.* 279(3):58–63
4. Roux W. 1885. The problems, methods, and scope of developmental mechanics. Introduction to *Archiv für Entwickelungsmechanik der Organismen*. Transl. WM Wheeler, 1895, in *Wood's Hole Biol. Lect.* pp. 149–90
5. D'Arcy Thompson W. 1942. *On Growth and Form*. Cambridge, UK: Cambridge Univ. Press
6. Harris AK. 1994. Multicellular mechanics in the creation of anatomical structures. In *Biomechanics of Active Movement and Division of Cells*, ed. N. Akkas, pp. 87–129. Berlin/Heidelberg: Springer Verlag
7. Bard J. 1990. *Morphogenesis*. Dev. Cell Biol. Ser. Vol. 23. Cambridge, UK: Cambridge Univ. Press
8. Newman SA, Müller GB. 2000. Epigenetic mechanisms of character origination. *J. Exp. Zool. (Mol. Dev. Evol.)* 288:304–17
9. Chalmers J, Ray RD. 1962. The growth of transplanted foetal bones in different immunological environments. *J. Bone Joint Surg.* 44B:149–64
10. Goodship AE, Cunningham JL. 2001. Pathophysiology of functional adaptation of bone in remodeling and repair *in vivo*. See Ref. 100, pp. 26-1–26-31
11. Jepsen KJ, Akkus O, Majeska RJ, Nadeau JH. 2003. Hierarchical relationship between bone traits and mechanical properties in inbred mice. *Mamm. Genome* 14: 97–114
12. Tommasini SM, Morgan TG, van der Meulen MCH, Jepsen KJ. 2003. Genetic variation in vertebral mechanical properties determined by the relationship between morphological and compositional bone traits. *Trans. Orthop. Res. Soc.* 28: 112
13. Turing AM. 1952. The chemical basis of morphogenesis. *Philos. Trans. R. Soc. Lond. B* 23:37–72
14. Murray JD. 1993. *Mathematical Biology*. New York: Springer Verlag

15. Newman SA, Frisch HL. 1979. Dynamics of skeletal pattern formation in developing chick limb. *Science* 205:662–68
16. Oster GF, Murray JD, Harris AK. 1983. Mechanical aspects of mesenchymal morphogenesis. *J. Embryol. Exp. Morph.* 78: 83–125
17. Harris AK, Wild P, Stopak D. 1980. Silicone rubber substrata: a new wrinkle in the study of cell locomotion. *Science* 208:177–79
18. Wolpert L, Beddington R, Brockes J, Jessel T, Lawrence P, Meyerowitz E. 1998. *Principles of Development.* Oxford, UK: Oxford Univ. Press
19. Keller EF. 2002. *Making Sense of Life.* Cambridge, MA: Harvard Univ. Press
20. Steinberg M. 1962. Mechanism of tissue reconstruction by dissociated cells. II. Time-course of events. *Science* 137:762–63
21. Steinberg M. 1964. *Cell Membranes in Development.* San Diego, CA: Acad. Press
22. Mombach J, Glazier JA, Raphael R, Zajac M. 1995. Quantitative comparison between differential adhesion models and cell sorting in the presence and absence of fluctuations. *Phys. Rev. Lett.* 75:2244–47
23. Alber MS, Kiskowski MA, Glazier JA, Jiang Y. 2002. On cellular automaton approaches to modeling biological cells. In *Mathematical Systems Theory in Biology, Communication, and Finance*, ed. J Rosenthal, DS Gilliam, *IMA*, 142:1–40. New York: Springer-Verlag
24. Beysens DA, Forgacs G, Glazier JA. 2000. Cell sorting is analogous to phase ordering in fluids. *Proc. Natl. Acad. Sci. USA* 97:137–45
25. Harris AK. 1976. Is cell sorting caused by differences on the work of intracellular adhesion? A critique of the Steinberg hypothesis. *J. Theor. Biol.* 61:267–85
26. Wolff J. 1892. *Das Gesetz der Transformation der Knochen.* Berlin: Hirschwald
27. Wolff J. 1986. *The Law of Bone Remodelling.* Berlin: Springer
28. Cowin SC. 2001. The false premise in Wolff's law. See Ref. 100, pp. 30-1–15
29. Roux W. 1885. Beiträge zur Morphologie der funktionellen Anpassung. *Arch. Anat. Physiol. Anat. Abt.* 1:120–85
30. Green PB. 1999. Expression of pattern in plants: combining molecular and calculus-based biophysical paradigms. *Am. J. Bot.* 86:1059–76
31. Green PB, Steele CR, Rennich SC. 1996. Phyllotactic patterns: a biophysical mechanism for their origin. *Ann. Bot.* 77:515–27
32. Dumais J, Steele CR. 2000. New evidence for the role of mechanical forces in the shoot apical meristem. *J. Plant Growth Regul.* 19:7–18
33. Silver FH, Freeman JW, Seehra GP. 2003. Collagen self-assembly and the development of tendon mechanical properties. *J. Biomech.* 36:1529–54
34. Cowin SC, Moss ML. 2000. Mechanosensory mechanisms in bone. In *Textbook of Tissue Engineering*, ed. R Lanza, R Langer, W Chick, pp. 723–38. San Diego, CA: Academic
35. Cowin SC, Moss-Salentijn L, Moss ML. 1991. Candidates for the mechanosensory system in bone. *J. Biomech. Eng.* 113:191–97
36. Weinbaum S, Cowin SC, Zeng Y. 1994. A model for the excitation of osteocytes by mechanical loading-induced bone fluid shear stresses. *J. Biomech.* 27:339–60
37. Cowin SC, Weinbaum S, Zeng Y. 1995. A case for bone canaliculi as the anatomical site of strain generated potentials. *J. Biomech.* 28:1281–96
38. Zhang D, Cowin SC, Weinbaum S. 1998. Electrical signal transmission in a bone cell network: the influence of a discrete gap junction. *Ann. Biomed. Eng.* 26:644–59
39. Cowin SC. 1999. Bone poroelasticity. *J. Biomech.* 32:218–38
40. Wang L, Fritton SP, Cowin SC, Weinbaum

S. 1999. Fluid pressure relaxation mechanisms in osteonal bone specimens: modeling of an oscillatory bending experiment. *J. Biomech.* 32:663–72
41. Wang L, Cowin SC, Weinbaum S, Fritton SP. 2000. Modeling tracer transport in an osteon under cyclic loading. *Ann. Biomed. Eng.* 28:1200–9
42. You L, Cowin SC, Schaffler M, Weinbaum S. 2001. A model for strain amplification in the actin cytoskeleton of osteocytes due to fluid drag on pericellular matrix. *J. Biomech.* 34:1375–86
43. Smit TH, Huyghe JM, Cowin SC. 2002. A double poroelastic model of cortical bone: estimation of the linear isotropic parameters. *J. Biomech.* 35:829–36
44. Wang L, Fritton SP, Weinbaum S, Cowin SC. 2003. On bone adaptation due to venous stasis. *J. Biomech.* 36:1439–51
45. Cowin SC. 2002. Mechanosensation and fluid transport in living bone. *JMNI* 2: 256–60
46. Cowin SC. 1984. Modeling of the stress adaptation process in bone. *Calcif. Tissue Int.* 36:S99–104
47. Guyton AC. 1976. *Medical Physiology.* Philadelphia, PA: WB Saunders
48. Rodriguez EK, Hoger A, McCulloch AD. 1994. Stress-dependent finite growth in soft elastic tissues. *J. Biomech.* 27:455–68
49. Tabor LA. 1995. Biomechanics of growth, remodeling and morphogenesis. *Appl. Mech. Rev.* 48:487–545
50. Omens JH. 1998. Stress and strain as regulators of myocardial growth. *Prog. Biophys. Mol. Biol.* 69:559–72
51. Taber LA, Keller BB, Clard EB. 1992. Cardiac mechanics in the stage-16 chick embryo. *J. Biomech. Eng.* 114:427–34
52. Lin IE, Taber LA. 1995. A model for stress-induced growth in the developing heart. *J. Biomech. Eng.* 117:343–49
53. Taber LA, Eggers DW. 1996. Theoretical study of stress-modulated growth in the aorta. *J. Theor. Biol.* 180:343–57
54. Taber L. 1998. A model for aortic growth based on fluid shear and fiber stresses. *J. Biomech. Eng.* 120:348–54
55. Cowin SC. 1996. Strain or deformation rate-dependent finite growth in soft tissues. *J. Biomech.* 29:647–49
56. Kamiya A, Bukhari R, Togawa T. 1984. Adaptive regulation of wall shear stress optimizing vascular tree function. *Bull. Math. Biol.* 46:127–73
57. Luo GM, Cowin SC, Sadegh AM, Arramon Y. 1995. Implementation of strain rate as a bone remodeling stimulus. *J. Biomech. Eng.* 117:329–38
58. Skalak R, Dasgupta G, Moss M, Otten E, Dullemeijer P, Vilmann H. 1982. Analytical description of growth. *J. Theor. Biol.* 94:555–77
59. Skalak R, Netti P, Jain R, Zargarian S, Hoger A. 1996. Compatibility and the genesis of residual stress by volumetric growth. *J. Math. Biol.* 34:889–914
60. Skalak R, Farrow DA, Hoger A. 1997. Kinematics of surface growth. *J. Math. Biol.* 35:869–907
61. Cowin SC, Hegedus DM. 1976. Bone remodeling I: a theory of adaptive elasticity. *J. Elast.* 6:313–25
62. Hegedus DM, Cowin SC. 1976. Bone remodeling II: small strain adaptive elasticity. *J. Elast.* 6:337–52
63. Cowin SC, Nachlinger RR. 1978. Bone remodeling III: uniqueness and stability in adaptive elasticity theory. *J. Elast.* 8:285–95
64. Hart RL. 2001. Bone modeling and remodeling: theories and computation. See Ref. 100, pp. 31-1–42
65. Lanyon LE, Rubin CT. 1984. Static vs dynamic loads as an influence on bone remodelling. *J. Biomech.* 17:897–905
66. O'Connor JA, Lanyon LE, MacFie H. 1982. The influence of strain rate on adaptive bone remodeling. *J. Biomech.* 15:767–81
67. Rubin CT, Lanyon LE. 1984. Regulation of bone formation by applied dynamic loads. *J. Bone Joint Surg.* 66A:397–402

68. Cowin SC. 2003. Adaptive elasticity: a review and critique of a bone tissue adaptation model. *Eng. Trans.* 51:1–79
69. Bookstein FL. 1978. The measurement of biological shape and shape change. In *Lecture Notes in Biomathematics*, vol. 24. New York: Springer. 189 pp.
70. Kröner E. 1960. Allgemeine Kontinuumstheorie der Versetzungen und Eigenspannugen. *Arch. Ration. Mech. Anal.* 4:273–334
71. Lee EH. 1969. Elastic-plastic deformation at finite strains. *J. Appl. Mech.* 36:1–8
72. Casey J, Naghdi PM. 1981. A remark on the use of the decomposition $\mathbf{F} = \mathbf{F}_e\mathbf{F}_p$ in plasticity. *J. Appl. Mech.* 47:672–75
73. DiCarlo A, Quiligotti S. 2002. Growth and balance. *Mech. Res. Commun.* 29:449–56
74. Deleted in proof
75. Rodríguez J, Goicolea J, García JC, Gabaldón F. 2003. Finite element models for mechanical simulation of coronary arteries. Prepr. E.T.S.I. Caminos, Canales y Puertos, Dep. Mec. Medios Continuos, Univ. Politéc. Madrid
76. Rodríguez JS. 2003. *Modelos numéricos para mecanica cardiovascular de las paredes arteriales y sus procesos de adaptacíon.* PhD thesis. Univ. Politéc. Madrid, Esc. Téc. Super. Ing. Caminos, Canales y Puertos
77. Viashnav RN, Vossoughi J. 1983. Estimation of residual strains in aortic segments. In *Recent Developments in Biomedical Engineering*, ed. CW Hall, pp. 330–33. New York: Pergamon Press
78. Viashnav RN, Vossoughi J. 1987. Residual stress and strain in aortic segments. *J. Biomech.* 20:235–39
79. Choung CJ, Fung YC. 1986. Residual stress in arteries. In *Frontiers in Biomechanics*, ed. GW Schmid-Schoenbein, SL Woo, BW Zweifach, pp. 117–29. New York: Springer-Verlag
80. Liu SQ, Fung YC. 1988. Zero-stress states of arteries. *J. Biomech. Eng.* 110:82–84
81. Xie JP, Liu SQ, Yang RF, Fung YC. 1991. The zero-stress state of rat veins and vena cava. *J. Biomech. Eng.* 113:36–41
82. Omens JH, Fung YC. 1990. Residual strain in rat left ventricle. *Circ. Res.* 66: 37–45
83. Rodriguez EK, Omens JH, Waldman LK, McCulloch AD. 1993. Effect of residual stress on transmural sarcomere length distribution in rat left ventricle. *Am. J. Physiol. Heart Circ. Physiol.* 264:H1048–56
84. Han HC, Fung YC. 1991. Residual strains in porcine and canine tracheas. *J. Biomech.* 24:307–15
85. Fung YC. 1990. *Biomechanics: Motion, Flow, Stress, and Growth.* New York: Springer-Verlag
86. Skalak R. 1981. Growth as a finite displacement field. In *Proc. IUTAM Symp. on Finite Elasticity*, ed. DE Carlson, RT Shield, pp. 348–55. Hague/Boston/London: Martinus Nijhoff
87. Fung YC, Liu SQ. 1989. Relationship between hypertension, hypertrophy, and opening angle of zero-stress state of arteries following aortic constriction. *J. Biomech. Eng.* 111:325–35
88. Liu SQ, Fung YC. 1989. Change of residual strains in arteries due to hypertrophy caused by aortic constriction. *Circ. Res.* 65:1340–49
89. Hoger A. 1997. Virtual configurations and constitutive equations for residually stressed bodies with material symmetry. *J. Elast.* 48:125–44
90. Johnson BE, Hoger A. 1998. The use of strain energy to quantify the effect of residual stress on mechanical behavior. *Math. Mech. Solids* 4:447–70
91. Chen YC, Hoger A. 2000. Constitutive function of elastic materials in finite growth and deformation. *J. Elast.* 59:175–93
92. Lubarda VA, Hoger A. 2002. On the mechanics of solids with a growing mass. *Int. J. Solids Struct.* 39:4627–64
93. Epstein E, Maugin GA. 2000. Thermomechanics of volumetric growth in uniform bodies. *Int. J. Plast.* 16:951–78

94. Taber LA, Perucchio R. 2001. Modeling heart development. *J. Elast.* 61:165–97
95. Taber LA. 1998. Mechanical aspects of heart development. *Prog. Biophys. Mol. Biol.* 69:225–54
96. Taber LA. 1998. Biomechanical growth laws for muscle tissue. *J. Theor. Biol.* 193: 201–13
97. Heegaard JE. 1999. Dynamics of joint morphogenesis. In *IUTAM Syposium on Synthesis in Bio-Solid Mechanics*, ed. P Petersen, MP Bendsøe, pp. 103–14. Dordrecht: Kluwer
98. Heegaard JH, Beaupre GS, Carter DR. 1999. Mechanically modulated cartilage growth may regulate joint surface morphogenesis. *J. Orthop. Res.* 17:509–17
99. Wolfram S. 2002. *A New Kind of Science*. Champaign, IL: Wolfram Media
100. Cowin SC. 2001. *Bone Mechanics Handbook*. Boca Raton, FL: CRC Press

Annu. Rev. Biomed. Eng. 2004. 6:109–30
doi: 10.1146/annurev.bioeng.6.040803.140032

First published online as a Review in Advance on February 26, 2004

# BREAST TISSUE ENGINEERING

Charles W. Patrick, Jr.
*Laboratory of Reparative Biology & Bioengineering, Department of Plastic Surgery, The University of Texas M.D. Anderson Cancer Center and The University of Texas Center for Biomedical Engineering, Houston, Texas 77030;*
*email: cpatrick@mdanderson.org*

**Key Words** adipogenesis, adipose tissue engineering, biomaterial, breast reconstruction, fat tissue

■ **Abstract** Tissue engineering has the potential to redefine rehabilitation for the breast cancer patient by providing a translatable strategy that restores the postmastectomy breast mound while concomitantly obviating limitations realized with contemporary reconstructive surgery procedures. The engineering design goal is to provide a sufficient volume of viable fat tissue based on a patient's own cells such that deficits in breast volume can be abrogated. To be sure, adipose tissue engineering is in its infancy, but tremendous strides have been made. Numerous studies attest to the feasibility of adipose tissue engineering. The field is now poised to challenge barriers to clinical translation that are germane to most tissue engineering applications, namely scale-up, large animal model development, and vascularization. The innovative and rapid progress of adipose engineering to date, as well as opportunities for its future growth, is presented.

CONTENTS

# INTRODUCTION

Tissue engineering has emerged over the past 15 years as a multidisciplinary field focused on the development of bioengineered, living tissue constructs. To date, prototypes of numerous tissues and organs have emerged on the biomedical landscape, and some have even translated to the clinical bedside, yet only recently has attention been focused on the engineering of adipose tissue to restore soft tissue defects. The clinical impetus to develop rational and translatable adipose tissue engineering strategies is enormous. Table 1 highlights soft tissue defects in the dermis and underlying subcutaneous tissue that result from resections of various tumors of the head and neck, breast, and bone, as well as trauma, congenital abnormalities, changes associated with aging, and a myriad of other medical conditions. These defects and resulting contour deformities can impair the aesthetic

**TABLE 1** Indications for a tissue engineered adipose strategy (updated from 24)

| Category | Application | Specifics | Incidence or Number of Procedures/Year |
|---|---|---|---|
| Reconstructive | Oncologic resection | Mastectomies | 81,729 breast reconstructions |
| | | Parotidectomies | |
| | Complex trauma | Soft tissue deficits | |
| | Congenital abnormalities | Hemifacial microsomia | 1 in 4000 to 1 in 5600 |
| | | Poland's syndrome | 1 in 20,000 to 1 in 32,000 |
| | | Romberg's syndrome | |
| | Other | | 44,147 reconstructions |
| Cosmetic | Augmentation | Breast | 219,883 breast augmentations (augmentation mammoplasty) |
| | | | 55,176 breast lifts (mastoplexy) |
| | | Cheek, chin, jaw | 8494 cheek implants (malar augmentation) |
| | | | 28,736 chin augmentations (mentoplasty) |
| | | Lips | |
| | | Buttocks | 1339 buttock lifts |
| | Rejuvenation | Wrinkles | 2495 fibril injections |
| | | | 796,526 collagen injections |
| | | | 855,846 botox injections |
| | Nonspecific revision/resculpting | Various locations | 72,632 fat injections |
| Correctional | Implant removal | Breast | 62,861 removals |
| | Bulking agent | Stress urinary incontinence | 1,500,000 |
| | | Vesicoureteral reflex | |
| | | Intrinsic sphincter deficiency | |
| | | Vocal cord insufficiency | |
| | Orthotic-related | Atrophied "cushion" in ball/heel of aged foot | |
| | Augmentation | Soft tissue deficits | |

appearance, function, and psychological well-being of patients. This review focuses on one subset of clinical indications, namely breast reconstruction following tumor resection.

Breast cancer is the second leading type of cancer in women (after skin cancer), affecting one in every eight women in America and one in every three women with cancer (1). Owing to the large number of clinical occurrences, breast reconstruction following lumpectomy (partial removal of breast tissue) or radical mastectomy (total removal of the breast) has become the sixth most common reconstructive procedure performed in the United States (2). Lumpectomy defects less than 25% of the total breast volume can typically be corrected by rearranging the local breast tissue (3). Larger lumpectomies and mastectomies require more drastic reconstruction modalities. Studies show that many women who have had a mastectomy tend to suffer from a syndrome "marked by anxiety, insomnia, depressive attitudes, occasional ideas of suicide, and feelings of shame and worthlessness" (4). Reconstruction of the breast mound following a mastectomy has proven to alleviate the sense of mutilation and suffering that women experience postsurgery (5). As a result, breast reconstruction is offered as an option to any woman undergoing surgery for breast cancer. Breast reconstruction was performed on 74,090 patients in 2002, with 50% of patients having the procedure concomitant with a mastectomy. Furthermore, 236,888 breast augmentation procedures were performed in 2002, being the third most common surgical cosmetic procedure (2).

This review presents the state of the art of adipose tissue engineering applied to breast reconstruction, discusses limitations realized with current strategies, and rationally speculates on the future. Space limitations necessarily abrogate a detailed presentation of the molecular and cellular mechanisms that dictate adipogenesis and fat cell proliferation. The reader is referred to the wealth of literature available on these subjects, largely from the obesity and diabetes research disciplines (6–21). Moreover, the restricted focus on breast reconstruction obviates discussion of adipose tissue engineering for small volume defects, such as skin contour deformities caused by trauma and aging, and the reader is directed to References 22–25 for this subject.

## ENGINEERING CHALLENGE DEFINED

### Anatomy of the Breast

A brief discussion of breast anatomy is required to properly frame engineering design constraints, as well as to introduce necessary clinical terminology (22). The female breast is a specialized organ composed of glandular, ductal, connective, and adipose tissue (26) (Figure 1). Each breast contains 15–25 lobes of compound glands that are embedded in fibrous and adipose tissue (27). These lobes, each containing an excretory duct that drains into the lactiferous sinus, radiate from a central nipple-areolar complex. The breasts are typically the most prominent superficial structures of the anterior thoracic wall, overlying the pectoral muscles and extending from the clavicle superiorly to the sixth rib inferiorly, and from the

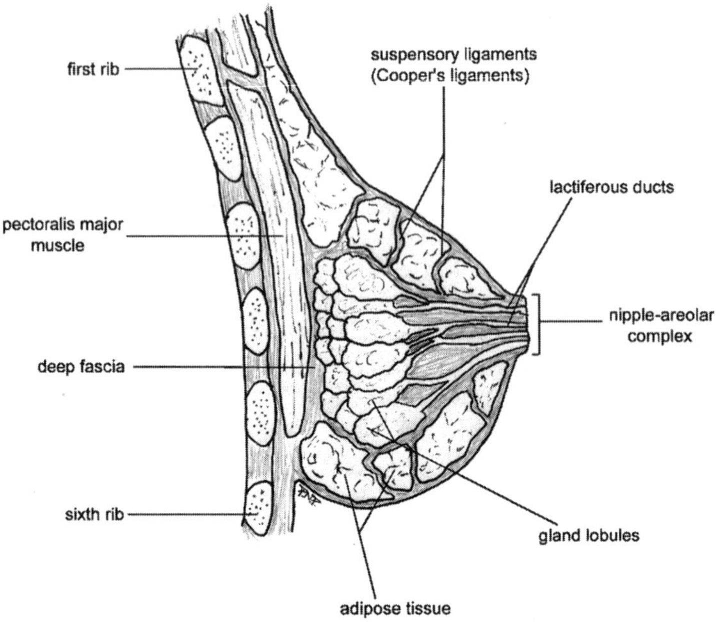


**Figure 1** Anatomy of the female breast (adapted from 25).

midsternal line medially to the axilla laterally, forming the axillary tail of Spence. The size and shape of a breast is determined by the bounding skin envelope and the adipose tissue surrounding the glandular structures. The presence of adipose tissue lobules interspersed between fibrous and glandular components of the breast help determine the bulk, softness, and contour of the breast mound. The deep aspect of the breast is separated from the underlying pectoralis major muscle by the deep fascia. Between the breast and this deep fascia is a thin layer of loose connective tissue (within the retromammary space) devoid of adipose tissue, which allows the breast to move freely over the deep fascia. The breast is firmly attached to the skin and underlying structures by fibrous bands referred to as suspensory ligaments (Cooper's ligaments), which provide additional support and also contribute to determining the shape and contour of the breast (28).

The minimal essential unit of adipose tissue is the fat lobule. Lobules are morphologically independent units of adipocytes consisting of $10^2$–$10^3$ cells (29). Each lobule is separated by fibrous septa and possesses terminal circulation. The size of a fat lobule is on the order of millimeters and the cytoplasm of each mature adipocyte is ~90% lipid. Adipose is highly vascular, even more than skeletal muscle when one corrects for the amount of active cytoplasm. In addition, adipose tissue is unlike the majority of adult tissues in that the tissue is constantly adapting or changing. Adipose tissue volume and vascular supply can decrease and increase over multiple length scales. Mature adipocytes can increase in size but

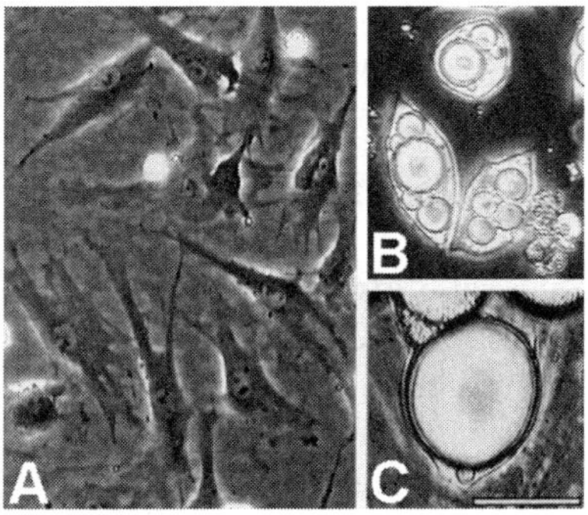


**Figure 2** Morphology of differentiating preadipocyte. (*A*) Preadipocyte in fibroblast-like morphology. (*B*) Preadipocyte that is lipid loading (phase bright intracellular inclusions). (*C*) Mature adipocyte exhibiting a signet ring structure. The cell is largely lipid surrounded by a thin border of active cytoplasm. The small circle at the bottom is the cell nucleus. Phase contrast microscopy. Bar denotes 50 $\mu$m.

not in cell number owing to terminal differentiation. However, the precursor to a mature adipocyte, the preadipocyte, can readily proliferate. As shown in Figure 2, preadipocytes differentiate from a fibroblast-like spindle morphology with small lipid inclusions; to a multilocular stage with numerous large inclusions; and finally to a state of a single, large lipid inclusion (mature adipocyte). The molecular and signaling events of preadipocyte differentiation are fairly well understood and the reader is invited to review the wealth of literature available in this area (6–21).

## Engineering Problem

Postmastectomy reconstruction involves replacing missing skin and soft tissue volume to recreate the appearance of the breast. Owing to the volume often involved and relative paucity of adequate fill, large breast tissue deficits can be particularly challenging to repair. The overall design goal is to restore the patient's breast mound while maintaining tactile sensation if possible. Breast function (i.e., lactation) is not currently an objective. The mass and organization of the breast must be addressed for individual patients because the size and shape of the breast varies from person to person. This is an important constraint as the majority of tissue engineering constructs can be fabricated as "one size fits all." Adipose constructs for breast reconstruction must be patient-specific. In addition, the designed construct cannot be a steady-state solution, rather, it must adapt with the patient. A breast naturally changes shape and size with age as the breast's architecture (e.g., skin elasticity and thickness, adipose tissue volume, ligaments) changes with time (28). As an engineering problem, designing a breast mound is ill posed. For example, Tebbetts lists at least 34 tissue and surgical factors affecting soft tissue dynamics and cosmesis subsequent to breast reconstruction using implants (30).

In the following sections, we explore the current and tissue engineering strategies for restoring the breast mound.

## ACELLULAR BREAST RESTORATION STRATEGIES

Prior to the development of tissue transfer techniques, women with breast cancer faced a choice between no breast restoration, wearing an external prosthesis, or the implantation of prosthetic devices. The latter choice is still widely used as a reconstructive option. There are two basic types of prosthetic devices available: fixed-volume breast implants and tissue expanders. Advantages of using an implant or expander are that these devices can be manufactured in a broad range of sizes, contours, profiles, and textures. Fixed-volume implants possess an outer layer or envelope of vulcanized silicone and are usually filled with a saline solution (3, 31). Implants filled with silicone gel are also available, but on a limited basis owing to the controls placed by the FDA in 1992 (32, 33). Controversy still exists as to the health problems in women with silicone breast implants (34). Recent studies demonstrate that siloxanes and platinum can bleed out from silicone implants, but a direct link of these contaminants has not yet been made to the observed health problems in women possessing silicone implants (35). Tissue expanders are implants in which the volume can be altered after implantation. An inflatable silicone tissue expander is placed submuscularly and is gradually inflated by the injection of physiological saline over a duration of weeks to months (3, 31). When expansion is complete, the tissue expander is removed and is replaced with a permanent breast saline- or silicone-filled implant to provide the volume necessary for breast mound restoration. Both implants and expanders are available with a smooth or textured silicone surface. Textured surfaces result in a lower incidence of capsular contracture following implantation than smooth surface implants (36). Textured surfaces also serve to stabilize the implant and facilitate tissue expansion. One drawback to a textured envelope, however, is that these implants possess a slightly thicker vulcanized silicone shell that may be more visible, exhibiting a rippled appearance through the skin, in some patients who possess a thin skin envelope (3, 31, 37). The thicker shell may also contribute to the implant folding and potentially deflating following insertion (3, 31).

The most common complication resulting from implants and expanders is capsular contracture (3, 31) (Figure 3). Inserting an implant into the body inevitably leads to the formation of a capsule of firm, fibrous scar tissue around the implant owing to a foreign body reaction (38–41). The implant capsule constricts over time, making the augmented breast feel harder and firmer than desired (3, 31, 33, 42). Capsular contracture often results in a spherical breast appearance (3, 31, 33), chronic chest wall discomfort, and restricted shoulder or arm movement (3, 31). Although capsule formation is normal after breast reconstruction with prosthetic devices, not all capsules result in severe contraction (43). Capsular contracture is graded on the Baker scale of I–IV (Table 2), where I denotes a breast that looks and feels soft and IV denotes a breast that feels firm, is beginning to become distorted in shape, and causes pain to the patient. Capsular contracture is related

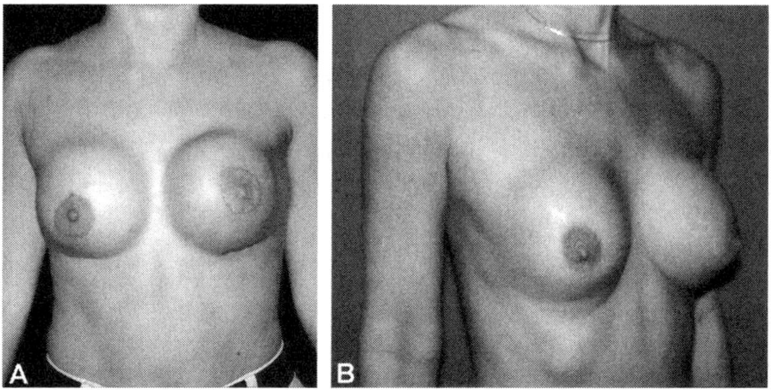

**Figure 3** Examples of capsular contracture around breast implants. (*A*) Patient possesses capsular contracture of both breasts, resulting in breast hardness, an unnatural spherical profile, and breast asymmetry. (*B*) Similarly, this patient possesses capsular contracture of her right breast. (Photographs are courtesy of Elisabeth Beahm, M.D., Department of Plastic Surgery, University of Texas M.D. Anderson Cancer Center.)

to implant duration, capsule thickness, patient age, and inflammation (44). The potential for calcium deposits accumulating in the capsule can also interfere with tumor detection (3, 31).

Implants are also subject to other local complications, such as rupture, possible silicone or saline leakage (3, 31), displacement, deformation (3, 31, 45), chronic seroma, implant exposure (3, 31), hematoma, and loss of nipple sensation (41). Breast augmentation using tissue expanders also results in more complications than using fixed-volume implants alone. Infection is most common with expanders owing to the bacteria that can be introduced from the serial saline injections (46, 47). Fill-valve problems and skin loss are also problems associated with using tissue expanders (31).

## CELLULAR BREAST RESTORATION STRATEGIES

There are three methods of breast reconstruction that do not rely on prosthetic devices. One method (autologous tissue transfer) is currently used clinically and the remaining two are adipose tissue engineering strategies under development.

**TABLE 2** The Baker classification for capsular contracture

| Grade | Criteria |
|---|---|
| I | Normally soft and natural appearing breast |
| II | Naturally appearing breast despite palpable firmness |
| III | Firm breast with visible distortion |
| IV | Breast with obvious spherical distortion |

Adipose tissue engineering strategies (Figure 4, see color insert) have not reached the stage in which there has been clinical translation, but numerous in vivo proof-of-principle studies have been conducted. In vivo studies are generally of two types: (*a*) those in which cultured or isolated preadipocytes are transferred to tissue sites or (*b*) those in which de novo fat formation is induced by altering the tissue microenvironment to recruit resident preadipocytes. Each cell-based method of reconstruction is discussed.

## Autologous Tissue

Breast reconstruction considers the aesthetic and anatomic properties of the breast mound to achieve optimal clinical results. Early on, autologous adipose tissue was investigated as a virtually limitless source of material for soft tissue repair (48). It is easily harvested, readily available, and most patients possess excessive amounts that can be harvested without producing significant contour defects. Despite the theoretical advantages, however, autologous adipose tissue alone has demonstrated poor results (49), with a 50%–70% reduction in graft volume owing to resorption (50–53). Moreover, mature adipocytes do not proliferate because they are terminally differentiated (54). Additional problems with autologous adipose tissue grafts include microdeposits of serum calcium from fat resorption that result in obscure mammographies and interfere with tumor detection (48, 55). As a result of these limitations, contemporary autologous tissue reconstruction commonly uses composite of tissue flaps, namely skin, fat, and muscle.

Breast reconstruction using the patient's own tissues, rather than implantable devices, tends to produce better results (3) with fewer complications (31). The use of autologous tissues tends to produce a breast mound that better recreates the shape, contour, softness, and fullness of the natural breast than the use of implants (3). There are a number of sites for donor tissue for breast reconstruction. The primary areas include the abdomen [transverse rectus abdominis musculocutaneous (TRAM) flap] (3, 31) and the back (latissimus dorsi musculocutaneous flap). The buttocks (inferior gluteus maximus musculocutaneous flap) and the hips (Rubens flap) are seldom used to reconstruct the breast mound. Tissue availability must be considered for each donor site based on the patient (31).

Abdominal flap reconstruction is the most common, yet technically demanding, procedure performed for breast reconstruction using autologous tissues (3). The TRAM flap conveniently provides abdominal wall skin, rectus abdominus muscle, and subcutaneous adipose tissue, along with the blood vessels that supply these tissues to reconstruct the breast. The tissue may be transferred with its blood supply intact by maintaining the superior attachment of the rectus abdominis muscle or by sacrificing the blood supply and performing microvascular anastomoses in the chest to the internal mammary blood vessels or in the axilla to the thoracodorsal blood vessels. The skin and fat can then be reshaped to take on the appearance of a breast. Breasts reconstructed using the TRAM flap uphold symmetry over time. Patients also view the accompanying abdominoplasty, or tummy tuck, as

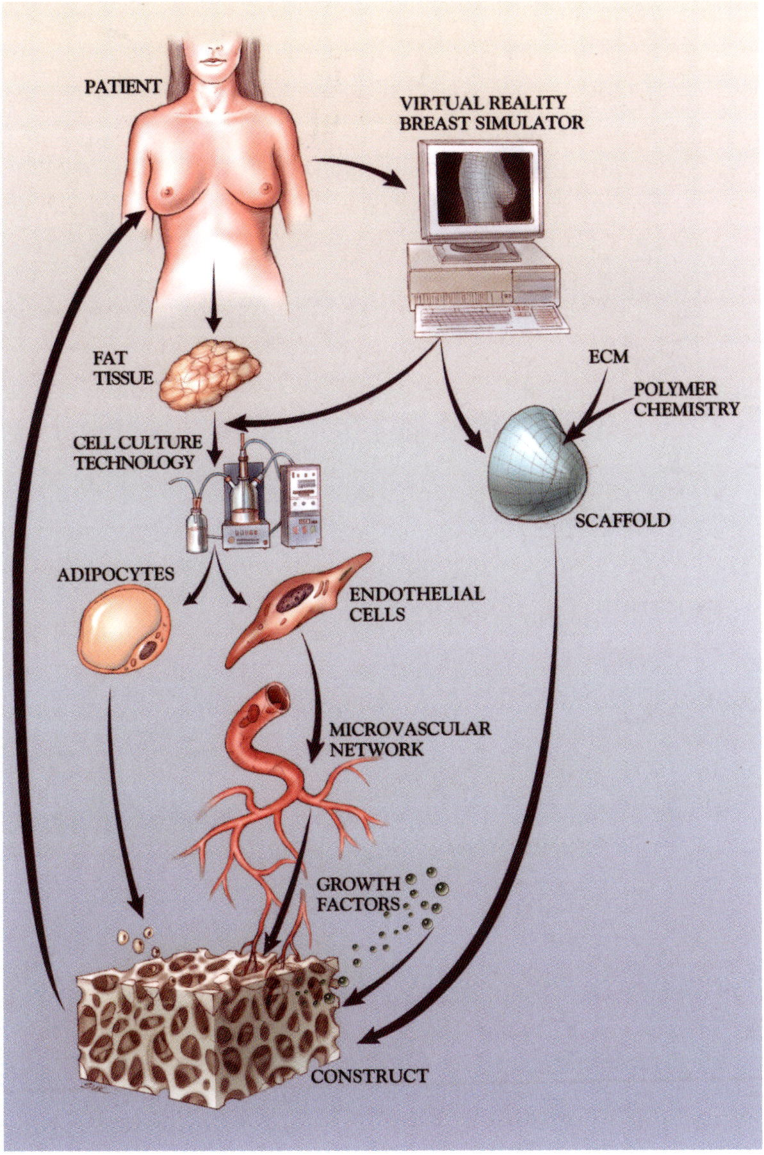


**Figure 4** A proposed strategy for breast tissue engineering is illustrated. Adipose tissue is obtained from the patient via liposuction or fat biopsy. From the tissue sample, preadipocytes and capillary endothelial cells are isolated and cultured using cell culture technologies. The capillary endothelial cells are finessed to form microvascular networks. The preadipocytes and microvascular network are later placed, along with appropriate angiogenic and adipogenic growth factors, within a biodegradable polymer scaffold. The patient-specific scaffold shape, volume, and the number of cells required are obtained from a virtual breast simulator using patient imaging data. (Image from 23.)

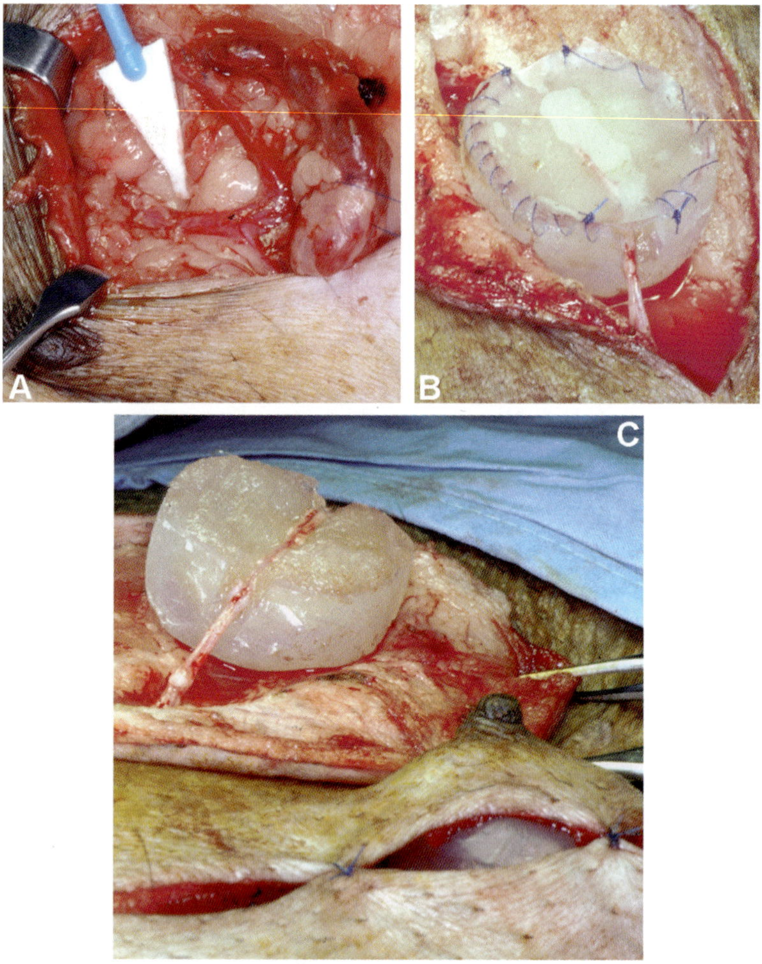


**Figure 7** Porcine animal model development. (*A*) Isolation of mammary vessel using microsurgical technique. (*B*) The vessel is placed within the tissue engineering construct to promote vascularization. The interior of the construct contains a polymer scaffold and a permissive environment for preadipocyte migration, proliferation, and differentiation into mature adipose tissue. (*C*) In lower right corner, the construct has been rotated and placed in the chest wall to create a "breast" mound on the pig. In the top, left corner, the construct is shown without its top so as to visualize the vessel placement. Vessel flow is checked with a pencil Doppler prior to closing.

an added benefit to having reconstruction using the TRAM flap. A disadvantage to having this surgery performed is that additional procedures to reconstruct the nipple-areola and to refine the breast mound are required. Additionally, owing to the complexity of the TRAM flap procedure, complications such as prolonged pain, abdominal weakness, an extended period of recovery, and occasional areas of necrosis accompany the surgery (31). Finally, contour abnormalities of the abdomen may result after TRAM flap reconstruction, including upper and lower abdominal bulge, upper fullness, and hernia (56–58). The latissimus dorsi muscle is a large triangular muscle that extends over the lower half of the thorax and lumbar region. Although the procedure involving the latissimus dorsi flap is less involved than the TRAM flap procedure, the long-term results of the latissimus dorsi flap procedure are inferior. The muscle tends to atrophy over time and there is typically a volume discrepancy in the back from the donor site (31). The desire to perform natural tissue reconstructions without the trauma of surgery or complications at the donor site realized with contemporary procedures provides the impetus for finding a tissue-engineered soft tissue alternative that may be used in postmastectomy breast reconstructions.

## Bioengineering In Situ Adipogenesis

Acellular tissue engineering constructs that elicit recruitment of surrounding resident preadipocytes are being investigated for de novo adipose tissue growth. For example, the reconstituted basement membrane of a mouse tumor, or Matrigel, has been shown by several investigators to induce migration, proliferation, and differentiation of preadipocytes when supplemented with fibroblast growth factor-2 (FGF-2) (59–62). It is speculated that when Matrigel plus FGF-2 is injected into a subcutaneous space, preadipocytes residing in the adjacent connective tissue migrate into the extracellular matrix gel. Results demonstrate that endothelial cells are also recruited (59, 60). It remains unclear whether the observed angiogenesis drives the adipogenesis or vice versa. When gelatin microspheres loaded with FGF-2 are coimplanted with Matrigel, similar results are obtained (61, 62). Matrigel, which consists largely of collagen IV, perlecan, and laminin, is thought to prevent degradation of the FGF-2. Investigators have hypothesized that the laminin molecule in Matrigel may be the predominant matrix component responsible for the observed adipogenesis. Although this conclusion is speculation at this point, recent studies have shown that integrin molecules mediate preadipocyte adhesion to and migration on laminin substrata (63).

Beahm and colleagues have demonstrated recruitment of resident preadipocytes and formation of de novo adipose tissue using a vascular pedicle model in athymic nude rats (64–66). Briefly, the superficial inferior epigastric blood vessels are isolated, and inert silicone molds of various shapes (sheet, hemisphere, sphere) are sutured around the vessels. The molds are packed with poly(glycolic acid) (PGA) fibers. Subsequently, Matrigel and FGF-2 are injected into the packing fibers. Qualitative assessment over 4–20 weeks demonstrated de novo adipogenesis in both young and old animals. This approach is currently being translated to a large animal model (Yucatan MicroPig) to assess adipose tissue engineering strategies.

Poly(L-lactic-coglycolic-acid)/polyethylene glycol (PLGA/PEG) microspheres have been investigated as growth factor delivery vehicles in the absence of Matrigel. Insulin, insulin-like growth factor-1 (IGF-1), and FGF-2 have been administered to the muscular fascia of the rat abdominal wall via these PLGA/PEG microspheres (67, 68). At the four weeks harvest, adipose tissue is grossly observed at the site of implantation. Histological and image analysis show that the microspheres loaded with both insulin and IGF-1 demonstrated statistically greater increases in adipose tissue (composed of fibroblasts and adipocytes) than did empty microspheres or microspheres loaded with insulin, IGF-1, or FGF-2 alone or with all three growth factors. This de novo generation of adipose tissue may result from one of three mechanisms. Stem cells present in the fascia may be stimulated to differentiate into preadipocytes and subsequently adipocytes. Another possible explanation is that preadipocytes residing in the fascia are stimulated to differentiate into adipose tissue. The third explanation, and the most speculative, is that the fibroblasts in the fascia dedifferentiate and then differentiate into preadipocytes and subsequently adipocytes.

## Bioengineering De Novo Adipogenesis

As mentioned above, autologous fat transplantation has demonstrated poor results. The adipose tissue resorption is postulated to be related to insufficient revascularization and mechanical damage. Some limited success has been obtained by using small-diameter "pearls" of fat tissue where mass transport occurs readily via diffusion (69, 70). However, this strategy is not viable for the majority of clinically sized defects, especially the breast. The advent of liposuction led investigators to attempt using single-cell suspensions of mature adipocytes. However, because adipocytes possess a cytoplasm composed of 80%–90% lipid, they tend to be traumatized by the mechanical forces of aspiration, resulting in approximately 90% damaged cells. The remaining 10% tend to form cysts or localized necrosis after injection. Moreover, mature adipocytes cannot be expanded ex vivo to obtain enhanced cell numbers because they are terminally differentiated. However, preadipocytes, precursor cells that differentiate into mature adipocytes, can be seeded onto a scaffold where they readily proliferate and differentiate to promote the formation of adipose tissue (71, 72). Preadipocytes are a preferred cell source over mature adipocytes because they can be readily expanded in culture, are mechanically stable, and can be obtained from fat biopsies or liposuction aspirates (22–24, 64, 73, 74). Preadipocytes have successfully been induced to form de novo adipose tissue in a low shear bioreactor on the order of millimeters (Figure 5).

A number of scaffolds have been utilized to support preadipocytes and facilitate adipogenesis, and all of these studies demonstrated the generation and the short-term support of adipose tissue (25). However, long-term persistence of

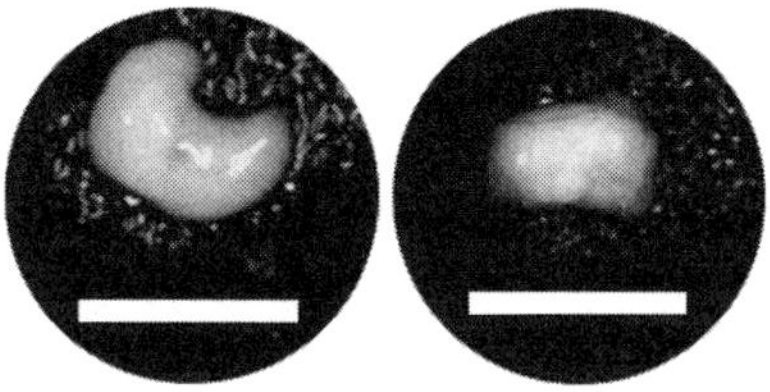

**Figure 5** De novo avascular adipose tissue grown within a low shear bioreactor seeded with preadipocytes. Bar is 5.0 mm.

generated adipose tissue remains elusive. Rigid PLGA polymer foams seeded with rat preadipocytes have been implanted subcutaneously into male Lewis rats in an effort to generate de novo adipose tissue. Results from short-term (2–5 weeks) and long-term (1–12 months) studies demonstrate the successful formation of adipose tissue for up to 2 months (71, 72). The volume of generated adipose tissue then begins to decrease and is completely resorbed by 5 months. The etiology of the resorption may be related to a number of widely divergent causes. The timing of the resorption correlates with the half-life of the scaffold, an event that has been frequently reported to occur over a spectrum of tissue engineering experiments. Only one study, utilizing fibrin glue to support the very small construct, has demonstrated stability on a long-term (12 months) basis in rats (75). Although different polymeric compounds with a longer half-life may alter the longevity of constructs, the issue of persistence of the tissue construct likely has a more complex and/or multifactorial etiology. Local factors, such as physical deformation from pressure of overlying tissues, or limitations of the chosen model owing to an unfavorable microenvironment for adipose tissue (i.e., implantation of the adipose tissue into an anatomic area that is naturally devoid of large amounts of fat, such as the subcutaneous tissue in rats) may inhibit adipose growth. Clearly, untoward or unanticipated events, such as infection and foreign body/inflammatory response, may adversely affect the outcome.

Fluortex monofilament-expanded polytetrafluoroethylene (52 $\mu$m pore size) has also been studied in vitro as a potential scaffold for adipose tissue engineering. Preadipocytes do not attach to uncoated polytetrafluoroethylene, and, hence, human collagen, albumin, and fibronectin coatings were studied to optimize seeding efficiency. Fibronectin coating results in a significantly higher number of attached human preadipocytes than the collagen or albumin coatings. Human preadipocytes are able to proliferate and differentiate into adipocytes on the fibronectin-coated expanded polytetrafluoroethylene in vitro over a period of 120 h. In vivo studies have not been conducted (76).

Von Heimburg and colleagues have studied porous collagen scaffolds and two types of hyaluronan-based devices for adipose tissue engineering (77–79). The collagen scaffolds are constructed based on a directional solidification method followed by freeze-drying to obtain a uniformly porous structure (77, 78). The hyaluronic acid-based devices are manufactured into sponges or scaffolds composed of nonwoven fibers. The sponges demonstrate open, interconnecting pores ranging from 50–340 μm, whereas the nonwoven mesh has an interfiber distance of 100–300 μm. In vivo studies conducted in mice show that the hyaluronan sponge proves to be a better scaffold than the freeze-dried collagen construct or the hyaluronan nonwoven carrier owing to the larger, interconnected pores. After eight months, a greater number of adipocytes are found in the sponge compared to the nonwoven mesh. The large pore size is important for the preadipocytes to incorporate lipids and enlarge during differentiation. Pore size was also found to be a factor in adipogenesis in several proprietary Johnson & Johnson biodegradable polymer sponges and nonwoven fibers (80).

Synthetic polymer hydrogels are also actively being studied as potential tissue engineering scaffolds because of the ability to derivatize the polymers with bioactive functional groups and, thereby, control molecular and cell function. Hydrogels are viscoelastic polymeric structures that contain a significant volume fraction of water (usually >90%). The three-dimensional polymeric structures of the hydrogel are held together primarily by cross-linking. Currently, hydrogels are being employed in biomedicine for controlled drug release, soft tissue augmentation, cell separations, and biosensors. In the tissue engineering arena, hydrogels can be used as nascent materials or they can be modified with bioactive peptides that aid them in mimicking cell adhesion properties of the extracellular matrix. Proteolytically degradable peptides can be incorporated into the backbone of the polymer to form hydrogels that are degraded by cell-secreted enzymes (81–85). For instance, PEG can be modified with the peptide sequence leucine, glycine, proline, and alanine (LGPA) to form a polymer degradable by collagenase. Preadipocyte adhesion sites can also be coupled to PEG using the peptides tyrosine, isoleucine, glycine, serine, and arginine (YIGSR) (25). YIGSR is a cell-binding peptide found on laminin. Wu & Patrick have shown that preadipocytes bind preferentially to laminin-1 and that cell adhesion to and migration on laminin-1 is mediated by the $\alpha_1\beta_1$ integrin (63). Combining the degradable PEG with the polymer coupled with cell adhesion sites produces a synthetic hydrogel that has been shown to be adequate scaffold material in vitro. The preadipocytes can be mixed into a PEG solution and then photopolymerized into a hydrogel. The clinical benefit of having a polymerizable hydrogel such as PEG is that the cell-polymer solution can easily be injected into soft tissue defects then photopolymerized in situ into a hydrogel.

Porous alginate material (a naturally derived hydrogel) has also been investigated as a construct for soft tissue engineering. Halberstadt et al. modified the alginate material with the peptide sequence arginine, glycine, and aspartic acid (RGD) to allow cells to adhere to the construct (86). In vitro studies demonstrate that the porous alginate-RGD material supports cell attachment, adhesion, and proliferation (87). Small animal studies performed over six months show that the implanted material is also conducive to tissue ingrowth and does not elicit major inflammatory responses (86). In a large animal model (sheep), the material is seeded with preadipocytes and injected into the nape of the neck. Well-defined adipose tissue is identified within the hydrogel at one and three months. Unfortunately, it cannot be determined whether the adipose tissue growth resulted from the previously seeded preadipocytes in the material or from resident preadipocytes (88).

Collagen hydrogels have also been investigated as a three-dimensional biological matrix upon which preadipocytes are cocultured with human mammary epithelial cells in order to form tissue that closely resembles the normal human breast. Histological analysis of the collagen gels from in vitro studies indicates a pattern of ductal structures of human mammary epithelial cells within clusters of adipocytes similar to the architecture of breast tissue. These findings indicate that there is a potential for breast tissue to be regenerated in vitro on a three-dimensional scaffold and later implanted for breast reconstruction purposes (89).

## SPECIAL CHALLENGES

### Blood Supply

The close interrelationship between adipose tissue and vascular tissue in vivo has been demonstrated on a number of levels: embryologic, developmental, anatomic, and metabolic. This interaction includes a critical interplay between the processes of angiogenesis and adipogenesis. It is important to note that angiogenesis precedes adipogenesis (90). This relationship is noted in embryologic growth and development as well as wound healing and has repeatedly been demonstrated experimentally. Our own studies (71, 72, 80) and those of others (91) demonstrate de novo adipogenesis in perivascular tissue around polymer implants. Moreover, the presence of adipose cells follows after the foundation of a vascular network has been established, and fat deposition is common after involution of a capillary hemangioma. Microvascular endothelial cells and preadipocytes are not, however, in direct apposition, as they do not possess cognate cell-cell adhesion molecules. Intercellular signaling instead occurs through secreted or matrix-bound factors. A host of such factors from microvascular endothelial cells has been shown to promote preadipocyte proliferation and differentiation during adipogenesis (90, 92–95). Conversely, established adult adipose tissue is proangiogenic, primarily owing to its secretion of growth factors and hormones (96–105). Adipogenesis is intimately coupled to angiogenesis and both processes must be considered in development of a clinically translatable strategy for adipose tissue engineering.

On a pragmatic level, adipose tissue is highly vascular, possessing resting values of blood flow and capillary filtration coefficients two to three times higher than those in skeletal muscle. This suggests that a rich vascular network is crucial to support the demands of an adipose construct. Although capillary ingrowth accompanies adipose cells, the initial vascular network is thin and tenuous, with the transport of oxygen and nutrients provided primarily by diffusion. Physiological diffusion of nutrients within tissue is limited to a distance of approximately 150 $\mu$m from an adjacent capillary (106). Distances greater than this result in oxygenation that is insufficient to maintain metabolic function. It would therefore seem logical that to successfully engineer a tissue construct of any size significant enough to approach clinical relevance, diffusion alone would be an inadequate means of vascular support. A discrete, well-established blood supply would seem to be most appropriate to maintain and nourish any sizeable, metabolically active tissue composite, as well as provide a means for subsequent microsurgical transfer to the reconstructive site.

Several different strategies to develop a vascular network capable of supporting adipose tissue or other tissues have been pursued. One method involves the concomitant induction of angiogenesis and adipogenesis. Utilizing a soft tissue model of human adipose stromal cells and endothelial cells placed in an in vitro fibrin-microcarrier scaffold, capillary-like structures are noted after addition of vascular endothelial growth factor, a potent angiogenic factor (107). Unfortunately, although supplementation with IGF-1 (known to indirectly stimulate angiogenesis by stimulating growth and maturation of smooth muscle cells and pericytes) is noted to maximize stabilization of these capillary-like structures, they cannot be sustained long term.

An alternative approach is the in vivo application of a defined vascular pedicle to the adipose construct. As early as 1969, vascularized conduits have been utilized in flap prefabrication and tissue engineering to enhance vascularization. A defined vascular pedicle has been utilized clinically to vascularize skin grafts and composite tissue constructs (108). A discrete vascular pedicle would appear significant in the engineering of tissues, providing not only a means for microsurgical transfer of the engineered construct, but a vascularized base that might enhance construct stability and perhaps the maintenance of a larger construct. Although a number of vascular pedicles have been utilized to promote neovascularization in both alloplastic and autogenous tissues, the optimal configuration for a vascular conduit has not been characterized (109, 110). Our studies suggest that an intact artery and vein provide the most optimal configuration for neovascularization of target tissues (65, 66). These findings are in agreement with previous studies of a spectrum of vascular conduits, which note that a number of artery-vein loop configurations, as well as a native flow-through pedicle, may lead to neovascularization, whereas long-vein grafts are generally ineffective to induce neovasculariztion (108, 109). The success of these vascularized constructs to support adipose tissue (as opposed to fibrous tissue) is encouraging, but sparse, and no long-term data are yet available. Additionally, the use of a pre-existing, defined vascular pedicle in vivo provides the potential ability to transfer the engineered construct microsurgically to a remote site. Although the mechanism of the vascular response demonstrated in these experimental constructs may be a function of a foreign body and/or wound healing response, and long-term studies are lacking, this appears to be a pragmatic and well-founded approach to the issues of construct maintenance and permanence.

Vascular support of the construct is likely to be one of the most profound if not the most critical factors limiting the size, maintenance, and quality of an engineered construct. Whereas angiogenesis and capillary ingrowth accompany adipogenesis, in the latter stages of wound healing vascular ingrowth regresses. As previously discussed, a defined vascular pedicle, analogous to the axial blood vessel of a flap, may be one of the ingredients necessary to ensure long-term support of the construct.

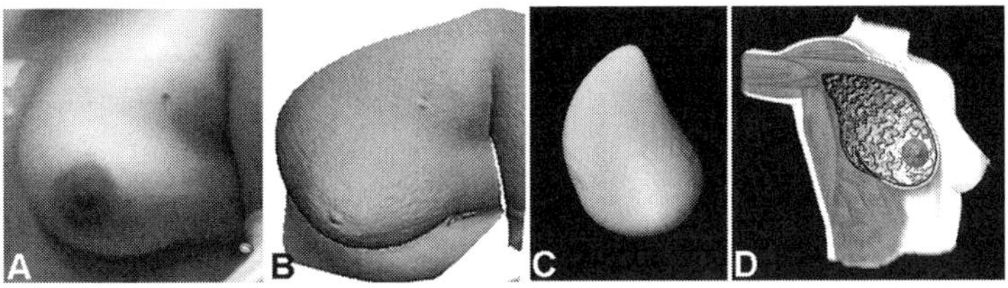


**Figure 6** (*A*) Photograph of a patient's breast. (*B*) Image scan of breast's (*A*) topography. (*C*) Virtual reality model result of breast scaffold required to restore the original breast shape in (*A*). The model gives a volume of 987 mL and surface area of 453 $cm^2$ as engineering design parameters. (*D*) Illustration depicting how the tissue engineered construct can then be placed in the patient to restore cosmesis.

## Matching Skin Envelope with Volume

As previously highlighted, adipose tissue engineering for breast reconstruction must be patient-specific in terms of size and shape. Given a bounding, fixed-skin envelope, the shape and volume of any implantable material (i.e., implant, autologous tissue, tissue engineered construct) determine the final shape of the breast. For proper engineering design, the volume of tissue required to restore the breast mound to a proper cosmesis must be known a priori. This currently does not occur with reconstructive techniques. That is, surgeons must make educated estimates as to what breast implant size or free autologous tissue is required to restore the proper breast shape. This process is unavoidably dependent on surgeon experience and often necessitates multiple revisions to the breast. With tissue engineering, we have the potential opportunity to determine ahead of time the required design parameters (e.g., scaffold shape and cell number) required for a restorative strategy. Investigators from the University of Texas M.D. Anderson Cancer Center and the University of Houston have created patient-specific virtual reality models of breasts based on three-dimensional patient imaging data that provides engineering design parameters (111–113) (Figure 6). The initial finite element breast model is composed of two components, skin and fat, and is capable of handling large deformation under gravity loading. The model in its current form can provide information as to the exact shape and volume of a tissue-engineered construct required to produce a specific cosmesis. Further refinements of the models are underway to include breast tissue biomechanics stratified by various parameters such as age, race, and ethnicity.

## Large Animal Model

To a large extent, the majority of infant tissue engineering strategies relies on small animal models to demonstrate proof of concept. Numerous investigators have demonstrated in small animal models the feasibility of adipose tissue engineering. It is critical that the scientific community begin to develop appropriate

**TABLE 3** Design criteria for large animal model

| |
|---|
| Blood vessels must be of sufficient diameter to permit anastamosis using standard microsurgery techniques |
| Animal size must be large enough to reflect convection- and diffusion-dependent mass transport |
| Animal's tissue structure must permit the harvest, isolation, and culture of preadipocytes |
| Animal's anatomy must permit placement of constructs without impairing the animal's mobility or quality of life, and provide protection from mechanical damage owing to animal's lifestyle |
| Animal's growth rate must permit long-term studies in that the animal must not become too large or reach the end of its natural life expectancy |
| Animal's soft tissue and cardiovascular physiology should be similar to human |

large animal models. Establishing a large animal model with quantitative metrics is required to achieve the goal of restoring the human breast mound subsequent to mastectomy.

The criteria for an adipose tissue engineering large animal model are listed in Table 3. Investigators at the University of Texas M.D. Anderson Cancer Center have selected Yucatan MicroPigs as a model system because they satisfy these criteria (Figure 7, see color insert). MicroPigs, specifically, offer the advantages of being pure breed (less in vivo variation); hairless; gentle and tractable; used extensively as wound healing and cardiovascular models; and have a slow, defined growth rate and desirable size (14–20 kg at sexual maturity/5–6 months and 40–60 kg at adult/12–14 months) (114–116). Moreover, preadipocytes have been successfully cultured from swine (117, 118). Early studies suggest that this model is appropriate, but further detailed characterization is required.

## CONCLUSION AND FUTURE DIRECTIONS

A few surgeons have just begun to apply tissue engineering in the clinical setting, designing composite flaps by isolating small amounts of fascia to a vascular pedicle, delaying the reconstruction, and then returning to harvest the construct. The field of adipose tissue engineering offers great potential in abrogating limitations realized with soft tissue augmentation after tumor resection and trauma. The development and practical application of an engineered adipose tissue construct remains a futuristic goal. This review has discussed the state-of-the-art techniques in adipose tissue engineering. Several options for engineering a fat construct have been postulated, including seeding a prefabricated, biocompatible, and degradable scaffold that will slowly and predictably reabsorb over time, leaving only the living tissue behind. Alternatively, a biological delivery system could be used to deliver hormonal and mitogenic factors over a prescribed time and location to cause the desired cell growth from the local endogenous tissues. These concepts are in the preliminary stages of investigation.

For engineered fat constructs to be a viable option, they must be as reliable as currently available reconstructive techniques are. The constructs must be biocompatible and maintain their three-dimensional shape over time. Concerns will focus on whether the fat produced is normal (although histological studies of engineered fat to date have indicated this to be the case) and on the reliability of the control of the process. The constructs must establish equilibrium and mature at the recipient site, and most importantly, they must not pose an oncologic risk. Transforming adipose tissue engineering strategies into a reality using the paradigms presented in this review will require the continued active partnership between clinicians, bioengineers, and life scientists.

## ACKNOWLEDGMENTS

This work was funded by grants from Cancer Fighters of Houston, U.S. Department of Defense Breast Cancer Research Program, and The University of Texas M.D. Anderson Cancer Center.

**The *Annual Review of Biomedical Engineering* is online at http://bioeng.annualreviews.org**

## LITERATURE CITED

1. American Cancer Society. 2002. Breast cancer statistics for 2002. http://www.cancer.org/docroot/STT/stt_0_2002.asp?sitearea=STT&level=1
2. American Society of Plastic Surgeons. 2002. 2001 National clearinghouse of plastic surgery statistics. http://www.plasticsurgery.org/public_education/2002statistics.cfm
3. Robb GL. 2001. Reconstructive surgery. In *Breast Cancer*, ed. KK Hunt, GL Robb, EA Strom, NT Ueno, pp. 223–53. New York: Springer-Verlag
4. Renneker R, Cutler M. 1952. Psychological problems of adjustment to cancer of the breast. *JAMA* 148:834
5. Jacobson N. 1998. The socially constructed breast: breast implants and the medical construction of need. *Am. J. Public Health* 88:1254–61
6. Lau DC, Shillabeer G, Li Z, Wonf KL, Tough SC, Russell JC. 1990. Paracrine interactions in adipose tissue and development and growth. *Int. J. Obes.* 20:16–25
7. Sorisky A. 1999. From preadipocyte to adipocyte: differentiation-directed signals of insulin from the cell surface to the nucleus. *Crit. Rev. Clin. Lab. Sci.* 36:1–34
8. Sul HS, Smas CM, Wang D, Chen L. 1998. Regulation of fat synthesis and adipose differentiation. In *Progress in Nucleic Acid Research and Molecular Biology*, pp. 317–45. Berkely, CA: Academic
9. Cinti S. 2002. Adipocyte differentiation and transdifferentiation: plasticity of the adipose organ. *J. Endocrinol. Invest.* 25: 823–35
10. Cornelius P, MacDougald OA, Lane MD. 1994. Regulation of adipocyte development. *Annu. Rev. Nutr.* 14:99–129
11. Harp JB, Franklin D, Vanderpuije AA,

Gimble JM. 2001. Differential expression of signal transducers and activators of transcription during human adipogenesis. *Biochem. Biophys. Res. Commun.* 281:907–12
12. Holst D, Grimaldi PA. 2002. New factors in the regulation of adipose differentiation and metabolism. *Curr. Opin. Lipidol.* 13:241–45
13. Loftus TM, Lane MD. 1997. Modulating the transcriptional control of adipogenesis. *Curr. Opin. Genet. Dev.* 7:603–8
14. MacDougald OA, Lane MD. 1995. Transcriptional regulation of gene expression during adipocyte differentiation. *Annu. Rev. Biochem.* 64:345–73
15. MacDougald OA, Mandrup S. 2002. Adipogenesis: forces that tip the scales. *Trends Endocrinol. Metab.* 13:5–11
16. Maeda K, Okubo K, Shimomura I, Mizuno K, Matsuzawa Y, Matsubara K. 1997. Analysis of an expression profile of genes in the human adipose tissue. *Genes* 190:227–35
17. Mandrup S, Lane MD. 1997. Regulating adipogenesis. *J. Biol. Chem.* 272:5367–70
18. Ntambi JM, Kim Y-C. 2000. Adipocyte differentiation and gene expression. *J. Nutr.* 130:3122S–26
19. Nakajima I, Yamaguchi T, Ozutsumi K, Aso H. 1998. Adipose tissue extracellular matrix: newly organized by adipocytes during differentiation. *Differentiation* 63:193–200
20. Ross SE, Hemati N, Longo KA, Bennett CN, Lucas PC, et al. 2000. Inhibition of adipogenesis by Wnt signaling. *Science* 289:950–53
21. Smas CM, SookSul HS. 1995. Control of adipocyte differentiation. *Biochem. J.* 309:697–710
22. Patel P, Robb GL, Patrick CW Jr. 2003. Soft tissue restoration using tissue engineering. *Semin. Plast. Surg.* 17:99–105
23. Patrick CW Jr. 2000. Tissue engineering of fat. *Surg. Oncol.* 19:302–11
24. Patrick CW Jr. 2001. Tissue engineering strategies for soft tissue repair. *Anat. Rec.* 263:361–66
25. Patel PN, Patrick CW Jr. 2004. Materials employed for breast augmentation and reconstruction. In *Scaffolding in Tissue Engineering*, ed. PX Ma, J Elisseeff. New York: Marcel Dekker
26. Dunnington GL, Andriole DA, Kaiser S. 2000. Breast. In *Essentials of General Surgery*, ed. S PF Lawrence, pp. 368–85. Philadelphia, PA: Williams & Wilkins
27. Junqueira LC, Carneiro J, Kelley RO. 1989. Female reproductive system. In *Basic Histology*, pp. 461–65. Norwalk, CT: Appleton & Lange
28. Moore KL. 1992. *Clinically Oriented Anatomy*. Baltimore, MD: Williams & Wilkins. pp. 45–48
29. Peer LA. 1977. Transplantation of fat. In *Reconstructive Plastic Surgery: Principles and Procedures in Correction, Reconstruction, and Transplantation*, ed. JM Converse, pp. 251. Philadelphia, PA: Saunders
30. Tebbetts J. 2002. A system for breast implant selection based on patient tissue characteristics and implant-soft tissue dynamics. *Plast. Reconstr. Surg.* 109:1396–409
31. Bostwick J III. 2000. *Plastic and Reconstructive Surgery*. St. Louis, MO: Qual. Med. Publ. 1606 pp.
32. Zuckerman D. 2002. Commentary: are breast implants safe? *Plast. Surg. Nurs.* 22:66–71
33. Gerszten PC. 1999. A formal risk assessment of silicone breast implants. *Biomaterials* 20:1063–69
34. Muzaffar A, Rohrich R. 2001. The silicone gel-filled breast implant controversy: an update. *Plast. Reconstr. Surg.* 109:742–47
35. Flassbeck D, Pfleiderer B, Klemens P, Heumann K, Eltze E, Hirner A. 2003. Determination of siloxanes, silicon, and platinum in tissues of women with silicone gel-filled implants. *Anal. Bioanal. Chem.* 375:356–62

36. Spear S, Elmaraghy M, Hess C. 1999. Textured-surface saline-filled silicone breast implants for augmentation mammaplasty. *Plast. Reconstr. Surg.* 105:15–42
37. Bronz G. 1999. How reliable are textured implants used in breast surgery? A review of 510 implants. *Aesth. Plast. Surg.* 23:424–27
38. Pollock H. 1993. Breast capsular contracture: a retrospective study of textured versus smooth silicone implants. *Plast. Reconstr. Surg.* 91:404–7
39. Peters W, Pritzker K, Smith D, Fornasier V, Holmyard D, et al. 1998. Capsular calcification associated with silicone breast implants: incidence, determinants, and characterization. *Ann. Plast. Surg.* 41:348–60
40. Coleman DJ, Foo ITH, Sharpe DT. 1991. Textured or smooth implants for breast augmentation? A prospective controlled trial. *Br. J. Plast Surg.* 44:444–48
41. Baran CN, Peker F, Ortak T, Sensoz O, Baran NK. 2001. A different strategy in the surgical treatment of capsular contracture: leave capsule intact. *Aesth. Plast. Surg.* 25:427–31
42. Bosetti M, Navone R, Rizzo E, Cannas M. 1998. Histochemical and morphometric observations on the new tissue formed around mammary expanders coated with pyrolytic carbon. *J. Biomed. Mater. Res.* 40:307–13
43. Pandya AN, Dickson MG. 2002. Capsule within a capsule: an unusual entity. *Br. J. Plast. Surg.* 55:455–56
44. Siggelkow W, Faridi A, Spiritus K, Klinge U, Rath W, Klosterhalfen B. 2003. Histological analysis of silicone breast implant capsules and correlation with capsular contracture. *Biomaterials* 24:1101–9
45. Clough KB, O'Donoghue JM, Fitoussi AD, Nos C, Falcou MC. 2001. Prospective evaluation of late cosmetic results following breast reconstruction: I. Implant reconstruction. *Plast. Reconstr. Surg.* 107:1702–9
46. Brown M, Markus Y, Belchetz B, Vearncombe M, Semple J. 2002. Microbial growth in saline breast implants and saline tissue expanders. *Plast. Reconstr. Surg.* 109:2242–44
47. Young V, Hertl M, Murray P, Jensen J, Witt H, Schorr M. 1997. Microbial growth inside saline-filled breast implants. *Plast. Reconstr. Surg.* 100:182–96
48. Coleman WP III. 1999. Fat transplantation. *Dermatol. Clin.* 17:891–98
49. Ellenbogen R. 1990. Invited comment. *Aesth. Plast. Surg.* 24:197
50. de la Fuente A, Tavora T. 1988. Fat injection for the correction of facial lipodistrophies: a preliminary report. *Aesth. Plast. Surg.* 12:39–43
51. Chajchir A, Benzaquen I. 1986. Liposuction fat grafts in face wrinkles and hemifacial atrophy. *Aesth. Plast. Surg.* 10:115–17
52. Matsudo P, Toledo L. 1988. Experience of injected fat grafting. *Aesth. Plast. Surg.* 12:35–38
53. Niechajev I, Sevcuk O. 1994. Long term results of fat transplantation: clinical and histologic studies. *Plast. Reconstr. Surg.* 94:496–506
54. Robb G, Miller M, Patrick CW Jr. 2001. Breast reconstruction. See Ref. 119, pp. 881–89
55. Ersek RA, Chang P, Salisbury MA. 1998. Lipo layering of autologous fat: an improved technique with promising results. *Plast. Reconstr. Surg.* 101:820–26
56. Hartrampf CR Jr. 1984. Abdominal wall competence in transverse abdominal island flap operations. *Ann. Plast. Surg.* 12:139–46
57. Lejour M, Dome M. 1991. Abdominal wall function after rectus abdominis transfer. *Plast. Reconstr. Surg.* 87:1054–68
58. Feller AM. 1994. Free TRAM: results and abdominal wall function. *Clin. Plast. Surg.* 21:223–32
59. Kawaguchi N, Toriyama K, Nicodemou-Lena E, Inou K, Torii S, Kitagawa Y. 1998. De novo adipogenesis in mice at the

site of injection of basement membrane and basic fibroblast growth factor. *PNAS* 95:1062–66
60. Tabata Y, Miyao M, Inamoto T, Ishii T, Hirano Y, et al. 2000. De novo formation of adipose tissue by controlled release of basic fibroblast growth factor. *Tissue Eng.* 6:279–89
61. Kimura Y, Ozeki M, Inamoto T, Tabata Y. 2002. Time course of de novo adipogenesis in Matrigel by gelating microspheres incorporating basic fibroblast growth factor. *Tissue Eng.* 8:603–13
62. Kimura Y, Ozeki M, Inamoto T, Tabata Y. 2003. Adipose tissue engineering based on human preadipocytes combined with gelatin microspheres containing basic fibroblast growth factor. *Biomaterials* 24:2513–21
63. Patrick CW Jr, Wu X. 2003. Integrin-mediated preadipocyte adhesion and migration on laminin. *Ann. Biomed. Eng.* 31:505–15
64. Beahm E, Walton R, Patrick CW Jr. 2003. Progress in adipose tissue construct development. *Clin. Plast. Surg.* 30:547–58
65. Beahm E, Wu L, Walton RL. 2000. *Lipogenesis in a vascularized engineered construct.* Presented at Am. Soc. Reconstruct. Microsurg., San Diego, CA
66. Walton RL, Beahm EK, Wu L. 2004. De novo lipogenesis in a vascularized construct. *Microsurgery.* In press
67. Yuksel E, Weinfeld AB, Cleek R, Wamsley S, Jensen J, et al. 2000. Increased free fat-graft survival with the long-term, local delivery of insulin, insulin-like growth factor-I, and basic fibroblast growth factor by PLGA/PEG microspheres. *Plast. Reconstr. Surg.* 105:1712–20
68. Yuksel E, Weinfeld AB, Cleek R, Waugh JM, Jensen J, et al. 2000. *De novo* adipose tissue generation through long-term, local delivery of insulin and insulin-like growth factor-1 by PLGA/PEG microspheres in an *in vivo* rat model: a novel concept and capability. *Plast. Reconstr. Surg.* 105:1721–29
69. Coleman SR. 1997. Facial recontouring with lipostructure. *Clin. Plast. Surg.* 24: 347–67
70. Coleman SR. 1995. Long-term survival of fat transplants: Controlled demonstrations. *Aesth. Plast. Surg.* 19:421–25
71. Patrick CW Jr, Zheng B, Johnston C, Reece GP. 2002. Long-term implantation of preadipocyte seeded PLGA scaffolds. *Tissue Eng.* 8:283–93
72. Patrick CW Jr, Chauvin PB, Reece GP. 1999. Preadipocyte seeded PLGA scaffolds for adipose tissue engineering. *Tissue Eng.* 5:139–51
73. Patrick CW Jr, Chauvin PB, Robb GL. 1998. Tissue engineered adipose. In *Frontiers in Tissue Engineering*, ed. CW Patrick Jr, AG Mikos, LV McIntire, pp. 369–82. Oxford: Elsevier Sci.
74. Patrick CW Jr, Wu X, Johnston C, Reece GP. 2001. Epithelial cell culture—breast. See Ref. 119, pp. 143–54
75. Wechselberger G, Russell RC, Neumeister MW, Schoeller T, Piza-Katzer H, Rainer C. 2002. Successful transplantation of three tissue-engineered cell types using capsule induction technique and fibrin glue as a delivery vehicle. *Plast. Reconstr. Surg.* 110:123–29
76. Kral JG, Crandall DL. 1999. Development of a human adipocyte synthetic polymer scaffold. *Plast. Reconstr. Surg.* 104:1732–38
77. von Heimburg D, Lemperle G, Dippe B, Kruger S. 1994. Free transplantation of fat autografts expanded by tissue expanders in rats. *Br. J. Plast. Surg.* 47:470–76
78. von Heimburg D, Zachariah S, Heschel I, Kuhling H, Schoof H, et al. 2001. Human preadipocytes seeded on freeze-dried collagen scaffolds investigated in vitro and in vivo. *Biomaterials* 22:429–38
79. von Heimburg D, Zachariah S, Low A, Pallua N. 2001. Influence of different biodegradable carriers on the in vivo behavior of human adipose precursor cells. *Plast. Reconstr. Surg.* 108:411–20
80. Roweton S, Freeman L, Patrick CW Jr,

Dempsey K, Zimmerman M. 2000. *Pre-adipocyte-seeded absorbable matrices*. Presented at Johnson & Johnson Excellence Sci. Symp., New Jersey
81. Mann B, Gobin A, Tsai A, West J. 2001. Smooth muscle cell growth in photopolymerized hydrogels with cell adhesive and proteolytically degradable domains: synthetic ECM analogs for use in tissue engineering. *Biomaterials* 22:3045–51
82. Mann BK, Tsai AT, Scott-Burden T, West JL. 1999. Modification of surfaces with cell adhesion peptides alters extracellular matrix deposition. *Biomaterials* 20:2281–86
83. Mann BK, Schmedlen RH, West JL. 2001. Tethered-TGF-$\beta$ increases extracellular matrix production of vascular smooth muscle cells. *Biomaterials* 22:439–44
84. Gobin AS, West JL. 2004. Cell migration through defined, synthetic ECM analogs. *FASEB J.* 16:751–53
85. Patel PN, Patrick CW Jr. 2002. *Cytocompatibility of preadipocytes in diacrylated polyethylene glycol crosslinked with various UV light photoinitiating systems*. Presented at Second Joint EMBS/BMES Conf., Houston, Texas
86. Halberstadt CR, Mooney DJ, Burg KJL, Eislet P, Rowley JA, et al. 2000. *The design and implentation of an alginate material for soft tissue engineering*. Presented at Sixth World Biomater. Congr., Kamuela, Hawaii
87. Eiselt P, Yeh J, Latvala RK, Shea LD, Mooney DJ. 2000. Porous carriers for biomedical applications based on alginate hydrogels. *Biomaterials* 21:1921–27
88. Halberstadt C, Austin C, Rowley J, Culberson C, Loebsack A, et al. 2002. A hydrogel material for plastic and reconstructive applications injected into the subcutaneous space of a sheep. *Tissue Eng.* 8:309–19
89. Huss FRM, Kratz G. 2001. Mammary epithelial cell and adipocytes co-culture in a 3-D matrix: the first step towards tissue-engineered human breast tissue. *Cells Tissues Organs* 169:361–67
90. Crandall DL, Hausman GJ, Kral JG. 1997. A review of the microcirculation of adipose tissue: anatomic, metabolic, and angiogenic perspectives. *Microcirculation* 4:211–32
91. Xaymardan M, Gibbins JR, Zoellner H. 2002. Adipogenic healing in adult mice by implantation of hollow devices in muscle. *Anat. Rec.* 267:28–36
92. Hutley LJ, Herington AC, Shurety W, Cheung C, Vesey DA, et al. 2001. Human adipose tissue endothelial cells promote preadipocyte proliferation. *Am. J. Physiol. Endocrinol. Metab.* 281:E1037–44
93. Knutson VP. 2000. The release of lipoprotein lipase from 3T3-L1 adipocytes is regulated by microvessel endothelial cells in an insulin-dependent manner. *Endocrinology* 141:693–701
94. Varzaneh FE, Shillabeer G, Wong KL, Lau DCW. 1994. Extracellular matrix components secreted by microvascular endothelia cells stimulate preadipocyte differentiation in vitro. *Metabolism* 43: 906–12
95. Smahel J. 1985. Failure of adipose tissue to heal in the capsule preformed by a silicone implant. *Chir. Plast.* 8:109–15
96. Zhang QX, Magovern CJ, Mack CA, Budenbender KT, Ko W, Rosengart TK. 1997. Vascular endothelial growth factor is the major angiogenic factor in omentum: mechanism of the omentum-mediated angiogenesis. *J. Surg. Res.* 67: 147–54
97. Silverman KJ, Lund DP, Zetter BR, Lainey LL, Shahood JA, et al. 1988. Angiogenic activity of adipose tissue. *Biochem. Biophys. Res. Commun.* 153: 347–52
98. Ouchi N, Kihara S, Arita Y, Maeda K, Kuriyama H, et al. 1999. Novel modulator for endothelial adhesion molecules: adipocyte-derived plasma protein adiponectin. *Circulation* 100:2473–76
99. Mick GJ, Wang X, McCormick K.

2002. White adipocyte vascular endothelial growth factor: regulation by insulin. *Endocrinology* 143:948–53

100. Lucarelli E, Sangiorgi L, Benassi S, Donati D, Gobbi GA, et al. 1999. Angiogenesis in lipoma: an experimental study in the chick embryo chorioallantoic membrane. *Int. J. Mol. Med.* 4:593–96
101. Claffey KP, Wilkison WO, Spiegelman BM. 1992. Vascular endothelial growth factor: regulation by cell differentiation and activated second messenger pathways. *J. Biol. Chem.* 267:16317–22
102. Castellot JJJ, Karnovsky MJ, Spiegelman BM. 1980. Potent stimulation of vascular endothelial cell growth by differentiated 3T3 adipocytes. *Cell Biol.* 77:6007–11
103. Castellot JJJ, Karnovsky MJ, Spiegelman BM. 1982. Differentiation-dependent stimulation of neovascularization and endothelial cell chemotaxis by 3T3 adipocytes. *Dev. Biol.* 79:5597–601
104. Bouloumie A, Lolmede K, Sengenes C, Galitzky J, Lafontan M. 2002. Angionenesis in adipose tissue. *Ann. Endocrinol.* 63:91–95
105. Sierra-Honigmann MR, Nath AK, Murakami C, Garcia-Cardena G, Papapetropoulos A, et al. 1998. Biological action of leptin as an angiogenic factor. *Science* 281:1683–86
106. Folkman J, Hochberg M. 1973. Self regulation of growth in three dimensions. *J. Exp. Med.* 138:745–53
107. Frerich B, Lindemann N, Kurtz-Hoffmann J, Oertel K. 2001. In vitro model of a vascular stroma for the engineering of vascularized tissues. *Int. J. Oral. Maxillofac. Surg.* 30:414–20
108. Erol OO, Spira M. 1990. Reconstructing the breast mound employing a secondary island omental skin flap. *Plast. Reconstr. Surg.* 86:510–18
109. Walton RL, Brown RE. 1993. Tissue engineering of biomaterials for composite reconstruction: an experimental model. *Ann. Plast. Surg.* 30:105–10
110. Morrison W. 2001. *Founders lecture*. Presented at Assoc. Reconstruct. Microsurg., San Diego, CA
111. Chen DT, Kakadiaris IA, Miller MJ, Loftin RB, Patrick C. 2000. Modeling for plastic and reconstructive breast surgery. In *Medical Image Computing and Computer-Assisted Intervention*, ed. SL Delp, AM DiGioia, B Jaramaz, pp. 1040–50. Pittsburgh, PA: Springer Verlag
112. Kakadiaris I, Chen D, Miller MJ, Loftin B, Patrick CW Jr. 2000. Simulation-base determination of breast tissue engineering design parameters. *Tissue Eng.* 6:662
113. Sarh K, Kakadiaris IA, Ravi-Chandar K, Miller M, Patrick CW Jr. 2001. *Towards a biomechanical model of the breast: a simulation-based study*. Presented at Am. Soc. Mech. Eng., New York, NY
114. Lavker RM, Dong G, Zheng P, Murphy GF. 1991. Hairless micropig skin: a novel model for studies of cutaneous biology. *Am. J. Pathol.* 138:687–97
115. Maas CS, Eriksson T, McCalmont T, Mabry D, Cooke D, Schindler R. 1998. Evaluation of expanded polytetrafluoroethylene as a soft-tissue filling substance: an analysis of design-related implant behavior using the porcine skin model. *Plast. Reconstr. Surg.* 101:1307–14
116. Panepinto LM, Phillips RW. 1986. The Yucatan miniature pig: characterization and utilization in biomedical research. *Lab. Anim. Sci.* 36:344–47
117. Hausman GJ, Richardson RL. 1998. Newly recruited and pre-existing preadipocytes in cultures of porcine stromal-vascular cells: morphology, expression of extracellular matrix components, and lipid accretion. *J. Animal Sci.* 76:48–60
118. Yu ZK, Hausman GJ. 1998. Preadipocyte screening by laminin in porcine stromal vascular cell culture. *Obes. Res.* 6:299–306
119. Atala A, Lanza R, eds. 2001. *Methods in Tissue Engineering*. San Diego, CA: Academic

Annu. Rev. Biomed. Eng. 2004. 6:131–56
doi: 10.1146/annurev.bioeng.6.040803.140037


# Tissue Engineering of Ligaments

G. Vunjak-Novakovic,[1] Gregory Altman,[2,3] Rebecca Horan,[2] and David L. Kaplan[2]

[1]*Massachusetts Institute of Technology, Harvard-MIT Division of Health Sciences and Technology, Cambridge, Massachusetts 02139; email: gordana@mit.edu*

[2]*Department of Biomedical Engineering, Tufts University, Medford, Massachusetts 02155; email: gregory.altman@tufts.edu, david.kaplan@tufts.edu, rebecca.horan@tufts.edu*

[3]*Tissue Regeneration, Inc., Medford, Massachusetts 02155*

**Key Words** bioreactor, scaffold, silk, human mesenchymal stem cells, mechanical loading

■ **Abstract** Tissue engineering is emerging as a significant clinical option to address tissue and organ failure by implanting biological substitutes for the compromised tissues. As compared to the transplantation of cells alone, engineered tissues offer the potential advantage of immediate functionality. Engineered tissues can also serve as physiologically relevant models for controlled studies of cells and tissues designed to distinguish the effects of specific signals from the complex milieu of factors present in vivo. A high number of ligament failures and the lack of adequate options to fully restore joint functions have prompted the need to develop new tissue engineering strategies. We discuss the requirements for ligament reconstruction, the available treatment options and their limitations, and then focus on the tissue engineering of ligaments. One representative tissue engineering system involving the integrated use of adult human stem cells, custom-designed scaffolds, and advanced bioreactors with dynamic loading is described.

CONTENTS

# INTRODUCTION

The incidence of tissue failures and repairs is already high and continues to increase owing to increased life spans and the improved quality of life. The risk for transmission of diseases has imposed additional restrictions on the already limited availability of human transplants. The anterior cruciate ligament (ACL), which serves as the primary stabilizer of the knee motion, is susceptible to ruptures or tears that can cause pain and discomfort, joint instability, and eventually degenerative joint diseases (1). An estimated 200,000 Americans required reconstructive surgery of ligaments in 2002 with a price tag exceeding five billion dollars (2, 3).

Three options have been utilized for the repair or replacement of damaged ligaments using biological substitutes: autografts, allografts, and xenografts. *Autografts* (patellar tendon with bony attachments, or two of four hamstring tendons harvested from the patient at the time of surgery) have produced the most satisfactory long-term results and are referred to as the "gold standard" (4). Donor site morbidity remains the limiting factor of patellar tendon grafts, because it is often associated with pain, muscle atrophy, and tendonitis, resulting in prolonged rehabilitation periods (5). Frozen *allografts* of ligaments with bony attachments frequently result in an immunological foreign-body response (6) that hinders tissue remodeling (7, 8). The risks of disease transmission, a lack of donors, and donor-recipient compatibility are significant problems. Bovine *xenografts* cross-linked with glutaraldehyde have been used with an initial success, but more recent studies have not reproduced these early findings (8). Bovine xenografts failed to obtain Food and Drug Administration (FDA) approval owing to occasional recurrent effusion, graft failure, and synovitis. Synthetic materials were popular in the 1980s, but their implantation frequently led to implant degeneration and failure (9).

In addition, a variety of synthetic materials have been used for ligament replacement (e.g., Versigraft, Dacron, Gore-Tex, Leeds-Keio polyester, polypropylene-based Kennedy Ligament-Augmentation Device), but with limited success (10–12) (Table 1). Of 855 prosthetic ligaments tracked for 15 years, 40% to 78% failed owing to wear debris, tissue reactions, and mechanical limitations (13). Experience with these synthetic ligament grafts replacement are particularly instructive from the perspective of tissue engineering. The first generation of ACL prostheses included polytetrafluorethylene (Gore-Tex®), polyester (Dacron®), carbon fibers, and ligament-augmentation devices (LAD) made of polypropylene. True (permanent) prostheses were designed to have high initial and sustained strength characteristics as well as an increased resistance to fatigue failure in order to withstand forces associated with continuous cyclic joint loading. In contrast, scaffolds for tissue-engineered ligaments must have high initial strength, but they must be designed to gradually transfer the load-bearing responsibilities to the maturing

**TABLE 1** Synthetic materials historically utilized for ligament replacement (5)

| | **Advantages** | **Disadvantages** | **Ultimate tensile strength (N)** | **Stiffness (N/mm)** | **Elongation at break (%)** |
|---|---|---|---|---|---|
| **Gore-Tex®** | High strength and fatigue life, limited particulate debris | Lack of tissue ingrowth, fraying at bone tunnels, chronic effusions, ultimate longevity | 5300 | 322 | 9 |
| **Dacron®** | High strength, supported collagenous ingrowth | Stress-shielding of collagenous in-growth, rupture of the femoral or tibial insertion, rupture of the central body, elongation | 3631 | 420 | 18.7 |
| **Carbon fiber** | Synthetic material | Particulate matter, foreign body response in synovium | 660 | $230 \times 10^9$ | 1 |
| **LAD** | Protects graft during maturation | Inflammatory reaction, high complication rate | 1730 | 56 | 22 |

tissue while allowing for autogenous cell and tissue ingrowth, which in turn contributes to the required mechanical properties. Augmentation devices (stents) are temporary prostheses designed to increase the immediate strength of the graft and augment the graft-host tissue fixation (14, 15). The Gore-Tex® ACL is made of a single strand of expanded polytetrafluorethylene that is wound into multiple loops. The prosthesis has been implanted in more than 18,000 patients worldwide (14). This prosthesis was designed to give immediate fixation with early load-bearing capabilities, thus promising early mobilization and return to activity (16). The Gore-Tex® graft ultimately failed from material fatigue owing to the lack of tissue ingrowth, likely the result of both the graft design and material properties; fraying at the bone tunnels and chronic effusions were observed (14). The graft eventually fatigued because it was unable to withstand the cyclic loads in active individuals without reinforcement of the in vivo environment; it was approved by the FDA for use only in previously failed autogenous reconstructions. The Gore-Tex II® prosthesis is currently being tested in Canada.

The Dacron® ligament was designed as a hybrid prosthesis to solve the problems of stiffness (i.e., stress shielding) that led to high failure rates in previous devices (10). The Dacron® prosthesis consists of a core of four tightly woven Dacron® tapes that are encased by a sleeve of loosely woven Dacron® velour, which promotes abundant tissue ingrowth. Complications resulting from the Dacron® prosthesis included rupture of the femoral or tibial insertion of the ligament, rupture of the central body of the prosthesis, and elongation of the ligament, possibly resulting from the permeation of synovial fluid and connective tissue (17). Although tissue ingrowth was significant, the graft did not provide knee stability because organized collagenous ingrowth was not observed, likely owing to stress shielding and the nondirectionality of the sheath covering.

The carbon fiber device was designed as a scaffold that would support rapid ingrowth of fibroblastic tissue and produce new collagen (14). The carbon fiber prosthesis is formed from carbon fiber (Plastafil®) bundles that are coated with biodegradable medical grade gelatin. The predominant complication associated with carbon fibers was the presence of particulates due to the choice of biomaterials. An immediate foreign-body response was observed in the synovium (18), and free carbon fibers were found within the joint and the regional lymph nodes (19). To reduce shedding of particulates, the carbon fiber implants were coated with polylactic acid, but this modification never received an approval by the FDA.

The Kennedy Ligament-Augmentation Device® was designed to provide protection to a weak portion of the quadriceps patellar tendon autograft using an over-the-top reconstruction as well as to the primary repair of the (e.g., partially torn) ACL. The LAD is composed of a ribbon of polypropylene woven from eight braids, and it is mostly of historic interest because the primary repair of the ACL is not routinely performed and because the over-the-top reconstruction has been displaced by newer techniques. LADs had high rate of complications in primary ACL reconstructions (up to 63%) and experienced a delay in maturation because of stress shielding (20).

## ANTERIOR CRUCIATE LIGAMENT

### Structure-Function Relationships

Ligaments have a unique combination of molecular, structural, and mechanical properties, but there is no single unique marker that can be used to distinguish between ligaments and other tissues. In addition, ligament properties vary with the anatomic location, age, and many factors associated with an injury or disease. On the structure-function level, the unique helical organization of collagen fiber bundles is thought to be essential for ligaments to perform their stabilizing function. During the rotation of the human knee ($\sim$140° in extension/flexion), the mode of attachment results in a 90° twist of the ACL and the peripheral fiber bundles. During flexion, ACL fibers remain isometric in length, allowing equal distribution in load to all fiber bundles, and thereby maximize its strength. It is this particular feature that allows the ACL to sustain high loading through all degrees of knee joint motion. A prosthesis that does not account for the isometric nature of the ACL fibers would result in a large increase in the length of fibers and the high risk for rupture. The opposite is observed for a fiber bundle attached posterior-posterior, which would become lax and unable to stabilize the load.

The complex ACL geometry and function are in part responsible for the difficulty encountered in developing suitable surgical replacements. Prosthesis design must consider the ultimate tensile strength and the stress-strain behavior of native ligaments (21). The biomechanical basis for many of the synthetic graft failures lies in the mismatches between the mechanical properties of synthetic materials and native tissues. Of particular importance is the high linear stiffness of the prosthesis that can lead to stress shielding of host tissue that tends to place the majority of the physiological load on the prosthesis alone. For example, the lack of collagen alignment can shift the dynamics of continuous ligament remodeling toward degradation and reduce the load-bearing capacity of the newly formed tissue.

The rigors of the intra-articular environment also include a rather unique biochemical environment. The cruciate ligaments (anterior and posterior) are encapsulated by synovium-containing fluid designed to lubricate the joint and prevent clots. As a result, the intra-articular environment has very low capacity for healing, leaving a torn ACL incapable of self-repair. A vascular network extending from the femoral and tibial bone attachment sites through the ligament provides long-term nourishment of the cruciate ligaments. Immediately following ACL reconstruction and prior to angiogenesis [occurring within $\sim$12 weeks of implantation (22)], the graft is dependent on the synovial fluid for nutrient and metabolite exchange. Because of the diffusional limitations of transport, the interior of the tissue is often necrotic, leading to alterations in mechanical properties. Jackson and coworkers (6) showed that even after a prolonged healing time of 6 months autologous patellar tendon grafts regained only 61% of their initial strength.

Human ACLs range in length from 27–32 mm. The fiber crimp pattern allows for 7% to 16% of creep prior to permanent deformation and ligament damage. The

ACL withstands cyclic loads of approximately 300 N about 1–2 million times per year, and it is regularly exposed to tensile forces ranging from 67 N (for ascending stairs) to 630 N (for jogging) (23). The mechanical and viscoelastic properties of the human ACL are well known (7, 21, 24–27). The established standards for ACL grafts are 1730 N for the tensile strength (26), 182 N/mm for linear stiffness (26), and 12.8 N-m for energy absorbed at failure (21).

## Molecular Markers

There is no unique marker for ACL fibroblasts. Ligaments (native and engineered, normal, and disrupted) have been evaluated on the presence of a combination of factors (Table 2):

- Extracellular matrix components (e.g., collagen types I and III, elastin, fibronectin, decorin, and biglycan) (12, 28–30)
- The relative ratio of collagen type I to type III (~88% Type I: 12% Type III) (28, 29, 31)
- Types and amounts of reducible cross-links (29)
- Cell morphology within distinct regions of the ACL (29, 32)
- The ultrastructure of collagen network (e.g., crimp pattern, collagen fibril diameter) (29, 30).

These specific features are used to distinguish the ACL from other ligaments, tendons, and tissues in general. Available data on ACL repair, embryonic development, and composition indicate that collagen types I and III, fibronectin, tenascin-C, elastin, laminin, and tissue inhibitor metalloproteinase-1 (TIMP-1) are present within the ACL (28, 29, 33–35). Furthermore, the study of the mechanical stimulation of cultured ACL fibroblasts suggests that the type I and type III collagen, tenascin-C, and vimentin all respond to mechanical loading (36–39).

**TABLE 2** Phenotypic differences between some ligaments and tendons based on biochemical analyses (29)

| | **Percent total collagen (mg collagen/g dry tissue)** | **Ratio collagen Type I to collagen Type III proteins** | **Total glycosaminoclycans (mg hexosamine/g dry tissue)** |
|---|---|---|---|
| Cruciate ligaments (ACL and PCL combined) | 80.3 +/− 1.0 | 7.3 +/− 1.4 | 9.89 +/− 0.56 |
| Medial collateral ligament | 79.7 +/− 1.1 | 10.1 +/− 2.6 | 4.56 +/− 0.26 |
| Patellar tendon | 86.7 +/− 0.9 | >19 | 3.92 +/− 0.16 |
| Achilles tendon | 86.8 +/− 1.0 | >19 | 2.75 +/− 0.20 |

Recent work quantifies eight specific proteins in torn human ACLs: collagen type I and III, fibronectin, tenascin-C, elastin, laminin, vimentin, and TIMP-1. In order to better understand the mechanisms of ACL healing, the expression of matrix metalloproteinases (MMPs) and the amount of the extracellular matrix (ECM) in ruptured human ACLs has been measured and a genetic baseline characterizing ACL tissue and behavior has been generated (40). Marker expression correlates to several predictors, such as age, gender, postinjury period, and the site of tissue scarring. A concise quantitative baseline of genotypic selected markers in ACL is essential for assessing mesenchymal stem cells (MSC) differentiation toward the ligament lineage in cell-based restoration strategies, such as tissue engineering. Importantly, establishment of such a baseline would allow the design of biomimetic culture environments for tissue engineering of functional ligaments.

## LIGAMENT TISSUE ENGINEERING

### Functional Tissue Engineering

Cells, biomaterial scaffolds, and biochemical and physical regulatory signals can be utilized in a variety of ways to engineer tissues in vitro and in vivo. In most cases, the goal is to replicate some aspects of the environment present in vivo during normal tissue development. Tissue engineering generally involves the presence of reparative cells, a structural template, facilitated transport of nutrients and metabolites, and a provision of molecular and mechanical regulatory factors. An envisioned scenario of clinically relevant tissue engineering involves the use of autologous cells, biodegradable scaffolds (designed to serve as a temporary structural and logistic template of tissue development), and bioreactors (designed to control the cellular environment).

Scaffold structure, mechanical properties, and the rate of degradation largely determine the mass transport and mechanotransduction at the cellular and tissue levels. For engineering of load-bearing tissues, the maintenance of mechanical properties of the scaffold until the new tissue becomes mechanically competent is an important requirement for scaffold design.

Tissue *engineering bioreactors* are generally designed to support physiologic concentrations of attached cells within clinically sized scaffolds and to control the environmental conditions via enhanced mass transfer (41). The provision of mechanical regulatory signals that are normally present in native tissues (e.g., a combination of dynamic strain and torsion for ligaments) is thought to be essential for the proper development of functional tissue properties (42, 43).

Despite the great potential of tissue engineering, human clinical trials with tissue-engineered ligaments have not been completed, perhaps owing to the lack of:

- Readily available autologous cell sources that do not result in donor site morbidity

- Biomaterial scaffolds with adequate composition, structure, and mechanical properties, capable of supporting ligament development in vitro (in a bioreactor) and remodeling in vivo (in a joint)
- Advanced bioreactor systems capable of mechanical conditioning of the cultured tissues, such that the engineered constructs are already functional to some extent at the time of implantation.

One approach to the engineering of ligaments, tissues that serve a predominantly biomechanical function, is based on the paradigm of functional tissue engineering. The set of principles recently defined by Butler et al. (43) stressed the importance of the mechanical properties of skeletal tissues and recognized the need to define mechanical requirements for tissue-engineered grafts and to utilize physical signals to direct cellular activity and phenotype toward functional tissue assembly, and thereby to achieve mechanically competent tissue repair.

## Approaches to Ligament Tissue Engineering

The shift from synthetic to biologically based ACL replacements was seen in early studies in which reconstituted type I collagen fibers were embedded in a type I collagen matrix, combined with polymethylmethacrylate bone fixation plugs, and used as ACL replacement tissues in rabbits (44). Subsequent studies utilized ligament analogs consisting of ligament fibroblasts seeded onto cross-linked collagen scaffolds (45, 46). Implantation of prestressed collagen sutures seeded with MSC repaired critical-size tendon defects (47). The collagen-fibroblast system was subsequently modified by using ligament fibroblasts seeded in noncross-linked collagen that was prestressed between the bone anchors (48). Passive tension within the engineered ligament induced fibroblast elongation and alignment and induced structural reorganization of the extracellular matrix (48). The application of cyclic mechanical loading during cultivation promoted the proliferation of smooth muscle cells and the assembly of newly synthesized ECM (49) as well as the synthesis of type I collagen by ACL fibroblasts (37). The cultivation of human ACL fibroblasts in collagen gel attached to two bone anchors and exposed to cyclic stretching resulted in ligament-like tissue architectures that depended on the application of mechanical stimuli (50, 51).

One advanced model system that has been used to engineer functional autologous ACLs in vitro involves an integrated use of three components:

- Adult MSC (isolated from bone marrow)
- Tissue formation template (collagen or silk fiber matrix designed to mimic structural and mechanical properties of a native ACL)
- Advanced bioreactors (providing environmental control and multidimensional dynamic loading).

The approach uses the directed differentiation and functional assembly of cultured MSC into engineered tissues that have the architecture and mechanical properties resembling those of native ligaments, in an environment designed to resemble some aspects of that in developing native ligaments (e.g., 42, 52). Engineered ligaments can be monitored in culture (magnetic resonance imaging), and characterized in vitro (molecular, structural, and mechanical properties) and in vivo (phenotype stability, capacity for survival, and vascularization). The ultimate goal of functional tissue engineering is to generate mechanically competent grafts for improved tissue repair.

## Key Requirements—Clinical Aspects

Tissue-engineered ligaments with appropriate biological and mechanical properties already established at the time of implantation would eliminate the limitations associated with present day surgical techniques. The following requirements for clinically relevant tissue engineering of ligaments have been identified (5):

- No additional surgical procedure for tissue harvest
- Minimal patient morbidity: no requirement for tendon graft harvest for use in ACL reconstruction
- Simple surgical technique for implantation with reliable fixation methods, enabling the graft to withstand aggressive rehabilitation
- Immediate stabilization of the knee to allow patients to rapidly return to their preinjury functions
- Minimal risk for infection or disease transmission
- Biocompatibility of the graft material
- Support of host tissue ingrowth without causing stress shielding (through the design of matrix geometry, porosity, and mechanical properties)
- Biodegradation at a rate providing adequate mechanical stability following implantation and during the transition to functional replacement tissue during remodeling in vivo
- Mechanical integrity for a duration sufficient to allow host tissue ingrowth

## Key Requirements—Tissue Engineering Aspects

The above requirements for clinically relevant tissue engineering can be translated into the following set of in vitro culture requirements:

- Autologous cell source (e.g., MSCs from adult human bone marrow that can be obtained by needle biopsy, selected, and expanded in vitro)
- Biomaterial scaffold (e.g., fibrous silk matrix custom designed for ligament tissue engineering, wire-rope structure, mechanical properties matching those of native ligaments, high porosity to allow cell infiltration, and biodegradation at a rate matching that of tissue formation)
- Bioreactor system (e.g., with medium perfusion to control the cellular microenvironment and with mechanical loading to induce/enhance functional tissue assembly)

- Biochemical regulation of MSC differentiation (e.g., by supplemental growth factors, bioinductive matrices, or at the genetic level)
- Biophysical regulation of MSC differentiation (e.g., by mechanical loading that is physiologic for ligaments: dynamic axial tension and torsion with periods of loading and rest)
- Quantitative methods of characterization in vitro (molecular, structural, and mechanical properties) and in vivo (phenotype stability, survival, vascularization, and mechanical function).

## Cell Source

Ideally, the patient should be treated with her/his own cells to eliminate concerns associated with the use of allograft cells (e.g., immunorejection and transmission of disease). ACL fibroblasts were shown to respond to specific growth factors, dynamic mechanical stimulation, and static tension (37, 48, 53). However, functional integration of allogeneic grafts has been delayed by a foreign-body response of the host (6), whereas a suitable source of autologous ACL fibroblasts is not yet available.

One candidate source of cells for engineering skeletal tissues is adult human bone marrow, which maintains a pool of MSCs capable both of some degree of self-renewal and of differentiation into cells of various mesenchymal lineages. MSCs have several distinct features that make them an obvious choice for engineering a variety of tissues:

- Marrow cells are routinely collected from adults using a needle biopsy and do not pose ethical concerns inherent in using embryonic or fetal tissue.
- Mesenchymal cells form discrete colonies of fibroblasts that can be isolated on the basis of their adherence to a solid surface and expanded to achieve large total cell numbers (54–58).
- The number of MSCs in bone marrow decreases as a function of age (54), but the cell potential to proliferate and differentiate is comparable in newborns and older individuals (59, 60).
- Culture conditions can be designed to direct MSC differentiation into a desired mesenchymal phenotype, including bone-forming osteoblasts, cartilage-forming chondrocytes, fat-storing adipocytes, and tendon/ligament-forming cells (47, 61–64).
- Engineered ligaments formed from MSCs could serve as suitable autografts without the need for additional surgery (involved in conventional autografts) and without the risk of immune reaction (seen with allografts).

## Regulatory Factors

Biochemical factors are essential for inducing and/or supporting the manifestation of specific mesenchymal cell lineages. Oxygen can markedly affect ECM synthesis

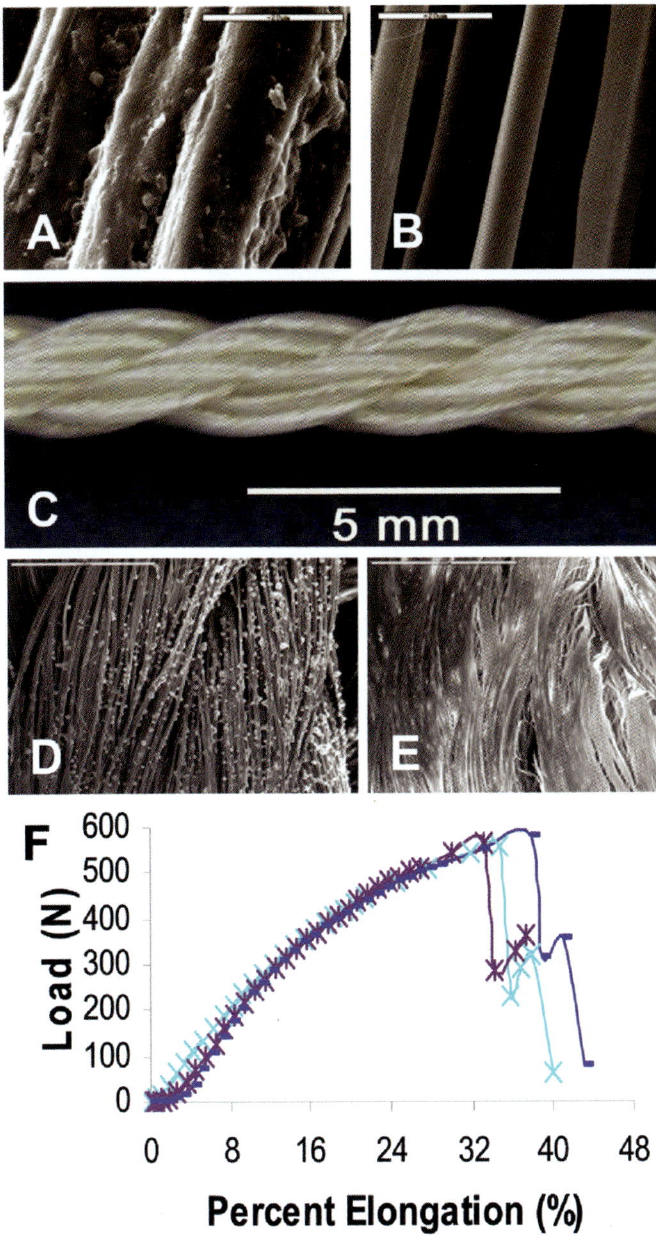


**Figure 1** Custom-designed silk scaffolds. (*A*) Virgin silk containing a sericine coat, (*B*) processed silk fibers, (*C*) 6-cord wire-rope silk scaffold, (*D*,*E*) scanning electron micrographs of human MSC (*D*) after 30 min of seeding on scaffolds and (*E*) after 14 days of cultivation. (*F*) Load-elongation curves for three independently made scaffolds [from Altman et al. (80), with permission of Elsevier Ltd.].

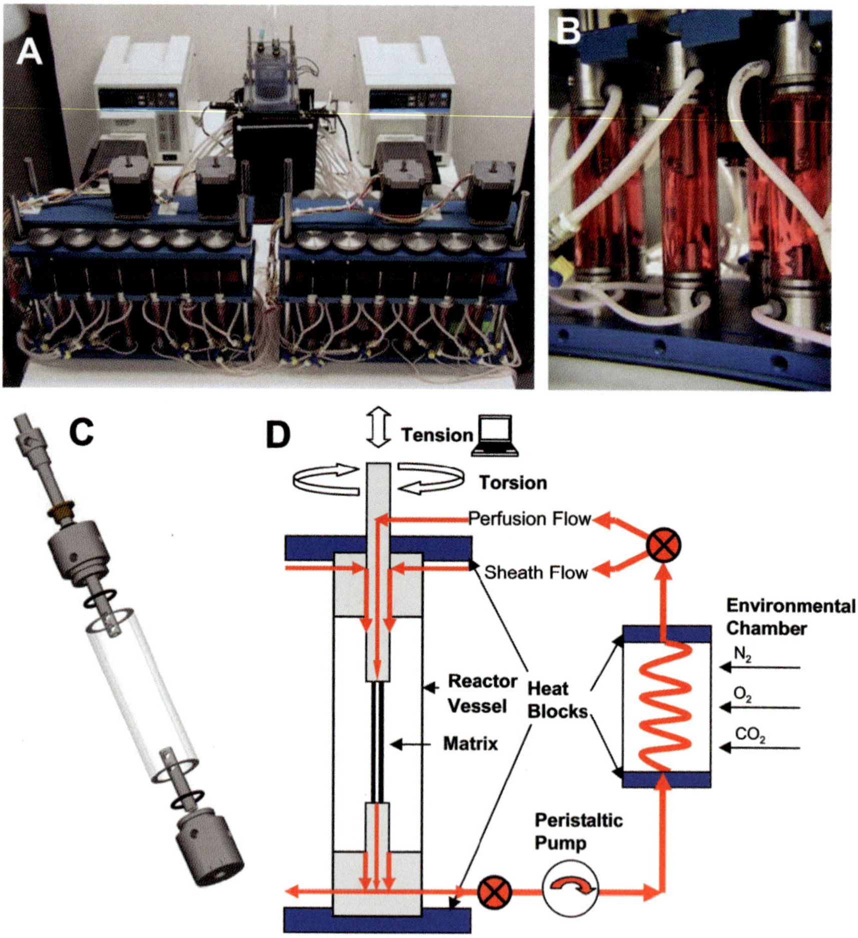


**Figure 2** Bioreactor system for ligament tissue engineering. (*A*) Functioning bioreactor system consisting of two units, each with 12 cartridges that can be used concurrently (e.g., 12 with loading, 12 without loading). (*B*) Cartridges containing an anchored silk scaffold during culture with human MSC. (*C*) Exploded view of the cartridge assembly. (*D*) Schematic illustration of one cartridge with its flow loop and anchors for the transmission of mechanical forces (from Altman et al. (52), with permission of ASME).

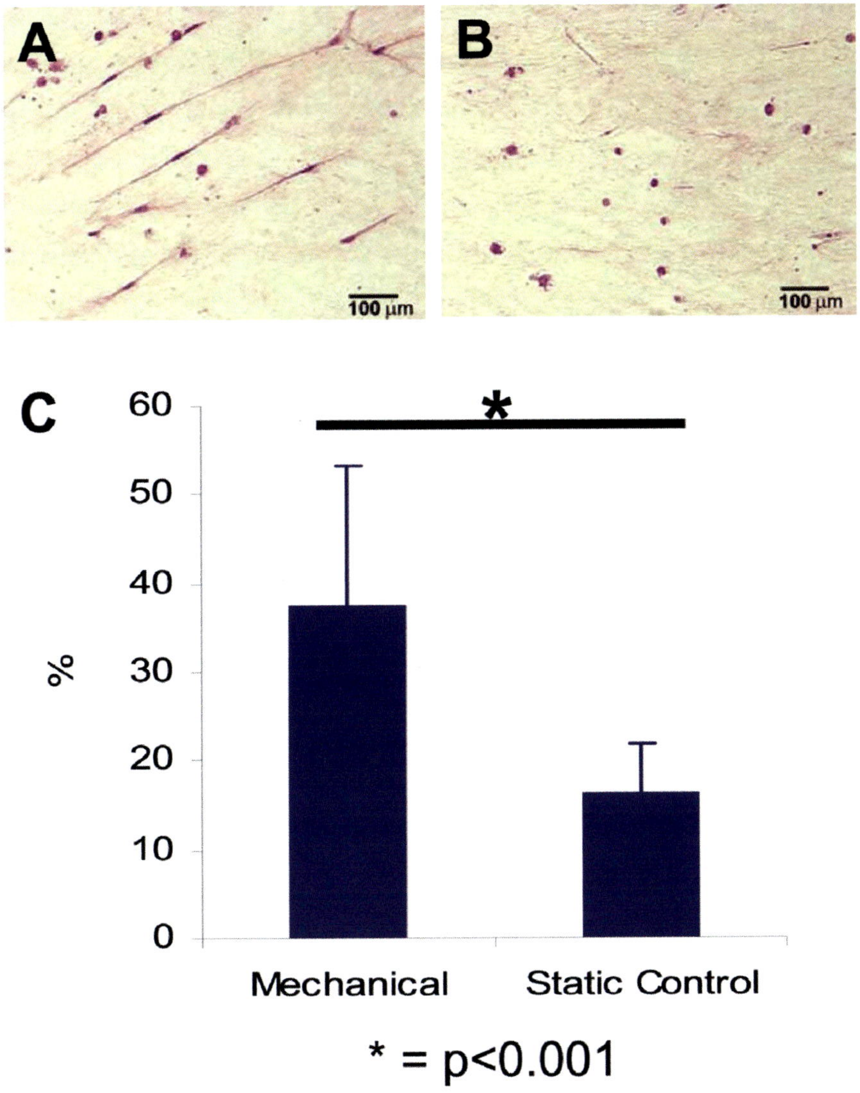


**Figure 3** Mechanical stimulation fostered cell alignment. Dynamic tension and torsion applied over 21 days of culture induced MSC in collagen gel to align in the direction of force. (*A*,*B*) H&E of stimulated and nonstimulated constructs, respectively. (*C*) Mechanical stimulation caused a 2.5-fold increase ($p < 0.001$) in cell alignment. From Reference 42.

rates and the in vitro development of engineered tissues (65, 66). Little is known about the effects of oxygen on stem cell differentiation into ligament fibroblasts. Fermor et al. (67) showed that high oxygen tensions (21%) supported optimal ACL fibroblast proliferation, whereas lower tensions (10%) enhanced ECM collagen synthesis. Ascorbate-2-phosphate, a long-acting derivative of vitamin C, enhanced cell growth in vitro and supported the maintenance of connective tissues (67, 68). Growth factors, such as epidermal growth factor (EGF), basic fibroblast growth factor (bFGF), insulin-like growth factor-II (IGF-II), and transforming growth factor-beta (TGF-$\beta$) have the capacity to increase cell proliferation (31, 69–74). Additionally, insulin, TGF-$\beta$, and IGF-II promote protein expression and the generation of ECM in soft connective tissues (72, 73, 75, 76). TGF-$\beta$ and EGF, as well as TGF-$\beta$ and insulin, act in concert to stimulate normal proliferation of fibroblasts and mesenchymal cells (73, 77, 78). Serum contains potent stimulators of in vitro cell growth and differentiation, including amino acids, growth factors, vitamins, proteins, hormones, lipids, and minerals, as well as protein inhibitors of cell differentiation.

Mechanical signals that affect the growth and development of native ligaments in vivo are likely to play similar roles during the in vitro cultivation of engineered ligaments. The application of loading can affect tissue development in at least two ways, by (*a*) enhanced mass transport, and (*b*) direct stimulation of the cells. Mechanical stimulation of cultured ligament fibroblasts upregulated the expression of collagens type I and type III, fibronectin, and tenascin-C (37–39, 79). Human MSC, in the absence of specific ligament growth and regulatory factors, could be directed to differentiate into ligament-like cells through the application of physiologically relevant cyclic strain (42, 80). Loading can cause changes to the extracellular environment both in native and in engineered ligaments by direct effects on cell shape and interfibrillar spacing or by fluid flow that can enhance the rate of mass transport to and from the cells.

Our knowledge about the effects of mechanical factors applied during cultivation (e.g., torsion and tension; frequency, amplitude, and regime of stimulation) on tissue structure and function at various hierarchical levels is limited. Controlled studies of mechanical factors affecting tissue-engineered ligaments can greatly benefit from the use of controllable physiologically relevant tissue models that can be studied with the application of dynamic loading in situ. Experimental studies of mechanotransduction are further complicated by the interactions between physical signals (associated with joint loading) and molecular factors (genetic expression, soluble and matrix-immobilized regulatory molecules). Experiments conducted more than 40 years ago suggested that mechanical factors and regulatory molecules acting in concert can determine the type of connective tissue that forms in a culture of MSCs (81).

## Biomaterial Matrix

Biomaterial scaffolds provide a structural and logistic template for cell attachment and tissue development, and they biodegrade in parallel with the accumulation of tissue components. Most studies suggest that a scaffold is essential for promoting orderly tissue repair (82–86). Scaffold structure determines the transport of nutrients, metabolites, and regulatory molecules to and from the cells, whereas its mechanical properties determine mechanotransduction at cellular and tissue levels. Ideally, a scaffold should be made of biocompatible, biodegradable material and degrade at a rate matching the rate of new tissue deposition (87). Biomaterials have been explored for use in skeletal tissue engineering (88–93), in some cases in conjunction with the delivery of regulatory molecules (56, 94–101). Regulatory molecules are usually supplemented to culture medium (102–106); they have also been incorporated into biomaterial scaffolds to provide localized delivery (107–114). Tissue engineering can greatly benefit from the new generation of bioinductive biomaterial scaffolds, for example those capable of delivering multiple growth factors (115) or capable of releasing growth factors in response to mechanical loading (116).

Collagen and silk have been used clinically for decades (e.g., hemostats and surgical sutures) and more recently for tissue engineering (52, 117–121). Collagen type I gel provided a three-dimensional environment for seeded ligament fibroblasts to proliferate and organize in response to mechanical stimulation (42, 48). However, the utility of collagen gels was limited by their inferior mechanical properties. Fibrous silk and collagen scaffolds were subsequently adopted in order to provide the necessary mechanical competence of the developing ligaments throughout the in vitro cultivation and following implantation in vivo.

COLLAGEN SCAFFOLDS Commercially available highly purified type I collagen has been used in form of gel and bundles of parallel fibers. Collagen was selected on the basis of its demonstrated ability to support the growth of ligament fibroblasts under static tension (48). Cross-linked collagen fibers were seeded with human MSCs. Fibrous collagen supported cell attachment, spreading, and fiber coverage with extracellular matrix deposition.

After one day of culture, the cells formed focal contacts, adopted a spindle-like morphology, and aligned along the scaffold fibers. After three days of culture, a smooth cell sheet was formed, and the number of cells increased with time in culture. Unfortunately, the capacity of the engineered construct to support mechanical loading decreased with time in culture, and as a result, the scaffold fibers could not impart repeatable stresses to the attached MSCs as previously observed (44–46). The poor mechanical integrity of the fibers created further concerns regarding anchoring of the fibers both in vitro (in the bioreactor) and in vivo (in the knee). The mechanical deficiencies, the bioburden associated with the use of bovine collagen products and leaching of chemical cross-linking agents, combined with the poor mechanical integrity of the collagen fibers prompted the search for improved biomaterials.

SILK SCAFFOLDS Silk has been used clinically for decades and has gained renewed interest as a biomaterial for tissue engineering (52, 80, 118–121). Initially, two problems were associated with the use of silk fibers: (*a*) native silkworm silk fibers were allergenic because of the glue-like protein coating, sericin (119), whereas spider silk fibers that are not coated with sericin are not abundant enough for use, and (*b*) silk fibers have high linear stiffness and, if organized in a parallel geometry, would fail to mirror the tensile strength and linear stiffness of native ACLs.

We have extensively explored the potential of native silk fibers for ligament tissue engineering from both the mechanical and biological perspective (52, 117). The processed silk does not have bio-burden risks associated with bovine-derived collagen; it is inexpensive and biocompatible, biodegrades at a slow rate in vitro and in vivo, and has outstanding and tailorable mechanical properties. Virgin silk is processed to extract sericin, the potential allergen (122–124). For the fabrication of surgical sutures, the fibers are coated with wax or silicone to obtain black braided silk (e.g., Perma-Hand™). To obtain highly purified silk, we developed a specialized extraction process for the treatment of silk fibers under static tension (117). Figure 1*A* and 1*B* (see color insert), respectively, show silk fibers before and after the sericin coat is removed.

Silk undergoes proteolytic degradation (125–128) at a rate that depends on the environmental conditions (125, 128–131). Silk fibers lose their tensile strength within one year in vivo and degrade completely within two years. Degradation half-lives of six weeks were reported for subcutaneous implantation in rats (128, 129). In vitro, silk can be degraded by protease (121) and chymotrypsin (132). Importantly, for silk to degrade, proteolytic attack that typically coincides with the onset of angiogenesis is needed. Overall, silk is a slowly degrading biomaterial with biocompatibility comparable to that of most materials in clinical use (e.g., polyglycolic acid (PGA) used to make degradable sutures, collagen).

Silk fibroin, when organized into an appropriate wire-rope geometry, exhibits mechanical properties similar to a functional ACL (80). In particular, the scaffold stiffness could be decreased without impacting the tensile strength of scaffold fibers by specific modifications of scaffold architecture. The six-cord wire-rope silk fiber matrix (Figure 1*C*) was designed to meet four important requirements of ligament tissue engineering:

- Enhance tissue infiltration (>90% void volumes)
- Minimize mass-transport limitations
- Increase surface area for cell attachment and extracellular matrix deposition
- Decrease the linear stiffness to match that of a native ligament and thereby avoid stress shielding.

Mechanical testing of a series of single cords from the wire-rope scaffold showed consistent load-elongation behavior (Figure 1*F*). Fatigue testing revealed a scaffold life in excess of 10 million cycles at a physiological load. As a result of silk's high tensile strength and the wire-rope design, the matrix provided significant void volume for cell seeding in vitro and tissue ingrowth in vivo. Compared to a native human ACL (per equivalent length), the silk matrix occupies only ~12%

of the volume of a human ACL (determined for an ACL 27 mm in length and 8 mm in diameter).

Silk scaffolds also support cell attachment and spreading by providing an appropriate 3-D culture environment. Cells readily attached to scaffolds, as evidenced by scanning electron micrographs (SEM) taken 30 min post seeding (Figure 1*D*). The cells spread after 1 h of culture, formed confluent cell sheets by day 7, and accumulated a ligament tissue matrix by day 14 (Figure 1*E*).

## Bioreactor System

Recent studies support the notion that bioreactors providing dynamic loading are essential for meeting the complex requirements of in vitro engineering of functional skeletal tissues (Tables 3 and 4). Various commercial bioreactor systems are available. However, the applicability of these systems to ligament engineering is limited owing to either the generality of the device, which lacks the specificity needed to mimic an in vivo ligament environment, or the design of the device tailored to meet the requirements of another tissue type other than ligaments.

An advanced bioreactor system with medium perfusion and mechanical loading was used to engineer ligaments starting from MSCs (52). The bioreactor was specifically designed for ligament tissue engineering to provide the application of multidimensional mechanical strains (axial tension/compression and torsion) to MSC cultured in a hydrogel or on a fibrous scaffold (Figure 2, see color insert).

**TABLE 3** Overview of selected commercial bioreactor systems

| Commercially Available Systems | | | |
|---|---|---|---|
| **Manufacturer** | **Product** | **Defining features** | **Limiting factors** |
| Synthecon | Rotary Culture Max | Perfusion, rotating wall vessel | Incubator required, one vessel, no environmental or mechanical control |
| Synthecon | RCCS | Rotating wall vessel | Incubator required, one vessel, no environmental or mechanical control |
| Synthecon | RCCS-4 | Four rotating wall vessels | Incubator required, no environmental or mechanical control |
| FlexCell International | FX-4000T<br>FX-4000C | Tension, 24 dishes, vacuum driven<br>Compression, 24 dishes, pump driven | Incubator required, no environmental, compression or perfusion control, limiting actuation and force monitoring systems, limited number of tissue geometries and sizes able for culture |
| FlexCell International | FlexFlow | Shear stress applied via fluid flow | Incubator required, no environmental or mechanical control |

**TABLE 4** Overview of selected bioreactor systems for which results have been published

| Group (Reference) | Tissue | Defining features | Constraints |
|---|---|---|---|
| Georgia Institute of Technology (138) | Blood vessel constructs | Dynamic conditioning through inflation and deflation of silicon tubing | Incubator required, no environmental control, limited mechanical control |
| Department of Anesthesiology and Biomedical Engineering, Duke University (139) | Arteries | Precise pulsatile radial stress and luminal flow | Incubator required, no environmental or mechanical control |
| M.E. for Biomechanics, University of Bern, Switzerland (140) | Cartilage | Samples compressed with sinusoidal dynamic displacement | Incubator required, no environmental or perfusion control |
| Lab for Tissue Engineering, German Heart Institute, Berlin (141) | Cardiovascular structures | Perfusion system, shear stress from .2–10 $dyne/cm^2$ | Incubator required, no environmental or mechanical control |
| University of Ferrara, Italy, School of Medicine (142) | Liver | Constant perfusion from 2 ml/min to 4 ml/min | Incubator required, no environmental or mechanical control |
| Department of Chemical Engineering, Zurich, Switzerland (143) | Epidermal autografts | Computer-controlled medium and gas exchange | Each chamber is 1-cm thick, no environmental or mechanical control |
| Division of Bioengineering, Massachusetts Institute of Technology (144) | Cartilage | Dynamic control of displacement, load, shear angle, or torque | Incubator required, no individual cassettes |

The bioreactor is computer controlled and consists of (*a*) 12 individual cartridges containing one engineered ligament apiece, each within a separate perfusion loop; (*b*) a gas exchanger to control medium pH and oxygen levels, (*c*) a 12-channel peristaltic pump, and (*d*) a strain-control system for mechanical stimulation of cultured constructs. Two bioreactors are operated in parallel, allowing concurrent cultivation of 24 ligaments, e.g., 12 with loading and 12 with unloaded controls (Figure 2*A*).

Each bioreactor cartridge is comprised of top and bottom mounts, a tube (an inside diameter of 0.75″, length sized to accommodate various ligaments, e.g., for knee joint or a temporomandibular joint), and two anchor shafts (Figure 2*B*,*C*). Cartridges are designed to allow for quick assembly and disassembly, and all parts can be steam sterilized. Each cartridge is operated within a separate flow loop with medium recirculation via one channel of a multichannel peristaltic pump and with an environmental chamber for oxygen and carbon dioxide exchange (52). Medium flow minimized diffusional distances around the growing ligament (Figure 2*D*). Axial strain (1%–10%) and torsional strain (up to 90°) could be applied via the top platen at frequencies of 0.01–1 Hz, with preset periods of loading and rest (52). Key functions of the bioreactor system include

- precise control of the applied mechanical strain (axial: $<0.1\ \mu$m, torsion: $<0.01°$);
- control of medium flow rate (0.17–17 ml/min per cartridge) and pathway (perfusion through and around the constructs);
- precise control over oxygen concentration in culture medium (0% to 95% saturation, $\pm 0.5\%$) and pH ($\pm 0.05$); and
- bench-top design that eliminates the need for housing within an incubator.

Mechanical stimulation induced cell alignment in the direction of the resulting force (concurrent axial and torsional strain over 21 days of culture) (Figure 3*A*, see color insert), in contrast to random cell orientation in unstimulated controls (Figure 3*B*) (42), and fostered the expression of collagen type I and type III and tenascin C (Figure 4). At the same time, neither upregulation of bone nor cartilage-specific cell markers was observed. Importantly, tension and torsion, without specific inducers of ligament differentiation, directed MSC differentiation into a ligament cell lineage in preference to alternative paths (i.e., bone or cartilage).

Cell function (e.g., proliferation rate, differentiation), ligament structure (e.g., amounts and distributions of tissue components, ultrastructural organization), mechanical behavior, and expression of ligament-specific markers are expected to change over the course of tissue cultivation. These changes are likely to depend on the developmental stage of the tissue and the environmental conditions (i.e., biochemical and mechanical signals) during cultivation. The model system allows systematic variation and quantitative assessment of environmental conditions and cell/tissue responses, thus enabling quantitative studies of in vitro tissue development.

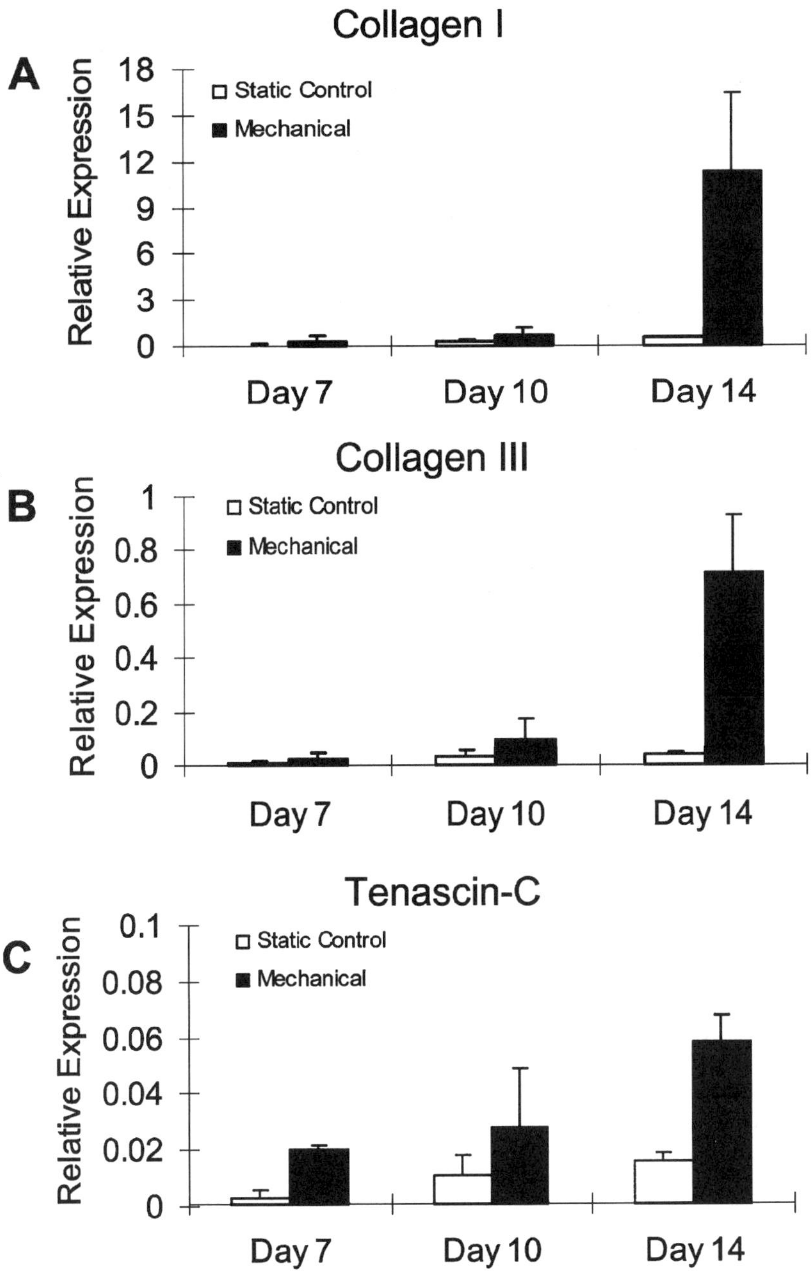


**Figure 4** Mechanical stimulation fostered cell differentiation: reverse transcription–polymerase chain reaction (RT-PCR) marker transcripts for (*A*) collagen I, (*B*) collagen III, and (*C*) tenascin C increased with time in culture and were higher for stimulated than nonstimulated ligaments.

Ligament-specific marker transcripts (collagen types I and III, tenascin C) increased with time in culture and were at all times higher in mechanically stimulated than nonstimulated ligaments, as determined by real-time RT-PCR (Figure 4). Maximum cell density was achieved 10 days post seeding, whereas maximum ligament-specific matrix transcription was observed after 14 days of culture, suggesting a transition from a proliferative into a differentiation state. Importantly, cells and extracellular matrix of mechanically stimulated ligaments aligned in the direction of loading and infiltrated the scaffold forming a multilayered tissue. Quantitative real-time RT-PCR of collagen types I and III and tenascin-C normalized to glyceraldehyde-3-phosphate dehydrogenase-indicated ligament-specific responses of MSC cultured on the six-cord matrix for 14 days (42). Expression of collagen type I was approximately one third of that in torn human ACLs. Furthermore, the ratio of collagen I to III exceeded that of normal and torn human ACLs, indicating a ligament-specific response and not that of scar tissue (e.g., high levels of collagen type III transcription).

The application of mechanical stimuli prior to uniform matrix coverage inhibited cell growth and matrix deposition. In contrast, dynamic axial and torsional strains applied after five days of static culture increased cell density and enhanced the alignment of cells and extracellular matrix along the scaffold fibers. This is consistent with previous results for other engineered tissues. For example, mechanical compression enhanced the synthesis of cartilaginous tissue matrix by chondrocytes cultured in agarose gels by amounts that increased as more matrix deposits occurred around the cells (133, 134). The effects of the same load can thus differ for different developmental stages of engineered ligaments and different regions within the same tissue sample.

In Femor et al. (67), a transition of cultured ACL fibroblasts from proliferation to collagen matrix synthesis occurred at days 7–9. Because of these findings and the data presented in Figure 4, in which we observed a 20-fold increase in collagen type I production in 14 days as well as upregulation of ligament specific markers, the development of structural and functional properties of engineered ligaments should be studied at 7-, 14-, and 28-day periods to gauge the time-dependent influences on proliferation (1 week), marker expression and differentiation (2 weeks), and the development of ligament integrity, structure, and function (4 weeks).

## SUMMARY

Tissue engineering is emerging as a significant clinical option to address tissue and organ failure by implanting biological substitutes of the compromised tissues. When compared to the transplantation of cells alone, engineered tissues offer the potential advantage of immediate functionality. The high incidence of ACL failures, lack of capacity for self-repair, and limitations of current treatment options have driven the research into ligament tissue engineering as a new option. An envisioned scenario of clinically relevant tissue engineering of ligaments involves the use of autologous cells, biodegradable scaffolds designed to serve as structural and logistic templates of tissue development, and bioreactors designed to control the cellular environment and provide the necessary biophysical regulatory signals. Engineered tissues can also serve as high-fidelity models for controlled studies of cell function and tissue development under normal and pathological conditions. We discussed the requirements for the ACL reconstruction, the available treatment options and their limitations, and focused on one advanced cell-scaffold-bioreactor system for tissue engineering of ligaments. When cultured on biomaterial scaffolds with architectural and mechanical properties resembling those of native ligaments, and with the application of dynamic loading, human bone marrow–derived mesenchymal stem cells were induced to assemble ligament-like tissue structures. The possibility of using biophysical regulatory signals to direct and modulate cell differentiation and tissue assembly can form a basis for tissue engineering of custom-designed, functional ligaments. However, a lot remains to be learned, and several risks and uncertainties surround the development of an autologous human tissue-engineered ACL. It is expected that coordinated in vitro and in vivo studies, involving the use of systems similar to those described in this article, will help define the exact conditions and duration of ligament cultivation for a clinically optimal outcome.

## ACKNOWLEDGMENT

The authors thank Dr. Paul Weitzel, Dr. Jingsong Chen, Jodie Moreau, Adam Collette, and Diah Bramono for their valuable contributions during the preparation of this article and Sue Kangiser for her expert help with manuscript preparation. Funding for the authors' studies of ligament tissue engineering has been provided by the NIH, NASA, NSF, and Tissue Regeneration, Inc.

**The *Annual Review of Biomedical Engineering* is online at http://bioeng.annualreviews.org**

## LITERATURE CITED

1. Woo SL-Y, Hildebrand K, Watanabe N, Fenwick JA, Papageorgiou CD, Wang JH. 1999. Tissue engineering of ligament and tendon healing. *Clin. Orthop. Relat. Res.* Oct. (367 Suppl.):S312–23
2. Pennisi E. 2002. Tending tender tendons. *Science* 295:1011
3. Albright JC, Carpenter JE, Graf BK, Richmond JC. 1999. Knee and leg: Soft-tissue trauma. In *Orthopaedic Knowledge Update 6*: Am. Acad. Orthop. Surg.
4. Fu FH, Bennett CH, Lattermann C, Menetrey J, Lattermann C. 1999. Current trends in anterior cruciate ligament reconstruction, part I. Biology and biomechanics of reconstruction. *Am. J. Sports Med.* 27: 821–30
5. Weitzel PP, Richmond JC, Altman GA, Calabro T, Kaplan DL. 2002. Future direction of the treatment of ACL ruptures. *Orthop. Clin. North Am.* 33:653–61
6. Jackson DW, Grood ES, Goldstein JD, Rosen MA, Kurzweil PR, et al. 1993. A comparison of patellar tendon autograft

and allograft used for anterior cruciate ligament reconstruction in the goat model. *Am. J. Sports Med.* 21:176–85

7. Noyes FR, Butler DL, Grood ES, Zernicke RF, Hefzy MS. 1984. Biomechanical analysis of human ligament grafts used in knee-ligament repairs and reconstructions. *J. Bone Jt. Surg.* 66:344–52
8. Woo SLY, Buckwalter JA, eds. 1988. *Injury and Repair of the Musculoskeletal Soft Tissues*, pp. 45–101. Park Ridge, IL: Am. Acad. Orthop. Surg.
9. Olson EJ, Kang JD, Fu FH, Georgescu HI, Mason GC, Evans CH. 1988. The biochemical and histological effects of artificial ligament wear particles: in vitro and in vivo studies. *Am. J. Sports Med.* 16:558–70
10. Richmond JC, Manseau CJ, Patz R, McConville O. 1992. Anterior cruciate reconstruction using a Dacron ligament prosthesis. A long-term study. *Am. J. Sports Med.* 20:24–28
11. Moyen BJ, Jenny J-Y, Mandrino AH, Lerat JL. 1992. Comparison of reconstruction of the anterior cruciate ligament with and without a Kennedy Ligament-Augmentation Device. *J. Bone Jt. Surg.* 74:1313–19
12. Amiel D, Billings E Jr, Akeson WH. 1990. Ligament structure, chemistry, and physiology. In *Knee Ligaments: Structure, Function, Injury, and Repair*, ed. DM Daniel, WH Akeson, JJ O'Connor, pp. 77–91. New York: Raven
13. Frank BC, Jackson DW. 1997. The science of reconstruction of the anterior cruciate ligament. *J. Bone Jt. Surg.* 79:1556–76
14. McCarthy DM, Tolin BS, Schwenderman L. 1993. *Anterior cruciate ligament: Current and future concepts*, pp. 343–56. New York: Raven
15. Weiss AB, Blazina ME, Goldstein AR, Alexander H. 1985. Ligament replacement with an absorbable copolymer carbon fiber scaffold–early clinical experience. *Clin. Orthop. Relat. Res.* 196:77–85
16. Markolf KL, Pattee GA, Strum GM, Gallick GS, Sherman OH, Dorey FJ. 1989. Instrumented measurements of laxity in patients who have a Gore-Tex anterior cruciate ligament substitute. *J. Bone Jt. Surg.* 71:887–93
17. Lopez-Vazquez E, Juan JA, Vila E, Debon J. 1991. Reconstruction of the anterior cruciate ligament with a Dacron prothesis. *J. Bone Jt. Surg.* 73:1294–300
18. Parsons JR, Bhayani S, Alexander H, Weiss AB. 1985. Carbon fiber debris within the synovial joint. A time-dependent mechanical and histological study. *Clin. Orthop. Relat. Res.* 196:69–76
19. Denti M, Arosio A, Monteleone M, Peretti G. 1990. Preliminary assessment of anterior cruciate reconstruction with the Leeds-Keio artificial ligament. *Am. J. Knee Surg.* 3:181–86
20. Kumar K, Maffulli N. 1999. The ligament augmentation device: an historical perspective. *Arthroscopy* 15:422–32
21. Woo SL-Y, Adams DJ. 1990. The tensile properties of human anterior cruciate ligament (ACL) and ACL graft tissues. See Ref. 135. pp. 279–89
22. Arnoczky S, Tarvin G, Marshall J. 1982. Anterior cruciate ligament replacement using patellar tendon. *J. Bone Jt. Surg.* 64A:217–24
23. Chen EH, Black J. 1980. Materials design analysis of the prosthetic anterior cruciate ligament. *J. Biomed. Mater. Res.* 14:567–86
24. Woo SL-Y, Hollis JM, Adams DJ, Lyon RM, Takai S. 1991. Tensile properties of human femur-anterior cruciate ligament-tibia complex: the effects of specimen age and orientation. *Am. J. Sports Med.* 19:217–25
25. Rauch G, Allzeit B, Gotzen L. 1987. *Tensile strength of the anterior cruciate ligament in dependence on age*. Presented at Proc. Eur. Soc. Biomech., Ulm, West Ger.
26. Noyes FR, Grood ES. 1976. The strength of the anterior cruciate ligament in

humans and Rhesus monkeys. *J. Bone Jt. Surg.* 58:1074–82
27. Woo SL-Y, Young E, Kwan M. 1990. Fundamental studies in knee ligament mechanics. See Ref. 135, pp. 115–34
28. Lo YY, Conquer JA, Grinstein S, Cruz TF. 1998. Interleukin-1 beta induction of c-fos and collagenase expression in articular chondrocytes: involvement of reactive oxygen species. *J. Cell. Biochem.* 69:19–29
29. Amiel D, Frank C, Harwood F, Fronek J, Akeson W. 1984. Tendons and ligaments: a morphological and biochemical comparison. *J. Orthop. Res.* 1:257–65
30. Arnoczky SP, Matyas JR, Buckwalter JA, Amiel D. 1993. Anatomy of the ACL. In *The Anterior Cruciate Ligament: Current and Future Concepts*, ed. DW Jackson, pp. 5–22. New York: Raven
31. Ross SM, Joshi R, Frank CB. 1990. Establishment and comparison of fibroblast cell lines from the medial collateral and anterior cruciate ligaments of the rabbit. *In Vitro Cell. Dev. B.* 26:579–84
32. Murray MM, Spector M. 1999. Fibroblast distribution in the anteromedial bundle of the human anterior cruciate ligament: the presence of alpha-smooth muscle actin-positive cells. *J. Orthop. Res.* 17:18–27
33. Mackie EJ, Ramsey S. 1996. Expression of tenascin in joint-associated tissues during development and postnatal growth. *J. Anat.* 188:157–65
34. Neurath MF, Stofft E. 1992. Structure and function of matrix components in the cruciate ligaments. An immunohistological, electron-microscopic, and immunoelectron-microscopic study. *Acta Anat.* 145:387–94
35. Neurath MF. 1993. Expression of tenascin, laminin and fibronectin following traumatic rupture of the anterior cruciate ligament. *Z. Ortho. Grenzgeb.* 131:168–72
36. Eckes B, Dogic D, Colucci-Guyon E, Wang N, Maniotis A, et al. 1998. Impaired mechanical stability, migration and contractile capacity in vimentin-deficient fibroblasts. *J. Cell Sci.* 111:1897–907
37. Toyoda T, Matsumoto H, Fujikawa K, Saito S, Inoue K. 1998. Tensile load and the metabolism of anterior cruciate ligament cells. *Clin. Orthop. Relat. Res.* 353:247–55
38. Chiquet M, Matthisson M, Koch M, Tannheimer M, Chiquet-Ehrisman R. 1996. Regulation of extracellular matix synthesis by mechanical stress. *Biochem. Cell Biol.* 74:737–44
39. Chiquet-Ehrismann R, Tannheimer M, Koch M, Brunner A, Spring J, et al. 1994. Tenascin-C expression by fibroblasts is elevated in stressed collagen gels. *J. Cell Biol.* 127:2093–101
40. Bramono DS, Richmond JC, Weitzel PP, Chernoff H, Martin I, et al. 2004. Characterization of mRNA levels for matrix molecules and proteases in ruptured human anterior cruciate ligaments utilizing quantitative real-time RT-PCR. *Int. Symp. Ligaments Tendons, 4th, San Francisco*, 4:34
41. Freed LE, Vunjak-Novakovic G. 2000. Tissue engineering bioreactors. See Ref. 136, pp. 143–56
42. Altman GH, Horan R, Martin I, Farhadi J, Stark P, et al. 2001. Cell differentiation by mechanical stress. *FASEB J.* 16:270–72
43. Butler DL, Goldstein SA, Guilak F. 2000. Functional tissue engineering: The role of biomechanics. *J. Biomech. Eng.* 122:570–75
44. Dunn MG, Tria AJ, Kato YP, Bechler JR, Ochner RS, et al. 1992. Anterior cruciate ligament reconstruction using a composite collagenous prosthesis. A biomechanical and histologic study in rabbits. *Am. J. Sports Med.* 20:507–15
45. Dunn MG, Liesch JB, Tiku ML, Zawadsky JP. 1995. Development of fibroblast-seeded ligament analogs for ACL reconstruction. *J. Biomed. Mater. Res.* 29: 1363–71
46. Dunn KJ, Perez-Polo JR, Wood TG. 1996. Rapid neurite formation in a human

cortical neuronal cell line. *Int. J. Dev. Neurosci.* 14:61–68

47. Young RG, Butler DL, Weber W, Caplan AI, Gordon SL, Fink DJ. 1998. Use of mesenchymal stem cells in a collagen matrix for Achilles tendon repair. *J. Orthop. Res.* 16:406–13
48. Goulet F, Germain L, Rancourt D, Caron C, Normand A, Auger FA. 1997. Tendons and ligaments. See Ref. 137, pp. 633–43
49. Kim BS, Nikolovski J, Bonadio J, Mooney DJ. 1999. Cyclic mechanical strain regulates the development of engineered smooth muscle tissue. *Nat. Biotechnol.* 17:979–83
50. Goulet F, Rancourt D, Cloutier R, Germain L, Poole AR, Auger FA. 2000. See Ref. 136, pp. 711–22
51. Langlier E, Rancourt D, Bouchard S, Lord C, Stevens P-P, et al. 1999. Cyclic traction machine for long-term culture of fibroblast-populated collagen gels. *Ann. Biomed. Eng.* 27:67–72
52. Altman GH, Lu HH, Horan RL, Calabro T, Ryder D, et al. 2002. Advanced bioreactor with controlled application of multi-dimensional strain for tissue engineering. *J. Biomech. Eng.* 124:742–49
53. Murray MM, Spector M, Martin SD. 2000. The migration of cells from the human anterior cruciate ligament explants into collagen-glycosaminoglycan scaffolds. *J. Orthop. Res.* 18:557–64
54. Bruder SP, Jaiswal N, Haynesworth SE. 1997. Growth kinetics, self-renewal, and the osteogenic potential of purified human mesenchymal stem cells during extensive subcultivation and following cryopreservation. *J. Cell. Biochem.* 64:278–94
55. Caplan AI, Bruder SP. 1997. Cell and molecular engineering of bone regeneration. See Ref. 137, pp. 603–17
56. Jaiswal N, Haynesworth SE, Caplan AI, Bruder SP. 1997. Osteogenic differentiation of purified, culture-expanded human mesenchymal stem cells in vitro. *J. Cell. Biochem.* 64:295–312
57. Ohgushi H, Caplan AI. 1999. Stem cell technology and bioceramics: from cell to gene engineering. *J. Biomed. Mater. Res.* 48:913–27
58. Simmons PJ, Torok-Storb B. 1991. CD34 expression by stromal precursors in normal human adult bone marrow. *Blood* 78:2848–53
59. Haynesworth SE, Reuben D, Caplan AI. 1998. Cell-based tissue engineering therapies: the influence of whole body physiology. *Adv. Drug Deliv. Rev.* 33:3–14
60. Turgeman G, Pittman DD, Muller R, Kurkalli BG, Zhou S, et al. 2001. Engineered human mesenchymal stem cells: a novel platform for skeletal cell mediated gene therapy. *J. Gene Med.* 3:240–51
61. Caplan AI. 1991. Mesenchymal stem cells. *J. Orthop. Res.* 9:641–50
62. Bruder SP, Jaiswal N. 1996. The osteogenic potential of human mesenchymal stem cells is not diminished after one billion-fold expansion in vitro. *Trans. Orthop. Res. Soc.* 21:580
63. Dennis JE, Merriam A, Awadallah A, Yoo JU, Johnstone B, Caplan AI. 1999. A quadripotential mesnchymal progenitor cell isolated from the marrow of an adult mouse. *J. Bone Miner. Res.* 14:700–9
64. Prockop DJ. 1997. Marrow stromal cells as stem cells for non-hematopoietic tissues. *Science* 276:71–74
65. Obradovic B, Carrier RL, Vunjak-Novakovic G, Freed LE. 1999. Gas exchange is essential for bioreactor cultivation of tissue engineered cartilage. *Biotechnol. Bioeng.* 63:197–205
66. Carrier RL, Papadaki M, Rupnick M, Schoen FJ, Bursac N, et al. 1999. Cardiac tissue engineering: cell seeding, cultivation parameters and tissue construct characterization. *Biotechnol. Bioeng.* 64:580–89
67. Fermor B, Urban J, Murray D, Pocock A, Lim E, et al. 1998. Proliferation and collagen synthesis of human ACL cells in vitro: effects of ascorbate-2-phosphate, dexamethasone and oxygen tension. *Cell Biol. Int.* 22:635–40

68. Murray MM, Rice K, Wright RJ, Spector M. 2003. The effect of selected growth factors on human anterior cruciate ligament cell interactions with a three-dimensional collagen-GAG scaffold. *J. Orthop. Res.* 21:238–44
69. Attisano L, Wrana JL. 2002. Signal transduction by the TGF-beta superfamily. *Science* 296:1646–47
70. Blakesley VA, Scrimgeour A, Esposito D, Le Roith D. 1996. Signaling via the insulin-like growth factor-I receptor: does it differ from insulin receptor signaling? *Cytokine Growth Factor Rev.* 7:153–59
71. Clemmons DR. 1997. Insulin-like growth factor binding proteins and their role in controlling IGF actions. *Cytokine Growth Factor Rev.* 8:45–62
72. Deie M, Marui T, Allen CR, Hildebrand KA, Georgescu HI, et al. 1997. The effects of age on rabbit MCL fibroblast matrix synthesis in response to TGF-beta 1 or EGF. *Mech. Ageing Dev.* 97:121–30
73. Lo IK, Marchuk L, Hart DA, Frank CB. 2003. Messenger ribonucleic acid levels in disrupted human anterior cruciate ligaments. *Clin. Orthop. Relat. Res.* Feb. (407):249–58
74. Marui T, Niyibizi C, Georgescu HI, Cao M, Kavalkovich KW, et al. 1997. Effect of growth factors on matrix synthesis by ligament fibroblasts. *J. Orthop. Res.* 15:18–23
75. Murakami S, Takayama S, Ikezawa K, Shimabukuro Y, Kitamura M, et al. 1999. Regeneration of periodontal tissues by basic fibroblast growth factor. *J. Periodontal Res.* 34:425–30
76. Sakai T, Yasuda K, Tohyama H, Azuma H, Nagumo A, et al. 2002. Effects of combined administration of transforming growth factor-beta1 and epidermal growth factor on properties of the in situ frozen anterior cruciate ligament in rabbits. *J. Orthop. Res.* 20:1345–51
77. Jin HJ, Chen J, Karageorgiou V, Altman GH, Kaplan DL. 2004. Human bone marrow stromal cell responses on electrospun silk fibroin mats. *Biomaterials* 25:1039–47
78. Scherping SC Jr, Schmidt CC, Georgescu HI, Kwoh CK, Evans CH, Woo SL. 1997. Effect of growth factors on the proliferation of ligament fibroblasts from skeletally mature rabbits. *Connect. Tissue Res.* 36:1–8
79. Trachslin J, Koch M, Chiquet M. 1999. Rapid and reversible regulation of collagen XII expression by changes in tensile stress. *Exp. Cell Res.* 247:320–28
80. Altman GH, Horan RL, Lu HH, Moreau J, Martin I, et al. 2002. Silk matrix for tissue engineered anterior cruciate ligaments. *Biomaterials* 23:4131–41
81. Bassett CAL, Herrmann I. 1961. Influence of oxygen concentration and mechanical factors on differentiation of connective tissues in vitro. *Nature* 190:460–61
82. Chu CR, Coutts RD, Yoshioka M, Harwood FL, Monosov AZ, Amiel D. 1995. Articular cartilage repair using allogeneic perichondrocyte-seeded biodegradable porous polylactic acid (PLA): a tissue-engineering study. *J. Biomed. Mater. Res.* 29:1147–54
83. Hunziker EB. 1999. Biologic repair of articular cartilage. Defect models in experimental animals and matrix requirements. *Clin. Orthop. Relat. Res.* 367(Suppl.): S135–46
84. Schaefer D, Martin I, Jundt G, Seidel J, Heberer M, et al. 2002. Tissue engineered composites for the repair of large osteochondral defects. *Arthritis Rheum.* 46:2524–34
85. Caplan AI, Elyaderani M, Mochizuki Y, Wakitani S, Goldberg VM. 1997. Principles of cartilage repair and regeneration. *Clin. Orthop. Relat. Res.* 342:254–69
86. Freed LE, Vunjak-Novakovic G, Biron R, Eagles D, Lesnoy D, et al. 1994. Biodegradable polymer scaffolds for tissue engineering. *Biotechnology* 12:689–93
87. Yannas IV. 2001. *Tissue and Organ*

*Regeneration in Adults*. New York: Springer-Verlag
88. Hubbell JA. 1995. Biomaterials in tissue engineering. *Biotechnology* 13:565–76
89. Hollinger JO, Brekke J, Gruskin E, Lee D. 1996. Role of bone substitutes. *Clin. Orthop. Relat. Res.* 324:55–65
90. Bennett S, Connolly K, Lee DR, Jiang Y, Buck D, et al. 1996. Initial biocompatibility studies of a novel degradable polymeric bone substitute that hardens in situ. *Bone* 19:S101–7
91. Attawia MA, Herbert KM, Laurencin CT. 1995. Osteoblast-like cell adherence and migration through 3-dimensional porous polymer matrices. *Biochem. Bioph. Res. Commun.* 213:639–44
92. Cook AD, Hrkach JS, Gao NN, Johnson IM, Pajvani UB, et al. 1997. Characterization and development of RGD-peptide-modified poly(lactic acid-co-lysine) as an interactive, resorbable biomaterial. *J. Biomed. Mater. Res.* 35:513–23
93. Kim KJ, Itoh T, Kotake S. 1997. Effects of recombinant human bone morphogenetic protein-2 on human bone marrow cells cultured with various biomaterials. *J. Biomed. Mater. Res.* 35:279–85
94. Gomi K, Davies JE. 1993. Guided bone tissue elaboration by osteogenic cells in vitro. *J. Biomed. Mater. Res.* 27:429–31
95. Callen BW, Sodhi RNS, Shelton RM, Davies JE. 1993. Behavior of primary bone cells on characterized polystyrene surfaces. *J. Biomed. Mater. Res.* 27:851–59
96. Rogers JJ, Young HE, Adkison LR, Lucas PA, Black AC. 1995. Differentiation factors induce expression of muscle, fat, cartilage, and bone in a clone of mouse pluriopotent mesenchymal stem cells. *Am. Surgeon* 61:231–36
97. Locklin RM, Williamson MC, Beresford JN, Triffitt JT, Owen ME. 1995. In vitro effects of growth factors and dexamethasone on rat marrow stromal cells. *Clin. Orthop. Relat. Res.* 313:27–35
98. Reddi AH. 1995. Bone morphogenetic proteins, bone marrow stromal cells, and mesenchymal stem cells: Maureen Owen revisited. *Clin. Orthop. Relat. Res.* 313:115–19
99. Reddi AH. 1998. Role of morphogenic proteins in skeletal tissue engineering and regeneration. *Nat. Biotechnol.* 16:247–52
100. Honda Y, Knutsen R, Strong DD, Sampath TK, Baylink DJ, Mohan S. 1997. Osteogenic protein-1 stimulates mRNA levels of BMP-6 and decreases mRNA levels of BMP-2 and -4 in human osteosarcoma cells. *Calcif. Tissue Int.* 60:297–301
101. Mason JM, Grande DA, Barcia M, Grant R, Pergolizzi RG, Breibart AS. 1998. Expression of human bone morphogenic protein 7 in primary rabbit periosteal cells: potential utility in gene therapy for osteochondral repair. *Gene Ther.* 5:1098–104
102. Lecanda F, Avioli LV, Cheng S-L. 1997. Regulation of bone matrix protein expression and induction of differentiation of human osteoblasts and human bone marrow stromal cells by bone morphogenetic protein-2. *J. Cell. Biochem.* 67:386–98
103. Martin I, Shastri VP, Padera RF, Yang J, Mackay AJ, et al. 2001. Selective differentiation of mammalian bone marrow stromal cells cultured on three-dimensional polymer foams. *J. Biomed. Mater. Res.* 55:229–35
104. Martin I, Padera RF, Vunjak-Novakovic G, Freed LE. 1998. In vitro differentiation of chick embryo bone marrow stromal cells into cartilaginous and bone-like tissues. *J. Orthop. Res.* 16:181–89
105. Pei M, Seidel J, Vunjak-Novakovic G, Freed LE. 2002. Growth factors for sequential cellular de- and re-differentiation in tissue engineering. *Biochem. Bioph. Res. Commun.* 294:149–54
106. Gooch KJ, Blunk T, Courter DL, Sieminski AL, Bursac PM, et al. 2001. IGF-I and mechanical environment interact to modulate engineered cartilage development. *Biochem. Bioph. Res. Commun.* 286:909–15
107. Massia SP, Hubbell JA. 1991. Human

endothelial cell interactions with surface-coupled adhesion peptides on a non-adhesive glass substrate and two polymeric biomaterials. *J. Biomed. Mater. Res.* 25:223–42
108. Ito Y, Liu SQ, Imanishi Y. 1991. Enhancement of cell growth on growth factor-immobilized polymer film. *Biomaterials* 12:449–53
109. Liu SQ, Ito Y, Imanishi Y. 1992. Cell growth on immobilized cell-growth factor; 4: interaction of fibroblast cells with insulin immobilized on poly(methyl methacrylate) membrane. *J. Biochem. Biophys. Methods* 25:139–48
110. Zheng J, Ito Y, Imanishi Y. 1994. Cell growth on immobilized cell-growth factor. *Biomaterials* 15:963–68
111. Laffargue P, Frayssinet P, Rtaimate M, Hildebrand HF, Marchandise X. 2000. Adsorption and release of insulin-like growth factor-I on porous tricalcium phosphate implant. *J. Biomed. Mater. Res.* 49:415–21
112. Lam XM, Duenas ET, Daugherty AL, Levin N, Cleland JL. 2000. Sustained release of recombinant human insulin-like growth factor-I for treatment of diabetes. *J. Control. Release* 67:281–92
113. Mann BK, Schmedlen RH, West JL. 2001. Tethered-TGF-b increases extracellular matrix production of vascular smooth muscle cells. *Biomaterials* 22:439–44
114. Kuhl PR, Griffith-Cima LG. 1996. Tethered epidermal growth factor as a paradigm for growth factor-induced stimulation from the solid phase. *Nat. Med.* 2:1022–27
115. Richardson TP, Peters MC, Ennett AB, Mooney DJ. 2001. Polymeric system for dual growth factor delivery. *Nat. Biotechnol.* 19:1029–34
116. Lee KY, Peters MC, Anderson KW, Mooney DJ. 2000. Controlled growth factor release from synthetic extracellular matrices. *Nature* 408:998–1000
117. Altman GH, Diaz F, Jakuba C, Calabro T, Horan R, et al. 2003. Silk-based biomaterials. *Biomaterials* 24:401–16
118. Sofia S, McCarthy MB, Gronowicz G, Kaplan DL. 2001. Functionalized silk-based biomaterials for bone formation. *J. Biomed. Mater. Res.* 54:139–48
119. Santin M, Motta A, Freddi G, Cannas M. 1999. In vitro evaluation of the inflammatory potential of the silk fibroin. *J. Biomed. Mater. Res.* 46:382–89
120. Inouye K, Kurokawa M, Nishikawa S, Tsukada M. 1998. Use of Bombyx mori silk fibroin as a substratum for cultivation of animal cells. *J. Biochem. Biophys. Methods* 37:159–64
121. Minoura N, Tsukada M, Nagura M. 1990. Physico-chemical properties of silk fibroin membrane as a biomaterial. *Biomaterials* 11:430–34
122. Hollander AP, Heathfield TF, Webber C, Iwata Y, Bourne R, et al. 1994. Increased damage to type II collagen in osteoarthritic articular cartilage detected by a new immunoassay. *J. Clin. Invest.* 93:1722–32
123. Wen CM, Ye ST, Zhou LX, Yu Y. 1990. Silk-induced asthma in children: a report of 64 cases. *Ann. Allergy* 65:375–78
124. Kurosaki S, Otsuka H, Kunitomo M, Koyama M, Pawankar R, Matumoto K. 1999. Fibroin allergy. IgE mediated hypersensitivity to silk suture materials. *Nippon Ika Daigaku Zasshi* 66:41–44
125. Lam KH, Nijenhuis AJ, Bartels H, Postema AR, Jonkman MF, et al. 1995. Reinforced poly(L-lactic acid) fibres as suture material. *J. Appl. Biomater.* 6:191–97
126. Rossitch E Jr, Bullard DE, Oakes WJ. 1987. Delayed foreign-body reaction to silk sutures in pediatric neurosurgical patients. *Childs Nerv. Syst.* 3:375–78
127. Soong HK, Kenyon KR. 1984. Adverse reactions to virgin silk sutures in cataract surgery. *Ophthalmology* 91:479–83
128. Bucknall TE, Teare L, Ellis H. 1983. The choice of a suture to close abdominal incisions. *Eur. Surg. Res.* 15:59–66

129. Greenwald D, Shumway S, Albear P, Gottlieb L. 1994. Mechanical comparison of 10 suture materials before and after in-vivo incubation. *J. Surg. Res.* 56:372–77
130. Salthouse TN, Matlaga BF, Wykoff MH. 1977. Comparative tissue response to six suture materials in rabbit cornea, sclera, and ocular muscle. *Am. J. Ophthalmol.* 84:224–33
131. Postlethwait R. 1969. Tissue reaction to surgical operation. In *Repair and Regeneration*, ed. J Dumphy, W Van Winkle, pp. 263–85. New York: McGraw-Hill
132. Asakura T, Demura M, Date T, Miyashita N, Ogawa K, Williamson MP. 1997. NMR study of silk I structure of Bombyx mori silk fibroin with N-15- and C-13-NMR chemical shift contour plots. *Biopolymers* 41:193–203
133. Buschmann MD, Gluzband YA, Grodzinsky AJ, Hunziker EB. 1995. Mechanical compression modulates matrix biosynthesis in chondrocyte/agarose culture. *J. Cell Sci.* 108:1497–508
134. Seidel JO, Pei M, Gray ML, Langer R, Freed LE, Vunjak-Novakovic G. 2004. Long-term culture of tissue engineered cartilage in a perfused chamber with mechanical stimulation. *Biorheology.* In press
135. Daniel D, Akeson W, O'Connor J, eds. 1990. *Knee Ligaments: Structure, Function, Injury, and Repair*. New York: Raven
136. Lanza RP, Langer R, Vacanti J, eds. 2000. *Principles of Tissue Engineering*. San Diego: Academic
137. Lanza RP, Langer R, Chick W, eds. 1997. *Principles of Tissue Engineering*. San Diego: Landes/Academic
138. Seliktar D, Black R, Vito R, Nerem R. 2000. Dynamic mechanical conditioning of collagen-gel blood vessel constructs induces remodeling in vitro. *Ann. Biomed. Eng.* 28:351–62
139. Niklason LE, Gao J, Abbot WM, Hirschi KK, Houser S, et al. 1999. Functional arteries grown *in vitro*. *Science* 284(5413):489–93
140. Buschmann MD, Kim Y, Wong M, Frank E, Hunziker E, Grodzinsky A. 1999. Stimulation of aggrecan synthesis in cartilage explants by cyclic loading is localized to regions of high interstitial fluid flow. *Arch. Biochem. Biophys.* 366(1):1–7
141. Sodian R, Lemke T, Loebe M, Hoerstrup S, Potapov E, et al. 2001. New pulsatile bioreactor for fabrication of tissue-engineered patches. *J. Biomed. Mater. Res.* 58:401–5
142. Morsiani E, Brogli M, Galavotti D, Bellini T, Ricci D, et al. 2001. Long-term expression of highly differentiated functions by isolated porcine hepatocytes perfused in a radial-flow bioreactor. *Artif. Organs* 25(9):740–48
143. Prenosil J, Villeneuve PE. 1998. Automated production of cultured epidermal autografts and sub-confluent epidermal autografts in a computer controlled bioreactor. *Biotech. Bioeng.* 59(6):679–83
144. Grodzinsky A, Levenston M, Jin M, Frank E. 2000. Cartilage tissue remodeling in response to mechanical forces. *Annu. Rev. Biomed. Eng.* 2:691–713

Annu. Rev. Biomed. Eng. 2004. 6:157–84
doi: 10.1146/annurev.bioeng.6.040803.140017

First published online as a Review in Advance on April 8, 2004

# ADVANCES IN HIGH-FIELD MAGNETIC RESONANCE IMAGING

Xiaoping Hu[1] and David G. Norris[2]
[1]*Coulter Department of Biomedical Engineering, Georgia Tech and Emory University, Atlanta, Georgia 30322; email: xhu@bme.emory.edu*
[2]*FC Donders Center for Cognitive Neuroimaging, Trigon, 6525 EK Nijmegen, The Netherlands; email: David.Norris@FCDonders.kun.nl*

■ **Abstract** Among advances in magnetic resonance imaging (MRI), the increase of the magnetic field strength is perhaps one of the most significant. The use of high magnetic fields for in vivo magnetic resonance is motivated by a number of considerations. Advantages are increases in signal-to-noise ratio, blood-oxygenation level–dependent contrast, and spectral resolution, while disadvantages include potential reduction of contrast in anatomic imaging owing to lengthening of $T_1$ and effects of susceptibility of high fields. To address these challenges, technical advances have been made in various aspects of MRI, allowing high-field MRI to provide exquisite morphological and functional details in clinical and research settings. This review provides an overview of technical issues and applications of high-field MRI.

CONTENTS



## INTRODUCTION

Magnetic resonance imaging (MRI) is one of the most significant developments in medical imaging in the twentieth century. Since its inception in the early 1970s (1), MRI has evolved into an indispensable modality for routine clinical diagnosis as well as a widely used tool for in vivo biomedical research. MRI is attractive in clinical medicine because it provides images with exquisite soft tissue contrast and it is completely noninvasive. Whereas in its early days MRI was used primarily for anatomic imaging, its role in biomedical research has expanded significantly in the past 15 years owing to its ability to provide physiological and functional measures. Even though MRI is becoming more and more mature, advances are still being made and are promising to further expand the utility of MRI to many previously unimaginable applications.

Throughout the history of MRI, its development has been intimately related to the increase of the strength of magnets used for in vivo magnetic resonance (MR). In fact, the past three decades have seen an approximately 700-fold rise (i.e., 0.015 T to 7 T) in the strength of magnets used for in vivo MR applicable to human studies. When MRI was in its infancy, magnetic fields for human use were on the order of 1/10 T or less. These early systems, made of mainly permanent or resistive magnets, dominated the market until the introduction of superconducting magnets, which pushed the field strength for clinical systems to the Tesla range and at the same time greatly improved the stability and homogeneity of the resultant magnetic field. The move toward higher fields continued in the past 15 years. Although 1.5 T systems were the state of the art for clinical imaging two decades ago, several experimental human systems with fields between 3 and 4 T were introduced and put to research use 15 years ago (2, 3). Despite initial doubts about the feasibility and utility of these systems in human subjects, it quickly became clear that high fields have benefits for a variety of applications, particularly functional brain imaging and spectroscopy.

Although the initial high-field research systems were not optimized and required highly trained individuals for their operation, advances in imaging hardware, physics, and software in the past decade have brought the high-field human MR systems into the main stream. At present, major MR manufacturers (General Electric, Siemens, and Phillips) have received clearance from the Food and Drug Administration (FDA) for marketing their whole-body 3 T systems. Around the globe, scores of 3 T systems, intended for both clinical and research applications, have been installed, with more than 100 additional 3 T systems being ordered or built. While 3 T is becoming the state of the art for clinical MRI, ultrahigh systems have been established for research in humans. These include a number of 7 T systems, with three systems operational or in the final stage of installation (one at the University of Minnesota operational since 1999, one at Massachusetts General Hospital, and one at the National Institutes of Health). Other systems are being ordered and systems above 7 T are the 8 T whole-body system operational at the Ohio State University since 1999 and a 9.4 Tesla system at the University of Illinois at Chicago.

In parallel with the increase in the magnetic field for human applications, the field strength used for small-animal research has also been rising. Two decades ago, the state-of-the-art system for animal research had a field strength of 2.0 T or 4.7 T. Today, the highest horizontal bore system for animal research is now at a field strength of 11.7 T, while 9.4 T systems are becoming the standard.

The impetus for this steady rise in the magnetic field is the anticipated increases in signal-to-noise ratio (SNR), blood oxygenation–dependent contrast, and spectral resolution. Such increases have been largely demonstrated experimentally and lead to significant improvement in both diagnostic imaging and biomedical research. Of course, the move toward higher field strength also comes with some technical issues. A major drawback of the high field is the increased radiofrequency (RF) field inhomogeneity (4–6), which arises from the reduced penetration and the shortened wavelength if studying protons. Other limitations include the increased RF power deposition (7) and increased susceptibility effects. Much progress has been made in addressing or circumventing these problems as well as in establishing applications at high fields. This review provides an overview of technical aspects and applications of high-field MRI.

# TECHNICAL ISSUES AND ADVANCES

## Magnetic Field

Access to high magnetic field strengths for biomedical MRI and spectroscopy has only been made possible by advances in design and construction of superconducting magnets. In this section, the properties of these magnets are summarized and safety aspects are examined.

DESIGN COST AND SITING It is generally true that as the main magnetic field strength of a magnet increases, so do its length, weight, stray field, and helium consumption. The first very high-field magnets installed, namely the 8 T, 80 cm system at Ohio State University and the 7 T, 90 cm system at the University of Minnesota, were over 3 m long, weighed approximately 30 tons, and stored approximately 80 MJ of energy. These magnets are both unshielded solenoids, whereas magnets of 3 T and less will tend to be self-shielded and of similar design to their lower-field counterparts. At lower fields it is easier to accommodate correction coils for the finite length of the main winding. As the field strength increases, either the length of the magnet has to increase or the homogeneity decreases. Helium consumption is determined largely by radiative loss mechanisms; therefore, helium consumption will increase with the surface area of the dewar. If magnet homogeneity is maintained in going from 1.5 T to 3 T, typical helium consumption is roughly doubled, the extent of the stray field is increased by approximately 50%, and the weight of the magnet alone is increased by a factor of more than two. The stray field of very high-field systems depends on the passive shielding that is installed, but the 5 Gauss line may not be expected to go under approximately 8 m axially and 3 m radially. The requirement to purchase and install a shield of several hundred tons imposes significant extra cost and severe siting limitations on these systems. However, it is expected that self-shielded 7 T systems will become available within a few years. An upper limit to $B_0$ for whole-body magnets is at approximately 11 T, above which the superconducting niobium titanium alloy approaches its critical field. Fields higher than 11 T depend on the use of niobium tin magnet wire, which is expensive and requires special care in winding, but can become available in future magnets.

SAFETY If the mundane but ever-present risk of projectiles is excluded from discussion with the self-evident remark that such dangers will generally increase with increasing $B_0$, then there are three areas that warrant consideration. Furthermore, it is prudent to note that devices that may be MR compatible at 1.5 T may no longer be at 3 T and higher.

*Electromagnetic and magnetohydrodynamic effects* All of the suggested mechanisms are related in some way to the Hall effect. First, it was postulated that the Lorentzian force exerted on current carriers could affect the action-potential propagation in myelinated nerve fibers and muscle tissue. However, it could be shown that even an external field of 24 T would only give a 10% reduction in nerve transmission velocity (8).

In a similar fashion, flowing ionic fluids, such as blood, or moving objects, where the velocity vector is perpendicular to that of the static magnetic field, will experience charge separation owing to Faraday's law, and hence the establishment of an electric field. Because this electric field will extend beyond the boundaries of the object in question, it is theoretically possible that a field generated in the aorta could result in cardiac fibrillation. It has been calculated that a static magnetic field of 5 T will only give a current density of approximately 100 mA $m^{-2}$ at the sinuatrial node (9), a value that is approximately 10% of the maximum current density occurring naturally.

The electric field caused by flow in the aorta can be detected by electrocardiogram (ECG) monitoring. The flow in the aorta is at its greatest during the T-wave of the ECG. The ECG trace will be distorted at this time, giving the well-known phenomenon of T-wave swell. This is of course a purely transitory effect and the ECG trace returns to normal as soon as the subject leaves the external field. However, this phenomenon makes it extremely difficult to obtain high-quality ECGs with increasing field.

In the process of charge separation, a current will flow until the electrical field resulting from the charge accumulation is sufficiently strong to prevent it. This current produces a retarding force that opposes the direction of flow. The cardiac system will hence have to perform additional work in order to overcome this force. However, precise analytical calculations have shown that even for an external field of 10 T, the increase in vascular pressure is less than 0.2% (10). The practical effect of these forces in major blood vessels can consequently be neglected.

Therefore, there will be no significant effects on the cardiovascular system for exposures to static magnetic fields up to the maximum values currently available.

*Transient phenomena* A number of transient phenomena were reported for human subjects in the first 4 T whole-body systems, including vertigo, difficulty in balancing after leaving the magnet, nausea, headache, numbness or tingling, magnetophosphenes, and an unusual metallic taste in the mouth (11, 12). Of these, vertigo, nausea, magnetophosphenes, and the metallic taste have been linked to the presence of the magnetic field. The presence of headache and numbness or tingling was not statistically significant in this study. All of these effects disappear rapidly upon leaving the field. The first two of these have been postulated to arise from magnetohydrodynamic forces within the inner ear. Motion of the head within a magnetic field gives rise to magnetohydrodynamic forces that are misinterpreted by the brain as arising from an angular rotation. This conflicts with the information received from the visual system, giving rise to similar effects as those found in travel sickness.

Magnetophosphenes are generally only observed in conditions of darkness during which the eyes are rapidly moved. In this situation, faint light flashes are seen. The phenomenon is caused by the diamagnetism of the retinal rods, which when rotated experience a slight torque that is responsible for the illusory stimulation (13). Similar effects can be expected for both dia- and paramagnetic objects. However, in most situations in vivo, the forces causing an alignment with the main magnetic field are insufficient to overcome the viscosity of the medium.

The metallic-taste phenomenon is also associated with movement in the magnetic field; the mechanism for this is believed to be electrical currents that are introduced on the surface of the tongue.

*Lack of carcinogenic effect* One natural concern is that the static main field may have a carcinogenic effect. A number of studies have been conducted that have examined a range of potential carcinogenic effects. Chromosome aberrations could not be detected in human lymphocytes exposed to fields of up to 1 T (14), nor could mutations be observed in cultured mammalian cells (15). The embryonic development of frogs was not affected even by exposure to an 8 T field (16). In conclusion, no convincing evidence exists that a static magnetic field in isolation has a carcinogenic effect.

## RF Field

At main magnetic field strengths higher than approximately 3 T, quasistatic solutions (17) may no longer be employed, and the propagation of the magnetic field through the object has to be considered. The strength and phase of the $\mathbf{B}_1$ field vary as a function of position within the object and are determined by its form, permittivity, and conductivity. Analytical solutions are difficult to obtain even for simple geometrical configurations (18), and realistic situations can only be modeled numerically, for example, using the finite difference time domain method (7). Using experimental results and theoretical work, we examine in this section the main RF characteristics for this complex situation.

SENSITIVITY The sensitivity increases in a linear fashion with increasing main-field strength (19). This is unequivocally true for main magnetic field strengths up to approximately 3 T. However, at higher field strengths the problem is complicated by the inhomogeneity in the $B_1$ field that makes the gain in sensitivity position dependent. In a comparison between 4 T and 7 T brain imaging, an average increase of 1.76 in SNR was recorded (5) in near perfect accordance with direct proportionality. However, significant regional variations of 1.3–2.0 were recorded in this study.

POWER DEPOSITION In accordance with theoretical calculations (20, 21), the square-law dependence of RF-power on field strength is weakened at higher field strengths at above approximately 200 MHz. The reduction in the rate of increase in the required RF-power with $B_0$ has been confirmed experimentally (5, 22). The increase in RF-power requirement is not as steep as may have been expected: For example, it increases by a factor of approximately 1.8 in going from 4 T to 7 T (5), rather than the factor of 3 predicted by the standard square-law. However, this still represents a significant restriction for many pulse sequences, particularly those relying on multiple refocusing RF pulses.

$B_1$ HOMOGENEITY From 3 T upward, head images are generally characterized by a hyper intense region at the center of the image (5, 23, 24), as shown in Figure 1. This originates from the dielectric properties of brain tissue; for example, an oil-filled phantom will give a homogeneous image. The effect has been termed field focusing (18) and is distinct from true dielectric resonances, which are now generally believed to be unsustainable in the human head (4, 25) owing to the conductivity of brain tissue and the geometry of the boundaries between regions of differing electrical properties. With some pulse sequences, quite significant variations in signal intensity can be found across the image, and it is not to be expected that these can be corrected by improved coil design.

PARALLEL IMAGING The use of multiple radio frequency receiver coils to independently encode spatial information has proven to be one of the major technological advances of recent years. In the SMASH (simultaneous acquisition of spatial harmonics) family of methods (26) the additional information from the receiver coils is used to complete the data set in *k*-space, whereas in the SENSE (sensitivity encoding)-based approaches (27) linear algebra in the image domain is used to the same effect. These techniques are capable of accelerating data acquisition by a factor of approximately two to three at 1.5 T, which gives a corresponding reduction in the echo train length for fast imaging experiments. In EPI (echo planar imaging), this results in a significant reduction in the degree of distortion, whereas for RARE/FSE/TSE (rapid acquisition with relaxation enhancement/fast spin echo/turbo spin echo) sequences, the main advantage is a reduction in radiofrequency power deposition. Theoretical considerations have shown (28) that the maximum acceleration factor consistent with an acceptable SNR increases linearly with main magnetic field strength, implying that if the technical limitations of constructing multiple receiver coils at very high field strength can be overcome, many of the problems that currently beset fast imaging sequences can be resolved.

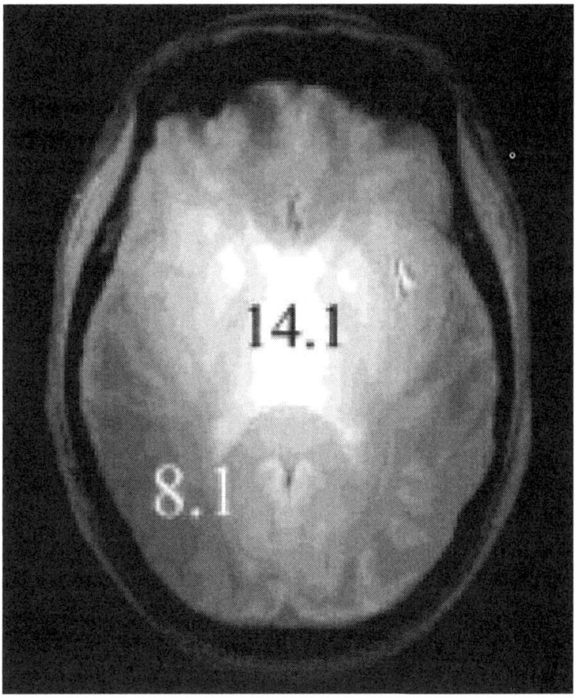


**Figure 1** $B_1$ inhomogeneity at 7 T. The image was obtained using a gradient echo sequence and a homogeneous TEM (transverse electromagnetic) transmission coil. The pulse angle was calibrated to give a 90° pulse at the center of the image. Adapted from figure 5 of Reference 5 with permission of the authors.

## Gradient Field

In MRI, spatial encoding is achieved with magnetic field gradients. Higher magnetic fields demand higher gradient performance and lead to louder acoustic noise associated with gradient switching. These aspects related to gradients are discussed below.

PERFORMANCE Magnetic field gradient performance is, of course, independent of the main magnetic field strength employed. However, the point spread function in both EPI and RARE/FSE is determined by the degree of signal relaxation during the echo train. As $T_2$, and more critically $T_2^*$, shorten appreciably with increasing $B_0$, the demands placed on magnetic field gradient performance increase accordingly. During the past fifteen years magnetic field gradient systems have been rapidly advanced, so that the current generation of whole-body systems is capable of delivering gradient strengths in excess of 40 mT $m^{-1}$ at magnetic field switching rates of approximately 200 T $s^{-1}$. Since the development of self-shielded magnetic field gradients (29, 30), there has been incremental progress in gradient design, and for many years gradient performance was limited by the availability of suitable power supplies, which were required to deliver voltages of the order of 1 kV and currents of approximately 500 A. Progress has been achieved by a combination of improved power supplies and the willingness of some manufacturers to sacrifice gradient linearity in the interest of more rapid switching: The nonlinearity is then corrected in the image reconstruction program. The performance of whole-body gradient sets is now more restricted by the limitations of physiological stimulation than by technical constraints. More rapid switching rates may be attained by the use of smaller gradient sets, for example, in head-only systems. The potential for muscle stimulation and the level of acoustic noise are issues that are now relevant for investigations with many systems.

PHYSIOLOGICAL LIMITATIONS There was considerable concern as NMR imaging was being developed that the electric field induced as a result of Faraday's law could produce not only stimulation of muscle but also stimulate the myocardium with potentially lethal consequences. The exact mechanism by which the electrical field in the body is induced is open to some discussion. The overwhelming majority of workers in the field consider inductive mechanisms to be responsible. However, surface charge accumulation (31) and capacitative coupling between the subject and the gradient coil (32) have also been invoked.

The dependence of the threshold on the duration of the stimulus is of some interest. It was found that for short stimulations, the threshold depends only on the absolute value of the magnetic field reached and not on the switching time, whereas for longer stimulations, the latter is also important. It was shown by Irnich & Schmitt (33) that the hyperbolic form first proposed by Lapicque (34) was appropriate and could provide a good fit to the experimental data of Budinger et al. (35) and to that of Mansfield & Harvey (32).

Fortunately, the threshold for muscle stimulation lies well below that for stimulating the myocardium, so even magnetic field switching, which is sufficient to cause painful muscle stimulation, is unlikely to have serious consequences. In the United States, the latest recommendation of the FDA is that gradient switching should not result in "severe discomfort or painful nerve stimulation" (FDA guidance from July 2003 http://www.fda.gov/cdrh/ode/guidance/793.pdf).

ACOUSTIC NOISE Current-carrying conductors in a magnetic field B will experience a force that is given by

$$F = I \oint d_1 \times B.$$

In the case of magnetic field gradients, these forces can be considerable, and as the equation shows, will increase in proportion to the main magnetic field strength. The current carriers are embedded in a solid matrix, so changes in the strength of current will lead to compressive waves in the matrix and hence to sound waves. EPI in particular can produce sound levels well in excess of 100 dB(A), and indeed at 3 T, values as high as 132 dB(A) have been reported (35). Various strategies have been proposed for reducing the sound level, including acoustic liners, active noise cancellation, and modifications to the gradient design (36, 37). Apart from the simple use of ear plugs and headphones, none of these has enjoyed widespread use; although, recent reports indicate that Toshiba has developed a very low-noise gradient set by vacuum sealing the gradient coil.

## Imaging Contrast and Quality

An increase in main magnetic field strength implies not only an increase in sensitivity, but also for many experiments a change in contrast. In this section, the nature of the contrast changes and the consequences for experimental design are examined.

RELAXATION TIME CHANGES As the main magnetic field increases, $T_1$ for different tissue types lengthens and converges, whereas $T_2$ and $T_2^*$ get shorter. Consequently, repetition times get longer and acquisition bandwidths have to increase. Currently, no $T_1$ values have been reported at very high fields, but measurements have been performed at 4 T (23, 39, 40), 3 T (41), and numerous studies at 1.5 T. The experimental values for gray matter $T_1$ as a function of Larmor frequency should be predicted by the empirical formula of Fischer et al. (42). This equation has the form

$$\frac{1}{T_1} = \frac{1}{T_{1w}} + D + \frac{A}{1 + (f/f_c)^{\beta}},$$

where $f$ is the Larmor frequency, $T_{1w}$ is the relaxation time of pure water, $D$ the baseline, $A$ is the height of the dispersion, $f_c$ the inflection frequency, and $\beta$ a parameter reflecting the steepness of the dispersion step. A good agreement is indeed found for the values given in table 2 of Fischer et al. (42) of $T_{1w} = 4.35$ s, $D = 0.105\ s^{-1}$, $A = 11.66\ s^{-1}$, $f_c = 0.059$ MHz, and $\beta = 0.42$. This equation predicts gray matter $T_1$ values of approximately 1.5 s at 7 and 8 T. However, any expectation that the difference in $T_1$ values between white and gray matter would become negligible has not been supported by experience (see below). For many experiments, it is also of relevance that the $T_1$ of arterial blood lengthens appreciably with increasing main magnetic field strength.

The presence of paramagnetic deoxyhemoglobin in the venous compartment ensures that brain tissue has an intrinsic $T_2^*$ value independent of any macroscopic gradients ascribable to bulk susceptibility gradients or imperfections of the main field. The strength of these susceptibility induced gradients is proportional to $\mathbf{B}_0$. It is, however, important to note that the $T_2^*$ values fall more slowly than if they were inversely proportional to $\mathbf{B}_0$.

The standard Bloemberg, Purcell, and Pound theory of relaxation does not predict any field strength dependency of $T_2$. However, possibilities of cross-relaxation with macromolecules and chemical exchange (43), as well as of dynamic averaging, exist (40), all of which show a dependence on field strength. The dynamic averaging effect occurs because of the motion of the water in the same static gradients that are responsible for $T_2^*$ relaxation. As the susceptibility gradients increase linearly in strength with the main magnetic field and the diffusion term responsible for dynamic averaging scales with the second power of the gradient strength, this effect will increase with $\mathbf{B}_0^2$. It was recently shown that dynamic averaging represents the dominant $T_2$ relaxation mechanism for water at 7 T (44); therefore, a further rapid reduction in $T_2$ can be expected at even higher field strengths.

The deoxyhemoglobin in venous blood causes a strong dependency of $T_2$ on $\mathbf{B}_0$. The mechanism for this is the rapid exchange of water between the erythrocytes and the surrounding plasma, which, owing to the presence of deoxyhemoglobin, have markedly different susceptibilities (45). Experimental values of $T_2$ are 109 ms (46) and 180 ms (47) at 1.5 T, 20 ms at 4 T, and 6.7 ms at 7 T (48). Thus, the shortening of $T_2$ becomes significant at the highest field strengths of 7 T and higher.

IMPLICATIONS FOR SEQUENCE DESIGN The main contrasts for anatomical imaging are based on the $T_1$ and $T_2$ relaxation parameters. The lengthening and converging of $T_1$ relaxation times of various tissues diminishes $T_1$ contrast. The short TR, short TE spin-echo and the high flip angle FLASH (fast low angle shot)-type sequences, both commonly used to obtain $T_1$ contrast at lower $\mathbf{B}_0$, become progressively less effective, so magnetization-prepared sequences are essential. Apart from the classical saturation- and inversion-recovery sequences, attention should also be paid to the MDEFT (modified driven equilibrium Fourier transform) sequence [90°-$\tau$-180°-$\tau$-(49)], which offers a contrast intermediate between that of the other two and is insensitive to inhomogeneities in the $B_1$ field. Despite the somewhat lower contrast, the advantages of MDEFT are that no negative longitudinal magnetization is generated and that the repetition time can be made shorter than for inversion recovery. This makes the acquisition of three-dimensional (3-D) and multi-slice two-dimensional (2-D) images possible within acceptable durations. The use of multiple adiabatic inversion pulses for multi-slice $T_1$-weighted imaging can cause problems of power deposition, but methods have recently been developed by which it is possible to share a single inversion pulse between multiple slices that have the same contrast (50), allowing multi-slice acquisition even at 8 T (51).

Time-of-flight (TOF) angiography clearly benefits from high $\mathbf{B}_0$. The primary reason for this is the prolonged $T_1$ of tissue, which increases the contrast with inflowing blood. Combined with the general increase in sensitivity and the possibility of further suppressing stationary tissue with MTC (magnetization transfer contrast) without encountering problems of power deposition, at least up to a $\mathbf{B}_0$ of 3 T (52), a significant improvement in the sensitivity of TOF angiography in going from 1.5 T to 3 T can be expected.

The application of arterial spin labeling (ASL) techniques benefits from increased $\mathbf{B}_0$ for much the same reason that TOF angiography does. In a detailed comparison between 1.5 T and 4 T, Wang et al. (53) have shown that significant benefits accrue for pulsed and continuous ASL techniques at higher $\mathbf{B}_0$ values: Up to approximately 4 T, the sensitivity scales directly with $\mathbf{B}_0$; above 4 T, the slope of the curve is lower because of the effect of shortened $T_2^*$ values on the sensitivity. Experimental results agreed with the theoretical predictions.

The essential characteristic of single-shot EPI is that the echo train length is limited by $T_2^*$, which will generally vary locally. With present-day gradient technology, even at 3 T the spatial resolution is limited by $T_2^*$ effects rather than sensitivity. Indeed, at field strengths of 7 T and higher, whole-brain coverage with single-shot EPI has so far not been achieved. At 3 T, gradient-echo EPI images of the brain show marked signal voids in the inferior regions. Apart from the direct effects of susceptibility gradients [signal voids in gradient-echo EPI, shearing, scaling, and shifting (54)] motion can affect the signal intensity in $T_2^*$-weighted sequences by modifying the pattern of susceptibility gradient within the image: an effect that obviously increases with $\mathbf{B}_0$.

Following the initial suggestion of Cho et al. (55), MR venographic methods are based on the susceptibility difference between venous blood and surrounding tissue. The original suggestion of using tailored RF pulses to selectively excite venous blood has been supplanted by the simpler approach of using a long TE (echo time) gradient echo image, with the TE tailored to give the maximum contrast. The strength of the contrast will increase linearly with $\mathbf{B}_0$, and the optimum echo time should correspondingly decrease linearly with $\mathbf{B}_0$, which is in accordance with experimental results obtained in going from 1.5 to 3 T (56). The contrast is generally enhanced by utilizing the phase information to provide a phase-mask with which the magnitude data are multiplied. Venograms are then obtained by minimum-intensity projection over a number of slices, as shown in Figure 2. At 8 T, single-slice data shows strong effects from venous structures, and by using very high spatial resolution, vessels with a diameter of as little as 100 $\mu$m may become visible (57). Such techniques may have value in identifying draining veins in functional MRI (fMRI) and in assessing tumor malignancy (58).

FSE or RARE (59) already starts to encounter problems of RF power deposition at 3 T. As mentioned above, parallel imaging offers immediate and dramatic reductions in power deposition. This technology may further be combined with methods of varying the refocusing angle throughout the sequence that reduce power deposition significantly (60, 61) without necessarily reducing sensitivity (62). Even the simple expedient of reducing the refocusing pulse angle (63) has allowed RARE imaging at 8 T (64). Despite these difficulties, an improvement in SNR can be obtained in going from 1.5 T to 3 T, as shown in Figure 3, which shows FSE images obtained with similar parameters at these two field strengths.

# APPLICATIONS

## Functional MRI

fMRI is a revolutionary development of the past decade that makes it possible to use MRI to noninvasively map areas of increased neuronal activity in the human brain without the use of an exogenous contrast agent (65–67). The main technique for mapping brain function with MRI is based on the blood oxygenation

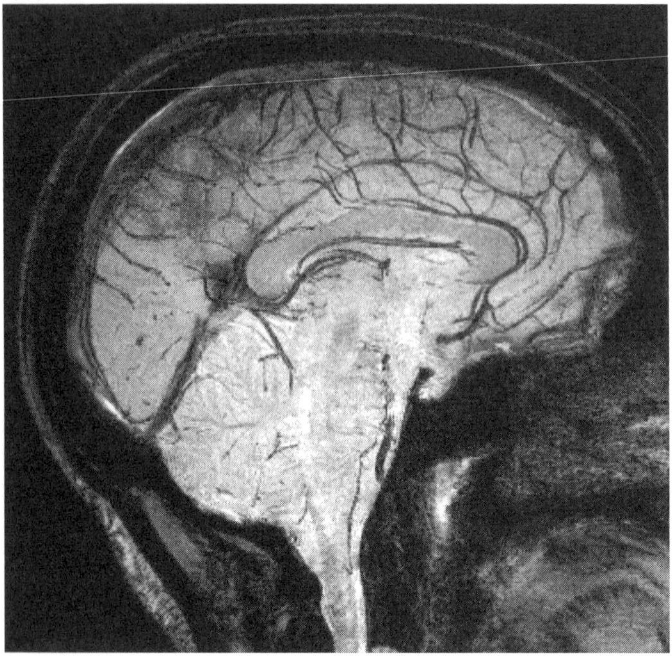

**Figure 2** Minimum intensity projection venogram obtained using a gradient echo sequence emphasizing susceptibility weighting. Image courtesy: Markus Barth, Alexander Rauscher, and Jürgen Reichenbach of the University of Vienna.

level–dependent (BOLD) contrast (68–70), which is derived from the fact that deoxyhemoglobin is paramagnetic, and changes in the local concentration of deoxyhemoglobin within the brain lead to alterations in the MR signal. Neuronal activation induces an increase in regional blood flow without a commensurate increase in the regional oxygen consumption rate ($CMR_{O_2}$) (71), such that the amount of oxygenated blood that is delivered to the tissue is greater than the oxygen extracted by the activated neurons. The net effect is a local increase in oxyhemoglobin and a local decrease in deoxyhemoglobin. Consequently, the decrease in paragmatic hemoglobin leads to an increase in $T_2^*$ and $T_2$ and a subsequent elevation of intensity in $T_2^*$- and $T_2$-weighted MR images. Therefore, to map neuronal function, $T_2^*$- or $T_2$-weighted images are acquired consecutively while the subject either rests or performs the function and the difference between the resting condition and performing the brain function is calculated.

For fMRI, it is desirable to have a high magnetic field because both the sensitivity and specificity increase with the magnetic field. In fact, the desire to improve the sensitivity and specificity of fMRI has been a major force driving the move toward higher and higher magnetic fields for in vivo MR. It is generally accepted that the SNR itself in MR images scales linearly with the field strength (72). Furthermore,

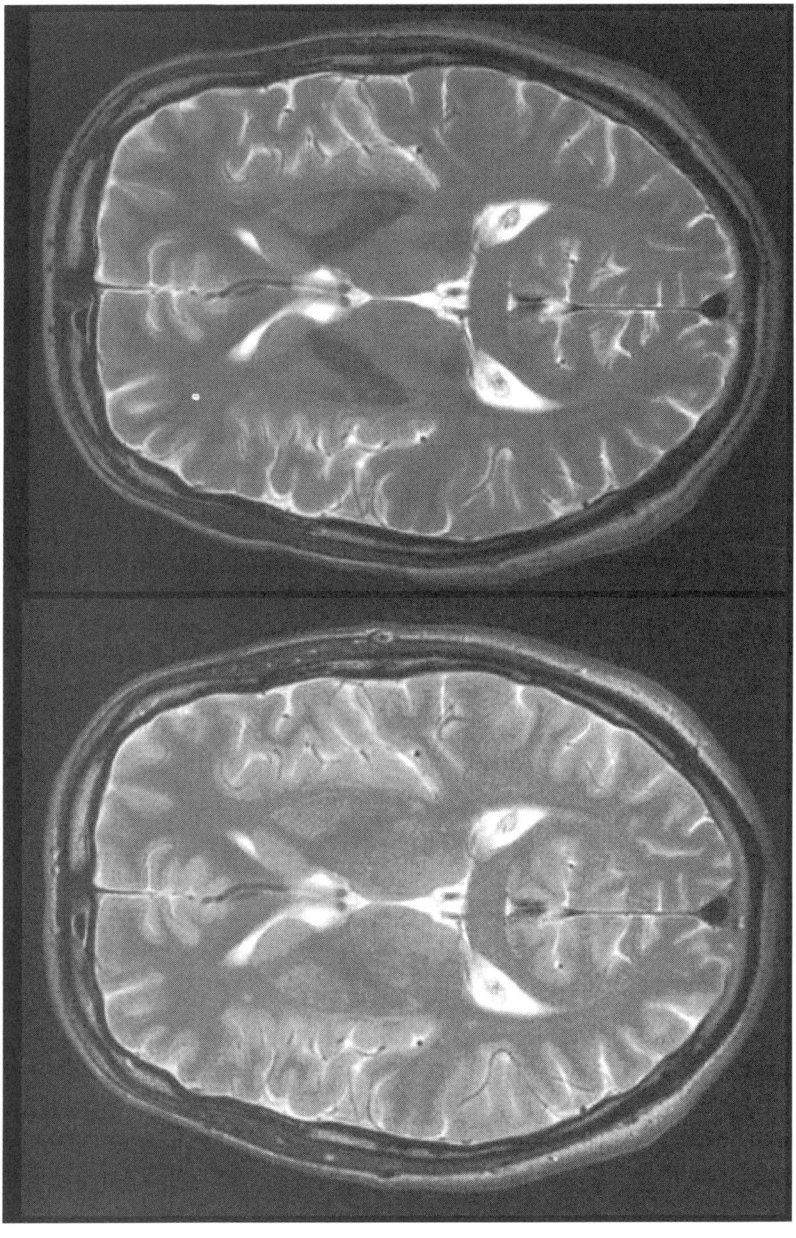

**Figure 3** FSE images obtained with a turbo factor of 9, FOV of 23 cm, slice thickness 4 mm, and TE of 81 ms (1.5 T, *left image*) and 88 ms (3 T). The data matrix was 512 × 384.

as a susceptibility phenomenon, BOLD contrast is expected to increase with field strength. In fact, theoretical considerations have revealed that the BOLD contrast increases supralinearly with the field strength, depending on contributions from static and dynamic averaging (73). Because both the raw SNR and the BOLD contrast increase with the field strength, the sensitivity of fMRI goes up with the field strength more than quadratically, despite a shortening in transverse relaxation times ($T_2$ and $T_2^*$) at high fields, as mentioned in the previous section. This has been experimentally demonstrated up to 7 T in humans (48, 74, 75). An example of this field dependence taken from a study comparing $T_2^*$-weighted fMRI at 4 T and 7 T (48) is illustrated in Figure 4 (see color insert). Except for the field strength, the imaging parameters and statistical methods used to obtain these maps were virtually identical, permitting a direct comparison of sensitivity. As can be seen in Figure 4, the active area seen at 7 T is much larger than that seen at 4 T as a result of increased sensitivity. A quantitative analysis by the authors (48) indicated that in the brain tissue, the BOLD contrast, quantified by $R_2^*$ ($= 1/T_2^*$) change, increased by a factor of two when going from 4 T to 7 T, clearly indicating a supralinear field dependence of the BOLD contrast. When noise is taken into account, a detailed study examining BOLD response in the motor area (74) revealed that the contrast-to-noise ratio (CNR) at 3.0 T is 1.8–2.2 times that at 1.5 T.

The increase in the sensitivity at high fields has been exploited to improve spatial resolution or temporal resolution or both (76). Several studies have used 4 T magnets to elucidate the columnar organization in the visual cortex in human subjects (77, 78). Another study (79) examined the fusiform face area using a shape from motion paradigm and demonstrated that the sensitivity (and specificity) available at 7 Tesla made it possible to reveal a spatial gradient in the response, which was otherwise undetectable at 1.5 T. More interestingly, a recent study of the rat sematosensory cortex performed at 11.7 T (80) has illustrated the ability of high-field fMRI in providing a map of layer-specific structure. An example of this layer-specific response, taken from the work of Silva et al. (80), is shown in Figure 5 (see color insert).

The high sensitivity of high-field fMRI has also been employed to study the temporal characteristics of the BOLD response. At 4 T, fMRI was used in one of first studies of event-related fMRI, exhibiting fMRI's ability to differentiate brain regions based their responses' temporal characteristics (81). In a true single-trial experiment at 4 T (82), the ability of fMRI to detect temporal information in individual trials, permitting the direct correlation with corresponding behavioral response, was demonstrated. Another interesting aspect of high-field fMRI is the detection of the initial dip (83–87), which is believed to arise from an initial increase in deoxyhemoglobin concentration before the hemodynamic response takes place and be more specific to the site of neuronal activation than the hyperemic BOLD response.

An elegant application of event-related fMRI, which relied on the increased sensitivity of high fields, was recently introduced by Ogawa et al. (88) using an ingenious design of the stimulation paradigm. The idea was to space two stimuli closely together in time, measure the BOLD response to the second stimulus, and monitor how that response changes with the interstimulus delay. Any effect of the first stimulus on the second stimulus, which may result owing to neuronal interaction, can be gauged at a timescale determined by the interstimulus delay (in millisecond range) rather than dictated by the hemodynamic response.

In addition to increase of the SNR and the BOLD contrast with the magnetic field strength, the dependence on the magnetic field is also a function of the size of the vessels contributing to the BOLD signal. Large vessel contributions scale linearly with the field, whereas small vessel contributions scale quadratically with the field strength. Consequently, microvascular contributions become more accentuated at high fields owing to its quadratic dependence on $\mathbf{B}_0$. This improves the spatial specificity of BOLD-based fMRI because capillaries are uniformly distributed in tissue and sufficiently high in density and close to the site of neuronal activation, whereas large vessels are not uniformly distributed and may be spatially removed from the activation. Although such an increase in sensitivity is present in $T_2^*$-weighted fMRI data as shown in Figure 4, this increase in sensitivity becomes more dramatic in $T_2$-weighted fMRI images, as discussed below.

$T_2^*$-based BOLD signals can arise from both intravascular and extravascular effects originating from large and small blood vessels. In a $T_2$-based BOLD fMRI map, the signal changes come from (*a*) intravascular blood $T_2$ changes from large and small blood vessels and (*b*) extravascular effect associated only with microvessels (capillaries and small postcapillary venules). Thus, extravascular BOLD effect in a $T_2$ image can only arise from the microvasculature, whereas in $T_2^*$ images it can originate from blood vessels of all sizes. It is often suggested that $T_2$-based fMRI avoids large vessel contribution. This claim is not strictly correct because it ignores the intravascular BOLD effect associated with changes in blood $T_2$. Such blood contribution can originate from large and small blood vessels. Fortuitously, at very high fields, e.g., 9.4 T and possibly 7 T, $T_2$-based BOLD fMRI may be largely associated with the capillaries because intravascular blood contributions are attenuated by the very short $T_2$ of blood (89, 90). Because large vessel contribution in $T_2$-weighted fMRI is mainly intravascular, it can be readily suppressed with diffusion gradients. This point has been demonstrated by several studies at high fields ranging from 4 to 9.4 T (90–92). An example of $T_2$-weighted functional map of the visual cortex obtained at 7 T in a human subject is shown in Figure 6 (see color insert). As can be seen, the activation is virtually restricted to the gray matter. It is also interesting to note that the $T_2$-BOLD contrast available at 7 T is sufficiently robust, allowing high-quality, high-resolution functional mapping.

## Clinical Applications

Whereas high-field systems for routine clinical applications have been available only for a few years, their potential in the clinical arena has already been extensively explored in conjunction with the technical development described in the previous section. Of particular interest to the clinical community is the increase in the SNR, which can be exploited either to improve the image quality, to shorten acquisition time, or to increase spatial resolution. The increase in SNR can lead to drastic improvement in image quality, as shown in Figure 7, where images of standard contrasts obtained at 1.5 T and 3.0 T are shown. In the following paragraphs, we highlight a few clinically relevant applications that have benefited from the availability of high fields.

In MRI, blood vessels can be imaged with MR angiography (MRA). One well-established approach is the TOF technique, which derives the vessel contrast based on the shortening of the effective $T_1$ of moving blood. In these types of images, vessels appear brighter than the background. High field provides an SNR advantage as well as a contrast advantage because it lengthens the $T_1$ of the stationary tissue (93). A remarkable example of improved MRA is shown in Figure 8, where 3-D TOF images obtained at 1.5 T and 3 T are compared. The 3 T images not only exhibit a substantial increase in the SNR but also an increase in the vessel contrast, allowing enhanced visualization of small vessels. Several systematic studies comparing MRA at 1.5 T and 3.0 T have been reported (93, 94). In the study performed by Bernstein et al. (94), a 3.0 T 3-D TOF intracranial imaging protocol with higher-order autoshimming was compared to a 1.5 T 3-D TOF protocol in 12 patients having cerebral aneurysms. According to rating by two radiologists, 3.0 T images are significantly better ($P < 0.001$) for visualizing the aneurysms. The same study also examined the feasibility of contrast-enhanced MRA at 3.0 T for cervical and intracranial examinations and found that 3.0 T is a favorable field strength for cervical contrast-enhanced MRA. Specifically, a high spatial resolution corresponding to a voxel volume of 0.62–0.73 $mm^3$ were readily achieved at 3.0 T, allowing the visualization of intracranial aneurysms, carotid dissections, and atherosclerotic disease, including ulcerations. Another study compared 1.5 T and 3.0 T TOF MRA with both numerical simulation and volunteer measurements (93). The simulations revealed enhanced superior blood-to-background contrast at 3 T over 1.5 T for typical 3-D TOF MRA parameters. In the volunteer data, 3 T provided better visualization of distal intracranial vessels and carotid arteries, with superior background suppression and excellent fat suppression. At 3 T, the combination of improved background suppression and increased SNR enabled high-resolution intracranial 3-D TOF MRA with voxel volumes as small as 0.14 $mm^3$ to be acquired.

Studies have also been performed to evaluate the advantage of high field in multiple sclerosis (MS). In an earlier study that compared the detection of white matter abnormalities in MS at 1.5 T and 4 T (95), 15 patients with clinically definite MS were imaged at both field strengths within a week, using a FSE long-TR sequence. According to evaluation by radiologists, images obtained at 4 T showed a mean of 88 more lesions as compared with images obtained at 1.5 T. MR imaging at 4 T depicted additional white matter abnormalities in MS patients not seen in 1.5 T images because 4 T images allowed higher spatial resolution with comparable SNR and imaging times. Another study (96) evaluated the relative sensitivity of MRI for MS at 1.5 T and 3.0 T. The study was performed in 25 patients, using

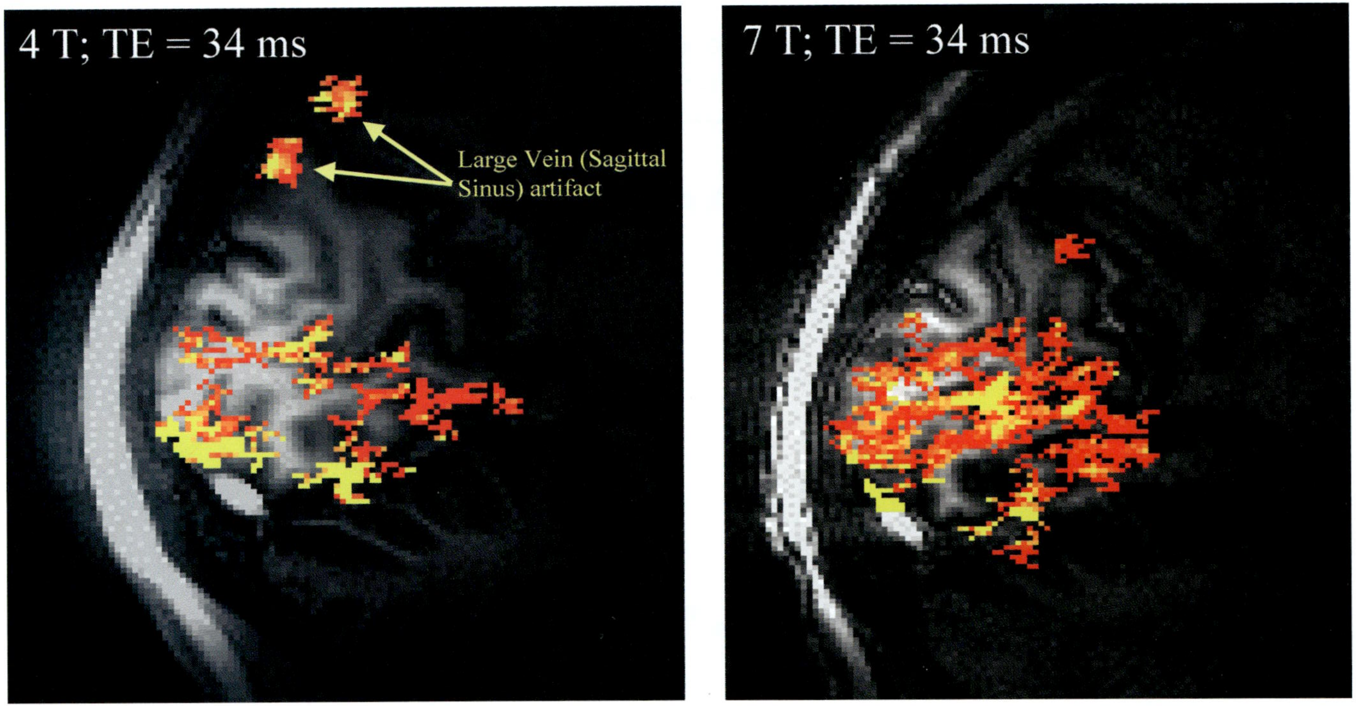


**Figure 4** Activation maps obtained at 4 T (*left*) and 7 T (*right*) using identical acquisition parameters and statistical analysis. The activated areas on the right are more widespread, indicating the sensitivity increase at 7 T. (Adapted from figure 2 of Reference 48 with permission).

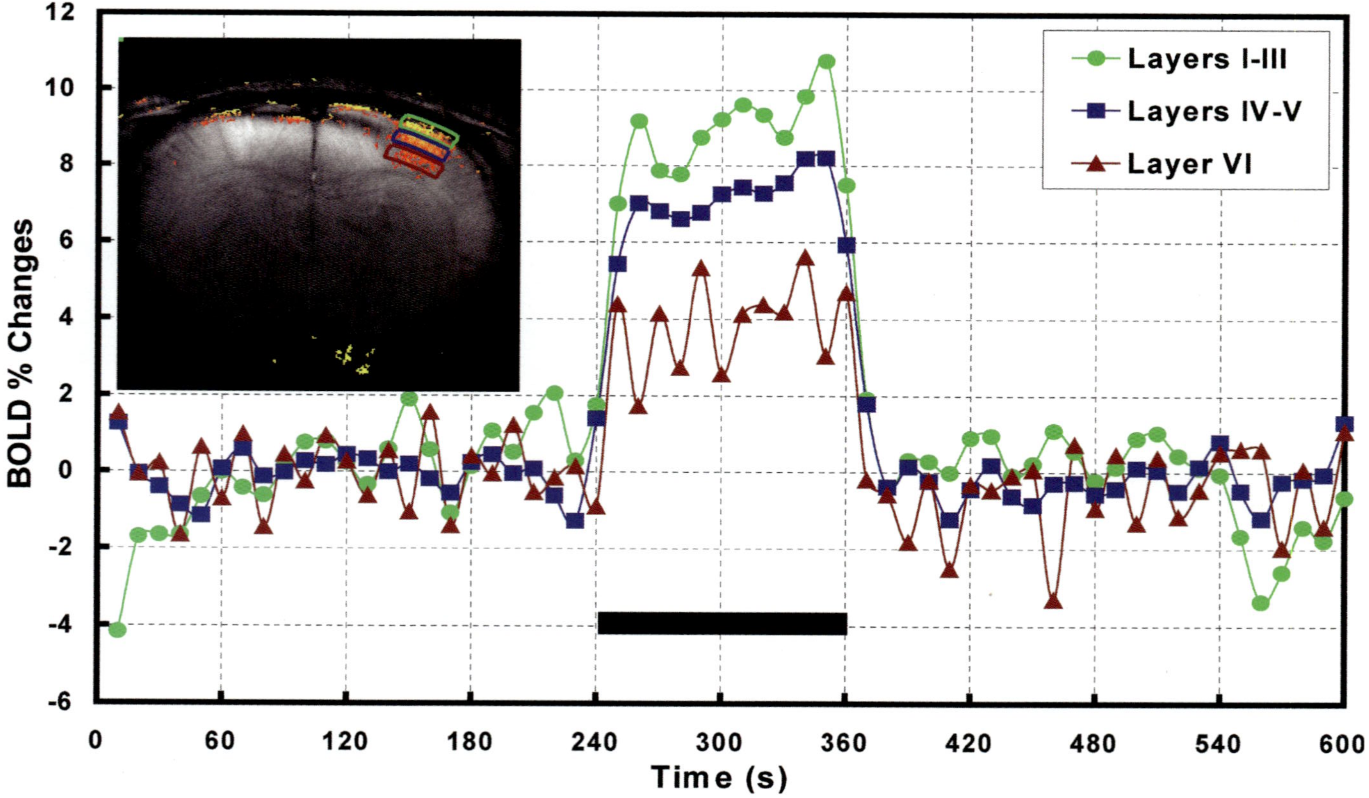


**Figure 5** Functional map (spatial resolution: 200 μm × 200 μm) of the somatosensory cortex of a rat in response to forepaw stimulation obtained at 11.7 T. Spatially separate activations are attributed to different cortical layers, whose amplitudes are distinctively different. Image courtesy of Afonso Silva and Alan Koretsky of NINDS, adapted from Figure 2 of Reference 80 with permission.

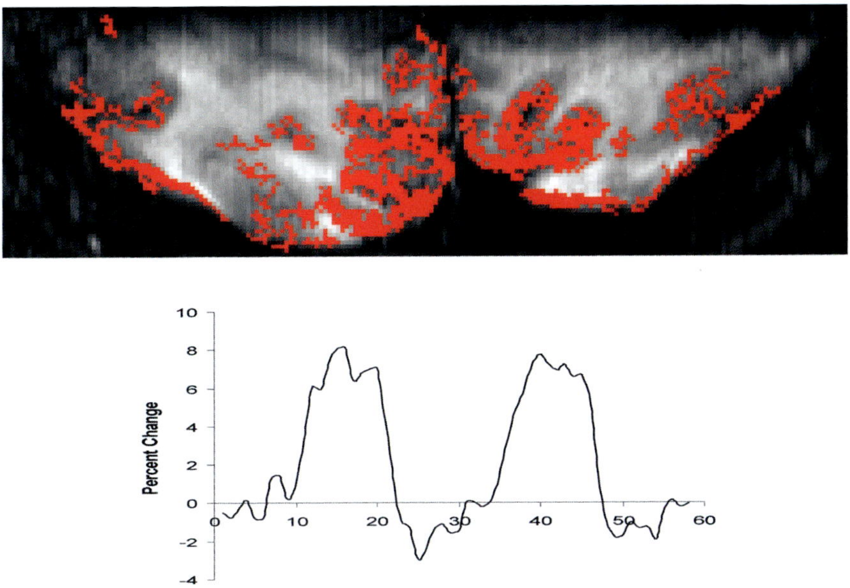


**Figure 6** Top: $T_2$-weighted functional map of the visual cortex in response to visual stimulation at 7 T. The spatial resolution of this map, $0.5 \leftrightarrow 0.5 \leftrightarrow 2\ \text{mm}^3$, is much higher than that in most fMRI studies. The activation is restricted in gray matter, demonstrating the increased spatial specificity of $T_2$-weighted fMRI at 7 T. In addition, the increased sensitivity at 7 T also allowed robust detection of the $T_2$-weighted signals as shown by the signal time course in the bottom.

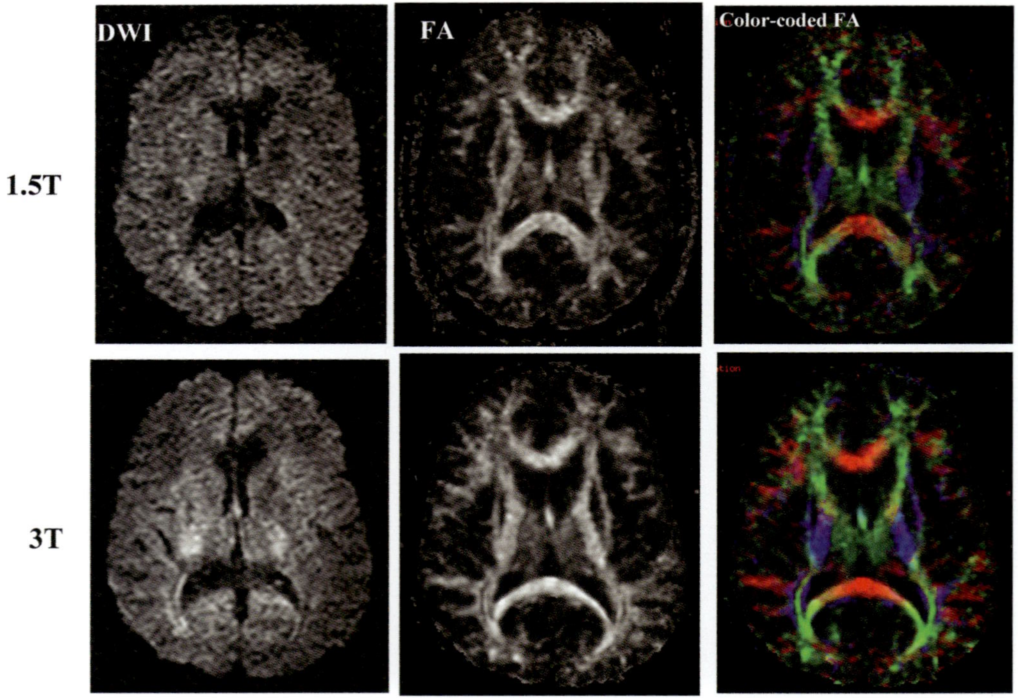


**Figure 9** An SNR comparison between 1.5 T (*top row*) and 3 T (*bottom row*) for diffusion tensor imaging. The two data sets at two fields were obtained with identical acquisition parameters. In each row, images correspond to diffusion-weighted image (*left*), fractional diffusion anisotropy map (*middle*), and color-coded fractional diffusion anisotropy map (*right*). Red, green, and blue represent fibers along the right/left, anterior/posterior, and inferior/superior directions, respectively. The SNR gain in the diffusion-weighted images is approximately 2.2-fold at 3 T. This higher SNR produced better quality fractional anisotropy maps. Image courtesy: X.J. Zhou, A.H. Poonawalla, University of Illinois at Chicago.

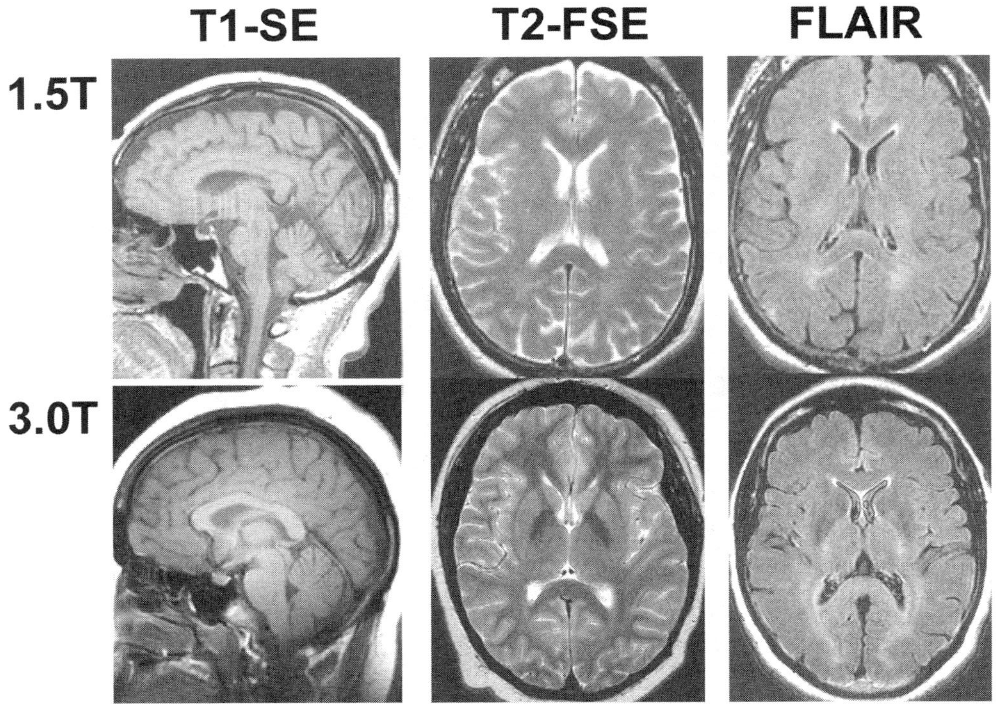


**Figure 7** Comparison of anatomic images obtained at 1.5 T and 3.0 T, all with a 5 mm slice thickness. 1.5 T images were reconstructed with 256 × 256 matrix with a field of view (FOV) of 20 cm. The TE/TR times were 465 ms/12 ms for T1-SE, 4000 ms/92 ms for T2-FSE, and 10,000 ms/158 ms for FLAIR (TI = 2200 ms). All 3.0 T images were reconstructed with 512 × 512 matrix with a FOV of 20 cm and slice thickness of 5 mm. The TE/TR times were 450 ms/8 ms for T1-SE, 4000 ms/98 ms for T2-FSE, and 10,000 ms/175 ms for FLAIR (TI = 2250 ms). The improved spatial resolution at 3.0 T provides more anatomic details for neuroradiological diagnoses. Image courtesy of K. Thulborn and X.J. Zhou, University of Illinois at Chicago.

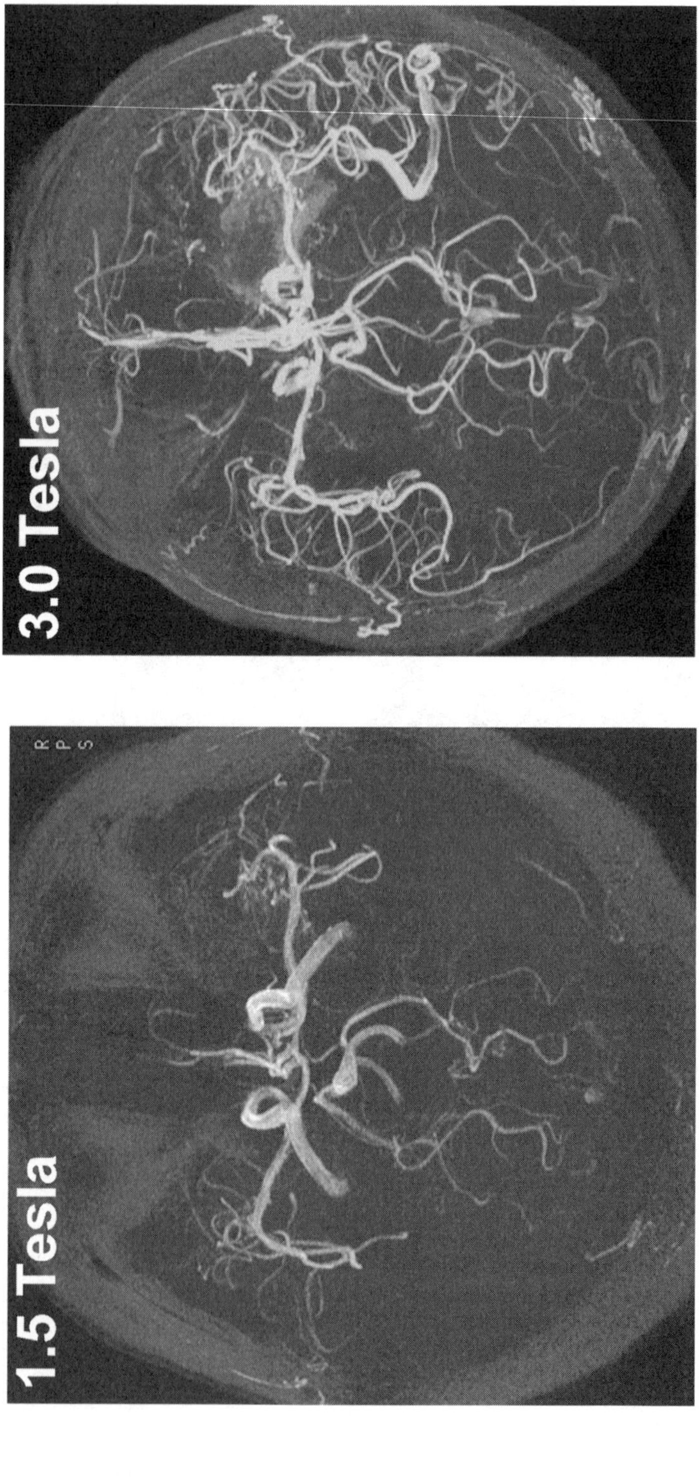


**Figure 8** MR angiograms obtained at 1.5 T and 3 T from a patient with an arteriovanous malformation (AVM). Both images were acquired with neither contrast agent nor magnetization transfer pulse. It is evident that 3 T offers better background tissue suppression, and improved resolvability of smaller vessels. Image courtesy of K. Thulborn and X.J. Zhou, University of Illinois at Chicago.

identical acquisition parameters with FSE and $T_1$-weighted spoiled gradient-echo sequences with and without gadolinium contrast injection. The resultant images were analyzed using automated segmentation and lesion counting. Compared with 1.5 T data, the 3.0 T images exhibited a 21% increase in the number of detected contrast-enhancing lesions, a 30% increase in enhancing lesion volume, and a 10% increase in total lesion volume, again indicating an increase in lesion detection with the higher field.

The increase in SNR at high fields has also been important for newly emerging applications where the SNR may be a limiting factor. One such application is diffusion tensor imaging (DTI), which acquires diffusion-weighted images along six or more noncolinear directions in space to map the directional dependence of water diffusion. DTI has generated a great deal of interest in both basic research and clinical medicine because it can be used to visualize microstructural tissue organization in the human brain (97). DTI provides a unique tool for the study of brain development and pathology of diseases associated with white matter damage. In addition, with fiber tracking techniques (90–100), DTI allows the exploration of neural connectivity and neural pathways in the human brain. In DTI data acquisition, to reduce sensitivity to subject motion and keep the acquisition time practical, raw images are usually acquired with diffusion-weighted EPI images, which are inherently low in SNR. SNR gain at high fields can significantly improve the quality of DTI. An example of improved DTI result is shown in Figure 9 (see color insert), which compares the DTI results of a patient obtained at 1.5 T and 3 T. A more detailed assessment of DTI at 3 T can be found in a study by Price et al. (101), where the potential of DTI at 3 T for assessing white matter tract invasion in brain tumors was investigated.

There have been a series of studies demonstrating the utility of an 8 T system for high-resolution imaging (57, 58, 102–104). Although systems at such a high magnetic field are far from routinely available, these studies do indicate the potential utility of ultrahigh fields for anatomic imaging. Further studies in this direction will be needed to fully establish their clinical utility. Furthermore, the prohibitively high cost associated with these systems may limit their availability to a few research sites at present.

Although early clinical applications of high-field MRI focused mainly on neuroimaging, it has been used in studying other parts of the body. Taking advantage of the SNR gain achieved by the combination of localized coils and the high field of 3 T, high resolution images of the knee (105) and microscopic images of the toe (106) were obtained. More recently, prostate images were obtained at 3.0 T for volumetric quantification using an external phased-array coil instead of an endorectal coil commonly used at 1.5 T, significantly reducing patient discomfort (107). Preliminary results of abdominal imaging at 4 T have also been recently reported (108). One aspect of body imaging that is of particular importance is cardiac imaging, which can greatly benefit from the increased SNR because imaging speed is critical. Using a phased-array setup, Noeke et al. (109) performed one of the early studies of the heart using 3.0 T, demonstrating the feasibility of cardiac

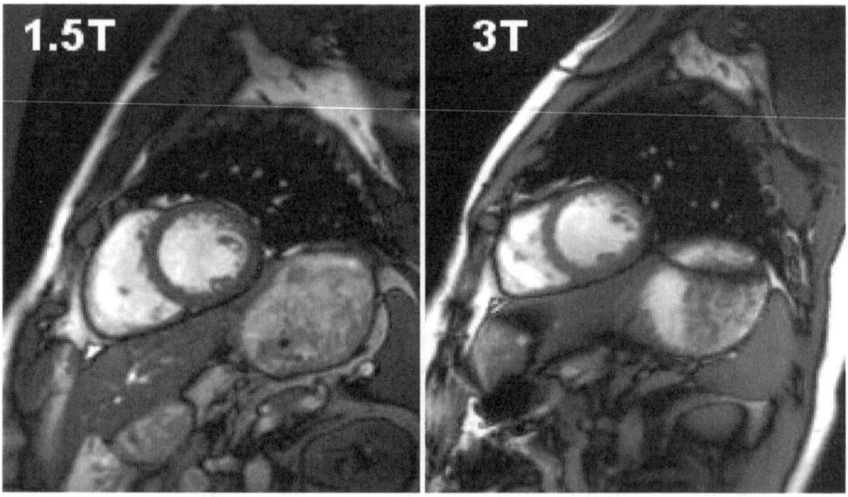


**Figure 10** End-diastolic frames from a short axis cine slice through the left ventricle of a normal volunteer at 1.5 T and 3.0 T. The cine was acquired with 20 time frames over the cardiac cycle using a steady-state free procession (SSFP) technique during a 14 s breath-hold. SNR is 35% higher at 3 T, but inhomogeneity artifacts are present in noncardiac structure at 3 T. Image courtesy of J. Oshinski and P. Sharma, Emory University.

imaging at high field. An example of cardiac cine imaging using a state-of-the-art cardiovascular coil array and a trueFISP type of sequence is shown in Figure 10; compared to 1.5 T, 3.0 T ~ 35% increase in SNR, although the increased susceptibility led to signal shading in regions outside the heart. It is interesting to note that because the relative relaxivity of paramagnetic contrast agents is higher, high fields may have a role to play in contrast agent-based perfusion studies. As shown in Figure 11, delayed enhancement of myocardial infarct can be readily detected at 3 T.

## Spectroscopy/Other Nuclei

Besides increased SNR, in vivo MR spectroscopy benefits from high magnetic fields from the increased spectral resolution. In NMR, the magnetic field experienced by a nucleus is not only determined by the applied magnetic field but also affected by its chemical environment. In particular, electron distribution of molecules may be perturbed by the external magnetic field, leading to a small but significant modification to the magnetic field at a nucleus surrounded by the electronic distribution, causing a shift in its resonance frequency. This shift is commonly known as chemical shift and is an important signature used in NMR spectroscopy for the identification of a specific nucleus. Because it is induced by the external magnetic field, it is proportional to the external field and scales

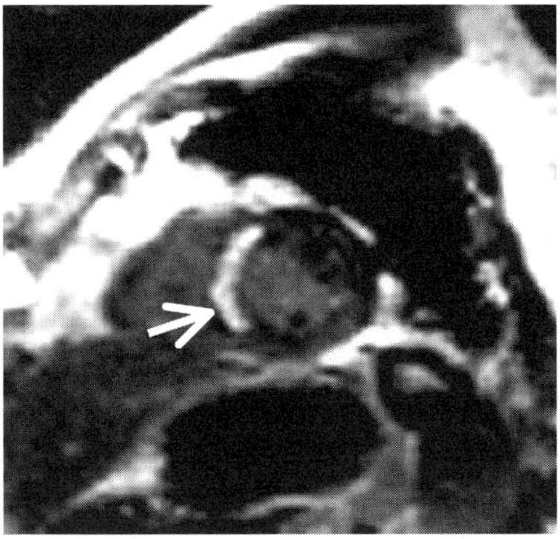

**Figure 11** A midventricular, short axis slice through the left ventricle showing post-contrast (0.3 mmol Gd-DPTA) delayed enhancement of a myocardial infarction in the septal wall (see *arrow*). Images were acquired with an ECG-gated turboFlash sequence and an inversion prepulse. Image courtesy of J. Oshinski and P. Sharma, Emory University.

up with the magnetic field, leading to an increase in spectral separation between chemically different nuclei and hence better spectral resolution.

The increased SNR and spectral resolution have been demonstrated and exploited in proton spectroscopy studies in both humans and animal models at high magnetic fields. In a study that compared 1.5 T with 4 T for a patient with hepatic encephalopathy (110), the improved sensitivity and spectral resolution allowed the detection of glutamine, which increased in the patient compared to that in a normal volunteer. In another study that used proton MR spectroscopy at 1.5 T and 3 T to study mild cognitive impairment and Alzheimer disease (111), (glutamine + glutamate)/creatine and glutamine/creatine ratios were readily detected only at 3 T. Other examples of high-field in vivo proton spectroscopy include the study of effect of insulin on cerebral glucose concentration, transport, and metabolism (112); the detection of gamma aminobutyric acid (113, 114); and the investigation of metabolic changes associated with brain activation (115).

In addition to the proton, there are other nuclei of biological interest, including $^{31}P$, $^{13}C$, $^{23}Na$, and $^{19}F$. These nuclei have a much lower in vivo sensitivity because of their low biological concentration and/or low natural abundance. The increase in SNR has proven to be tremendously beneficial for studying these nuclei in vivo. For example, $^{13}C$ studies have been successfully conducted at 7 T and 9.4 T, permitting the study of metabolism of cerebral carbohydrates (116), brain energetics during activation (117), and brain glycogen concentration and turnover (118, 119). Imaging with $^{23}Na$ at 3 T has also been shown to be sufficiently robust for evaluating cerebral tissue sodium concentration altered by brain tumors (120). With $^{31}P$, fast, direct imaging of phosphocreatine in the human myocardium was shown to be feasible at 4 T using a RARE type of sequence (121), providing a potentially important tool for the evaluation and management of myocardial ischemia. More recently, human brain $^{31}P$ spectroscopy at 7 T was reported, demonstrating the advantage of ultrahigh field for performing in vivo $^{31}P$ MR spectroscopy (122). Therefore, high fields can be of critical importance for in vivo MR spectroscopy, particularly with nuclei other than proton. The potential of high-field systems to clinical spectroscopy is yet to be fully revealed.

## SUMMARY

High field is changing the field of in vivo MR in many significant ways. Although there are inherent pitfalls associated with the high field, benefits, which have been indisputably demonstrated in many applications, certainly outweigh these pitfalls. With technical advances outlined in Technical Issues and Advances (above), numerous applications of high-field MRI have been established and are becoming routinely available in the clinical setting and research environment. Some examples of these applications are illustrated in Applications (above). Although researchers have enjoyed the benefits of high field for years, particularly in fMRI and spectroscopy, its advantages in the clinical arena are only emerging and yet to be fully exploited. With the current growth of the number of 3 T clinical systems, clinical applications of high field will become routine, improving both the throughput and quality of diagnostic imaging and providing enhanced patient care. Future efforts in high-field MRI include expanding body imaging capabilities, further technical advances, and development of new applications that can take advantage of high field.

### ACKNOWLEDGMENTS

The authors would like to thank Dr. Tuong Le for helpful suggestions, and various authors for contributing data to this chapter. Xiaoping Hu acknowledges the generous support by the National Institutes of Health and Georgia Research Alliance.

**The *Annual Review of Biomedical Engineering* is online at http://bioeng.annualreviews.org**

### LITERATURE CITED

1. Lauterbur PC. 1973. Image formation by induced local interactions: examples employing nuclear magnetic resonance. *Nature* 242:190–91
2. Barfuss H, Fischer H, Hentschel D, Ladebeck R, Vetter J. 1988. Whole-body MR imaging and spectroscopy with a 4-T system. *Radiology* 169:811–16

3. Barfuss H, Fischer H, Hentschel D, Ladebeck R, Oppelt A, et al. 1990. In vivo magnetic resonance imaging and spectroscopy of humans with a 4 T whole-body magnet. *NMR Biomed.* 3(1):31–45
4. Yang QX, Wang JH, Zhang XL, Collins CM, Smith MB, et al. 2002. Analysis of wave behavior in lossy dielectric samples at high field. *Magn. Reson. Med.* 47(5): 982–89
5. Vaughan JT, Garwood M, Collins CM, Liu W, DelaBarre L, et al. 2001. 7 T vs. 4 T: RF power, homogeneity, and signal-to-noise comparison in head images. *Magn. Reson. Med.* 46(1):24–30
6. Collins CM, Smith MB. 2001. Calculations of B-1 distribution, SNR, and SAR for a surface coil adjacent to an anatomically-accurate human body model. *Magn. Reson. Med.* 45(4):692–99
7. Collins CM, Smith MB. 2001. Signal-to-noise ratio and absorbed power as functions of main magnetic field strength, and definition of "90 degrees" RF pulse for the head in the birdcage coil. *Magn. Reson. Med.* 45(4):684–91
8. Wikswo JP, Barach JP. 1980. An estimate of the steady magnetic field strength required to influence nerve conduction. *IEEE Trans. Biomed. Eng.* 27:722–23
9. Kinouchi Y, Yamaguchi H, Tenforde TS. 1996. Theoretical analysis of magnetic field interactions with aortic blood flow. *Bioelectromagnetics* 17:21–32
10. Keltner JR, Roos MS, Brakeman PR, Budinger TF. 1990. Magnetohydrodynamics of blood flow. *Magn. Reson. Med.* 16:139–49
11. Schenck JF, Dumoulin CL, Redington RW, Kressel HY, Elliott RT, McDougall IL. 1992. Human exposure to 4.0-Tesla magnetic fields in a whole-body scanner. *Med. Phys.* 19:1089–98
12. Schenck JF. 1992. Health and physiological effects of human exposure to whole-body four-Tesla magnetic fields during MRI. *Ann. NY Acad. Sci.* 649:285–301
13. Budinger TF, Bristol KS, Yen CK, Wong P. 1984. Biological effects of static magnetic fields. *Proc. Meet. Soc. Magn. Reson. Med., 3rd,* pp. 113–14, New York
14. Cooke P, Morris PG. 1981. The effect of NMR exposure on living organisms II. A genetic study of human lymphocytes. *Br. J. Radiol.* 54:622–25
15. Schwartz JL, Crooks LE. 1982. NMR imaging produces no observable mutations or cytotoxicity in mammalian cells. *Am. J. Radiol.* 139:583–85
16. Ueno S, Iwasaka M, Shiokawa K. 1994. Early embryonic development of frogs under intense magnetic fields up to 8 T. *J. Appl. Physiol.* 75:7165–167
17. Hoult DI, Lauterbur PC. 1979. Sensitivity of the zeugmatographic experiment involving human samples. *J. Magn. Reson.* 34(2):425–33
18. Hoult DI. 2000. Sensitivity and power deposition in a high-field imaging experiment. *J. Magn. Reson. Imaging* 12(1):46–67
19. Edelstein WA, Glover GH, Hardy CJ, Redington RW. 1986. The intrinsic signal-to-noise ratio in NMR imaging. *Magn. Reson. Med.* 3(4):604–18
20. Bottomley PA, Andrew ER. 1978. RF magnetic-field penetration, phase-shift and power dissipation in biological tissue-implications for NMR imaging. *Phys. Med. Biol.* 23(4):630–43
21. Keltner JR, Carlson JW, Roos MS, Wong STS, Wong TL, Budinger TF. 1991. Electromagnetic-fields of surface coil in vivo NMR at high-frequencies. *Magn. Reson. Med.* 22(2):467–80
22. Robitaille PML, Abduljalil AM, Kangarlu A, Zhang X, Yu Y, et al. 1998. Human magnetic resonance imaging at 8 T. *NMR Biomed.* 11(6):263–65
23. Bomsdorf H, Helzel T, Kunz D, Roschumann P, Tschendel O, Wieland J. 1988. Spectroscopy and imaging with a 4 Tesla whole-body MR system. *NMR Biomed.* 1(3):151–58
24. Robitaille PM. 1999. Black body and transverse electromagnetic resonators

operating at 340 MHz: volume RF coils for ultra high field MRI. *J. Comput. Assist. Tomogr.* 23(6):879–90
25. Kangarlu A, Baertlein BA, Lee R, Ibrahim T, Yang LN, et al. 1999. Dielectric resonance phenomena in ultra high field MRI. *J. Comput. Assist. Tomogr.* 23(6):821–31
26. Sodickson DK, Griswold MA, Jakob PM. 1999. SMASH imaging. *Magn. Reson. Imaging Clin. N. Am.* 7(2):237–54,vii–viii
27. Pruessmann KP, Weiger M, Scheidegger MB, Boesiger P. 1999. SENSE: sensitivity encoding for fast MRI. *Magn. Reson. Med.* 42(5):952–62
28. Wiesinger F, Pruessmann KP, Boesiger P. 2002. Potential and limitations of parallel imaging at high field strength. *MAGMA* 15(Suppl. 1):447
29. Mansfield P, Chapman B. 1986. Active magnetic screening of coils for static and time-dependent magnetic field generation in NMR imaging. *J. Phys. E Sci. Instrum.* 19:540–45
30. Turner R. 1986. A target field approach to optimal coil design. *J. Phys. D Appl. Phys.* 19:L147–51
31. Roth BJ, Cohen LG, Hallett M, Friauf W. 1990. A theoretical calculation of the electric field induced by magnetic stimulation of a peripheral nerve. *Muscle Nerve* 13(8):734–41
32. Mansfield P, Harvey PR. 1993. Limits to neural stimulation in echo-planar imaging. *Magn. Reson. Med.* 29:746–58
33. Irnich W, Schmitt F. 1995. Magnetostimulation in MRI. *Magn. Reson. Med.* 33: 619–23
34. Lapicque L. 1909. Definition experimental de l'excitation. *CR Acad. Sci.* 67:280–5
35. Budinger TF, Fischer H, Hentshel D, Reinfelder HE, Schmitt F. 1991. Physiological effects of fast oscillating magnetic field gradients. *J. Comput. Assist. Tomogr.* 15: 609–14
36. Foster JR, Hall DA, Summerfield AQ, Palmer AR, Bowtell RW. 2000. Sound-level measurements and calculations of safe noise during EPI at 3 T. *J. Magn. Reson. Imaging* 12(1):157–63
37. Mansfield P, Chapman BL, Bowtell R, Glover P, Coxon R, Harvey PR. 1995. Active acoustic screening: reduction of noise in gradient coils by Lorentz force balancing. *Magn. Reson. Med.* 33:276–81
38. Mansfield P, Haywood B, Coxon R. 2001. Active acoustic control in gradient coils for MRI. *Magn. Reson. Med.* 46(4):807–18
39. Kim S-G, Hu X, Ugurbil K. 1994. Accurate $T_1$ determination from inversion recovery images: application to human brain at 4 Tesla. *Magn. Reson. Med.* 31: 445–49
40. Jezzard P, Duewell S, Balaban RS. 1996. MR relaxation times in human brain: measurement at 4 T. *Radiology* 199(3):773–79
41. Wansapura JP, Holland SK, Dunn RS, Ball WS. 1999. NMR relaxation times in the human brain at 3.0 Tesla. *J. Magn. Reson. Imaging* 9(4):531–38
42. Fischer HW, Rinck PA, Vanhaverbeke Y, Muller RN. 1990. Nuclear-relaxation of human brain gray and white matter-analysis of field-dependence and implications for MRI. *Magn. Reson. Med.* 16(2):317–34
43. Zhong JH, Gore JC, Armitage IM. 1989. Relative contributions of chemical-exchange and other relaxation mechanisms in protein solutions and tissues. *Magn. Reson. Med.* 11(3):295–308
44. Michaeli S, Garwood M, Zhu XH, DelaBarre L, Andersen P, et al. 2002. Proton T-2 relaxation study of water, n-acetylaspartate, and creatine in human brain using Hahn and Carr-Purcell spin echoes at 4T and 7T. *Magn. Reson. Med.* 47(4):629–33
45. van Zijl PCM, Eleff SM, Ulatowski JA, Oja JM, Ulug AM, Kauppinen RA. 1998. Quantitative assessment of blood flow, blood volume and blood oxygenation effects in functional magnetic resonance imaging. *Nature Med.* 4(2):159–67
46. Oja JME, Gillen JS, Kauppinen RA, Kraut

M, van Zijl PCM. 1999. Determination of oxygen extraction ratios by magnetic resonance imaging. *J. Cereb. Blood Flow Metab.* 19(12):1289–95
47. Barth M, Moser E. 1997. Proton NMR relaxation times of human blood samples at 1.5 T and implications for functional MRI. *Cell. Mol. Biol.* 43(5):783–91
48. Yacoub Y, Shmuel A, Pfeuffer J, Van de Moortele PVM, Adriany G, et al. 2001. Imaging brain function in humans at 7 Tesla. *Magn. Reson. Med.* 45:588–94
49. Ugurbil K, Garwood M, Hendrich K, Hinke R, Hu X, et al. 1993. Imaging at high magnetic fields: initial experiences at 4 Tesla. *Magn. Reson. Q.* 9:259–77
50. Norris DG. 2000. Reduced power multislice MDEFT imaging. *J. Magn. Reson. Imaging* 11:445–51
51. Norris DG, Kangarlu A, Schwarzbauer C, Abduljalil AM, Robitaille P-ML. 1999. MDEFT imaging of the human brain at 8 T. *MAGMA* 9:92–96
52. Thomas SD, Al-Kwifi O, Emery DJ, Wilman AH. 2002. Application of magnetization transfer at 3.0 T in three-dimensional time-of-flight magnetic resonance angiography of the intracranial arteries. *J. Magn. Reson. Imaging* 15(4): 479–83
53. Wang J, Alsop DC, Li L, Listerud J, Gonzalez-At JB, et al. 2002. Comparison of quantitative perfusion imaging using arterial spin labeling at 1.5 T and 4.0 Tesla. *Magn. Reson. Med.* 45:242–54
54. Schmitt F, Stehling MK, Turner R, eds. 1998. *Echo-Planar Imaging Theory, Technique and Application.* Berlin: Springer
55. Cho ZH, Ro YM, Lim TH. 1992. NMR venography using the susceptibility effect produced by deoxyhemoglobin. *Magn. Reson. Med.* 28(1):25–38
56. Reichenbach JR, Barth M, Haacke EM, Klarhofer M, Kaiser WA, Moser E. 2000. High-resolution MR venography at 3.0 Tesla. *J. Comput. Assist. Tomogr.* 24(6): 949–57
57. Christoforidis GA, Bourekas EC, Baujan M, Abduljalil AM, Kangarlu A, et al. 1999. High resolution MRI of the deep brain vascular anatomy at 8 Tesla: susceptibility-based enhancement of the venous structures. *J. Comput. Assist. Tomogr.* 23(6):857–66
58. Christoforidis GA, Grecula JC, Newton HB, Kangarlu A, Abduljalil AM, et al. 2002. Visualization of microvascularity in glioblastoma multiforme with 8-T high-spatial-resolution MR imaging. *Am. J. Neuroradiol.* 23(9):1553–56
59. Hennig J, Nauerth A, Friedburg H. 1986. RARE imaging: a fast imaging method for clinical MR. *Magn. Reson. Med.* 3:823–33
60. Le Roux P, Hinks RS. 1993. Stabilization of echo amplitudes in FSE sequences. *Magn. Reson. Med.* 30:183–91
61. Alsop DC. 1997. The sensitivity of low flip angle RARE imaging. *Magn. Reson. Med.* 37:176–84
62. Hennig J, Weigel M, Scheffler K. 2003. Multiecho sequences with variable refocusing flip angles: optimization of signal behavior using smooth transitions between pseudo steady states (TRAPS). *Magn. Reson. Med.* 49(3):527–35
63. Hennig J. 1988. Multiecho imaging sequences with low refocusing flip angles. *J. Magn. Reson.* 78(3):397–407
64. Kangarlu A, Abduljalil AM, Schwarzbauer C, Norris DG. 1999. Human rapid acquisition with relaxation enhancement imaging at 8 T without specific absorption rate violation. *MAGMA* 9:81–84
65. Ogawa S, Tank DW, Menon R, Ellermann JM, Kim S-G, et al. 1992. Intrinsic signal changes accompanying sensory stimulation: functional brain mapping with magnetic resonance imaging. *Proc. Natl. Acad. Sci. USA* 89:5951–55
66. Kwong KK, Belliveau JW, Chesler DA, Goldberg IE, Weisskoff RM, et al. 1992. Dynamic magnetic resonance imaging of human brain activity during primary

sensory stimulation. *Proc. Natl. Acad. Sci. USA* 89:5675–79
67. Bandettini PA, Wong EC, Hinks RS, Tifosky RS, Hyde JS. 1992. Time course EPI of human brain function during task activation. *Magn. Reson. Med.* 25:390–98
68. Ogawa S, Lee T, Nayak AS, Glynn P. 1990. Oxygenation-sensitive contrast in magnetic resonance image of rodent brain at high magnetic fields. *Magn. Reson. Med.* 14:68–78
69. Ogawa S, Lee TM, Kay AR, Tank DW. 1990. Brain magnetic resonance imaging with contrast dependent on blood oxygenation. *Proc. Natl. Acad. Sci. USA* 87:9868–72
70. Ogawa S, Lee TM, Barrere B. 1993. The sensitivity of magnetic resonance image signals of a rat brain to changes in the cerebral venous blood oxygenation. *Magn. Reson. Med.* 29:205–10
71. Fox PT, Raichle ME. 1986. Focal physiological uncoupling of cerebral blood flow and oxidative metabolism during somatosensory stimulation in human subjects. *PNAS* 83:1140–44
72. Edelstein WA, Glover GH, Hardy CJ, Redington RW. 1986. The instrinsic signal-to-noise ratio in NMR imaging. *Magn. Reson. Med.* 3:604–18
73. Ugurbil K, Ogawa S, Kim S-G, Hu X, Chen W, Zhu XH. 1999. Imaging brain activity using nuclear spins. In *Magnetic Resonance and Brain Function: Approaches from Physics*, ed. B Maraviglia, p. 261–310. Amsterdam: Ital. Phys. Soc. Press
74. Kruger G, Glover GH. 2001. Physiological noise in oxygenation-sensitive magnetic resonance imaging. *Magn. Reson. Med.* 46(4):631–37
75. Gati JS, Menon RS, Ugurbil K, Rutt BK. 1997. Experimental determination of the BOLD field strength dependence in vessels and tissue. *Magn. Reson. Med.* 38: 296–302
76. Pfeuffer J, van de Moortele PF, Yacoub E, Shmuel A, Adriany G, et al. 2002. Zoomed functional imaging in the human brain at 7 Tesla with simultaneous high spatial and high temporal resolution. *Neuroimage* 17(1):272–86
77. Menon RS, Ogawa S, Strupp JP, Ugurbil K. 1997. Ocular dominance in human V1 demonstrated by functional magnetic resonance imaging. *J. Neurophysiol.* 77:2780–87
78. Cheng K, Waggoner RA, Tanaka K. 1999. Patterns of human ocular dominance columns as revealed by high-field (4T) functional magnetic resonance imaging. *Soc. Neurosci. Annu. Meet., 29th*, Miami
79. Kim DS, Formisano E, van de Moortele P-F, Ugurbil K, Goebel R. 2001. Ultrahigh field (7T) mapping of the human ventral visual area for "head-from-motion." *NeuroImage* 13:6, S901
80. Silva A, Koretsky AP. 2002. Laminar specificity of functional MRI onset times during somatosensory stimulation in rat. *Proc. Natl. Acad. Sci. USA* 99(23):15182–87
81. Richter W, Andersen PM, Georgopoulos AP, Kim S-G. 1997. Sequential activity in human motor areas during a delayed cued finger movement task studied by time-resolved fMRI. *NeuroReport* 8:1257–61
82. Richter W, Andersen PM, Georgopoulos AP, Kim S-G. 1997. Time-resolved fMRI of mental rotation. *NeuroReport* 8:3697–702
83. Hu X, Le TH, Ugurbil K. 1997. Evaluation of the early response in fMRI in individual subjects using short stimulus duration. *Magn. Reson. Med.* 37(6):877–84
84. Menon RS, Ogawa S, Hu X, Strupp JS, Andersen P, Ugurbil K. 1995. BOLD based functional MRI at 4 Tesla includes a capillary bed contribution: echo-planar imaging mirrors previous optical imaging using intrinsic signals. *Magn. Reson. Med.* 33:453–59
85. Yacoub E, Shmuel A, Pfeuffer J, Van De Moortele P-F, Adriany G, et al. 2001.

Investigation of the initial dip at 7 Tesla. *NMR Biomed.* 14:408–12
86. Yacoub E, Le TH, Ugurbil K, Hu X. 1999. Further evaluation of the initial negative response in functional magnetic resonance imaging. *Magn. Reson. Med.* 41(3): 436–41
87. Yacoub E, Hu X. 2001. Detection of the early decrease in fMRI signal in the motor area. *Magn. Reson. Med.* 45:184–90
88. Ogawa S, Lee T-M, Stepnoski R, Chen W, Zhu XH, Ugurbil K. 2000. An approach to probe some neural systems interaction by functional MRI at neural time scale down to milliseconds. *Proc. Natl. Acad. Sci. USA* 97:11026–31
89. Ogawa S, Lee TM, Nayak AS, Glynn P. 1990. Oxygenation-sensitive contrast in magnetic resonance image of rodent brain at high magnetic fields. *Magn. Reson. Med.* 14:68–78
90. Lee SP, Silva AC, Ugurbil K, Kim SG. 1999. Diffusion-weighted spin-echo fMRI at 9.4 T: microvascular/tissue contribution to BOLD signal changes. *Magn. Reson. Med.* 42:919–28
91. Duong TQ, Yacoub E, Adriany G, Hu X, Ugurbil K, et al. 2002. High-resolution, spin-echo BOLD, and CBF fMRI at 4 and 7 T. *Magn. Reson. Med.* 48(4):589–93
92. Yacoub E, Duong TQ, Van De Moortele PF, Lindquist M, Adriany G, et al. 2003. Spin-echo fMRI in humans using high spatial resolutions and high magnetic fields. *Magn. Reson. Med.* 49(4):665–64
93. Al-Kwifi O, Emery DJ, Wilman AH. 2002. Vessel contrast at three Tesla in time-of-flight magnetic resonance angiography of the intracranial and carotid arteries. *Magn. Reson. Imaging* 20:181–87
94. Bernstein MA, Hutson J III, Lin C, Gibbs GF, Felmlee JP. 2001. High-resolution intracranial and cerical MRA at 3.0 T: technical considerations and initial experience. *Magn. Reson. Med.* 46:955–62
95. Keiper MD, Grossman RI, Hirsch JA, Bolinger L, Ott IL, et al. 1998. MR identification of white matter abnormalities in multiple sclerosis: a comparison between 1.5 T and 4 T. *Am. J. Neuroradiol.* 19:1489–93
96. Sicotte NL, Rhonda RV, Bouvier S, Klutch R, Cohen MS, Mazziotta JC. 2003. Comparison of multiple sclerosis lesions at 1.5 and 3.0 Tesla. *Invest. Radiol.* 38(7):423–27
97. Basser PJ, Jones DK. 2002. Diffusion-tensor MRI: theory, experimental design and data analysis—a technical review. *NMR Biomed.* 15(7–8):456–67
98. Basser PJ, Pajevic S, Pierpaoli C, Duda J, Aldroubi A. 2000. In vivo fiber tractography using DT-MRI data. *Magn. Reson. Med.* 44(4):625–32
99. Conturo TE, Lori NF, Cull TS, Akbudak E, Snyder AZ, et al. 1999. Tracking neuronal fiber pathways in the living human brain. *Proc. Natl. Acad. Sci. USA* 96:10422–27
100. Jones DK, Simmons A, Williams SC, Horsfield MA. 1999. Non-invasive assessment of axonal fiber connectivity in the human brain via diffusion tensor MRI. *Magn. Reson. Med.* 42:37–41
101. Price SJ, Burnet NG, Donovan T, Green HA, Pena A, et al. 2003. Diffusion tensor imaging of brain tumours at 3 T: a potential tool for assessing white matter tract invasion? *Clin. Radiol.* 58(6):455–62
102. Kangarlu A, Abduljalil AM, Robitaille EML. 1999. T1- and T2-weighted imaging at 8 Tesla. *J. Comput. Assist. Tomogr.* 23(6):875–78
103. Bourekas EC, Christoforidis GA, Abduljalil AM, Kangarlu A, Chakeres DM, et al. 1999. High resolution MRI of the deep gray nuclei at 8 Tesla. *J. Comput. Assist. Tomogr.* 23(6):867–74
104. Burgess RE, Yu Y, Christoforidis GA, Bourekas EC, Chakeres DM, et al. 1999. Human leptomeningeal and cortical vascular anatomy of the cerebral cortex at 8 Tesla. *J. Comput. Assist. Tomogr.* 23(6): 850–56
105. Peterson DM, Carruthers CE, Wolverton

BL, Meister K, Werner M, et al. 1999. Application of a birdcage coil at 3 Tesla to imaging of the human knee using MRI. *Magn. Reson. Med.* 42:215–21
106. Szeles JC, Csapo B, Klarhofer M, Balassy C, Hoda R, et al. 2001. In vivo magnetic resonance micro-imaging of the human toe at 3 Tesla. *Magn. Reson. Imaging* 19:1235–38
107. Sosna J, Rofsky NM, Gaston SM, DeWolf WC, Lenkinski RE. 2003. Determinations of prostate volume at 3 Tesla using an external phased array coil: comparison to pathologic specimens. *Acad. Radiol.* 10(8):846–53
108. Uematsu H, Dougherty L, Takashi M, Ohno M, Nakatsu M, et al. 2003. Abdominal imaging at 4 T MR system: a preliminary result. *Eur. J. Radiol.* 47(2):161–63
109. Noeske R, Seifert F, Rhein KH, Rinneberg H. 2000. Human cardiac imaging at 3 T using phased array coils. *Magn. Reson. Med.* 44:978–82
110. Gruetter R, Weisdorf SA, Rajanayagan V, Terpstra M, Merkle H, et al. 1998. Resolution Improvements in in vivo $^1$H NMR spectra with increased magnetic field strength. *J. Magn. Reson.* 135:260–64
111. Kantarci K, Reynolds G, Petersen RC, Boeve BF, Knopman DS, et al. 2003. Proton MR spectroscopy in mild cognitive impairment and Alzheimer disease: comparison of 1.5 and 3 T. *Am. J. Neuroradiol.* 24(5):834–39
112. Seaquist ER, Damberg GS, Tkac I, Gruetter R. 2001. The effect of insulin on in vivo cerebral glucose concentrations and rates of glucose transport/metabolism in humans. *Diabetes* 50(10):2203–9
113. Terpsta M, Ugurbil K, Gruetter R. 2002. Direct in vivo measurement of human cerebral GABA concentration using MEGA-editing at 7 Tesla. *Magn. Reson. Med.* 47(5):1009–12
114. Ke Y, Cohen BM, Bang JY, Yang M, Renshaw PF. 2000. Assessment of GABA concentration in human brain using two-dimensional proton magnetic resonance spectroscopy. *Psych. Res. Neuroimaging* 100(3):169–78
115. Chen W, Zhu X-H, Gruetter R, Seaquist ER, Adriany G, Ugurbil K. 2001. Study of tricarboxylic acid cycle flux changes in human visual cortex during hemifield visual stimulation using 1H-(13C) MRS. *Magn. Reson. Med.* 45:349–55
116. Gruetter R. 2002. In vivo 13C NMR studies of compartmentalized cerebral carbohydrate metabolism. *Neurochem. Int.* 41:143–54
117. Shulman RG, Hyder F, Rothman D. 2003. Cerebral metabolism and consciousness. *Comptes Rendus Biol.* 326(3):253–73
118. Oz G, Henry P-G, Seaquist ER, Gruetter R. 2003. Direct, noninvasive measurement of brain glycogen metabolism in humans. *Neurochem. Int.* 43:323–29
119. Choi I-Y, Gruetter R. 2003. In vivo 13C NMR assessment of brain glycogen concentration and turnover in the awake rat. *Neurochem. Int.* 43:317–22
120. Thulborn K, Davis D, Adams H, Gindin T, Zhou J. 1999. Quantitative tissue sodium concentration mapping of growth of focal cerebral tumors with sodium magnetic resonance imaging. *Magn. Reson. Med.* 41:351–59
121. Greenman RL, Axel L, Ferrari VA, Lenkinski RE. 2002. Fast imaging of phosphocreatine in the normal human myocardium using a three-dimensional RARE pulse sequence at 4 Tesla. *J. Magn. Reson. Imaging* 15:467–72
122. Lei H, Zhu X-H, Zhang XL, Ugurbil K, Chen W. 2003. In vivo 31P magnetic resonance spectroscopy of human brain at 7 T: an initial experience. *Magn. Reson. Med.* 49:199–205

Annu. Rev. Biomed. Eng. 2004. 6:185–208
doi: 10.1146/annurev.bioeng.6.040803.140130


# MICRO-COMPUTED TOMOGRAPHY—CURRENT STATUS AND DEVELOPMENTS

Erik L. Ritman
*Department of Physiology and Biomedical Engineering, Mayo Clinic College of Medicine, Rochester, Minnesota 55905; email: elran@mayo.edu*

**Key Words** X-ray, synchrotron, contrast agents, three-dimensional, small animal

■ **Abstract** The recent rapid increase in interest in tomographic imaging of small animals and of human (and large animal) organ biopsies is driven largely by drug discovery, cancer detection/monitoring, phenotype identification and/or characterization, and development of disease detection methods and monitoring efficacies of drugs in disease treatment. In biomedical applications, micro-computed tomography (CT) scanners can function as scaled-down (i.e., mini) clinical CT scanners that provide a three-dimensional (3-D) image of most, if not the entire, torso of a mouse at image resolution (50–100 $\mu$m) scaled proportional to that of a human CT image. Micro-CT scanners, on the other hand, image specimens the size of intact rodent organs at spatial resolutions from cellular (20 $\mu$m) down to subcellular dimensions (e.g., 1 $\mu$m) and fill the resolution-hiatus between microscope imaging, which resolves individual cells in thin sections of tissue, and mini-CT imaging of intact volumes.

CONTENTS



1523-9829/04/0815-0185$14.00

# INTRODUCTION

The rapid increase in interest in tomographic imaging of small animals and organ biopsies is conveyed in recent publications (1), the appearance of dedicated specialty meetings, the NIH call for a number of Request for Applications (RFA)-type grant proposals for developing small-animal imaging capabilities, and the growing number of newly emerging companies that build such specialty imaging scanners. Examples of the characteristics of some commercially available micro-computed tomography (CT) scanners are summarized in Table 1 and a representative scanner is illustrated in Figure 1. Note that these data are not exhaustive and their operational capabilities are also selected from the range of capabilities of each scanner. This selection of scanners and their characteristics will likely be improved in the next five years, but the physics and technological trade-offs that are involved in the design of a small-animal CT scanner are expected to be common to future systems.

The first clinically practical CT method was introduced in the early 1970s. The state of the art in clinical helical CT scanners now involves volume imaging with voxels that are of the order of 1 $mm^3$ over an axial height of several centimeters that is scanned within a half second. Although these scanners are also of some use for small-animal imaging, special purpose, high-resolution CT scanners are necessary for many studies of intact small animals and reasonably large ($>1$ $cm^3$) tissue specimens (2). A number of in-depth reviews of the technicalities and applications of micro-CT have been published since the late 1980s (e.g., 3–8).

In the early 1980s, the first micro-CT scanners were developed (9–14) using bench-top X-ray CT sources. With the introduction of synchrotron radiation sources (15) in a number of countries, material scientists used the high intensity and brightness of these X-ray sources to do CT at micrometer resolutions. Several landmark events occurred that laid the groundwork for the extension of the method to biological specimens. Grodzins (16) presented the value of adjusting the X-ray photon energy (E) to achieve an optimal, energy-dependent attenuation [$\mu(E)$] by the specimen [i.e., the X-ray pathlength or approximately the specimen diameter (D)] such that $\mu(E) \cdot D = 2$, which maximizes CT image signal-to-noise ratio. As illustrated in Figure 2, X-ray photons less than 25 keV interact mainly via the photoelectric effect, and their attenuation varies approximately as $E^{-3}$,

**TABLE 1** Summary of selected, manufacturer-supplied, performance characteristics of several commercially available micro-CT scanners. (Courtesy of data provided by G. Wang, University of Iowa.)

| | **BIR** | **EVS/GE** | **ImTek** | **Scanco** | **SkyScan** | **Stratec** |
|---|---|---|---|---|---|---|
| **Scanner Name** | ***ACTIS Volume CT*** | ***eXplore RS*** | ***MicroCAT II*** | ***VivaCT 40*** | ***SkyScan-1076*** | ***XCT Research M*** |
| **Micro-Focused Source** | 3 μm<br>10-225 kV<br>0.01-3 mA | 20-90 kVp<br>0.18 mA | 9 μm<br>80 kVp | 5, 7 μm<br>50-70 kVp<br>0.16 mA | 5 μm<br>20-100 kV<br>10W | 50 μm<br>45-60 kV<br>0.2-0.5 mA |
| **Detector Array** | 1408 by 1888 | $2048^2$ | $4096^2$ | 2048 by 255 | 4000 by 2300 | 12 detectors |
| **Field of View** | 300 mm | 40 mm | 35-110 mm | 20-40 mm | 35 or 68 mm | 50 mm |
| **Spatial Resolution** | 12.5 μm | 27-90 μm | 15 μm | 10 μm | 9-35 μm | 70-500 μm |
| **Scan Speed** | 1-30 fps | 180-900 s | 5 fps | 360 s<br>($1024^2$ by 100) | 5 fps | 80 s |
| **Remark** | Manipulators for part & detector | | Respiratory/cardiac-gating | | Physiological Monitoring | Narrow fanning |

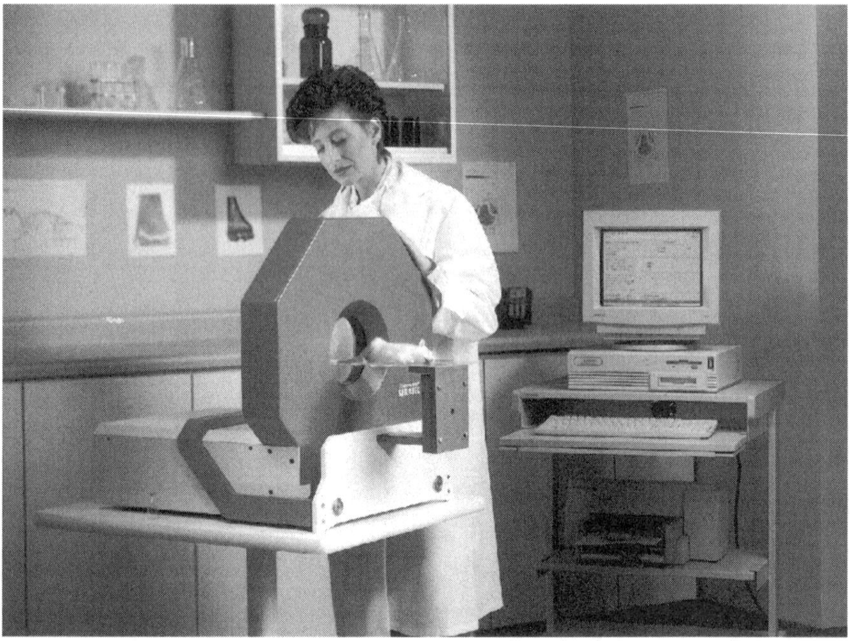

**Figure 1** Photograph of a commercially available micro-CT scanner with operator and mouse subject. This particular scanner is designed for in vitro scanning in preclinical and pharmaceutical research applications, especially for animal bone histomorphometry. It operates at 25–45 kV with anode current <0.6 mA, X-ray tube focal spot size 50 $\mu$m × 150 $\mu$m, measurement diameter up to 50 mm, and length of scout view up to 90 mm. Voxel size variable, from 30 $\mu$m to 300 $\mu$m with multislice capability, variable 1 to 99 slices. The scan duration is <80 seconds. Courtesy of Orthometrix, Inc., White Plains NY.

whereas at higher photon energies, at which Compton scatter is the main mechanism of X-ray interaction with matter, the attenuation varies as $E^{-0.5}$, indicating the greater tissue contrast that could be achieved at low photon energies. A number of investigators in physics and material sciences (18–24) published examples of early implementations that built on Grodzins' analysis. Another important landmark was the publication by Feldkamp (12), who was developing a CT scanner for structural analysis of ceramics in turbine engines. In 1981, he built a scaled-down CT scanner (L.A. Feldkamp, personal communication) using a microfocus X-ray source, a sensitive video camera, and a fluorescent screen. By modifying Herman's fan-beam reconstruction algorithm (25) he, together with Davis, advanced from fan beam to cone beam geometry. Davis subsequently formalized this approach (12). In 1984, Feldkamp started a collaboration with investigators at Henry Ford Hospital and at the University of Michigan resulting in several pioneering papers on the use of bench-top micro-CT applied to bone microarchitecture (25a). This

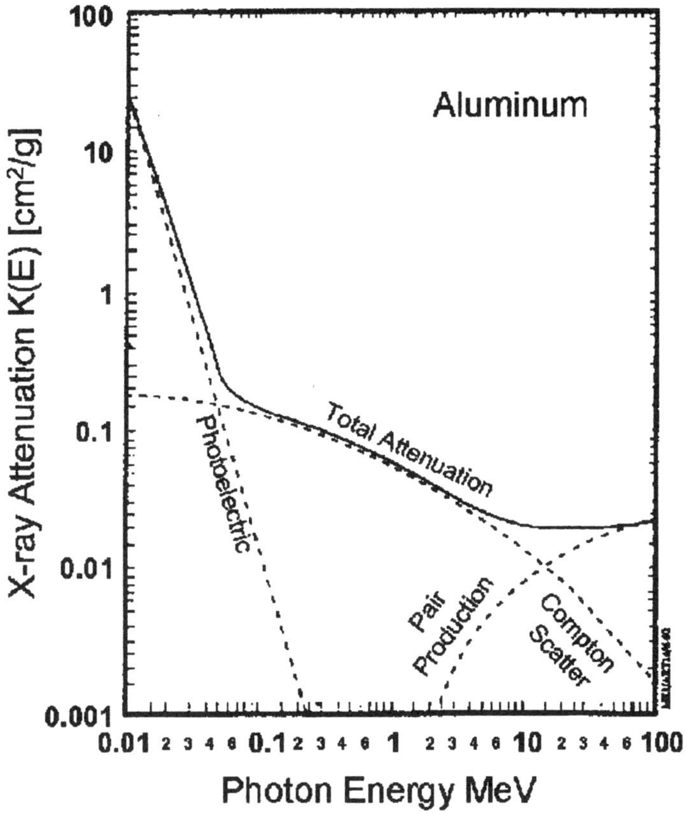


**Figure 2** Total mass attenuation coefficients, K(E), have several mechanism of X-ray/matter interaction, such as the photoelectric effect, Compton scatter, and pair production, each of which predominates over a defined energy band as shown here. These different mechanisms have different implications for CT image contrast and artifacts owing to beamhardening and scatter contamination. Reproduced with permission from Reference 17.

reconstruction algorithm was central in enabling the use of large-angle cone beam so that bench-top micro-CT scanners could now complete scans within reasonable time periods. This is because a number of contiguous slices can be scanned simultaneously as compared to scanning one slice at a time, moving the specimen along its axis of rotation by one slice thickness and repeating the scan and so forth until the volume of interest is scanned (26, 27).

The cone-beam method, however, limits the axial extent of the specimen that can be scanned in one scan. A third method, developed by Kalendar and others (28) involves continuously translating the specimen along its axis of rotation. The helical CT reconstruction algorithms are generalized versions of the cone beam algorithm (29). This results in "helical" scanning (30), which has the advantage that very long specimens (such as an intact mouse or arterial segments) can be scanned intact, independent of the imaging array's axial length.

The current phase of micro-CT development, which started in the mid 1990s, involves bench-top scanners that can scan intact small rodents in response to the rapidly developing need to screen small animals for drug discovery, cancer detection and monitoring, and genomics purposes (7, 8, 31–33). This need is well met by use of special-purpose microimaging methods because it has the potential for accurate measurement of organ anatomy and the spatiotemporal distribution of various functions within the organs in a minimally invasive manner. The minimally invasive aspect is required when longitudinal studies, which are statistically preferable to cross-sectional studies, are desired. Moreover, in genomics research, this capability is particularly important because once the genetically expressed modification of interest is identified, the (now) valuable animal is left intact for more detailed study, use as a disease model, and/or reproduction.

## BASIC COMPONENTS OF MICRO-COMPUTED TOMOGRAPHY

All micro-CT scanners follow the same general plan: an X-ray source, a specimen that is to be imaged, an X-ray-to-electronic signal-converting imaging array, and a device that either rotates the specimen within the stationary scanner or rotates the scanner around the stationary specimen. The method for providing high resolution generally falls into one of three approaches, as illustrated in Figure 3.

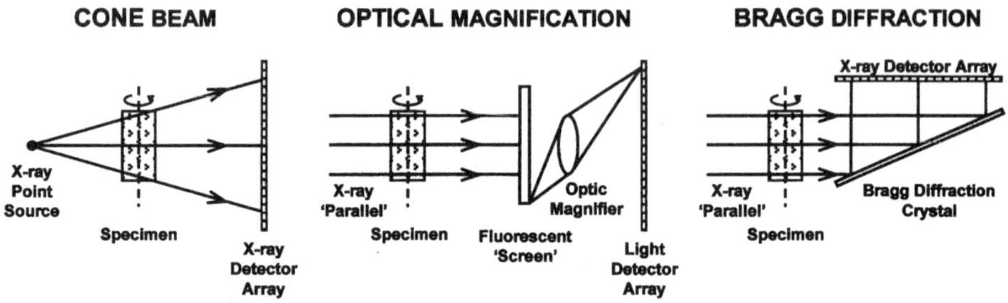


**Figure 3** All micro-CT scanners follow the same basic principle of X-ray source, specimen, and X-ray imaging device. There are three main approaches to achieving the magnification needed to exceed the inherent spatial resolution of the X-ray image conversion to signal system. Each method has its different advantages and limitations. The left panel shows the conventional use of the X-ray cone beam, which projects a magnified X-ray image onto a large-area X-ray imaging system. The middle panel shows how a nonmagnified X-ray image can be magnified by subsequent optical means either by a lens or by a tapered fiber-optic coupling (not shown here). The right panel shows the use of a Bragg interferometer that can be used to magnify the image by virtue of photon wavelength-specific diffraction rather than specular reflection.

## X-Ray Source

Bench-top X-ray sources are generally microfocus (i.e., focal spot diameter <100 μm). Line focus spectroscopy X-ray tubes can be used to produce a stack of parallel fan beam exposures (34) or, when held at an acute angle, for use as a "contact" illuminating system (35). The power output (P) of the microfocus tubes is limited (36) and follows $P_{max} = 1.4\ (x)^{0.88}$, where x equals the focal spot diameter in μm. X-ray scatter has not been as serious a problem in micro-CT as it is in clinical CT. However, to obtain maximum signal to noise, the scatter can be greatly reduced by use of a diffraction X-ray optic placed between the specimen and the detector when monochromatic radiation is used (37).

## X-Ray to Light Conversion Systems

A thin (<0.5 mm) fluorescent crystal plate [e.g., CsI(Tl)] that is cut from a large crystal (or it is built up via vapor deposition) is very efficient at converting X-rays to light. However, there are several trade-offs. A thicker crystal plate will convert more X-ray photons to light, but the thicker crystal plate provides more opportunity for the light to stray from the X-ray-to-light interaction site before it leaves the crystal; hence, poorer spatial resolution. Some very efficient crystalline materials have birefringence, which also degrades spatial resolution. Another concern of any fluorescent material is that of "lag," which is the duration during which fluorescence continues to be emitted from in the crystal after the X-ray exposure has ceased. This can result in superposition of different angles of view or in blurring owing to cardiogenic or respiratory motion during the X-ray exposure.

A fluorescent screen made up of a compressed layer of small granules of fluorescing material can be made very efficient as far as X-ray-to-light conversion is concerned. Although spatial resolution is limited essentially by the granule size, this medium is useful for conebeam-magnified images because the granule size has diminished importance the greater the magnification.

Fiber optics doped with fluorescent material and/or tipped with fluorescent material has great potential for increased efficiency owing to depth of fluorescent material, and the fibers result in constrained light transmission, i.e., maintain spatial resolution (38).

## The Light to Electron Coupling/Conversion System

Image intensifiers are still used, but most micro-CT scanners use a fluorescent image that is coupled to a charge-coupled device (CCD) imaging array [light to electrons (39)] via an optical lens or a fiber optic (40). The lens is relatively inefficient at optical coupling, but it has the advantage of variable magnification (20). The fiber-optic coupling is much more efficient, but magnification is fixed. The image intensifier does provide more rapid illumination of the imaging array (but not necessarily more X-ray photon statistics), which allows for more rapid bench-top CT scanning (41). The number of levels of analog-to-digital conversion needed depends on the noise in the image being digitized and the dynamic range of signal within the image (42).

## CAPABILITIES OF MINI- AND MICRO-CT

Of the three approaches to bench-top CT scanner design (Figure 3), the conebeam magnification approach is preferred in miniscanners where speed is an important factor, but the contact imaging approach has the advantage of high-resolution CT down to approximately 1 $\mu$m owing to the limit of X-ray-to-light conversion resolution (43). The Bragg diffraction approach magnifies the X-ray image (while maintaining near-parallel X-ray beams), which then allows for submicron resolution (44, 45).

### Resolution Requirements: Mini-CT Scanner

The volume of a mammal's internal organs scales with its body weight (46). Hence, if we wish to merely scale the current clinical images (an adult human is approximately 75 kg with CT image voxel dimensions of the order of 1 $mm^3$) to a mouse, we need to have a scanner that has voxels of the order of $(100\ \mu m)^3$ for a 25 g adult mouse or $(30\ \mu m)^3$ for a neonatal mouse. In addition to dimensional scaling, which, broadly speaking, is proportional to body mass $M^{0.3}$, the functional aspects, such as heart and respiratory cycle durations, scale as $M^{-0.25}$ so that scan aperture durations should be reduced from <300 ms in humans to <75 ms in mice if, for instance, the heart is to be imaged.

Because even small rodents have a large range in relative size as they mature from neonate to adult, it would seem reasonable to match the scan resolution to the smallest animal to be scanned, and then to retrospectively "bin" the CCD imaging pixels in proportion to the size of the larger animal. Another method is to adjust the angle of the detector array to the X-ray beam so that the projected, transverse dimension of each detector element (which we might call a dexel so as to distinguish it from the effective image pixel size) is reduced (47). The impact of the different resolutions is illustrated in Figure 4.

### Micro-CT Scanner

Although bench-top micro-CT scanners can achieve meaningful cubic voxel sizes as small as 5 $\mu$m, the synchrotron radiation-based scanners provide the highest resolution. This is because of the narrow bandwidth of the energy-selective X-ray and intensity is sufficient to permit rapid scanning (49). Organs' basic functional units (BFUs, the smallest aggregation of diverse cells within an organ that functions like the organ, such as an hepatic lobule or a nephron) are of the order of $(100\ \mu m)^3$ and are approximately the same size in humans and mice. Hence, with a voxel size of less than $(50\ \mu m)^3$ it is possible to obtain information not achievable in clinical scanners, such as the number, size, and packing of BFUs and membranes only

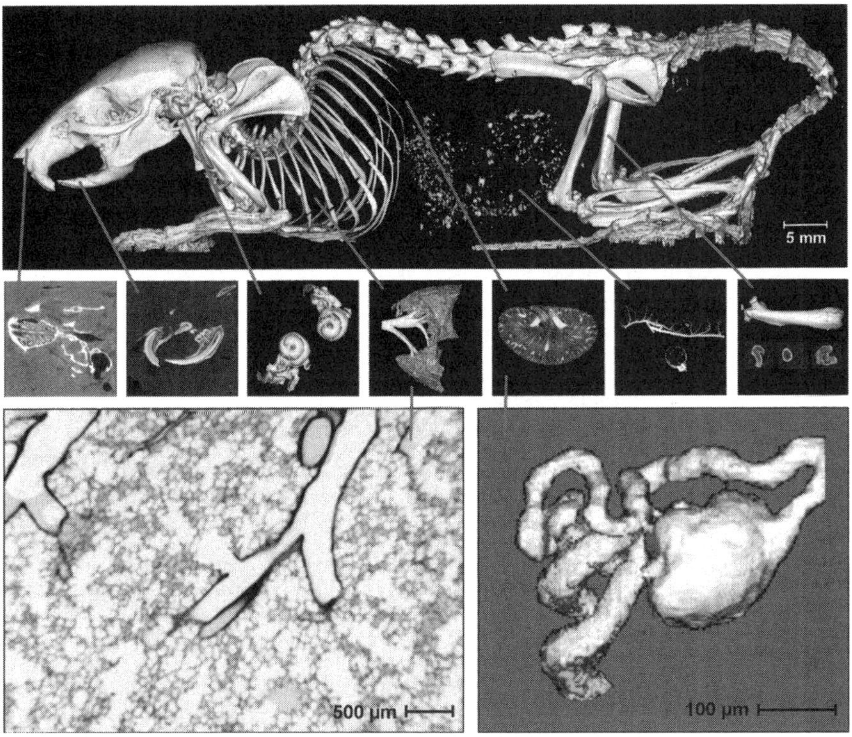


**Figure 4** Computer-generated displays of mini- and micro-CT image data. The upper two panels depict a resolution (40 $\mu$m) that might be expected from a mini-CT scanner, which is a clinical CT scanner scaled down to match the mouse. The lower panels depict higher-resolution (5 $\mu$m) micro-CT. These images clearly resolve the basic functional units (approximately 0.001 $mm^3$), the terminal bronchiole and its alveoli of the lung (*left*) and the glomerulus and associated arterioles and tubule in the kidney (*right*). Reproduced with permission from Reference 48.

a few cells thick (50). In addition to BFUs, there are structures, such as pores, trabeculi, ducts, and blood vessels, that have a range of dimensions. Kinney et al. (51) showed how CT voxel size plays a role in the ability to accurately measure such features. With voxel sizes less than $(10\ \mu m)^3$, even cellular dimensions, such as osteoclast erosions in the surface of bone (52) can be imaged, and with voxel sizes less than $(1\ \mu m)^3$, subcellular dimensions can be imaged (45, 53, 54).

## Physics and Technology

Although scaling down the voxel size involves machining the scanner components down to a smaller size (which has technological implications for precision tolerances and component packing), it also means that different aspects of the well-understood physics underlying CT scanning must be accommodated. Thus, as pointed out previously (16, 55), if the X-ray photon-energy used is less than 25 keV, the X-ray interaction with matter is predominated by the photoelectric effect, whereas in clinical scanners in which the photon energy generally exceeds 50 keV, it is predominantly Compton scatter (56). A desirable feature of the low photon energy is that the X-ray attenuation is up to two decades higher than it is in clinical CT images, thereby allowing better discrimination of soft tissue types. Another consequence is, however, that if maximum signal-to-noise ratio is to be achieved, the X-ray photon energy must be adjusted to match the object diameter, and the radiation should be essentially monochromatic if excessive imaging artifacts, such as X-ray beam hardening (57), are to be minimized. This has the implication that individual, scaled-down scanners must be used for individual mice because the simultaneous scanning of multiple mice within, for instance, a clinical scanner will result in suboptimal image signal-to-noise ratio and spatial resolution. In addition, synchronization of the cardio-respiratory movements if multiple small animals are being imaged at the same time is almost impossible.

In an attempt to generate quasi-monochromatic radiation in bench-top micro-CT scanners, some X-ray source anode materials can be selected for their characteristic $K_\alpha$ emission radiation (e.g., 8.0 keV for Cu, 17.5 keV for Mo, and 22.2 keV for Ag). This radiation output can then be filtered through a thin metal foil selected to have its K absorption edge at an energy just above the $K_\alpha$ of the respective anode material (e.g., 8.3 keV for Ni, 18.0 keV for Zr, and 24.4 keV for Pa), which predominantly attenuates the X-ray photons with energies above and below the $K_\alpha$ characteristic radiation energy. Some promising approaches to bench-top monochromatic X-ray sources suitable for micro-CT are in development, for example, the use of a powerful laser to elicit characteristic $K_\alpha$ emission (e.g., 17.5 keV for Mo) from a suitable target material, so that when combined with a suitable foil filter, little bremsstrahlung contamination occurs and $<400$ eV bandwidth at full width at half maximum (FWHM) of the spectrum of the $K_\alpha$ peak is possible (58).

For mini-CT scanners applied to living animals, the speed of scanning is critically important. This can be achieved by several mechanisms (49, 59, 60). One is by use of higher X-ray photon energies (e.g., $>50$ keV) usually generated with a tungsten anode with considerable filtering through an aluminum or a copper foil. At these higher energies, the bandwidth is not as critical as at lower keV because of the reduced impact of beamhardening, as indicated in Figure 2. This increased speed can also be enhanced by bringing the X-ray source closer to the object, thus increasing the cone beam angle together with all the difficulties that result (e.g., penumbral blurring owing to focal spot diameter and the reconstruction algorithm needed). Scan speed can be further increased by using multi X-ray source/detector array scanners so that the scan duration is proportionately decreased, such as the micro-CT system built by Bioimaging Research, Inc. (BIR) (61). Another approach to increasing the X-ray intensity at the specimen, and to some extent reducing the photon energy bandwidth, is the use of polycapillary-focused X-ray optics (62).

For the micro-CT scanners, specimens are generally rotated around a vertical axis within a fixed X-ray/detector system. However, anesthetized animals would be physiologically challenged if held in this vertical orientation for any extended period of time. Rotation of the animal horizontally around its cephalo-caudal axis would result in gross distortions and movements of the animal during the scan. Hence, in the mini-CT scanner, the torso of intact animals requires a fixed horizontal support table for the animal, and the X-ray/detector system should rotate around the animal, resulting in a true mini-clinical CT scanner, such as illustrated in Figure 1.

## Software-Based Extension of Micro-CT Capability

Mini- and micro-CT scanners are limited by financial as well as physical constraints. For example, the area of the X-ray imaging detector array that restricts the transverse diameter of the object that can be scanned, the size of the dexels that limit the spatial resolution of the CT image that can be generated, the nonuniformity of dexel characteristic exposure/output curves that results in CT image artifacts such as the so-called third generation ring artifact, and the limitations in use of large-angle conebeam geometry to do the image magnification. These limitations can, in part, be overcome by special scanning modifications and image processing techniques. Thus, to avoid incomplete scan data sets resulting from too small an imaging array, one approach is to place the axis of rotation at one edge of the detector array (instead of the usual central location) so that the full transverse profile can be recorded for a 180° range of angles of view from a 360° scan. If this is not possible then profile extension techniques (63) or local reconstruction algorithms can be used (64). Higher resolution can be achieved (than would be expected for the dexel size used) by shifting the detector array by a fraction of the dimension of a dexel in the transaxial direction, which can then be used to make CT images with resolution higher than would be possible without this trick (65). The third-generation CT ring artifacts can be minimized by shifting the detector array during the scan so that the self-reinforcing ring artifact mechanism is interrupted (66). High resolution obtained by use of conebeam magnification is limited by the focal spot size. If it is too small, the heat generated by the electron beam bombardment will melt the anode so that it needs to be operated at low flux (36), resulting in very slow data acquisition, but if it is too large, then the increased flux has to be traded-off against the penumbral blurring that occurs. The latter can be, in part, overcome by point spread function (PSF) deconvolution, but this requires that the PSF be measured at all dexels of the imaging array because it generally differs depending on location within the array (67).

## Extension of Micro-CT Capabilities by Non-Scanner Methods

When synchrotron radiation is used, which is very intense, rapid scanning is possible, so that in vivo scanning of limbs (68), lower torso, or head can be accomplished without significant motion blurring. With slower bench-top scanners, some cyclic motions owing to the heartbeat could be accommodated by acquiring the necessary scan data incrementally at the same phase of the cardiac cycle of sequential heart beats, such as achieved for micro-MRI scanners (69). However, noncyclic transient events, such as the progressive accumulation or washout of a contrast agent in or from a physiological space, cannot be scanned fast enough, even by the high-intensity synchrotron radiation or such a gated scanning method. The transient process can, however, be literally snap-frozen within the tissue of interest, and that frozen specimen can then be scanned at leisure while frozen (70, 71).

## Radiopaque Indicators of Physiological Spaces and Processes

Essentially, all current X-ray micro-CT scanners, and clinical CT scanners use the attenuation of the X-ray by tissues as the signal for generating the x-ray images. In micro-CT scanners, this means that for a given X-ray photon energy, the contrast signal is most closely related to the atomic number (Z) and the concentration of that element (72). At the X-ray exposures tolerated by living tissues, this means that the signal-to-noise ratio in the CT image is adequate primarily for differentiating air, fatty tissue (e.g., brain white matter), nonfatty tissue [e.g., muscle, brain gray matter (73)], and bone [within bone, several layers at different stages of mineralization can be distinguished (26)]. In some tissues, there are normally high concentrations of heavy elements (e.g., iodine in the thyroid and iron in hemoglobin and in the hemachromatotic liver) that just reach a level at which pathological increases, or decreases, can be detected by change in CT image contrast (19, 74).

The most commonly used clinical contrast agents are based on the highly attenuating elements iodine or barium. Iodine is attractive because it is readily attached to sugars, which are tolerated at relatively high concentrations in blood (75), and barium is used because it forms insoluble salts and is therefore useful for opacifying the gut or airway. Other elements, such as bromine (76) and xenon, which is useful for aeration of the lung and increased solubility in fatty tissue such as brain white matter (77), and for tissue perfusion. The relatively low sensitivity of X-ray attenuation imaging to these agents requires that relatively high concentrations are needed for quantitation of local concentrations of the contrast agent in small regions of interest. Clinical CT scanners need at least 10 mg iodine per cubic centimeter. This brings with it the problem of the physiological perturbation caused by the relatively high concentration of the indicator as well as the perturbation caused by the physical characteristics of the volume, viscosity, and specific gravity of the injected contrast agent (75).

The discrimination of physiological spaces, other than the intravascular, can be achieved by selectively opacifying those spaces with administered contrast agents. As a fraction of the intravascular contrast agent passes through the vascular endothelium (especially if it is impaired by reduced oxygen levels or because it is newly formed, as is often the case in malignancies) and remains in the extravascular space for up to several minutes, the extravascular space and endothelial permeability can also be estimated from the images as has been shown in clinical CT image analysis (78). Moreover, as these contrast agents are generally preferentially excreted through the kidney, the opacification of the nephrons (which occurs over many minutes) could be used to quantitate several aspects of renal function as well, as shown with clinical CT image analysis (79). An intraperitoneal injection of iodinated contrast agents has two effects: (*a*) the immediate ability to better delineate the gut and liver within the abdominal cavity, and (*b*) because of the slow transfer of the contrast medium to the blood stream, the cardiac chambers and large vessels, as well as the filtration by the kidneys, are subsequently opacified (2). Iodinated contrast agents encapsulated in micrometer-sized or submicrometer-sized liposomes can be used as markers of the intravascular space or to be conveyed into the lymphatic space (80, 81).

For micro-CT, it is also possible to use heavy elements that are physiological surrogates for the normal elements. For example, the use of strontium as a more radiopaque surrogate for calcium in bone deposition (52). In this case, a short duration of strontium loading, repeated at, for example, a month's interval, will provide two, separated, narrow bands of strontium laid down in the newly deposited calcium mineral in bone. This could be used to quantitate local bone growth or resorption and relate it to local 3-D microarchitecture. Another method, applied to isolated specimens, is the use of osmium tetroxide staining because it preferentially stains structures high in lipid content, such as cell walls, in high-resolution micro-CT images (48).

## X-Ray Micro-CT as a Complementary Methodology

No single imaging modality provides all the information about microstructure, function, and molecular processes in one image. Indeed, scanners of each modality need special emphasis of a particular aspect of physics to optimize the imaging of a particular aspect of organ microstructure and/or function. Consequently, no individual CT image is likely to provide even the full range of the applications that are possible for any one imaging modality. However, such limitations can often be mitigated by combined use of micro-CT with another imaging modality, thus greatly increasing the sensitivity and/or specificity of the resulting image data. A necessary aspect of this synergistic use of multiple modalities is that accurate spatial and temporal registration of the 3-D anatomy is achieved. This presents a challenging technological problem that can, in part, be solved by software registration algorithms that warp, rotate, and/or translate an image within the 3-D image, such as performed in the Gamma-Medica combined (but spatially sequential) micro-CT-SPECT scanner. Three examples of this combined approach follow.

## Radionuclide-Based Imaging

Radionuclide-based imaging methods have great strengths the very high specificity and sensitivity of the images (82, 83). This sensitivity allows the use of picomolar concentrations of the radionuclide-labeled biologically active molecules and labeling of relatively sparsely distributed specific cells. Unfortunately, the methods are limited by poor spatial resolution (>1 mm) and the poor photon statistics that can be achieved within a reasonable time interval. However, X-ray CT can provide the high spatial resolution distribution of X-ray attenuation coefficients, which can be used to improve the accuracy of the radionuclide-based imaging methods by enabling correction for the gamma-ray attenuation through tissues. Similarly, if there is a priori knowledge as to what physiological space the radionuclide is likely to accumulate in, then radionuclide activity can be constrained to that space (which is delineated by the X-ray CT image data so that the SPECT reconstruction process can restrict the backprojected activity to the confines of that space) so that the concentration of that radionuclide can be more accurately estimated.

## Histological Techniques

Histological techniques, with their broad spectrum of tissue element-specific stains and immunohistochemical methods, can provide useful information about molecular and cellular processes in cells and tissues. A weakness of the histological method alone is that preparation and sectioning can damage and distort the sections as well as destroy the specimen for subsequent analysis by other methodologies. Consequently, it provides isotropic 3-D microstructural information only with considerable difficulty. Figure 5 illustrates a 3-D micro-CT image of the

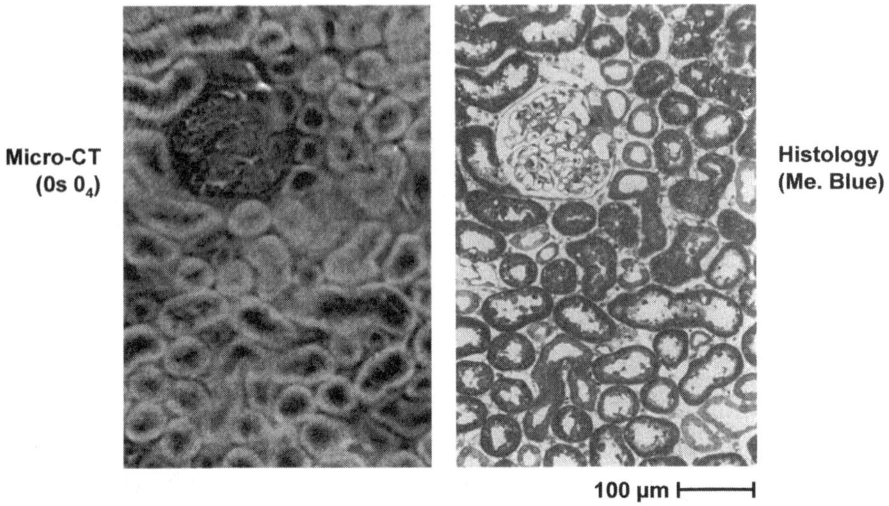


**Figure 5** Left panel: a micro-CT image of a gerbil kidney impregnated with osmium tetroxide. This particular section was found within the 3-D micro-CT image so as to match the (*right panel*) histological (Methylene blue-stained) section that was performed after the micro-CT scan was completed. The excellent registration enables us to integrate the histological information (e.g., cell type, immunological state) with the 3-D microarchitectural information obtained from the micro-CT image, something that is virtually impossible to obtain from any one imaging modality by itself. Courtesy of Dr. Michael D. Bentley, Minnesota State University, Mankato, MN.

microanatomy can be used to register the histological sections obtained after the micro-CT scan is completed. This could greatly extend the information content beyond that of either method used alone.

## Molecular Analysis Methods

Molecular analysis methods, such as immunohistochemistry or mRNA quantitation, often require fresh specimens and generally involve destruction of the specimen. Respectively, these methods provide either sparsely sampled information or values averaged over an entire tissue sample. Some tissue analysis methods can tolerate prior fixation, whereas others cannot. The 3-D microanatomy obtained via micro-CT can be used to determine the fraction of the tissue sample that has, and/or the likely location where, the molecule of interest accumulates so that a more meaningful comparison between animals can be made. The latter case can be dealt with by doing a micro-CT scan of the freshly frozen specimen, while frozen, so that the specimen can subsequently be processed for molecular analysis without loss of the 3-D microanatomic information (84). Here, too, the average value of the molecular concentration in the tissue sample can be corrected for the physiological space's volume. The 3-D micro-CT images can be used to direct where the biopsy within the specimen should be obtained so as to enhance the likelihood that the concentration of the molecule of interest is highest, or, conversely, how the concentration distribution is related to microarchitectural features.

## Data Processing

A major feature of the recent developments in genomics, drug discovery, and cancer research is the pressure to increase throughput, driven by the need to screen many animals. Some automated procedures are needed for managing the acquisition analysis and archiving of thousands of images per year. The logistics of the multitude of microimaging applications, however, may well be the Achilles' heel of the whole endeavor of rapid throughput mode of operation. With each image containing $10^8$–$10^{10}$ voxels, just transmitting and archiving the data is a challenge, let alone performing intelligent analysis within a reasonable time frame. Consequently, one might ask if a smaller image data set would provide a statistically adequate representation of the data for the entire organ or region within the body. Often, this is not sufficient because a single, localized deficiency may initiate the mechanical or functional breakdown of an organ (85, 86) and this means that the entire organ must be inspected at the resolution necessary to detect this microscopic nidus or weakest link (e.g., a hairline fracture). Similarly, the entire organ or part of the body must be inspected if the early appearance of a malignant tumor cell or some other cell is of interest.

It is also likely that the large number of animals to be investigated will require computer-aided procedures to analyze the image data. Matching the recorded images to a standard atlas seems to be one such approach, a process currently underway in the International Union of Physiological Sciences (IUPS) Physionome project (87). Additional quantifying tools also need to be designed to get accurate and specific quantification for different organs or structures within the organs. Thus, a tremendous effort has to be brought to bear on image analysis procedures (such as segmentation), which have to be defined in close interaction between computer science and biology investigators.

## ONGOING DEVELOPMENTS OF X-RAY MICRO-CT

For mini- and micro-CT there will likely be continued incremental improvements of the technology of the scanners, and there are several potential physics aspects that are being explored for the purposes of broadening the spectrum of contrast mechanisms that can be utilized. The synchrotron radiation source, with its brilliance and energy-selective and narrow bandwidth photon generation capabilities, provides a convenient and effective means to study nonattenuation-based X-ray imaging, such as phase delay, fluorescence and K-edge subtraction, and X-ray scatter-based micro-CT imaging. Much technological development is needed to make such approaches suitable for routine bench-top CT imaging use. The following physics principles are being explored for the purposes of extending the contrast and sensitivity, primarily of micro-CT, at this stage. A particular advantage of the fluorescent and scatter-based approaches is that the detected X-ray is the signal of interest (so-called dark field acquisition) as compared to attenuation-based methods in which the signal is a reduction in the bright-field acquisition.

For the purposes of comparison with the methods described below, note that attenuation-based CT using monchromatic synchrotron radiation has been shown to discriminate 1 mg I/cm$^3$ (74) and 30 mg Ca/cm$^3$ (24). Strictly speaking, this objective index of contrast resolution should be further normalized to the voxel volume.

### K-Edge Subtraction

K-edge subtraction has been explored by a number of investigators (72, 88, 89). The method is based on the fact that every element has a well-defined, up to tenfold, energy-dependent transition of X-ray attenuation value. Examples of K-edge transition energy use 7.1, 13.5, 15.2, 16.1, and 33.2 keV for Fe (hemoglobin), Br (Cl surrogate), Rb (K surrogate), Sr (Ca surrogate), and I (in thyroid, but also because it chemically binds readily to many organic compounds of interest), respectively. This characteristic can be utilized by making a CT image at an X-ray photon energy just below and again just above this transition photon energy. The small difference between the X-ray attenuation values of other elements in various tissues in these two images essentially eliminates the signal from these tissues if the two CT images, obtained at the two slightly different energies, are subtracted. The subtracted image therefore contains just the specific element that was selected for imaging. A concentration of 15 $\mu$g iodine/cm$^3$ has been detected with this method (74). This method has not been used as much as one might anticipate because of the difficulty generating the tuned, narrow-spectral-bandwidth X-ray photon energy with a bench-top X-ray source. Although synchrotron imaging can overcome this difficulty, routine access to synchrotron is typically limited for large-scale applications. This logistic bottleneck is being reduced somewhat by several new synchrotron radiation sources that have recently been, or are almost to be, added at several international locations. Another factor is that at the low photon energies involved in K edge subtraction imaging of most biologically relevant elements, only small-diameter specimens can be scanned at optimal image quality.

## X-Ray Phase Delay

X-ray phase delay can also be used for X-ray imaging (90–93). X-rays travel at slightly different velocities through different tissues, so that as an X-ray beam passes through a particular tissue, a phase delay (or advance) relative to an X-ray not passing through that tissue develops. Phase differences can be represented by interference patterns in the X-ray intensities, which in turn can be mathematically converted to actual phase delays. This method provides a tissue contrast higher than that achieved with attenuation-based X-ray imaging. The concentration of iodine that has been detected with this method is of the order of 250 $\mu g/cm^3$, which is four times more sensitive than attenuation-based, monochromatic synchronization photon detector.

## X-Ray Scatter

X-ray scatter at both small angle and large angle (to the direction of the X-ray beam) contains much information about lower atomic number elements, and to some extent, the molecule bonds along the X-ray beam path (94–97). As organic molecules have a characteristic angle-dependant X-ray intensity distribution, this becomes a signature for that molecule. For highly periodic molecules, such as collagen, distinct diffraction peaks can be identified (98–100). At >50 keV X-ray photon energy, the ratio of Rayleigh-to-Compton scanner can be used to achieve increased contrast for small changes in Z, such as 6 $mg/cm^{-3}$ for iodine, 8 $mg/cm^{-3}$ for iron, and 10 $mg/cm^{-3}$ for potassium (101). However, these data must be corrected for attenuation, which can be done with the concurrently recorded attenuation image. However, a difficulty with scatter imaging is the inefficient mechanisms currently available for measuring, and localizing, the source of the scattered radiation.

## X-Ray Fluorescence

X-ray fluorescence occurs when an electron that has been knocked out of its atomic orbit by an X-ray photon results in a secondary X-ray photon being generated. This photon's energy is characteristic for the specific element, for example, 6.4, 11.9, 13.4, 14.2, and 28.6 keV for Fe, Br, Ru, Sr, and I, respectively. Hence, the identity, concentration, and location of that element can be accurately derived, for example, a concentration of iodine down to 60 $\mu g/cm^3$ has been detected with fluorescence CT (73, 102, 103). A problem with this method is that the energy of fluorescent X-ray photons is less than that of the illuminating X-rays, and hence they are generally considerably more attenuated (104) and difficult to distinguish from photons that have been scattered by other physics mechanisms.

### Very High Resolution

X-ray optical methods, such as zone plates (53) or Bragg diffraction optics (19, 44, 45), can be used to magnify the X-ray projection image to the extent that sub-micrometer resolution can be achieved. At this magnification, additional physics aspects as well as sensitivity to small temperature changes of the optics become increasingly important issues.

## RADIATION DOSE LIMITATIONS

A major limitation of X-ray attenuation imaging is its ionizing effect, which can result in immediate radiation damage and long-term genetic damage (56). The signal-to-noise ratio of X-ray attenuation imaging depends largely on the number of X-ray photons detected per voxel of the 3-D image [i.e., the X-ray exposure has to increase with increasing spatial resolution (105)]; therefore, its sensitivity is ultimately limited by its potential for radiation damage. Grodzins showed that for constant signal-to-noise ratio, the radiation dose necessary for small samples was approximately proportional to the specimen diameter to the third power, so that an X-ray exposure of 0.01 Gy (0.1 Rad) for a 10 cm diameter specimen would require $10^2$, $5 \times 10^4$, and $2.5 \times 10^7$ Gy for water-like specimens 1, 0.1, and 0.01 cm diameter, respectively. An exposure of 6 Gy is generally considered lethal for a small rodent; therefore, exposures must be much less in animals required to undergo multiple sequential scans. For mini-CT applications, a dose of 0.5–1.0 Gy is generally required, which represents approximately 5% of LD 50/30 (50% of animals die by 30 days) in mature mice (2). But as longitudinal studies require repeated exposures, and dose accumulation will present increasing risks to the animal, efforts to achieve reduction in dose through instrumentation and algorithms are essential for repeated animal studies.

## SUMMARY AND CONCLUSIONS

Mini- and micro-CT imaging are rapidly developing fields stimulated by the recent increased demand for small-animal imaging. These imaging methods are useful because they nondestructively image a 3-D volume. However, they are limited by relatively poor contrast of most biologically important molecules, as well as by radiation damage. Current developments of micro-CT that are not based on X-ray attenuation have the potential to improve contrast. Synergistic use of micro-CT with radionuclide or histological imaging methods can greatly expand the role for micro-CT.

## ACKNOWLEDGMENTS

The author acknowledges Dr. Brian P. Flannery and Mr. John H. Dunsmuir of Exxon Mobil, who introduced him to the intricacies of micro-CT; the helpful input from Professor Ulrich Bonse of Dortmund University for his insights into synchrotron-based micro-CT; Dr. Ge Wang of the University of Iowa for providing the information about commercially available scanners (especially Table 1); and Dr. Lee Feldkamp of the Ford Motor Company for his information that lead up to the generation his conebeam algorithms. I also thank Ms. Julie M. Patterson and Mr. Steven M. Jorgensen for the preparation of several of the illustrations, and Ms. Delories C. Darling for typing this manuscript. The author's micro-CT research is supported by NIH grants EB000305 and HL65342, and research was carried out in part at the National Synchrotron Light Source, Brookhaven National Laboratory, which is supported by the US Department of Energy, Division of Materials Sciences, and Division of Chemical Sciences, Contract No. DE-AC02-98CH10886.

**The *Annual Review of Biomedical Engineering* is online at http://bioeng.annualreviews.org**

## LITERATURE CITED

1. Service RF. 1999. Scanners get a fix in lab animals. *Science* 286:2261–62
2. Paulus MJ, Sari-Sarraff H, Gleason SS, Bobreck M, Hicks JS, et al. 1999. A new X-ray computed tomography system for laboratory mouse imaging. *IEEE Trans. Nucl. Sci.* 46:558–64
3. Kinney JH, Johnson QC, Nichols MC, Bonse U, Saroyan RA, et al. 1988. Three dimensional X-ray computed tomography in material science. *MRS Bull.* XIII:13–17
4. Graeff W, Engelke K. 1991. Micro radiography and microtomography. In *Handbook on Synchrotron Radiation*, eds. S Ebashi, M Koch, E Rubinstein, pp. 361–405. Amsterdam: Elsevier
5. Graeff W. 1996. Biomedical application of microtomography. In *Proceedings of International School of Physics "Enrico Fermi" Course CXXVII, BiomedicalAapplications of Synchrotron Radiation*, eds. E Buratitni, A Baleran, pp. 155–170. Amsterdam: IOS Press
6. Bonse U, Busch F. 1996. X-ray computed microtomography ($\mu$CT) using synchrotron radiation (SR). *Prog. Biophys. Mol. Biol.* 65(1/2):133–69
7. Paulus MJ, Gleason SS, Kennel SJ, Hunsicker PR, Johnson DK. 2000. High resolution X-ray computed tomography: an emerging tool for small animal cancer research. *Neoplasia* 1–2:62–70
8. Holdsworth DW, Thornton MM. 2002. Micro-CT in small animal and specimen imaging. *Trends Biotech.* 20(8):S34–39
9. Kujoori MA, Hillman BJ, Barrett H. 1980. High resolution computed tomography of the normal rat nephrogram. *Invest. Radiol.* 15:148–54
10. Sato T, Chieda O, Yamakashi Y, Tsubouchi M. 1981. X-ray tomography for

microstructural objects. *Appl. Opt.* 20: 3880–83
11. Elliott JC, Dover SD. 1982. X-ray tomography. *J. Microsc.* 126(2):211–13
12. Feldkamp LA, Davis LC, Kress JW. 1984. Practical cone-beam algorithm. *J. Opt. Soc. Am.* A 1:612–19
13. Burstein P, Bjorkholm PJ, Chase RC, Seguin FH. 1984. The largest and the smallest X-ray computed tomography systems. *Nucl. Instrum. Methods Phys. Res.* 221:207–12
14. Bowen DK, Elliott JS, Stock SR, Dover SD. 1986. X-ray microtomography with synchrotron radiation. *Proc. SPIE* 691:94–98
15. Margaritondo G. 1988. *Introduction to Synchrotron Radiation.* New York: Oxford Univ. Press
16. Grodzins L. 1983. Optimum energies for X-ray transmission tomography of small samples. *Nucl. Instrum. Methods* 206(3):541–45
17. Tonner PD, Stanley JH. 1992. Supervoltage computed tomography for large aerospace structures. *Mater. Evol.* 50(12):1434–38
18. Cho ZH, Honmg KS, Nicioglu O. 1984. Three dimensional microtomography with synchrotron radiation using planar integral projection data. *Nucl. Instrum. Methods Phys. Res. A* 227(2):385–92
19. Bonse U, Johnson Q, Nichols M, Nußhardt R, Krasnicki S, et al. 1986. High resolution tomography with chemical specificity. *Nucl. Instrum. Methods Phys. Res. A* 246(1–3):644–48
20. Flannery BP, Deckman HW, Roberge WG, D'Amico KL. 1987. Three dimensional X-ray microtomography. *Science* 237:1439–44
21. Spanne P, Rivers M. 1987. Computerized microtomography using synchrotron radiation from the NSLS. *Nucl. Instrum. Methods Phys. Res. B* 24/25:1063–67
22. Kinney JH, Nichols MC, Bonse U, Stock SR, Breunig TM, et al. 1991. Non destructive imaging of materials microstructures using X-ray microscopy. *Mat. Res. Soc. Symp. Proc.* 217:81–95
23. Bonse U, Nußhardt R, Busch F, Pahl K, Kinney JH, et al. 1991. X-ray tomographic microscopy of fibre-reinforced materials. *J. Mater. Sci.* 26:4076–85
24. Salome M, Peyrin F, Cloetens P, Odet C, Laval-Jeantet A-M, et al. 1999. A synchrotron radiation microtomography system for the analysis of trabecular bone samples. *Med. Phys.* 26(10):2194–204
25. Herman GT. 1980. Image reconstruction from projection. *The Fundamentals of Computerized Tomography*, pp. 40–54. New York: Academic Press
25a. Feldkamp LA, Goldstein SA, Parfitt AM, Jesion G, Kleerekoper M. 1989. The direct examination of three-dimensional bone architecture in vitro by computed tomography. *J. Bone Miner. Res.* 4:3–11
26. Elliott JC, Dover SD. 1984. Three dimensional distribution of mineral in bone at resolution of 15 $\mu$m determined by x-ray microtomography. *Metab. Bone Rehab. Res.* 5:219–21
27. Rüegsegger P, Köller B. 1994. A micro CT system for the nondestructive analysis of bone samples. *Bone Miner.* 25:S4
28. Kalendar W, Klotz W, Vock E. 1990. Spiral volumetric CT with single-breathhold technique, continuous transport, and continuous scanner rotation. *Radiology* 176:181–83
29. Wang G, Lin TH, Cheng PC, Shinozaki DM, Kim HG. 1991. Scanning cone-beam reconstruction algorithms for X-ray microtomography. *Proc. SPIE* 1556:99–112
30. Corrigan NM, Chavez AE, Wisner ER, Boone JM. 1999. A multiple detector array helical X-ray microtomography system for specimen imaging. *Med. Phys.* 26(8):1708–13
31. Weber DA, Ivanovic M. 1999. Ultra-high-resolution imaging of small animals: implications for preclinical and research studies. *J. Nucl. Med.* 6:332–34
32. Wang G, Vannier MW. 2001. Micro-CT

scanners for biomedical applications. An overview. *Adv. Imaging* 16:18–27
33. Paulus MJ, Gleason SS, Easterly ME, Foltz CJ. 2001. A review of high resolution X-ray computed tomography and other imaging modalities for small animals. *Lab Anim.* 30:36–45
34. Kohlbrenner A, Hämmerle S, Laib A, Koller B, Rüegsegger P. 1999. Fast 3D multiple fan-beam CT systems. *Proc. SPIE* 3772:44–53
35. Jorgensen SM, Demirkaya O, Ritman EL. 1998. Three-dimensional imaging of vascular and parenchyma inintact rodent organs with X-ray micro-CT. *Am. J. Physiol. Heart Circ. Physiol.* 44:H1103–14
36. Flynn MJ, Hames, SM, Reimann DA, Wilderman SJ. 1994. Microfocus X-ray sources for 3D microtomography. *Nucl. Instrum. Methods Phys. Res. A* 352(1–3):312–15
37. Takeda T, Hai Y, Hayashi K, Nagata Y, Yamaji H, Hyodo K. 1994. High spatial resolution CT with a synchrotron radiation system. *J. Comp. Assist. Tomogr.* 18:98–101
38. Bueno C, Rairden RL, Betz RA. 1996. Hybrid scintilators for X-ray imaging. *Proc. SPIE* 2708:1–14
39. Reimers P, Goebbels J, Weise HP, Wilding K. 1984. Some aspects of industrial non-destructive evaluation by X-ray and gamma ray computed tomography. *Nucl. Instrum. Methods Phys. Res. A* 221:201–6
40. Castelli CM, Allinson NM, Moon KJ, Watson DL. 1994. High spatial resolution scintillator screens coupled to CCD detectors for X-ray imaging applications. *Nucl. Instrum. Methods Phys. Res.* A 348:649–53
41. Johnson RH, Karau KL, Molther RC, Dawson CA. 1999. Quantification of pulmonary arterial wall distensibility using parameters extracted form volumetric micro-CT images. *Proc. SPIE* 3772:15–23
42. Dunsmuir JH, Ferguson SR, D'Amico KL. 1992. Design and operation of an X-ray imaging X-ray detector for microtomography. *Proc. Conf. Photoelectron. Image Dev. Sect.* 3:257–64
43. Stamapanoni M, Borchert GL, Wyss P, Abela R, Patterson B, et al. 2002. High resolution X-ray detector for synchrotron-based microtomography. *Nucl. Instrum. Methods Phys. Res. A* 491:291–301
44. Nußhardt R. 1990. *Elementspezifische und hoch ortsauflösende mikrotomographie mit synchrotronstrahlung*. PhD thesis. Univ. Dortmund, Germany
45. Stampanoni M, Borchert G, Abela R, Rüegsegger P. 2002. Bragg magnifier: a detector for submicrometer X-ray computer tomography. *J. Appl. Phys.* 92: 7630–35
46. Calder WA III. 1984. *Size Function and Life History*. Cambridge: Harvard Univ. Press
47. DiBianca FA, Zou P, Jordan LM, Laughter JS, Zeman HD, Sebes J. 2000. A variable resolution X-ray detector for computed tomography. II. Imaging theory and performance. *Med. Phys.* 27(8):1875–80
48. Ritman EL. 2002. Molecular imaging in small animals—roles for micro-CT. *J. Cell. Biochem.* 39:116–24
49. Wang Y, DeCarlo F, Foster I, Insley J, Kesselman C, et al. 1999. A quasi-real time X-ray microtomography system at the advanced photon source. *Proc. SPIE* 3772:318–27
50. van Spaendonck MP, Cryns K, van de Heyning PH, Scheuermann DW, van Camp G, Timmermans JP. 2000. High resolution imaging of the mouse inner ear by microtomography: a new tool in inner ear research. *Anat. Rec.* 259:229–36
51. Kinney JH, Haupt DL, Nichols MC, Breunig TM, Marshall GW Jr, Marshall SJ. 1994. The X-ray tomographic microscope: three-dimensional perspectives of evolving microstructures. *Nucl. Instrum. Methods Phys. Res. A* 347(1–3):480–86
52. Ritman EL, Bolander ME, Fitzpatrick LA, Turner RT. 1998. Micro-CT imaging of structure-to-function relationship of bone

microstructure and associated vascular involvement. *Technol. Health Care* 6:403–12
53. Haddad WS, McNulty GI, Trebes JE, Anderson EH, Levesque RA, Yang L. 1994. Ultrahigh resolution X-ray tomography. *Science* 266:1213–15
54. Wang Y, Jacobson C, Maser J, Osanna A. 1999. Soft X-ray microcopy with cryoscanning transmission X-ray microscopc: II. Tomography. *J. Microsc.* 197(Pt. 1):80–93
55. Spanne P. 1989. X-ray energy optimization in computed tomography. *Phys. Med. Biol.* 34(6):679–90
56. Dowseth DJ, Kenny PA, Johnston RE. 1998. *The Physics of Diagnostic Imaging*. London: Chapman Hall Med.
57. Kak AC, Slaney M. 1988. *Principles of Computerized Tomographic Imaging*. New York: IEEE Press
58. Chen LM, Forget P, Toth R, Kieffer JC, Krol A, et al. 2003. Laser-based intense hard X-ray source for mammography. *Proc. SPIE* 5030:923–28
59. Kohlbrenner A, Koller B, Hammerle S, Ruegsegger P. 2001. In vivo microtomography. *Adv. Exp. Med. Biol.* 496:213–24
60. Sasov A. 2002. In vivo micro-CT for small animal imaging. *Proc. IEEE. Int. Symp. Biomed. Imaging,* Washington, DC, pp. 377–80
61. Bio-Imaging Research, Inc. (BIR). www.bio-imaging.com
62. Jorgensen SM, Reyes DA, MacDonald CA, Ritman EL. 1999. Micro-CT scanner with a focusing polycapillary x-ray optic. *Proc. SPIE* 3772:158–66
63. Lewitt RM. 1979. Processing of incomplete measurements data in computed tomography. *Med. Phys.* 6:412–17
64. Ritman EL, Dunsmuir JH, Faridani A, Finch DV, Smith KT, Thomas PJ. 1997. Local reconstruction applied to X-ray microtomography. *IMA Vol. Math. Appl. Inverse Probl. Wave Propag.* 90:443–52
65. Faridani A, Ritman EL. 2002. High-resolution computed tomography from efficient sampling. *J. Inverse Probl.* 16:635–50
66. Davis GR. 1997. Image quality in X-ray microtomography. *Proc. SPIE Dev. X-Ray Tomogr.* 3149:213–21
67. Witt ST, Riedel CH, Gössl M, Chmelik MS, Ritman EL. 2003. Point spread function deconvolution in 3D micro-CT angiography for multiscale vascular tree separation. *Proc. SPIE Med. Imag. Phys. Med. Imaging* 5030:720–27
68. Kinney JH, Lane NE, Haupt DL. 1995. In vivo three dimensional microscopy of trabecular bone. *J. Bone Miner. Res.* 10(2):264–70
69. Qui HH, Cofer GP, Hedlund LW, Johnson GA. 1997. Automated feedback control of body temperature for small animal studies with MR microimaging. *IEEE Trans. Biomed. Eng.* 44:1107–13
70. Kantor B, Jorgensen SM, Lund PE, Chmelik MS, Reyes DA, Ritman EL. 2002. Cryostatic micro-computed tomography imaging of arterial wall perfusion. *Scanning* 24:186–90
71. Gössl M, Beighley PE, Malyar NM, Ritman EL. 2004. Transendothelial solute transport in the coronary vessel wall—role of vasa vasorum: a study of cryogstatic micro-CT. *Am. J. Physiol.* In review
72. Torikoshi M, Tsumoo T, Sasaki M, Endo M, Noda Y, et al. 2003. Electron density measurement with dual energy X-ray CT using synchrotron radiation. *Phys. Med. Biol.* 7:673–85
73. Takeda T, Momose A, Hirano K, Haraoka S, Watannabe T, Itai Y. 2000. Human carcinoma, early experience with phase contrast X-ray CT with synchrotron radiation-comparative specimen study with optical microscopy. *Radiology* 214:298–301
74. Dilmanian FA. 1992. Computed tomography with monochromatic X-rays. *Am. J. Physiol. Imaging* 3/4:175–93
75. Paroz Z, Moncada R, Sovak M. 1987. *Contrast Media: Biological Effects and*

*Clinical Applications*, Vols. 1–3. Boca Raton, FL: CRC Press
76. Gonzalez CF, Osterholm JL, Triolo AJ, Bell RD, Menghetti RA. 1986. Fluorocarbon emulsion as a potential contrast medium in the subarachnoid space and brain tissue. Experiments in cats. *Acta Radiol. Suppl.* 369:554–57
77. Gur D, Yonas H, Jackson DL, Wolfson SK Jr, Rockette H, et al. 1985. Simultaneous measurements of cerebal blood flow by xenon/CT method and the microsphere method. A comparison. *Invest. Radiol.* 20:672–77
78. Ritman EL. 1994. Myocardial capillary permeability to iohexol: evaluation with fast X-ray computed tomography. *Invest. Radiol.* 29:612–17
79. Lerman LO, Rodriguez-Porcel M, Romero JC. 1999. The development of X-ray imaging to study renal function. *Kidney Int.* 55:400–16
80. Ketai LH, Muggenberg BA, McIntire GL, Bacon ER, Rosenberg R, et al. 1999. CT imaging of intrathoracic lymph nodes in dogs with bronchoscopically administrated iodinated nanoparticles. *Acad. Radiol.* 6:49–54
81. Kao C-Y, Hoffman EA, Beck KC, Billamkonda RV, Annapragada AV. 2003. Long residence time nano-scale liposomal iohexol for X-ray-based blood pool imaging. *Acad. Radiol.* 10:475–83
82. Williams MB, Guimin Z, More MJ, Goode AR, Majewski S, et al. 2000. Integrated CT-SPECT system for small-animal imaging penetrating radiation systems and application II. *Proc. SPIE* 4142: 265–74
83. Cherry SR, Shao Y, Silverman RW, Chatziioannou A, Meadors K. 1997. MicroPET: a high resolution PET scanner for imaging small animals. *IEEE Trans. Nucl. Sci.* 44:1161–66
84. Maran A, Khosla S, Riggs BL, Zhang M, Ritman EL, Turner RT. 2003. Measurement of gene expression following cryogenic $\mu$-CT scanning of human iliac crest biopsies. *J. Musculoskeletal. Neuronal. Interact.* 3:83–88
85. Müller R, Gerber SC, Hayes WC. 1998. Micro-compression: a novel technique for the nondestructive assessment of local bone failure. *Technol. Health. Care* 6:433–44
86. Suki B, Lutchen KR, Ingenito EP. 2003. On progressive nature of emphysema: roles of proteases, inflammation, and mechanical forces. *Am. J. Respir. Crit. Care Med.* 168:516–21
87. Cowley AW Jr. 1997. Genomics to physiology and beyond. How do we get there? *Physiologist* 40:205–11
88. Bonse U, Nußhardt R, Busch F, Pahl R, Johnson QC, et al. 1989. Optimizing of CCD-based energy-modulated X-ray micro-tomography. *Rev. Sci. Instrum.* 60(7, Pt. 2B):2478–81
89. Kinney JH, Johnson QC, Nichols MC, Bonse U, Nußhardt R. 1986. Elemental and chemical state imaging using synchrotron radiation. *Appl. Opt.* 25:4583–85
90. Momose A. 1995. Demonstration of phase-contrast X-ray computed tomography using an X-ray interferometer. *Nucl. Instrum. Methods Phys. Res. A* 352:622–28
91. Beckman F, Bonse U, Busch F, Gunnewig O. 1997. X-ray microtomography ($\mu$CT) using phase contrast for the investigation of organic matter. *J. Comput. Assist. Tomogr.* 21:539–53
92. Beckman F, Heise K, Kölsch, Bonse U, Rajewsky MF, et al. 1999. Three-dimensional imaging of nerve tissue by X-ray phase contrast microtomography. *Biophys. J.* 76:98–102
93. Takeda T, Momose A, Yu Q, Yuasa T, Dilmanian FA, et al. 2002. New types of X-ray computed tomography (CT) with synchrotron radiation, fluorescent X-ray CT and phase-contrast X-ray CT using interferometer. *Cell. Mol. Biol.* 46:1077–88
94. Harding G, Kosanetzky J. 1986. Chemical imaging with X-ray scatter. *Proc. SPIE* 671:81–88

95. Schlomka JP, Harding A, van Stevendaal U, Grass M, Harding G. 2003. Coherent scatter computed tomography—a novel medical imaging technique. *Proc. SPIE* 5030:256–65
96. Westmore MS, Fenster A, Cunningham IA. 1997. Tomographic imaging of the angular-dependant coherent scatter cross section. *Med. Phys.* 24:3–10
97. Wernick MN, Wirjadi O, Chapman D, Oltulu O, Zhong Z, Yang Y. 2002. Preliminary investigation of a multiple-image radiography method. *Proc. IEEE Int. Symp. Biomed. Imaging*, July 7–10, Washington, DC, pp. 129–132
98. Harding G, Kosanetzky J, Neitzel U. 1987. X-ray diffraction computed tomography. *Med. Phys.* 14(4):515–25
99. Stock SR, Barss J, Dohl T, Veis A, Almer JD. 2002. X-ray absorption microtomography (micro-CT) and small beam diffraction mapping of sea urchin teeth. *J. Instr. Biol.* 139:1–12
100. Jin H, Hm K, Chan JY, Butler LG, Kurtz RL, Thiam S, et al. 2002. High resolution three-dimensional visualization and characterization of coronary atherosclerosis by synchrotron radiation X-ray microtomography and highly localized X-ray diffraction. *Phys. Med. Biol.* 47:4345–56
101. Duvauchelle P, Peix G, Babot D. 1999. Rayleigh to Compton ratio computed tomography using synchrotron radiation. *Proc. SPIE* 3772:268–78
102. Takeda T, Tu Q, Yashiro T, Yuasa T, Hasegawa Y, et al. 1999. Human thyroid specimen imaging by fluorescent X-ray computed tomography with synchrotron radiation. *Proc. SPIE* 3772:258–67
103. Takeda T, Maeda T, Yuasa T, Itai K, Sakamoto K, et al. 1996. Fluorescent scanning X-ray tomographic image with monochromatic synchrotron X-ray. *Med. Image. Tech.* 14(2):183–94
104. Hogan JP, Gonsalves RA, Krieger AS. 1991. Fluorescent computed tomography: a model for correction of X-ray absorption. *IEEE Trans. Nucl. Sci.* 38:1721–27
105. Chesler DA, Riederer SJ, Pelc NJ. 1977. Noise due to photon counting statistics in computed X-ray tomography. *J. Comput. Assist. Tomogr.* 1:64–77

Annu. Rev. Biomed. Eng. 2004. 6:209–28
doi: 10.1146/annurev.bioeng.6.040803.140210

First published online as a Review in Advance on April 9, 2004

# OPTICAL PROJECTION TOMOGRAPHY

James Sharpe
*MRC Human Genetics Unit, Western General Hospital, Crewe Road South, EH4 2XU, United Kingdom; email: James.Sharpe@hgu.mrc.ac.uk*

**Key Words** 3-D imaging, reconstruction, gene expression, fluorescence, phenotyping

■ **Abstract** Optical projection tomography is a new approach for three-dimensional (3-D) imaging of small biological specimens. It fills an imaging gap between MRI and confocal microscopy, being most suited to specimens that are from 1 to 10 mm across. The tomographic principles of optical projection tomography (OPT) are explained, its most important applications in biomedical research explored, and comparisons drawn of its pros and cons compared to a number of alternative imaging technologies.

CONTENTS

# INTRODUCTION

## The Need for 3-D Imaging of Small Biological Specimens

UNDERSTANDING GENES AND DEVELOPMENT Understanding how networks of genes coordinate the myriad cellular processes involved in organogenosis remains one of the frontiers of modern science. Although various tools available for developmental biology (molecular biology, bioinformatics, theoretical biology) have combined to make great headway over the past decade or so, a lack of appropriate imaging technologies has meant that we are still surprisingly unfamiliar with the true three-dimensional (3-D) shapes of many of the vertebrate organs we study. An important first step in understanding these complex dynamic processes is simply to describe accurately what happens, so 3-D representations of these interacting shapes can be extremely helpful to embryologists.

The ability to map gene activity within these 3-D shapes is also useful, as knowledge of where genes are expressed gives us insight into their functions, and a gene's distribution relative to other genes gives us clues about which genes or proteins interact with each other. With the advent of complete genome sequences, microarray techniques, and biological databases, it is likely that comprehensive databases of gene expression information will become a reality (1, 2). A number of laboratories are already initiating projects to map gene expression patterns by the hundreds or thousands (3, 4). Fast 3-D imaging technology to digitize gene expression patterns could therefore provide a major boost to these bioinformatic approaches.

Beyond the use of imaging for populating databases, the ability to map gene activity within these 3-D shapes is potentially even more useful. Twelve years ago, the question was asked, "Is molecular biology yet a science?" (5). In the case of molecular biology, the complaint was made that quantitativeness was still lacking to such an extent that many kinds of scientific questions could not be addressed. What was asked of molecular biology then can certainly still be asked of developmental biology now. The daunting complexity of the systems we study sometimes provides little hope that we will one day understand them well enough to construct hypotheses and models that are rigorous, predictive, and accurate. Experimentally obtaining the amount of information necessary to fully describe these genetic systems at the molecular level (binding constants, dissociation rates, and diffusion rates for thousands of different biomolecules) is clearly beyond our current capabilities. However, preliminary results from a few computer modeling projects over the past decade (6) suggest that a viable alternative to gathering molecular-kinetic information about gene networks is to gather accurate, quantitative activity-state data (e.g., gene expression patterns and protein state distributions). A reliable 3-D imaging technique (coupled with high-performance computer modeling) might therefore prove to be an essential complement to more traditional biochemical approaches.

THE IMAGING GAP If we want to capture all this 3-D data for developing organs (or other small tissues), what are the available techniques? Serial-section reconstruction techniques have improved dramatically over the past five years, but for mapping gene expression patterns in whole embryos they are still laborious and time-consuming. Until recently, the alternatives to physical cutting were not ideal either; however, microscopic magnetic resonance imaging (MRI) shows promise for a number of applications, and in particular it is capable of imaging living *Xenopus* embryos and dynamic gene expression in 3-D during development (7, 8). However, it also suffers a number of drawbacks. As the intended resolution of MRI increases, so does the required strength of the magnet used, such that systems designed to image mouse embryos become too expensive for most laboratories. Also, the achievable resolution of MRI is often not sufficient to identify all the tissues or organs within the embryo. Additionally, because it is not an optical technique, it cannot image the distributions of commonly used staining techniques, such as histological stains, standard immunohistochemical protocols, or in-situ hybridization techniques used to visualize the RNA expression patterns of genes. These limitations have therefore meant that it has become particularly useful for capturing the anatomy of specimens approximately 1 cm in diameter (and over).

At the other end of the size scale is a well-established imaging technology, which is indeed optical but has not been developed to image anatomy. Confocal laser-scanning microscopy is very efficient at generating clear, 3-D images of specimens that have been fluorescently labeled (9). However, it is typically used on specimens up to only a few hundred microns in thickness, and usually much less than that. As such, it is often used for exploring the subcellular distributions of fluorochromes within small groups of cells. An imaging gap has therefore been left between confocal and MRI, and unfortunately for developmental anatomists, most vertebrate embryos fall precisely in that gap—too large for confocal imaging and too small for MRI. The technique described in this review, OPT, is most optimal for specimens of exactly this size range and is therefore proving to be of great use in developmental biology.

## Types of Tomography: Putting OPT into Context

The word tomography has commonly become associated with X-rays and the idea of imaging an object from many angles [as is the case in X-ray computed tomography (CT)]. In reality, the range of technologies that have been given the name tomography is broader than this and now includes measurements of many regions of the electromagnetic spectrum (10), electron beams (11), electrical resistance, capacitance and impedance (12), sound waves (13, 14), and magnetic fields (as distinct from MRI, which uses a quite distinct reconstruction principle) (15). The word is derived from the Greek tomos—a cut or section—and in a very general sense relates to the ability to recreate sections through a 3-D object. A suitably broad modern definition from *Merriam-Webster's Dictionary* is "a method of producing a three-dimensional image of the internal structures of a solid object (as the human body or the earth) by the observation and recording of the differences in the effects on the passage of waves of energy impinging on those structures." For many scientists tomography has specifically come to mean a form of imaging that involves solving an inverse problem—in other words, none of the pieces of raw data contain information about precisely where they come from within the specimen—and mathematical transformations or computer models must be used to predict how the 3-D structure of the specimen interacts with the imaging rays to cause the observed external measurements (16). This is in contrast to techniques that directly read out the internal structure by, for example, optically sectioning the specimen. However, as the following list demonstrates, an increasingly popular technique called optical coherence tomography (OCT) has recently expanded the meaning of tomography to include exactly this type of optical sectioning approach (17, 18).

The technologies labeled as tomography can be split into three broad categories (Table 1), the first two of which do involve solving an inverse problem:

1. The first category includes the well-known examples of CT, single-photon electron computed tomography (SPECT), positron emission tomography (PET), and electron tomography (ET) (see Table 1). In these techniques, various types of beams are either transmitted through the specimen or emitted from the specimen. The rays in question (high-energy photons for PET and SPECT, X-rays for CT, and electron beams for ET) pass through the specimen in more-or-less straight lines that approximate projections (10, 11). The principle of this type of imaging is to record either (*a*) how much the ray is attenuated or (*b*) how many photons are emitted along each projection and then use a back-projection algorithm (19) to reconstruct the distribution of either absorbance or emission. In these cases, because the projections are straight lines, one of the methods that can be used to help solve this inverse problem is the Radon transform (19).
2. The second group has many similarities with the first but does not involve straight-line projections. In diffuse optical tomography (DOT) and electrical resistance tomography (ERT), the measurements made record the quantity and/or timing of photons or electrons traveling through the specimen from one point on the surface to another (12, 20). These measurements are often made by attaching an array of sources and detectors to the periphery of the specimen. Unlike the first category above, the exact path traveled between each source and detector is not known—only the probabilities of various possible paths. In these cases, the inverse problem is solved using models of photon/electron transport through the material being imaged (for example, diffusion models).
3. The last category contains only a single technique—OCT. As mentioned above, it is very different from the previous two categories and is sometimes not considered to be a form of tomography. OCT is an optical equivalent of ultrasonic scanning—coherent light is focused into a specimen and interferometry is used to limit detection of reflected photons to a specific

time-of-flight that corresponds to a specific depth within the tissue (17, 18). The imaging is not performed at different orientations through the specimen, and each piece of raw data is associated with implicit depth information. As such, it is a form of optical sectioning and is more similar to confocal microscopy than to OPT. Its name, therefore, begs the question as to whether conventional B-scan ultrasound [as distinct from ultrasound tomography (14, 15)] and/or confocal imaging could also be labeled as forms of tomography.

Of the three categories just described, OPT falls into the first group (21). The specimen is rotated and optical images are captured that approximate straight-line projections through it. As a method of 3-D optical microscopy, it is therefore very different from the previous approaches—confocal and OCT—neither of which actually involve solving an inverse problem.

**TABLE 1** Relationships between different types of tomography*

| | **Tomography as an inverse problem** | | |
|---|---|---|---|
| | **Projections** | **Probabilities** | **Direct measurement** |
| Reflection | | | Optical coherence tomography (OCT)<br>Ultrasound biomicroscopy (UBM) |
| Emission | Positron emission tomography (PET)<br>Single-photon electron computed tomography (SPECT)<br>Optical projection tomography (OPT) | Diffuse optical tomography (DOT)<br>Fluorescent molecular tomography (FMT) | Confocal microscopy |
| Transmission | X-ray computed tomography (CT)<br>Electron tomography (ET)<br>Optical projection tomography (OPT)<br>Ultrasound tomography (UT) | Diffuse optical tomography (DOT)<br>Electrical resistance tomography (ERT)<br>Electrical capacitance tomography (ECT)<br>Electrical impedance tomography (EIT)<br>Magnetic induction tomography (MIT) | |

*The first category involves the measurement of straight-line projections—PET, SPECT, and CT (9), ET (10), OPT (21), and UT (12, 13). Techniques in the second category measure "fuzzy" paths through the specimen (so-called banana functions) and therefore cannot use the Radon transform—DOT and FMT (20), ERT, ECT, and EIT (11), and MIT (14). Techniques in the third category do not perform an inverse calculation, but instead directly measure properties within the specimen, usually sampled as a rasterized section—OCT (18), UBM (31), and confocal microscopy.

# OPT IMAGING

## Data-Capture

Our most common approach for OPT imaging is to suspend the specimen in an index-matching liquid to (*a*) reduce the scattering of light and (*b*) reduce heterogeneities of refractive index throughout the specimen. This means that light passes through the specimen in approximately straight lines and a standard back-projection algorithm can generate relatively high-resolution images. The liquid most often used is BABB or Murray's Clear [a mixture of benzyl alcohol and benzyl benzoate (21)]. Inside the OPT scanning device, the specimen is maintained within the liquid, rotated to a series of angular positions (usually less than 1° apart), and an image is captured at each orientation. The apparatus is carefully aligned to ensure that the axis of rotation is perpendicular to the optical axis so that projection data pertaining to each plane is collected by a linear row of pixels on the charge-coupled device (CCD) of the camera (Figure 1).

The fact that lenses are used to focus an image means that OPT suffers one technical drawback compared to its X-ray equivalent: As with all optical imaging-forming systems, there is only a limited depth of focus, and this usually cannot

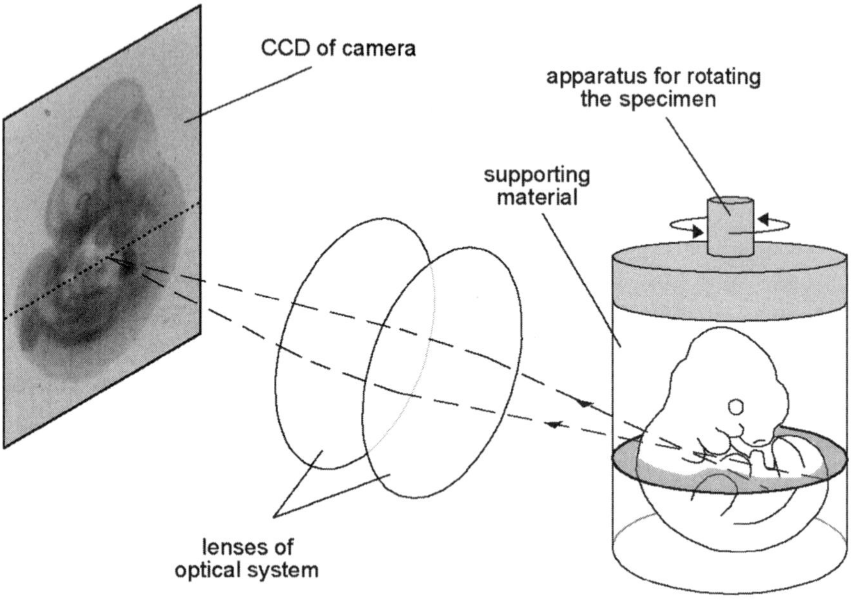


**Figure 1** Optical projection tomography. The specimen is supported in a transparent material (such as an agarose gel) and rotated to a series of angular positions. The axis of rotation is aligned so that a plane perpendicular to it is projected onto a single row of pixels on the CCD (*dotted line*).

encompass the entire specimen. In other words, whereas the shape of the sampled projections in CT can be approximated to long, thin cylinders whose cross-sections are roughly constant from one end to the other, in OPT the cross-sections vary—they are small near the focal plane and become larger further away from it (Figure 2). The most convenient scheme for OPT therefore employs the following compromise: The focal plane is positioned halfway between the axis of rotation and the edge of the specimen closest to the objective lens. This means that every image contains both focused data from the front half of the specimen (the half closest to the lens), and out-of-focus data from the back half of the specimen.

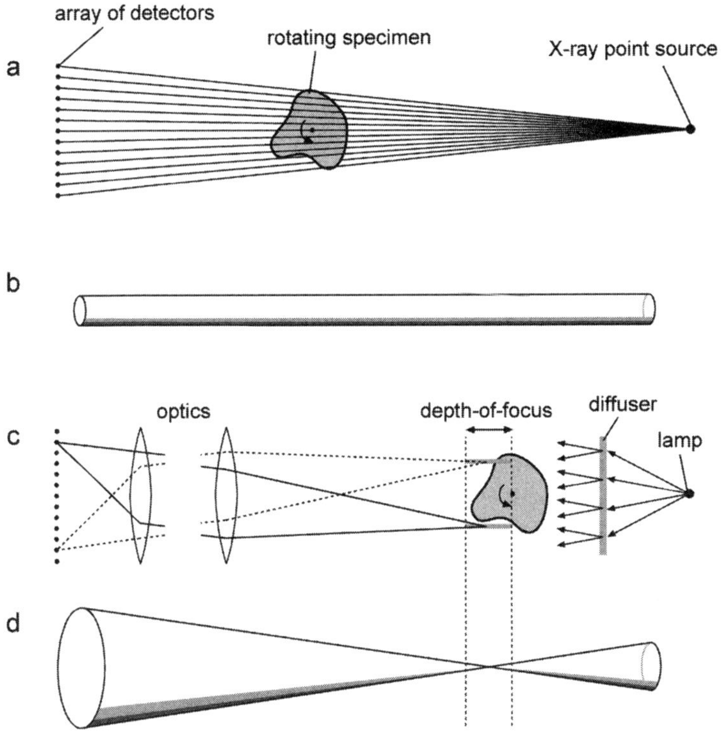


**Figure 2** Comparison between CT and OPT. (*a*) The ray geometry in a typical CT scanner—each projection is implicitly known as being a straight line between the point source and one of the detectors. (*b*) As such, each projection approximates a long, thin cylinder with a roughly constant cross-section along its length. (*c*) The light paths in OPT. The focal plane is positioned such that the depth of focus covers the front half of the specimen (*dashed vertical lines*). The brightfield illumination is provided by a diffuser (see Tomography Using Lenses: Transmission and Emission OPT, below). (*d*) The use of image-forming optics means that each sampled projection is actually the acceptance cone for a particular pixel and therefore has a changing cross-section along its length.

The back-projection algorithm can be slightly modified to take this into account (see below). This arrangement maximizes the focused information obtained from the specimen while avoiding the need to image at multiple depths. Of course, depending on the type of specimens being imaged, the technique may benefit from capturing a series of images at different depths for each angular position (for example, to accumulate an improved estimate of the projection), but so far, satisfactory results have been obtained without using this approach. An alternative is to reduce the numerical aperture of the system so that the depth of focus is larger; however, this cannot be pushed very far as the images soon become less sharp owing to the increased size of the overlapping airy discs (lower resolving power of the system).

In an idealized parallel-beam version of projection tomography, raw data is only required from orientations covering 180° because an image from one direction should be an exact mirror image of a view from the opposite direction and therefore contain exactly the same information (Figure 3). In X-ray CT, this is not the case because the beam geometry is usually fan-shaped or cone-shaped (i.e., the perspective from one angle is not the same as that from the opposite view). In OPT, this is not the case, although for different reasons: (*a*) The focusing scheme described above means that two opposite images will actually be focused on different regions of the specimen. (*b*) Even if the focal plane is positioned on the axis of rotation (such that the same region is in focus from any angle), the residual scattering and diffraction of light passing through the tissue means that deeper tissue will always be less resolved than tissue closer to the lens. This is particularly true for larger, more opaque tissues.

In our current OPT scanner design, 400 images are taken for the 360° rotation (one image every 0.9°); however, it is clear that a higher angular resolution will result in a higher image resolution. As with most imaging techniques, a compromise must therefore be reached between image resolution and speed, and for most practical purposes this is likely to be an angular resolution of approximately 0.5°. A good quality CCD camera is required, and the resulting images (12-bit or higher) must not be subjected to lossy compression before being reconstructed, so the volume of data generated can also become an issue (for transfer, storage, etc.). Two-by-two binning is therefore a useful feature of certain CCD cameras, meaning that the pixels on the imaging chip are divided into square blocks of four (2 × 2), and the total photon intensity summed across the four pixels is read out as a single larger pixel in the final image. The width and height of the resulting images are half the width and height of the pixel dimensions on the chip, so resolution is reduced. But the advantages are data capture that is four times faster (owing to the higher sensitivity), which is particularly useful for fluorescent imaging, and four times less data to process or store.

## Tomography Using Lenses: Transmission and Emission OPT

In general, when a photon is produced it can radiate away from its source in any direction; however, tomographic algorithms need to know the trajectories of any

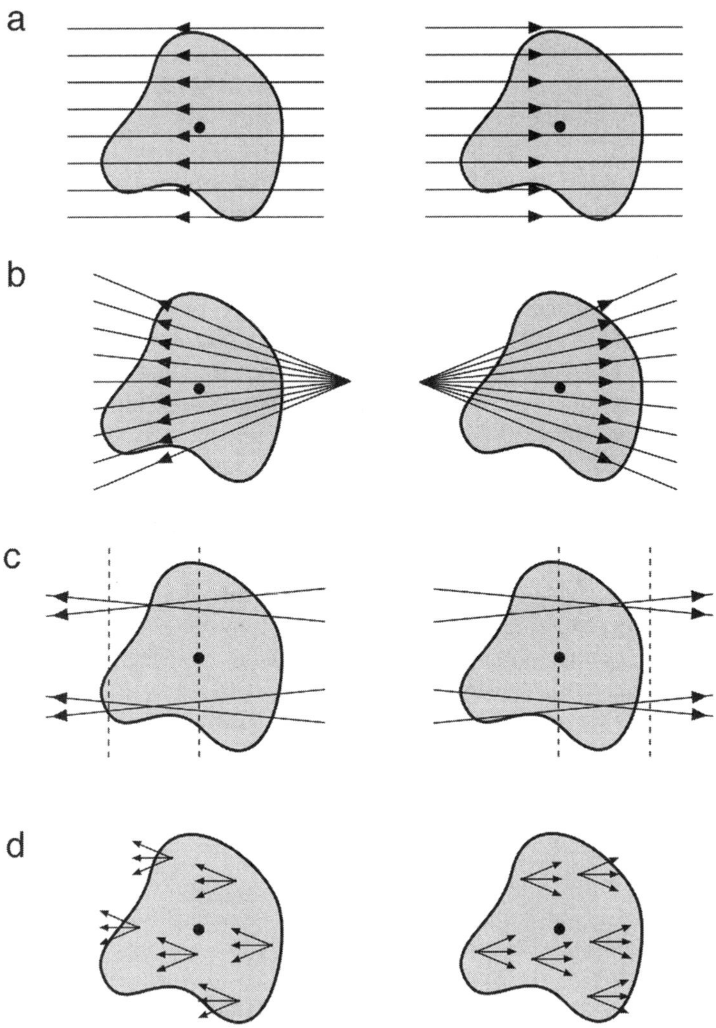


**Figure 3** The need for 360° imaging. In each panel, the specimen is shown at two angular positions during imaging that are 180° apart. In the first column, the detector is always to the left and the ray source to the right, whereas in the second column, this is reversed. (*a*) An idealized parallel tomography system (e.g., electron tomography). The two images contain exactly the same information. (*b*) In CT scanning, the two images are not identical because the beam is diverging in opposite directions. (*c*) In OPT, the opposite images are not mirror images because a different part of the specimen is in focus (focal depth indicated by *dashed vertical lines*). (*d*) Also, residual scattering can be significant in OPT, meaning that the part of the specimen closer to the objective lens has a greater chance of being sharply focused.

photons recorded. Photon detectors only measure the intensity of a signal, not the direction it was traveling before detection; therefore, all tomography technologies involve a strategy for determining this direction. In conventional transmission tomography (such as CT), this is simple because the position of the ray source is known, and the trajectories therefore lie on straight paths between it and the detectors (Figure 2*a*). In emission tomography, however, the source is distributed throughout the specimen. PET solves the problem by detecting a particular type of gamma-ray that is always produced as a pair of high-energy photons traveling in opposite directions. By placing detectors on both sides of the specimen and registering when two photons are detected within a few nanoseconds of each other, the system defines a straight line along which the original emission event must have occurred (10). SPECT, by contrast, does not produce pairs of photons—just single photons at a time. Its detectors are therefore fitted with collimators—slabs of lead containing narrow slits (10). Only photons traveling at the same angle as the slit will pass through to the detector, so the photon trajectory is implicitly known. The main drawback of this approach is that a high proportion of the photons have to be screened out by the lead and cannot therefore contribute to the image.

In effect, OPT employs a similar approach to SPECT. It uses the acceptance cone for each pixel (defined by the lenses of the system) as a virtual collimator, screening-out photons that are traveling at the wrong angle (Figure 2*c*). When performing emission OPT, the technique therefore works very similarly to a SPECT scanner—fluorescent molecules are excited throughout the specimen, and emitted photons are detected by the pixels of the CCD only if they emerge from the specimen at certain positions and angles. Usually, the excitation light is directed onto the specimen from the same side as the imaging lenses.

At first glance, transmission OPT appears superficially to be more like CT than SPECT. Light is shone into the back of the specimen, directly toward the objective lens, and the image formed records the attenuation of this beam. However, in reality, even specimens maintained in an index-matching liquid, such as BABB, still cause diffraction, refraction, and scattering of photons as they pass through. For this reason, successful OPT cannot be achieved using the same principle as CT (i.e., calculating the photon trajectories through knowledge of the relative positions of source and detector). Instead, as mentioned above, the lenses act in a similar way to the collimators in SPECT, only sampling rays that emerge from the specimen at specific positions and angles. As a result, the optimal lamp for OPT is not a point-source, but a wide-field illumination that, owing to the intrinsic scattering within the specimen, can in fact be a diffuse source (although more collinear beams provide higher definition results). For this reason, transmission OPT is usually referred to as brightfield OPT owing to its similarity with conventional two-dimensional (2-D) brightfield microscopy.

The choice of wavelength used for OPT can be important in obtaining a good image. As specimens become more opaque, or more heavily stained (more absorbing), shorter visible wavelengths penetrate less efficiently. However, shifting up toward the infrared end of the spectrum has proven to significantly improve the image quality. This is particularly useful for specimens stained with a colored precipitate (which are imaged using transmission mode) and for larger adult tissues, which tend to be more opaque owing to the more differentiated state of the cells.

## Computed Tomography Reconstruction

At the time of writing, OPT has been performed using standard tomographic algorithms (19, 21). The only modification tested so far relates to the limited depth of field mentioned above. Owing to the position of the focal plane relative to the axis of rotation (Figure 2*c*), two images taken 180° apart from each other will be focused on different parts of the specimen (Figure 3*c*). Whereas the standard algorithm back-projects the measurements across the whole image (Figure 4*b*), limiting the back-projection to the region corresponding to the focused part of the specimen (Figure 4*c*) does slightly improve the quality of the results (J. Sharpe, unpublished data). As data is accumulated for the various orientations through the specimen, a semidisc mask can be rotated to ensure that only focused data is back-projected (Figure 4*d*).

So far, a simple filtered back-projection algorithm such as this produces very good results, and it is not yet clear the degree to which more sophisticated programs will be able to improve on it. In particular, there may be inherent limitations of resolution, which have more to do with the residual scattering of photons through specimens rather than the principles of the reconstruction algorithm. With our own software, it currently takes a typical processor approximately 100 min to perform one reconstruction of roughly $512^3$ voxels; however, this is one area in which improvements are likely to be rapid. Optimized algorithms can already perform the calculation many times faster (J. Walls, personal communication), and future OPT setups are likely to employ multiple processors. It therefore seems certain that a future OPT device will provide the 3-D results almost immediately after having captured the data.

## Visualization

The 3-D voxel data sets from OPT are similar to those produced by other techniques, such as MRI, and as such, all the same visualization techniques can be used. Virtual sections through the data can be viewed at any orientation, and the specimen can also be rendered as a 3-D object—either as isosurfaces, volume renderings, or a combination of both. The major difference between OPT data and MRI or CT data is that multiple channels (different wavelengths) can be captured, so every voxel has a number of 16-bit data points associated with it. Interestingly, within the world of scientific 3-D visualization, there appears to be a rendering gap analogous to the imaging gap mentioned in the Introduction, above. Whereas expensive dedicated hardware can certainly cope with interactive-speed rendering of the large data sets produced by OPT, at the time of writing, affordable desktop computers cannot. Commercial software has therefore tended to focus on two important but distinct preexisting imaging markets: On one hand is the software for

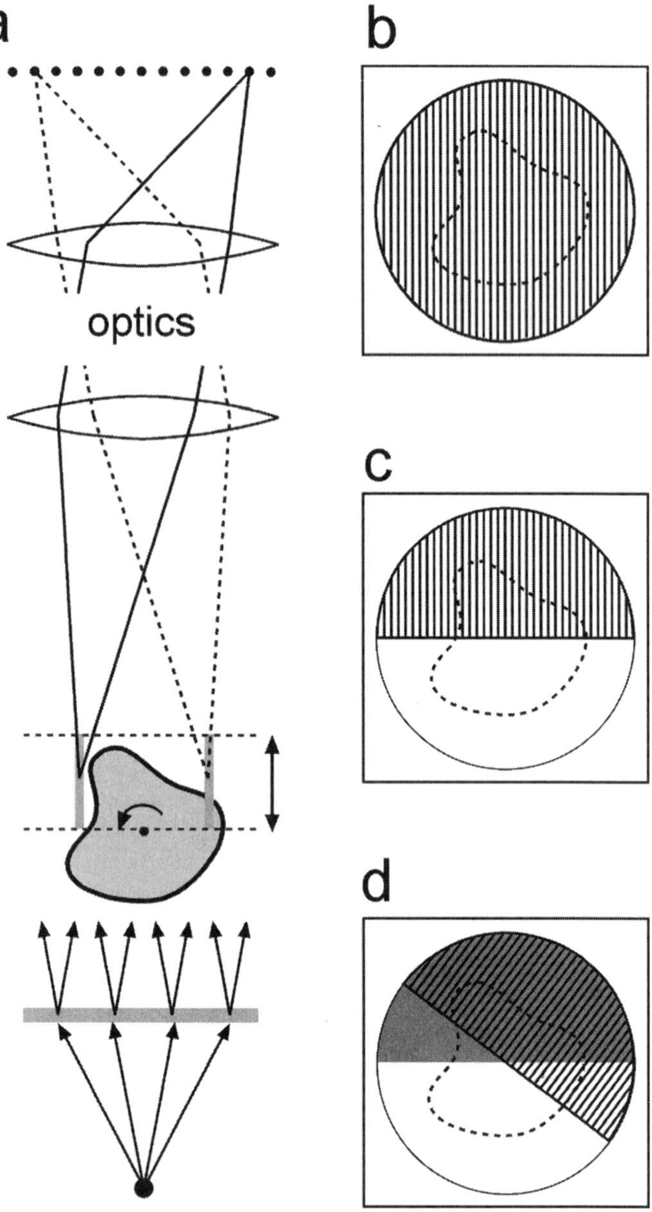


**Figure 4** Modified back-projection. (*a*) The specimen is imaged such that only its top half is fully in focus. (*b*) A normal algorithm would back-project this data across the whole image. (*c*) An improvement is to limit the back-projection to the region corresponding to the focused half of the specimen. (*d*) As the data for successive angles is accumulated, the semidisc mask is rotated to maintain back-projection in the correct region of the image.

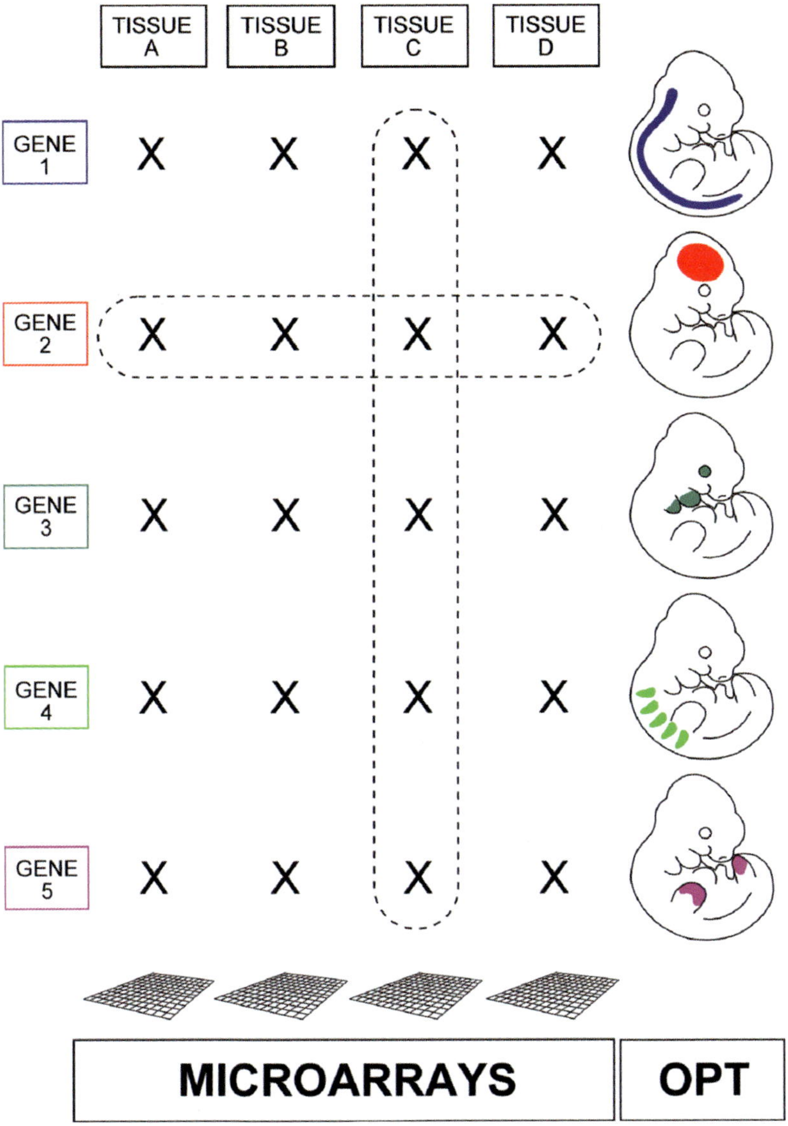


**Figure 5** Comparison of OPT data versus microarray data. Both techniques can be used to build up information about which genes are expressed in which tissue (or cell type). A single microarray experiment will sample many genes for a single cell type (*vertical dashed region*). Conversely, an OPT experiment samples many tissues for a single gene (*horizontal dashed region*). This illustrates how the two techniques act as orthogonal approaches for obtaining the same kind of information. If software can be developed that automatically identifies the tissues within OPT data, then this will prove an important complement to microarray data.

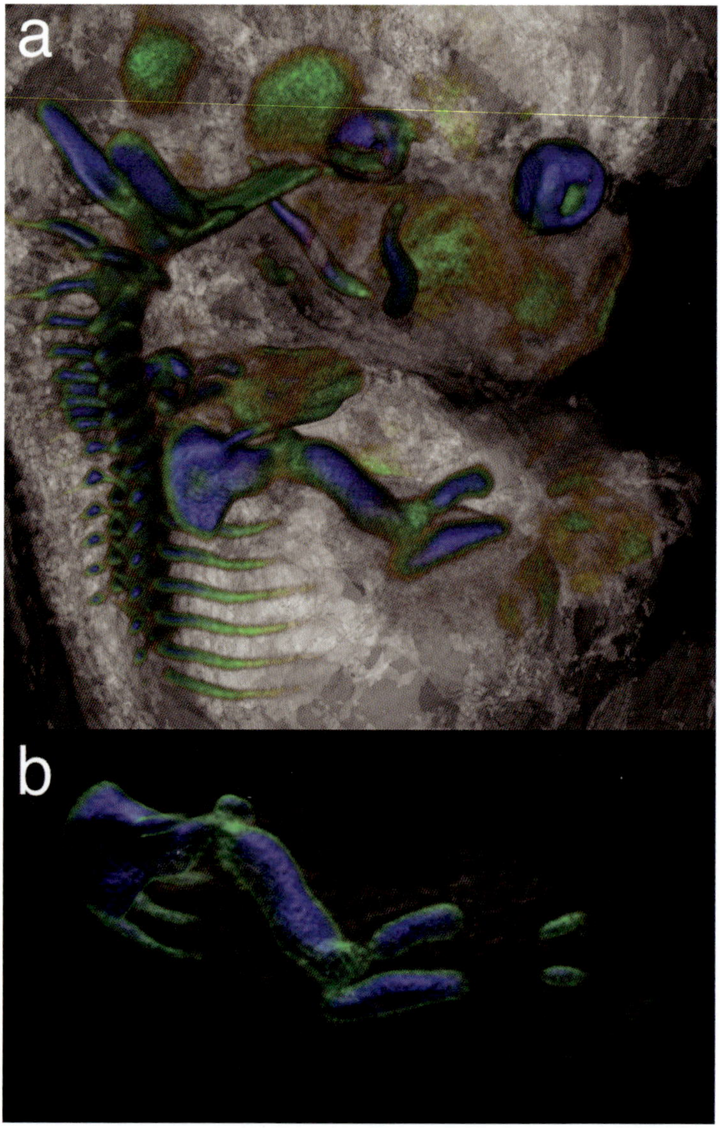


**Figure 6** Transmission OPT of the developing skeleton. This 12.5 dpc embryo was stained with Alcien blue, which labels cartilage. The embryo was then cleared through methanol into BABB and imaged using a wavelength over 750 nm (to aid photon penetration). These images show a combined surface and volume rendering of (*a*) the head and trunk of the embryo and (*b*) one of the forelimbs digitally dissected away from the rest of the body. The original images are monochromatic, but the rendering uses blue to show high optical density and green for medium density. In this example, the eyes are highlighted as blue because their pigmentation is also highly absorbing. (Specimen kindly provided by Seth Ruffins.)

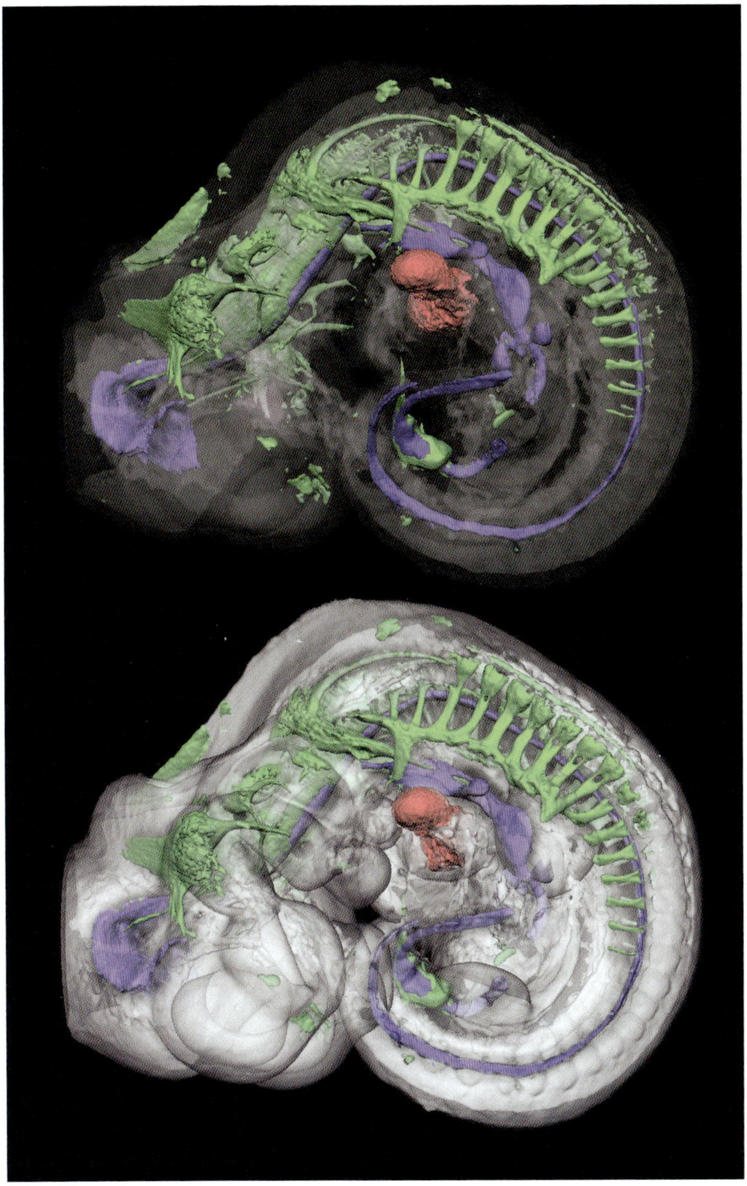

**Figure 7** Fluorescence emission OPT. This 10.5 dpc mouse embryo was labeled with fluorescently tagged antibodies to highlight the expression of two different proteins (21). In green is the expression of neurofilament, which labels the developing nervous system, and in blue is the expression of HNF3b, which labels the endoderm of the gut and the floorplate of the neural tube. The transparent surface represents the structure of the unlabelled regions of the embryo, and the red region indicates where high autofluorescence from the blood was recorded. The two images show the same data rendered with different degrees of transparency.

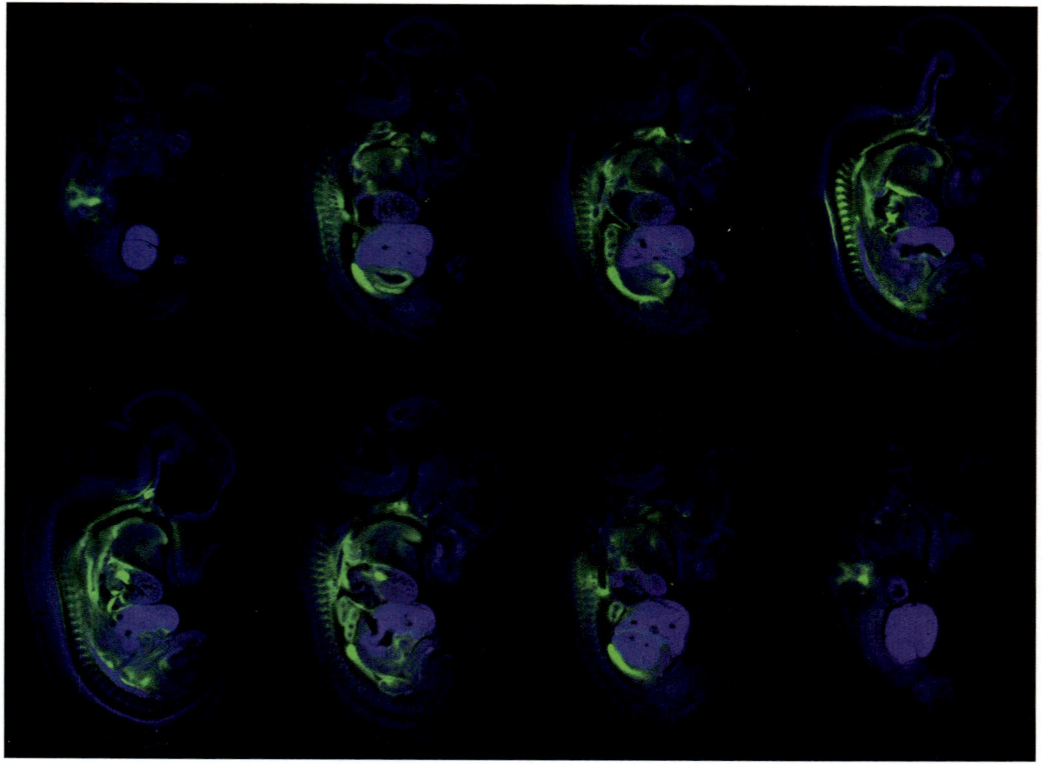

**Figure 8** Combined fluorescence and brightfield OPT. This specimen was stained for the pattern of a transgenic LacZ reporter gene using the substrate X-gal. The distribution of b-Gal activity was imaged by transmission OPT and highlights where light was absorbed by the blue precipitate (*shown in green*). The anatomy of the embryo itself was imaged by recording the autofluorescent signal emitted from the unstained tissue (*shown in blue*). Reproduced with kind permission of Sharon Mulroy and Richard Sanford.

large-volume data sets, such as MRI and CT. These algorithms allow a standard PC to rapidly volume-render large MRI data sets, but only for single channels. On the other hand is software for multichannel 3-D confocal data sets. Although these cope very well with many channels in the same space, computer speeds and memory sizes still make them frustratingly slow for interactive volume rendering of multichannel OPT data sets. For the moment, this means that good-quality rendering requires off-line precalculation of images (we currently use the package VTK); however, it must certainly not be too far in the future before affordable desktop computers will be able to cope with high-volume multichannel OPT data.

## APPLICATIONS OF OPT

### Gene-Expression Analysis

Because OPT can record both absorption and emission profiles, it is able to image the wealth of different staining techniques that exist to record the spatial distribution of gene activity. The most common assay for gene activity at the RNA level is still a protocol that produces a purple precipitate within the tissue (22, 23). Because this precipitate is not fluorescent, it cannot be imaged by confocal microscopy. However, in brightfield mode, OPT can recreate the 3-D distribution of this precipitate for a complete 11.5 dpc (days-post-coitum) mouse embryo. At the protein level, gene expression is usually detected using immunohistochemistry and therefore can be detected using fluorochromes. Using fluorescent approaches, OPT can record more than one gene activity within the same specimen through the selection of different fluorescent wavelength filters (Figure 5, see color insert).

For gene-expression experiments, the power of OPT lies in its ability to provide an overview of expression patterns for many specimens relatively fast. OPT does not provide subcellular resolution, but does allow the identification of which tissues are expressing at different levels. It is therefore particularly suited to experiments in which we wish to explore the patterns of, for example, 10 genes during 5 stages of development. If these are relatively unknown genes and we plan to study them by cutting serial sections, then almost every section from each embryo would have to be analyzed. This would mean hundreds of sections for each of 50 embryos. By contrast, with OPT the analysis could be achieved within a reasonable time.

Microarray technology has seen an explosion in popularity over the past few years because the ability to measure the expression levels for thousands of genes within a particular cell type or tissue type (2, 3) is a potentially very powerful tool for gene function studies. In many ways, an OPT scan that maps the expression pattern of a gene within an embryo is the inverse of a microarray experiment. Instead of measuring many genes for a particular tissue type, it measures the expression of one gene in many tissue types. In fact, the two types of data are orthogonal to each other, as seen in the Figure 6 (see color insert). In this context, the current advantage of microarrays is that the information about which point in the array relates to which gene has been programmed into computers so they can easily relate the detected expression levels to specific gene names. The equivalent function for an OPT scan does not yet exist. A human can look through the OPT data and observe that expression is high in tissue A and low in tissue B, but so far, computers by themselves cannot automatically identify which tissue is which. This will hopefully be solved in the future by projects such as the Edinburgh Mouse Atlas Project (eMAP), which should allow OPT scans to be mapped automatically into a standard 3-D framework (1). This could allow automatic assignment of every voxel from the OPT data to a named tissue. When this becomes possible, the close relationship between OPT data and microarrays will become apparent—the optimal approach to building comprehensive expression databases will then be to use each technique to support and verify the other.

## Screening for Abnormal Anatomy or Histology

Another important application for OPT is to help analyze normal and abnormal morphology (Figure 7, see color insert) (24). There are two particular areas in which this is likely to become important: First, for phenotyping mice, either from targeted knockout/transgenic experiments (Figure 8, see color insert) or from mutagenesis projects. Scientists are producing mouse mutants at an increasing rate; however, our ability to identify morphological changes is limited, and it is likely that many subtle phenotypes go unnoticed for lack of an appropriate and convenient imaging technology. We have found that the ability to generate 3-D reconstructions of a particular organ relatively fast for a number of specimens (for example, by immunohistochemistry) often highlights morphological defects that were never spotted before. A particular advantage of examining organ shapes interactively on a computer is that differences are much easier to spot than when examining histological sections. Features that appear insignificant on a 2-D section may become important once seen in the context of the surrounding 3-D tissue. The result is that differences between wild-type and mutant phenotype are easy to detect, even for researchers with little anatomical training.

The second area is in the growing field of animal models of disease. Mouse models for many diseases are generated with the aim of screening potential drugs that may either alleviate the symptoms or cure the disease. In many cases there are structural changes associated with these diseases. For example, in diabetes the number, size, and distribution of Islets of Langerhans may change within the pancreas, and in emphysema the shape and sizes of alveoli are affected. A technology to rapidly assess and quantify such structural changes within adult tissues could therefore be of great benefit to projects that are seeking therapies for these conditions.

## Pinpointing Cells Within a Tissue

Another useful function is the ability to localize where labeled cells are within a tissue. This has clear benefits in the field of developmental biology, but could also be useful in assessment of cell-therapy experiments in which genetically modified cells are injected into an animal model of a particular disease to accurately discover where these cells become localized. A developmental example of this application was recently published by Wilkie et al. (25) in which the distribution of small clones of cells expressing LacZ was examined within the developing mouse brain. Originally, the results from these experiments were being studied by serial sections; however, some of the early conclusions had to be modified upon viewing the clones in their true 3-D organization. This highlights again the usefulness of seeing organs in their correct 3-D context. In general, if a colored stain is used (such as X-gal staining of LacZ-expressing cells) then small clusters of cells can be detected, and possibly single cells. If a fluorescent dye is used (such as by fluorescent immunohistochemistry) then single cells can clearly be identified (J. Sharpe, unpublished data).

## COMPARISON OF OPT WITH OTHER 3-D MICROSCOPY TECHNOLOGIES

### Serial Sections

In terms of resolution, none of the whole-organ imaging techniques described here are able to compete with cutting real serial sections. Once tissue has been sliced into 10-micron sections, it can be imaged using high-power microscopes, and sub-micron resolutions are therefore trivial. However, there are drawbacks beyond the obvious problem of speed. If the aim is to reconstruct tissue morphology/histology alone, then the most efficient technique is block-face imaging. The specimen is embedded in a cutting medium, such as paraffin wax, and the microscope is focused on the face of the block. As cutting proceeds, images are captured of each section just before it is cut, while still part of the block. The most efficient example of this approach is episcopic fluorescence image capture (EFIC) in which contrast is provided by autofluorescence of the tissue (26). However, imaging assay-specific fluorescent signals, for example, from immunohistochemistry, has not yet been reported, and so the current method for imaging a signal is a negative one—the signal must be viewed using a light-absorbing stain that quenches the autofluorescence. An alternative that allows positive detection is the technique called external marker automatic congruencing (EMAC) (27). Because this uses glass-mounted sections, it can perform normal microscopy techniques and image colored stains and fluorescent dyes; however, because every section must be mounted on glass slides, the process has not been fully automated.

### Confocal Microscopy

Decades of research have provided us with a veritable battery of fluorescent dyes that can be used to label biologically significant molecular distributions. The biggest advantage of 3-D optical sectioning approaches, such as confocal microscopy and multiphoton microscopy (28), is therefore their ability to visualize many of these signals within a single specimen. In terms of resolution, they are unsurpassed; however, when it comes to imaging mouse organs or embryos, confocal microscopy has been unable to image the entire specimen intact (apart from the very earliest stages). It can generally produce good 3-D data from structures up to a few hundred microns in depth. There is, however, another drawback of these approaches that is sometimes overlooked: their inability to generate 3-D reconstructions of colored stains (as opposed to fluorescent dyes). There are still many common assays for which the most reliable signal-detection method is the production of a dark-colored precipitate—for example, the use of BCIP/NBT (5-bromo-4-chloro-3-indolyl phosphate and nitroblue tetrazolium chloride) to visualize whole-mount in situ hybridization. Although such precipitates can easily be detected on physically cut sections by brightfield microscopy, this particular assay for gene expression patterns cannot be imaged in 3-D by confocal. These patterns can, however, be imaged in 3-D using OPT (in transmission mode).

## X-Ray Micro-CT

Micro-CT displays a resolution that is ideal for embryos (less than 10 microns) (E. Buelens, personal communication). However, its main drawback relates to contrast: X-rays are hardly absorbed at all by soft tissue and optical colored stains (34). This means that it is difficult to image both standard gene expression assays and the structure of the tissue. Contrast for X-ray CT is often enhanced through the use of solutions containing heavy-metal atoms, so in the case of micro-CT, the same principle has successfully been applied (M. Henkelman, personal communication). However, developing this approach into a gene-activity assay has not been described.

## Microscopic MRI

This modality does display a big improvement over one of the problems of micro-CT—it is able to detect useful contrast between the tissues of untreated embryos (8). However, the achievable resolution of micro-MRI is significantly lower than micro-CT [approximately 25 microns in the studies by Schneider (29)]. A similar drawback to CT is the paucity of assays for molecule-specific labeling of the tissue compared to optical techniques. Arguably, the most important application for this technique will therefore be its ability to image dynamically changing gene expression patterns in 3-D within living embryos, using high-contrast agents that respond to transgene expression (7).

## Optical Coherence Tomography

OCT has recently been used in developmental studies (18, 30). This technique is an optical equivalent of ultrasound—photons are sent into the specimen in one direction, and those reflected by the tissue are detected and their time-of-flight calculated through interferometry. As explained in the Introduction (above), this technique is very different from all other approaches named as tomography because it does not require solving an inverse problem. One of OCT's advantages is that it can image living tissue, and can do so down to a depth of 2–3 mm. However, owing to its reliance on interferometry, this approach is more limited than confocal in terms of signal detection: Because the light reflected from the specimen must be coherent with a reference beam, it cannot detect fluorescence (as this requires the illumination and detected beams to be of different wavelengths). As such, it appears unsuitable for analysis of immunohistochemistry or other standard gene-expression assays.

### Ultrasonic Biomicroscopy

Real microscopic ultrasound imaging using high-frequency sound waves is actually better suited to whole-embryo imaging than OCT, as it displays far greater depth penetration. It can image an entire mouse embryo alive within the uterus of a pregnant female (31). Similar to OCT, its strength lies in its ability to image living embryos, but with more convenient access to embryos within a pregnant mouse compared to MRI, as the probe needs only to be held against the skin of the mouse. However, for fixed specimens, it does not display high resolution (achieving voxels approximately 50 microns across), nor does it currently feature convenient gene-expression assays.

## FUTURE DEVELOPMENTS

OPT is still in its early days. Over the next few years, we hope to see improvements in various aspects, such as speed and accuracy of the reconstruction algorithm, more dedicated optics, and improvements to the specimen-preparation protocols. However, in addition to these more general goals, we will be working on a few specific projects.

So far, all major OPT work has been done with fixed material. This allows the use of organic solvents to act as index-matching agents, which, in turn, allows for relatively high-resolution imaging. However, these solvents are generally toxic, so OPT in living material will have to cope with a much higher degree of photon scattering. For this reason, we are focusing our attempts on live OPT imaging of small embryonic tissue (such as the vertebrate limb bud) that are already fairly transparent. The ability to monitor in 4-D the development of complex shapes and dynamic gene expression patterns through the use of transgenic fluorescent proteins may transform our understanding of these complex events.

Various other incarnations of fluorescence imaging (such as confocal microscopy) have adopted the technique of multispectral imaging (32, 33). Whereas conventional fluorescence imaging employs a limited set of filters to select specific wavelengths of light to be detected, multispectral imaging detects a whole spectrum of wavelengths. Fluorochromes emit photons over a whole range of wavelengths, so rather than trying to distinguish the different molecules by recording the intensity at only a couple of wavelengths, multispectral imaging identifies them by calculating their relative contribution to the spectrum detected at each pixel. In this way, multispectral imaging is able to image many more signals from the same specimen. OPT should therefore benefit from this approach in the same way that any other fluorescence-based imaging technique does.

Another technological development that may improve OPT is the use of a scanning laser in place of a wide-field CCD. This should improve imaging in a manner analogous to the use of laser scanning in confocal imaging. Because a much smaller region of the tissue will be excited at any one time, there will be less noise at a given pixel. In a wide-field arrangement, some of the noise at each pixel is generated by multiply scattered photons that were emitted from regions of the tissue that do not lie on the intended projection for that pixel. The laser scanning approach may therefore be particularly useful for applications in which scattering is more of a problem, such as living tissues.

## ACKNOWLEDGMENTS

I wish to thank Mark Henkelman and Simon Arridge for useful discussion about tomography. All aspects of OPT development were funded by the Medical Research Council.

**The *Annual Review of Biomedical Engineering* is online at http://bioeng.annualreviews.org**

## LITERATURE CITED

1. Davidson D, Baldock R. 2001. Bioinformatics beyond sequence: mapping gene function in the embryo. *Nat. Rev. Genet.* 2: 409–417
2. Bono H, Yagi K, Kasukawa T, Nikaido I, Tominaga N, et al. 2003. Systematic expression profiling of the mouse transcriptome using RIKEN cDNA microarrays. *Genome Res.* 13:1318–23
3. The Mouse Atlas of Gene Expression. http://www.mouseatlas.org
4. Visel A, Thaller C, Eichele G. 2004. GenePaint.org: an atlas of gene expression patterns in the mouse embryo. *Nucleic Acids Res.* 1:D552–56
5. Maddox J. 1992. Is molecular biology yet a science? *Nature* 355:201
6. Reinitz J, Sharp DH. 1995. Mechanism of eve stripe formation. *Mech. Dev.* 49:133–58
7. Louie AY, Huber MM, Ahrens ET, Rothbacher U, Moats R, et al. 2000. In vivo visualization of gene expression using magnetic resonance imaging. *Nat. Biotechnol.* 18:321–25
8. Dhenain D, Ruffins S, Jacobs RE. 2001. Three-dimensional digital mouse atlas using high-resolution MRI. *Dev. Biol.* 232: 458–70
9. Hecksher-Sorensen J, Sharpe J. 2001. 3D confocal reconstruction of gene expression in mouse. *Mech. Dev.* 100:59–63
10. Massoud TF, Gambhir SS. 2003. Molecular imaging in living subjects: seeing fundamental biological processes in a new light. *Genes Dev.* 17:545–80

11. Midgley PA, Weyland M. 2003. 3D electron microscopy in the physical sciences: the development of Z-contrast and EFTEM tomography. *Ultramicroscopy* 96:413–31
12. Brown BH. 2003. Electrical impedance tomography (EIT): a review. *J. Med. Eng. Technol.* 27:97–108
13. Mather ML, Baldock C. 2003. Ultrasound tomography imaging of radiation dose distributions in polymer gel dosimeters: preliminary study. *Med. Phys.* 30:2140–48
14. Bronstein MM, Bronstein AM, Zibulevsky M, Azhari H. 2002. Reconstruction in diffraction ultrasound tomography using nonuniform FFT. *IEEE Trans. Med. Imaging* 21:1395–401
15. Korjenevsky A, Cherepenin V, Sapetsky S. 2000. Magnetic induction tomography: experimental realization. *Physiol. Meas.* 21: 89–94
16. Markel VA, Schotland JC. 2001. Inverse problem in optical diffusion tomography. I. Fourier-Laplace inversion formulas. *J. Opt. Soc. Am. A. Opt. Image Sci. Vis.* 18:1336–47
17. Huang D, Swanson E, Lin C, Schuman J, Stinson W, et al. 1991. Optical coherence tomography. *Science* 254:1178–81
18. Yelbuz TM, Choma MA, Thrane L, Kirby ML, Izatt JA. 2002. Optical coherence tomography: a new high-resolution imaging technology to study cardiac development in chick embryos. *Circulation* 106:2771–74
19. Kak AC, Slaney M. 1988. *Principles of Computerized Tomographic Imaging*. Piscataway, NJ: IEEE Press
20. Ntziachristos V, Chance B. 2001. Probing physiology and molecular function using optical imaging: applications to breast cancer. *Breast Cancer Res.* 3:41–46
21. Sharpe J, Ahlgren U, Perry P, Hill B, Ross A, et al. 2002. Optical projection tomography as a tool for 3D microscopy and gene expression studies. *Science* 296:541–45
22. Hammond KL, Hanson IM, Brown AG, Lettice LA, Hill RE. 1998. Mammalian and Drosophila dachsund genes are related to the Ski proto-oncogene and are expressed in eye and limb. *Mech. Dev.* 74:121–31
23. Ariza-McNaughton L, Krumlauf R. 2002. Non-radioactive in situ hybridisation: simplified procedures for use in whole-mounts of mouse and chick embryos. *Int. Rev. Neurobiol.* 47:239–50
24. Sharpe J. 2003. Optical projection tomography as a new tool for studying embryo anatomy. *J. Anat.* 202:175–81
25. Wilkie AL, Jordan SA, Sharpe JA, Price DJ, Jackson IJ. 2004. Widespread tangential dispertion and extensive cell death during early neurogenesis in the mouse neocortex. *Dev. Biol.* 267:109–18
26. Weninger WJ, Mohun T. 2002. Phenotyping transgenic embryos: a rapid 3-D screening method based on episcopic fluorescence image capturing. *Nat. Genet.* 30: 59–65
27. Streicher J, Donat MA, Strauss B, Sporle R, Schughart K, Muller GB. 2000. Computer-based three-dimensional visualization of developmental gene expression. *Nat. Genet.* 25:147–52
28. Potter SM, Fraser SE, Pine J. 1996. The greatly reduced photodamage of 2-photon microscopy enables extended 3-dimensional time-lapse imaging of living neurons. *Scanning* 18:147
29. Schneider JE, Bamforth SD, Grieve SM, Clarke K, Bhattacharya S, Neubauer S. 2003. High-resolution, high-throughput magnetic paragraph sign resonance imaging of mouse embryonic paragraph sign anatomy using a fast gradient-echo sequence. *MAGMA* 16:43–51
30. Boppart S, Brezinski M, Bouma B, Tearney G, Fujimoto J. 1996. Investigation of developing embryonic morphology using optical coherence tomography. *Dev. Biol.* 177:54–63
31. Foster FS, Zhang M, Duckett AS, Cucevic V, Pavlin CJ. 2003. In vivo imaging of embryonic development in the mouse eye by ultrasound biomicroscopy. *Invest. Ophthalmol. Vis. Sci.* 44:2361–66

32. Dickinson ME, Bearman G, Tille S, Lansford R, Fraser SE. 2001. Multi-spectral imaging and linear unmixing add a whole new dimension to laser scanning fluorescence microscopy. *Biotechniques* 31:1272, 1274–76, 1278
33. Hadjantonakis AK, Dickinson ME, Fraser SE, Papaioannou VE. 2003. Technicolour transgenics: imaging tools for functional genomics in the mouse. *Nat. Rev. Genet.* 4(8):613–25
34. Ritman EL. 2002. Molecular imaging in small animals—roles for micro-CT. *J. Cell Biochem. Suppl.* 39:116–24

Annu. Rev. Biomed. Eng. 2004. 6:229–48
doi: 10.1146/annurev.bioeng.6.040803.140126

First published online as a Review in Advance on April 30, 2004

# MECHANICAL BIOEFFECTS OF ULTRASOUND

Diane Dalecki
*Department of Biomedical Engineering and the Rochester Center for Biomedical Ultrasound, University of Rochester, Rochester, New York 14627;*
*email: dalecki@bme.rochester.edu*

**Key Words** acoustics, cavitation, radiation force, diagnostic imaging, therapeutic ultrasound

■ **Abstract** Ultrasound is used widely in medicine as both a diagnostic and therapeutic tool. Through both thermal and nonthermal mechanisms, ultrasound can produce a variety of biological effects in tissues in vitro and in vivo. This chapter provides an overview of the fundamentals of key nonthermal mechanisms for the interaction of ultrasound with biological tissues. Several categories of mechanical bioeffects of ultrasound are then reviewed to provide insight on the range of ultrasound bioeffects in vivo, the relevance of these effects to diagnostic imaging, and the potential application of mechanical bioeffects to the design of new therapeutic applications of ultrasound in medicine.

CONTENTS

# INTRODUCTION

The use of ultrasound in medicine is wide ranging and continues to expand. Ultrasound is now an indispensable tool for noninvasive diagnostic imaging of the body. The development of sophisticated new imaging modalities continues to increase the role of ultrasound in diagnosis. Ultrasound is also well established as a means of providing noninvasive therapy. Ultrasound is used widely in physiotherapy. Lithotripsy employs high-amplitude acoustic shock waves to treat kidney stone disease. Emerging therapeutic applications are capable of using high-intensity focused ultrasound (HIFU) for noninvasive treatment of tumors. In addition, current research suggests promising new therapeutic applications of ultrasound in the delivery of drugs and genetic material, thrombolysis, and tumor therapy. Further progress in diagnostic and therapeutic applications of ultrasound will require a greater understanding of the mechanisms by which ultrasound interacts with tissues. Given the range of novel diagnostic and therapeutic applications of ultrasound now on the horizon, the advancement of biomedical ultrasound in medicine has never been more exciting.

# MEDICAL ULTRASOUND

## Diagnostic Imaging

Pulsed ultrasound is used extensively as a diagnostic imaging tool throughout many areas of medical practice. Ultrasound used for diagnostic imaging typically employs frequencies in the ~1–10 MHz range. Higher frequencies can be used for specialized imaging applications, such as imaging the eye and skin, or for imaging cellular structures using acoustic microscopy. Ultrasound offers several advantages as a noninvasive imaging modality because it provides real-time imaging capabilities and is widely available, cost effective, and easily portable. The use of ultrasound in diagnostic imaging continues to develop at a rapid pace. Many wide-ranging advances have been made in two- and three-dimensional (2-D and 3-D) imaging modalities, as well as in the use of ultrasound contrast agents.

Ultrasound has a long-standing record of safety and efficacy in diagnostic imaging. Currently, the U.S. Food and Drug Administration (FDA) regulates the acoustic output levels of diagnostic ultrasound imaging devices. The output display standard (1) provides a method to quantify output levels through the use of an on-screen thermal index (TI) and a mechanical index (MI). Three TIs are used to provide a reasonable estimate of temperature rise for conditions when ultrasound propagates through soft tissue (TIS), when the ultrasound beam impinges on bone (TIB), and when the transducer face is very close to bone, as occurs in transcranial applications (TIC) (1). The MI is defined as the derated in situ peak negative pressure (in MPa) (at the point of maximal pulse intensity integral) divided by the center frequency (in MHz) (1). The MI was originally developed as a relative indicator of the potential for mechanical bioeffects (1, 2). Currently, maximum output levels of diagnostic devices are limited to an MI of 1.9 and a spatial peak, temporal average intensity of 720 mW/cm$^2$. Continuing progress in our understanding of ultrasound bioeffects contributes to the excellent record of safety of diagnostic ultrasound.

Knowledge of the acoustic mechanisms of interaction of ultrasound propagation with tissues has facilitated the development of new imaging techniques. For example, the unique responses of microbubbles exposed to acoustic fields have resulted in new imaging techniques that employ gas-based ultrasound contrast agents to expand diagnostic imaging capabilities (see section below). Techniques, such as harmonic imaging, now exploit the nonlinear propagation of ultrasound to enhance diagnostic imaging. New imaging modalities, sometimes termed sonoelastography or elasticity imaging, can provide novel methods for imaging the elastic properties of biological tissues.

## Therapeutic Ultrasound

Ultrasound provides unique avenues for a variety of noninvasive therapies in medicine. Many of these therapeutic applications rely on the ability of ultrasound to focus within tissues and produce a therapeutic bioeffect noninvasively. Lithotripsy has dramatically changed the treatment of kidney stone disease. Lithotripsy procedures employ high-amplitude focused acoustic shock waves to fragment kidney stones. Stone fragmentation results from mechanical interactions of the acoustic waves with the kidney stones. Ultrasound is also used widely in physiotherapy. Low-intensity, pulsed ultrasound has been demonstrated clinically to accelerate the rate of fracture healing. The acoustic mechanism for this therapeutic interaction of ultrasound and bone is yet unknown. HIFU employs focused ultrasound at intensities that can exceed 1000 W/cm$^2$ to selectively heat tissue and produce necrosis. HIFU has promising applications for the nonsurgical treatment of tumors and for noninvasive hemostasis (see 3 for review). Although still in various stages of development, exciting new therapeutic applications of ultrasound in the areas of thrombolysis, drug delivery, gene therapy, and tumor therapy now appear on the horizon (4, 5).

## Ultrasound Contrast Agents

Ultrasound contrast agents can enhance the capabilities of diagnostic imaging and are also providing new avenues for the use of ultrasound in therapy. Ultrasound contrast agents are gas-filled microbubbles on the order of 1–10 $\mu$m in diameter that are stabilized from dissolution through the use of a protein, polymer, or lipid shell. The microbubbles are injected intravenously, and because of their large scattering cross-sections, are useful clinically to enhance diagnostic images. Imaging techniques, such as harmonic imaging and intermittent imaging, have been developed specifically for use with ultrasound contrast agents. The first contrast agent approved by the FDA was composed of a suspension of air-filled microbubbles stabilized with an albumin shell. Newer contrast agents contain gases with low solubility (e.g., perfluorocarbon gas) to increase the duration of effectiveness of the contrast agent for diagnostic imaging. Development of many other types of contrast agents is currently ongoing in various public and private sectors. Targeted contrast agents aim to provide site-specific localization of contrast agents, and they show promise in new applications of ultrasound in the areas of molecular imaging, drug delivery, and gene therapy (4, 5).

# ACOUSTIC MECHANISMS

## Thermal and Nonthermal Mechanisms

Ultrasound exposures used for diagnostic imaging are designed to minimize the interaction of the sound field with the tissue such that potential biological effects are avoided. In comparison, therapeutic applications of ultrasound depend on the direct interaction of the sound field with the tissue to produce the desired beneficial bioeffect. It is very important to recognize that the exposure parameters used for ultrasound therapies are often dramatically different than those used for diagnostic imaging. For example, the pressure amplitude of a typical lithotripter shock wave used to fragment kidney stones can be more than an order of magnitude greater than that used for diagnostic imaging. Also, the exposure intensities and pulse durations used to heat tissue with HIFU far exceed the outputs of diagnostic imaging devices. Knowledge of the acoustic mechanisms for the interaction of ultrasound with tissues is required to maintain the safe use of diagnostic ultrasound and to facilitate the design of new therapeutic applications of biomedical ultrasound.

Acoustic waves can interact with tissue through either thermal or nonthermal physical mechanisms. Absorption of ultrasound results in the conversion of ultrasonic energy to heat. Ultrasound-induced temperature rise is dependent on several factors, including tissue properties (e.g., absorption coefficient, density, perfusion, etc.), ultrasound exposure parameters [e.g., frequency, pressure amplitude, pulse duration, pulse repetition frequency (PRF), etc.], and beam and scanning configurations. Thus, the generation of heat in tissues can typically be controlled through proper exposure design. Biological effects of ultrasound that result solely from heat production are not the primary focus of this review article (see 6).

Ultrasound bioeffects also occur through nonthermal mechanisms. Acoustic cavitation is perhaps the most widely studied nonthermal mechanism, and a variety of biological effects, both in vitro and in vivo, can be attributed to activity associated with acoustic cavitation. Other nonthermal bioeffects result from radiation forces that are associated with ultrasound propagation. Fundamentals of key nonthermal mechanisms that are relevant to biological effects of ultrasound are summarized in the sections below.

## Acoustic Cavitation

Acoustic cavitation describes the interaction of a sound field with a gas bubble. The occurrence of cavitation thus requires the presence of a stabilized gas body or nucleus. Aside from tissues such as the lung and intestine, the presence of

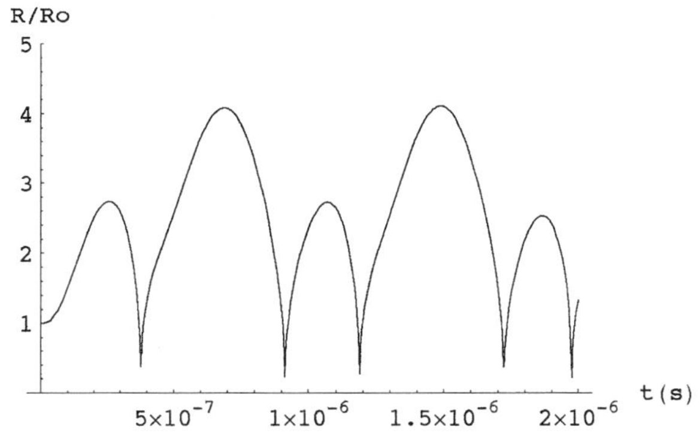


**Figure 1** Acoustic cavitation. Predicted response of an air microbubble (initial radius $R_o$ of 1 $\mu$m) in water exposed to 2.5 MHz ultrasound at a pressure amplitude of 0.4 MPa.

naturally occurring gas in tissues is typically rare. Microbubbles can be introduced intentionally into the body through the injection of gas-based ultrasound contrast agents. Several models exist to explain the stabilization of gas nuclei in fluids (7, 8). One model (the crevice model) assumes that gas nuclei are stabilized in crevices of hydrophobic impurities in the liquid. As the pressure in the liquid decreases, the gas in the crevice expands and may separate from the impurity to form a microbubble. If preexisting nuclei are present, gas bodies can be produced in tissues by a high-amplitude acoustic exposure, such as a lithotripter field (9) or HIFU exposure (10).

When exposed to an acoustic field, a bubble in a liquid will oscillate around an equilibrium radius (Figure 1). Various theoretical models can be used to predict the radius of a bubble as a function of time of exposure (see 7, 8, 11). The maximum response of a bubble to an acoustic field occurs when it is exposed at its resonance frequency. The resonance frequency is dependent on the initial size of the bubble, and for frequencies relevant to diagnostic ultrasound imaging, resonance size bubbles are on the order of a few micrometers in radius. Noninertial cavitation (sometimes termed stable cavitation in earlier literature) describes a repetitive oscillation of a bubble over many acoustic cycles (8, 12). The maximum expansion of a noninertial cavity typically does not exceed twice the equilibrium radius. The response of the bubble can be nonlinear and is dependent on variables, including the acoustic pressure amplitude, exposure frequency, and size of the bubble. Bubble oscillations can be damped through viscous dissipation, sound radiation, and thermal conduction (7, 8, 11).

A variety of physical phenomena can be associated with noninertial cavitation (6). Rectified diffusion describes the slow growth of an oscillating bubble owing to a net flow of gas into the bubble over many acoustic cycles. Acoustically driven bubble oscillations can result in heat production, microstreaming of fluid near the bubble, and localized shear stresses. In a traveling wave field, radiation forces can produce bubble translation, whereas in a stationary acoustic wave, field radiation forces can cause bubbles to collect at pressure minima and maxima depending on their size (7). Interactions between bubbles and particles in a sound field can result in bubble coalescence or the attraction of nearby particles or cells to an oscillating bubble (6).

At sufficiently high exposure amplitudes, a bubble may expand to a maximum radius greater than twice its initial radius and then collapse rapidly to a small fraction of its initial radius. This response of the bubble to the acoustic field is termed inertial cavitation (sometimes termed transient cavitation in earlier literature). Here, the motion of the bubble is highly nonlinear and the collapse is dominated by the inertia of the surrounding liquid medium (12). For appropriate exposure conditions, a single ultrasound pulse on the order of one microsecond in duration can cause a bubble to expand rapidly and collapse violently (12). The violence of the collapse of the inertial cavity is determined by various parameters, including acoustic frequency, pressure amplitude, and initial bubble radius. The response of an inertial cavity to an acoustic field is highly nonlinear, such that a small increase in acoustic pressure amplitude can change the bubble response from a noninertial cavity to an inertial cavity. The acoustic pressure at which the transition occurs is often called the threshold for inertial cavitation.

Extremely high temperatures and pressures can be achieved at the minimum radius of the inertial bubble collapse (e.g., 12). Some models predict maximum collapse temperatures exceeding thousands of degrees Kelvin (e.g., 2, 8, 12). These high temperatures and pressures are localized spatially near the collapsing bubble and are limited temporally to the duration of the collapse. In general, for a given bubble radius and pressure amplitude, as the frequency of exposure increases the maximum collapse pressure in the bubble decreases (12).

Several interesting physical phenomena are associated with inertial cavitation. The production of high temperatures and pressures during inertial collapse can lead to the formation of free radicals (6). The field of sonochemistry explores the application of inertial cavitation to generate chemical species or drive chemical reactions. Sonoluminescence describes the generation of light from activities associated with inertial cavitation. During inertial collapse, the motion of the bubble wall may become supersonic and generate a spherically diverging shock wave in the liquid medium surrounding the collapsing bubble. Bubbles undergoing inertial cavitation near solid boundaries can collapse asymmetrically. Asymmetric collapse can result in the formation of high-speed, fluid microjets that impinge on the solid boundary. Microjets can produce pitting of metals, such as aluminum foil, and likely play a role in the fragmentation of kidney stones with lithotripter shock waves (13).

## Radiation Force, Radiation Torque, and Acoustic Streaming

A steady, time-averaged force called the acoustic radiation force typically acts upon an object in an acoustic field. This force results from a transfer of momentum from the sound field to the object (14). Techniques that employ radiation force are frequently used in methods to calibrate ultrasonic fields (15–18). The magnitude of the radiation force depends on characteristics of both the sound field and the object in the field. For the case of a plane wave incident normally on a perfectly absorbing target, the radiation force is equal to $W/c$, where $W$ is the total acoustic power and $c$ is the speed of sound in the propagating medium. The radiation force exerted by a plane wave on a perfectly reflecting target is twice that of a perfectly absorbing target. These plane wave approximations provide adequate estimates of radiation force. However, actual ultrasonic fields have finite beam widths, can be focused, and may be distorted by nonlinear propagation, all of which can influence radiation force. Radiation forces exerted on cells in a stationary wave field are more complex and can result in the banding of red cells at one-half wavelength intervals in a blood vessel in vivo (19). Radiation forces can also displace contrast agents to the wall of blood vessels in laboratory animals (20).

Radiation force is the underlying mechanism for phenomena such as radiation torque, acoustic streaming, acoustic levitation, and acoustic fountain effects. Radiation torque can result in the rotation or spinning of symmetrical particles, whereas asymmetrical particles may rotate to a preferential orientation in the sound field. An acoustic field propagating in a fluid medium can give rise to a bulk fluid flow termed acoustic streaming. The streaming velocity is dependent on factors including the absorption coefficient, speed of sound, kinematic viscosity, intensity, beam geometry, and nonlinear propagation. The use of acoustic streaming produced by ultrasound may hold promise as a diagnostic technique to identify cysts noninvasively (21).

## Mechanical Bioeffects In Vivo

It is well documented that ultrasound can produce a wide variety of biological effects in vitro and in vivo, and the acoustic mechanisms responsible for some of these bioeffects have been identified (6, 22). Cavitation can occur in vivo if appropriate microbubbles are present, such as in the intestine or in tissues containing microbubble contrast agents. Radiation forces have been demonstrated to stimulate cardiac and neural tissues. Mechanisms for other effects of ultrasound, including acceleration of bone fracture healing and extravasation of red blood cells in the lung, are currently unknown and still under active investigation. The environment for some acoustic mechanisms, such as heating, cavitation, and acoustic streaming, is much different in vitro than in vivo. Therefore, this review concentrates on mechanisms of ultrasound bioeffects in vivo.

The sections that follow review several categories of bioeffects of ultrasound in vivo that result from nonthermal mechanisms. These sections provide insight on the range of mechanical bioeffects in vivo produced by ultrasound, the relevance of these effects to diagnostic and therapeutic applications of ultrasound, and in some instances also provide examples of avenues of investigations used by researchers to identify mechanisms for ultrasound bioeffects. Complete and extensive reviews of the biological effects of ultrasound in vitro and vivo have been published by the

National Council on Radiation Protection and Measurements (6) and the American Institute of Ultrasound in Medicine (22).

## TISSUES CONTAINING GAS NATURALLY

Tissues that contain gas bodies naturally, such as the lung and intestine, are susceptible to bioeffects from exposure to pulsed ultrasound and lithotripter fields. In laboratory mammals, damage to the microvasculature in the lung and intestine results from nonthermal mechanisms and is associated with the presence of gas in these tissues (23, 24). Although both organs contain gas, the effects of ultrasound on the lung and intestine likely result from different acoustic mechanisms (25).

### Lung

Ultrasound-induced damage to the vasculature of the lung is characterized by localized, extravasation of red blood cells from the capillaries into the alveolar space (26). This damage appears to repair with time without intervention (27). The first report of ultrasound-induced damage to the lung (28) indicated a pressure threshold of ~1 MPa in situ for exposure at 2 MHz (10 $\mu$s pulse duration, 100 Hz PRF, 3 min exposure). Similar results have been reported under diagnostically relevant exposure conditions using mice, monkeys, pigs, rabbits, and rats (e.g., 29–35). One study that looked specifically for the generation of lung hemorrhage in humans did not observe any lung hemorrhage after intraoperative transesophageal echocardiography (36). The sensitivity of the lung to ultrasound exposure is directly related to the presence of gas in this tissue because gas-free fetal lungs do not exhibit the lung damage observed in air-filled adult lungs (23). The degree of inflation of the lung influences the acoustic impedance difference between lung and intercostal tissues and also the extent of lung damage (37). One study reported detection of cavitation activity during ultrasound exposure of rat lung (32). The threshold for lung hemorrhage has been investigated as a function of frequency (28, 38), pulse duration (28, 39), pulse repetition frequency (28, 40), exposure duration (23, 40–42), beam characteristics (28, 43), and age (29–31, 44).

The acoustic mechanism by which damage to the lung vasculature occurs is nonthermal in origin. Although the presence of gas in the tissue is required to produce the effect, results of several studies do not clearly support inertial cavitation as the primary mechanism for this bioeffect (25). Thresholds for bioeffects more clearly related to cavitation (i.e., intestinal damage and damage to the microvasculature when microbubbles are present, see sections below) exhibit a much greater dependence on frequency than that observed for lung hemorrhage (28, 38). Furthermore, introduction of additional cavitation nuclei (i.e., microbubble ultrasound contrast agents) into the vasculature of mice does not increase the extent of lung hemorrhage (45). Although hydrostatic pressure is expected to decrease inertial cavitation activity, exposure of mice to pulsed ultrasound under hydrostatic pressure does not eliminate ultrasound-induced lung damage (46). Finally, exposure to negative acoustic pressures produces no greater lung damage than exposure to positive pressures, even though negative pressure exposures enhance inertial cavitation theoretically (47–49).

## Intestine

Intestine is another tissue that contains gas bodies naturally. It is reasonable to hypothesize that acoustic cavitation may occur in the intestinal environment because the intestine contains gas bodies spanning a wide range in size often located in a fluid-like medium. Although damage to the intestine can be caused by heat (50), ultrasound-induced intestinal hemorrhage has indeed occurred in laboratory mammals even when thermal effects have been minimized (24, 51–53). Intestinal petechiae can be produced in mice exposed to pulsed ultrasound at diagnostically relevant frequencies and pulse durations (53). The threshold for intestinal hemorrhage increases with exposure frequency, and the pressure threshold ranges from ~1 to 4 MPa over the frequency range of ~1 to 4 MHz (53). These thresholds are near the current upper limit of outputs of diagnostic imaging devices. The increase in threshold with increasing frequency is consistent with cavitation as a mechanism for this bioeffect.

Lithotripter fields can also produce petechial hemorrhage in the intestine of laboratory animals (51, 52, 54). The pressure threshold for intestinal damage in mice is ~1–3 MPa, and the extent of damage increases with increasing pressure amplitude and shock number (51, 52). One study, designed to test for the cavitation mechanism, demonstrated that the presence of gas in the intestine was necessary to produce intestinal petechiae with ultrasound (24). In this study, pregnant mice were exposed to a lithotripter field of pressure amplitude exceeding the threshold for intestinal damage in adult mice. Although the gas-containing maternal intestines were extensively damaged, the gas-free intestines of the fetal mice were not damaged by the exposure (24).

Further evidence of cavitation as a mechanism for effects of acoustic fields on intestine arises from several investigations employing ultrasound contrast agents. The presence of microbubble ultrasound contrast agents in the vasculature significantly increases the extent of damage to murine intestines exposed to pulsed ultrasound (55, 56). In one study, the threshold for production of intestinal petechiae when Albunex™ was present in the blood was ~3 MPa for exposure at 2.4 MHz (10 $\mu$s pulse duration, 1 kHz PRF) (56). In general, the threshold for the effect increases with increasing frequency and decreasing pulse duration (55, 56). Ultrasound-induced petechiae in the intestine were more extensive with contrast agents containing perfluorocarbon gases compared to those containing air (56). A further test of cavitation employed an electrohydraulic lithotripter to generate either a positive pressure pulse or a negative pressure pulse (48). Theoretically, the response of microbubbles to negative-pressure amplitudes is greater than the response to positive pressures. For mice exposed to these lithotripter fields, significantly more damage occurred in the intestine (as well as other tissues) for exposure to negative pressures compared to positive pressures when contrast agents were present (48). The results from all investigations summarized above are consistent with cavitation as a mechanism for production of intestinal petechiae with ultrasound.

## CARDIAC EFFECTS

Single pulses of high-amplitude ultrasound can produce effects on cardiac rhythm. Premature ventricular contractions can result from lithotripter fields (57, 58). The most sensitive phase of the cardiac cycle for producing a premature contraction with an acoustic pulse is during the T-P segment (i.e., diastole) (57, 59). When a single lithotripter pulse is delivered to the heart during this phase of the cardiac cycle, the threshold pressure amplitude for producing a premature contraction is on the order of 5 MPa (57, 58). Interestingly, a series of repetitive pulses delivered to the heart can capture and pace the heart in laboratory animals (57). The threshold for the production of premature cardiac contractions is below pressure amplitudes used typically for clinical lithotripsy. However, in clinical practice, the delivery of lithotripter pulses is synchronized with the electrocardiogram (ECG) to avoid producing effects on cardiac rhythm.

Premature cardiac contractions can also be produced by exposure to single pulses of ultrasound (59, 60). In frogs and mice, the threshold for producing a premature contraction with a single 5-ms pulse of ultrasound at 1.2 MHz is ~2–5 MPa (59, 60). The threshold for the effect increases with decreasing pulse duration and increasing frequency (59, 60). The long pulse durations and relatively high-pressure amplitudes necessary to produce premature contractions are not characteristic of exposures used for diagnostic ultrasound imaging.

Investigations using ultrasound contrast agents suggest that gas bodies or acoustic cavitation may play a role in the generation of premature cardiac contractions with ultrasound. When microbubble ultrasound contrast agents are present in the vasculature, the threshold for the production of premature contractions with ultrasound is significantly reduced, and short pulse durations are capable of producing the effect (Figure 2) (61–64). Premature ventricular contractions occurred in humans exposed to diagnostic ultrasound when an experimental contrast agent was present in the blood (64). In laboratory animals injected with contrast agents, the threshold for producing a premature contraction with a single, 10-$\mu$s pulse of 1-MHz ultrasound is on the order of 1 MPa (61, 62). Microvasculature damage has also been observed in hearts exposed to ultrasound with contrast agents present; however, the relationship between the generation of arrhythmia and the effects on the microvasculature is uncertain (62, 63).

In addition to producing premature cardiac contractions, a single pulse of high-amplitude ultrasound can affect cardiac contractility (59, 65, 66). In the frog heart, a pulse of ultrasound can produce either a decrease in the maximum aortic pressure, an abnormal relaxation, or a combination of the two effects (59). The aortic pressure

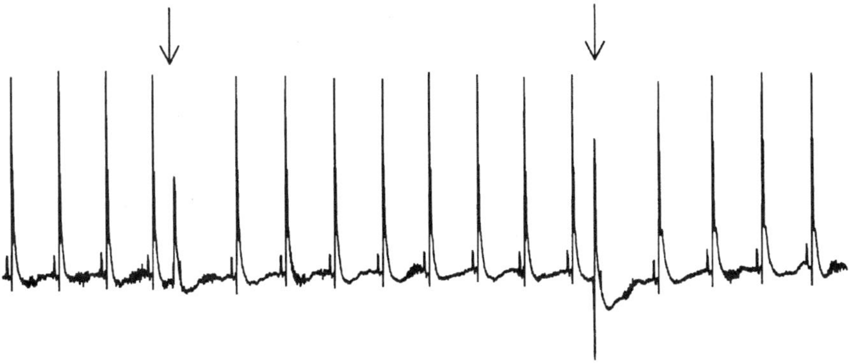

**Figure 2** ECG of a mouse depicts ultrasound-induced premature cardiac contractions when contrast agent microbubbles are present in the blood. An ultrasound pulse (10 $\mu$s, 1.2 MHz) at pressure amplitude above threshold is delivered at each arrow. Each resulting premature contraction is then followed by a return to normal rhythm.

returns to control values within one or two beats after the ultrasound exposure, suggesting that contractile components of the tissue are not damaged. For this effect, an ultrasound pulse is most effective when delivered to the heart during systole (59). In the frog heart, the threshold for this effect is ~5 MPa using a 5-ms pulse with a carrier frequency of 1.2 MHz (59). Again, the threshold increases significantly for shorter pulse durations such that this effect would not occur with pulse durations and outputs of diagnostic imaging devices.

A series of experimental investigations suggests that radiation force is the acoustic mechanism for this effect of ultrasound on cardiac contractility (66). Heat does not appear to be the primary mechanism for this effect on the heart (65). Results of two experiments indicated that the occurrence of effects of ultrasound on aortic pressure in the frog heart correlated directly with the magnitude of the radiation force exerted on the heart (66). In a third experiment, an acoustic reflector was placed on the surface of the heart to maximize the radiation force delivered to the heart and preclude the possibility of heating or cavitation in the tissue. Effects on aortic pressure were still observed with the reflector on the heart, confirming that radiation force alone is capable of producing this bioeffect (66).

## BLOOD AND MICROVASCULATURE

Hemolysis in vivo is not known to occur for exposure of normal mammals to diagnostic ultrasound. If cavitation nuclei are introduced into the blood through injection of ultrasound contrast agents, hemolysis can occur in laboratory animals in vivo for diagnostically relevant frequencies. One study reports the threshold for ultrasound-induced hemolysis in mice is ~2 MPa negative pressure for exposure at 1.1 MHz (10-$\mu$s pulse duration, 100 Hz PRF) when contrast agent microbubbles are present in the blood (67). The relatively high threshold for hemolysis in vivo, combined with a strong dependence of the threshold for the effect on ultrasound frequency, indicate little likelihood for significant hemolysis for diagnostic exposures (67, 68).

Evidence indicates that high-amplitude pressures associated with lithotripter pulses can produce cavitation in vivo (9, 69). Exposure to high-amplitude lithotripter fields can produce damage to the microvasculature in tissues such as the kidney and liver in laboratory animals (9, 54, 70–73). If contrast agents are introduced in the vasculature, the extent of damage to the microvasculature is significantly increased (74–76). In one study, injection of Albunex™ in mice during exposure to a piezoelectric lithotripter field with amplitude of only 2 MPa produced microvascular damage in most soft tissues, including muscle, mesentery, kidney, stomach, bladder, and fat (74, 75). The sensitivity of these tissues to lithotripter exposures can persist for hours after the initial injection of contrast agent (75). Without contrast injections, these soft tissues showed only minimal damage at exposure amplitudes up to 40 MPa. Observations that damage produced from negative-pressure pulses exceeds that produced by positive acoustic pulses provide further evidence that microvasculature damage from exposure to lithotripter fields when contrast agent is present results from inertial cavitation (48).

Pulsed ultrasound can also produce capillary damage when microbubbles are present in the blood. Exposure of laboratory animals to ultrasound under diagnostically relevant conditions can produce capillary rupture in muscle (77, 78), kidney (79), and cardiac tissues (62). These tissues show no damage from exposure to pulsed ultrasound alone, indicating again that the presence of cavitation nuclei in normal tissue is rare. In general, using higher frequencies of exposures, lower concentrations of contrast agents, and lower-pressure amplitudes minimizes the effects of ultrasound on tissues containing ultrasound contrast agents. For some therapeutic applications of contrast agents, such as site-specific drug delivery, localized capillary rupture may be particularly beneficial (78, 80). Some studies also indicate potential beneficial uses of ultrasound-induced capillary rupture for arteriogenesis (81) or localized tumor destruction (82). The ability of ultrasound to enhance membrane permeability in the presence of microbubble contrast agents provides the potential for new therapeutic methods for site-specific delivery of drugs or genetic material, as discussed below. A complete understanding of the interaction of ultrasound with contrast agents is needed for ultrasound contrast agents to achieve their full potential use in biomedical ultrasound.

## DELIVERY OF DRUGS AND GENETIC MATERIAL

Although still in various stages of development, ultrasound contrast agents show promise for potential applications of ultrasound for drug delivery (83), tumor therapy (82), thrombolysis (84, 85), and gene therapy (86, 87). Because cavitation activity is highly localized, the combination of ultrasound and microbubble contrast agents provides a means for noninvasive, site-specific therapies. Contrast agents can be passively localized in tissues through uptake by phagocytic cells. Targeted contrast agents are modified with ligands and specifically bind to cellular receptors to produce site-specific localization of contrast. Targeted ultrasound contrast agents are under investigation for therapeutic applications and molecular imaging (4, 5). Even without the use of specialized contrast agents, ultrasound can enhance transdermal delivery of drugs (i.e., sonophoresis). Ultrasound at frequencies of 20–100 kHz has been demonstrated to significantly increase transdermal delivery of topical anesthetics (88), insulin (89, 90), and high-molecular-weight proteins (90).

Ultrasound provides new opportunities for noninvasive thrombolysis enhancement. The combination of ultrasound and thrombolytic drugs can accelerate the rate of clot dissolution in vitro and in vivo (e.g., 91–94). Low-frequency ultrasound is reported to be more effective than higher frequencies (92, 95, 96). Although the mechanism for ultrasound-induced thrombolysis is not fully understood, cavitation, microstreaming, and direct mechanical effects may all contribute to clot lysis. Injection of microbubble contrast agents in the vasculature during exposure can further increase the rate of clot lysis with and without a thrombolytic agent (84, 85). Development of targeted contrast agents may further enhance the therapeutic applications of ultrasound for thrombolysis (97).

# INTERACTIONS WITH BONE

Low-intensity pulsed ultrasound can be used to accelerate the rate of bone fracture healing noninvasively. Early studies demonstrated that relatively low-intensity ultrasound significantly increased the rate of fracture repair in various animal models (e.g., 98–100). Since then, a wide range of investigations have studied the interaction of low-intensity pulsed ultrasound on fracture healing (see 101 for review). Typical exposures that are effective in accelerating fracture healing consist of pulsed ultrasound at a carrier frequency of 1.5 MHz; pulse duration of 200 $\mu$s; duty factor of 0.2; and spatial-average, temporal-average intensity of $\sim$30 mW/cm$^2$ (101). Several clinical trials have confirmed the efficacy of ultrasound in accelerating fracture healing in humans (e.g., 102, 103). Although a complete understanding of the mechanism for this therapeutic effect on bone healing is currently unknown, the effective exposures are of such a low intensity that thermal and cavitation mechanisms are unlikely.

At much higher-pressure amplitudes, lithotripter fields and pulsed ultrasound can have adverse effects on tissues near developing bone in small laboratory animals (104, 105). Lithotripter pulses with amplitudes less than 1 MPa can produce vascular damage to late-term murine fetuses (104). Hemorrhages occurred only in tissues near developing bone (head, limbs, and ribs), whereas soft tissues distant from bone were unaltered. No damage was observed to occur in murine fetuses exposed to lithotripter pulses at a stage of gestation prior to bone formation. Pulsed ultrasound, under appropriate exposure conditions, can also produce damage to tissues near developing bone in mice (105). The pressure threshold for exposure at 1 MHz (10-$\mu$s pulses, 100 Hz PRF) was ~2.5 MPa negative pressure, and the threshold increased with increasing frequency (105). This threshold is above the current output limits of diagnostic devices. Although this bioeffect does not result primarily from heat generation, the acoustic mechanism for this phenomenon is not yet fully understood.

## PERCEPTUAL SYSTEMS

Acoustic radiation force or radiation pressure resulting from ultrasound exposure appears capable of stimulating auditory and tactile responses. The production of auditory nerve responses in cat brain exposed to pulsed ultrasound has been reported to result from radiation pressure (106). Another study demonstrated that hearing is produced in humans when focused ultrasound is modulated at audible frequencies and directed at the middle ear (107). This phenomenon is attributed to modulated radiation pressure transmitted to the inner ear (107). Several studies have demonstrated that pulsed ultrasound can produce tactile sensations (108–111). Sensations of touch, temperature, and pain were produced in the hand from exposure to focused ultrasound at increasing exposure levels (109–111). Thresholds for tactile sensations were lowest for exposure to pulsed ultrasound modulated at frequencies of ~100–200 Hz (108). A series of experiments designed to test the radiation force mechanism demonstrated that the tactile perception of ultrasound results primarily from radiation force exerted on the tissue (108).

## SUMMARY

Ultrasound possesses unique capabilities for noninvasive diagnostic imaging and therapy. Ultrasound can interact with tissue to produce a variety of effects through both thermal and nonthermal mechanisms. Some of these bioeffects can be attributed to activity associated with either acoustic cavitation or radiation forces. However, the mechanisms for other bioeffects of ultrasound are unknown and currently under investigation. Expanding our knowledge of the physical mechanisms for ultrasound bioeffects, combined with efforts to elucidate the cellular and molecular events that mediate these effects, will provide vital information for advancing the use of ultrasound in medicine.

### ACKNOWLEDGMENTS

This work was supported in part by grants HL69824 and EB002282 from the National Institutes of Health.

The *Annual Review of Biomedical Engineering* is online at http://bioeng.annualreviews.org

## LITERATURE CITED


1. AIUM/NEMA. 1992. *Standard for Real-Time Display of Thermal and Mechanical Acoustic Output Indices on Diagnostic Ultrasound Equipment*. Laurel, MD: AIUM Publ.
2. Apfel RE, Holland CK. 1991. Gauging the likelihood of cavitation from short-pulse, low-duty cycle diagnostic ultrasound. *Ultrasound Med. Biol.* 17:179–85
3. Vaezy S, Andrew M, Kaczkowski P, Crum L. 2001. Image-guided acoustic therapy. *Annu. Rev. Biomed. Eng.* 3:375–90
4. Klibanov AL. 1999. Targeted delivery of gas-filled microspheres, contrast agents for ultrasound imaging. *Adv. Drug Deliv. Rev.* 37:139–57
5. Unger EC, Matsunaga O, McCreery T, Schumann P, Sweitzer R, Quigley R. 2002. Therapeutic applications of microbubbles. *Euro. J. Radiol.* 42:160–68
6. National Council on Radiation Protection and Measurements (NCRP). 2002. *Exposure Criteria for Medical Diagnostic Ultrasound: II. Criteria Based on All Known Mechanisms*. Bethesda, MD: Natl. Counc. Radiat. Prot.
7. Young F. 1989. *Cavitation*. New York: McGraw-Hill
8. Flynn HG. 1964. Physics of acoustic cavitation in liquids. In *Physical Acoustics*, ed. WP Mason, vol. 1B, chapter 9. New York: Academic
9. Delius M, Draener K, Aldiek Y, Liebich H-G, Jordan M, Brendel W. 1990. Biological effects of shock waves: cavitation by shock waves in piglet liver. *Ultrasound Med. Biol.* 16:467–72
10. Hynynen K. 1991. The threshold for thermally significant cavitation in dog's thigh muscle in vivo. *Ultrasound Med. Biol.* 17:157–69
11. Leighton TG. 1994. *The Acoustic Bubble*. London: Academic
12. Flynn HG. 1982. Generation of transient cavities in liquids by microsecond pulses of ultrasound. *J. Acoust. Soc. Am.* 72:1926–32
13. Bailey MR, Blackstock DT, Cleveland RO, Crum LA. 1999. Comparison of electrohydraulic lithotripters with rigid and pressure-release ellipsoidal reflectors. II. Cavitation fields. *J. Acoust. Soc. Am.* 106:1149–60
14. Rooney JA, Nyborg WL. 1972. Acoustic radiation pressure in a traveling plane wave field. *Am. J. Phys.* 40:1825–30
15. Kossoff G. 1965. Balance technique for the measurement of very low ultrasonic power outputs. *J. Acoust. Soc. Am.* 30:880–81
16. Rooney JA. 1973. Determination of acoustic power outputs in the microwatt-milliwatt range. *Ultrasound Med. Biol.* 1:13–16
17. Hasegawa T, Yosioka K. 1975. Acoustic radiation force on fused silica spheres and intensity determination. *J. Acoust. Soc. Am.* 58:581–85
18. Dunn F, Averbuch AJ, O'Brien WD. 1977. A primary method for the determination of ultrasonic intensity with the elastic sphere radiometer. *J. Acoust. Soc. Am.* 38:58–61
19. Dyson M, Woodward B, Pond JB. 1971. Flow of red blood cells stopped by ultrasound. *Nature* 232:572–73
20. Dayton A, Klibanov A, Brandenburger G, Ferrara K. 1999. Acoustic radiation force in vivo: a mechanism to assist targeting of microbubbles. *Ultrasound Med. Biol.* 25:1195–201
21. Nightingale KR, Kornguth PJ, Walker WF, McDermott BA, Trahey GE. 1995.

A novel ultrasonic technique for differentiating cysts from solid lesions: preliminary results in the breast. *Ultrasound Med. Biol.* 21:745–51
22. American Institute of Ultrasound in Medicine. 2000. Mechanical bioeffects from diagnostic ultrasound: AIUM consensus statements. *J. Ultrasound Med.* 19:68–153
23. Hartman C, Child SZ, Mayer R, Schenk E, Carstensen EL. 1990. Lung damage from exposure to the fields of an electrohydraulic lithotripter. *Ultrasound Med. Biol.* 16:675–79
24. Dalecki D, Raeman CH, Child SZ, Carstensen EL. 1996. A test for cavitation as a mechanism for intestinal hemorrhage in mice exposed to a piezoelectric lithotripter. *Ultrasound Med. Biol.* 22:493–96
25. Carstensen EL, Gracewski S, Dalecki D. 2000. The search for cavitation in vivo. *Ultrasound Med. Biol.* 26:1377–85
26. Penney DP, Schenk EA, Maltby K, Hartman-Raeman C, Child SZ, Carstensen EL. 1993. Morphologic effects of pulsed ultrasound in the lung. *Ultrasound Med. Biol.* 19:127–35
27. Zachary JF, Frizzell LA, Norrell KS, Blue JP, Miller RJ, O'Brien WD. 2001. Temporal and spatial evaluation of lesion reparative responses following superthreshold exposure of rat lung to pulsed ultrasound. *Ultrasound Med. Biol.* 27:829–39
28. Child SZ, Hartman CL, McHale LA, Carstensen EL. 1990. Lung damage from exposure to pulsed ultrasound. *Ultrasound Med. Biol.* 16:817–25
29. Baggs R, Penney DP, Cox C, Child SZ, Raeman CH, et al. 1996. Thresholds for ultrasonically induced lung hemorrhage in neonatal swine. *Ultrasound Med. Biol.* 22:119–28
30. Dalecki D, Child SZ, Raeman CH, Cox C, Penney DP, Carstensen EL. 1997. Age dependence of ultrasonically induced lung hemorrhage in mice. *Ultrasound Med. Biol.* 23:767–76
31. Dalecki D, Child SZ, Raeman CH, Cox C, Carstensen EL. 1997. Ultrasonically induced lung hemorrhage in young swine. *Ultrasound Med. Biol.* 23:777–81
32. Holland CK, Deng CX, Apfel RE, Alderman JL, Fernandez LA, Taylor KJ. 1996. Direct evidence of cavitation *in vivo* from diagnostic ultrasound. *Ultrasound Med. Biol.* 22:917–25
33. Tarantal AF, Canfield DR. 1994. Ultrasound-induced lung hemorrhage in the monkey. *Ultrasound Med. Biol.* 20:65–72
34. Zachary JF, O'Brien WD. 1995. Lung hemorrhage induced by continuous and pulsed wave diagnostic ultrasound in mice, rabbits and pigs. *Vet. Pathol.* 32:43–54
35. O'Brien WD, Zachary JF. 1997. Lung damage assessment from exposure to pulsed-wave ultrasound in the rabbit, mouse and pig. *IEEE Trans. Ultrasonics Ferroelectr. Freq. Control* 44:473–85
36. Meltzer RS, Adsumelli R, Risher WH, Hicks GL Jr, Stern DH, et al. 1998. Lack of lung hemorrhage in humans after intraoperative transesophageal echocardiography with ultrasound exposure conditions similar to those causing lung hemorrhage in laboratory animals. *J. Am. Soc. Echocardiogr.* 11:57–60
37. O'Brien WD, Krammer JM, Waldrop TG, Frizzell LA, Miller RJ, et al. 2002. Ultrasound-induced lung hemorrhage: role of acoustic boundary conditions at the pleural surface. *J. Acoust. Soc. Am.* 111:1102–9
38. Zachary JF, Sempsrott JM, Frizzell LA, Simpson DG, O'Brien WD Jr. 2001. Superthreshold behavior and threshold estimation of ultrasound-induced lung hemorrhage in adult mice and rats. *IEEE Trans. Ultrasonics Ferroelectr. Freq. Control* 48:581–92
39. O'Brien WD, Simpson DG, Frizzell LA, Zachary JF. 2003. Threshold estimates and superthreshold behavior of ultrasound-induced lung hemorrhage in

adult rats: role of pulse duration. *Ultrasound Med. Biol.* 29:1625–34
40. O'Brien WD, Frizzell LA, Schaeffer DJ, Zachary JF. 2001. Superthreshold behavior of ultrasound-induced lung hemorrhage in adult mice and rats: role of pulse repetition frequency and exposure duration. *Ultrasound Med. Biol.* 27:267–77
41. Raeman CH, Child SZ, Carstensen EL. 1993. Timing of exposures in ultrasonic hemorrhage of murine lung. *Ultrasound Med. Biol.* 19:507–12
42. Raeman CH, Child SZ, Dalecki D, Cox C, Carstensen EL. 1996. Effects of exposure time on threshold for murine lung hemorrhage. *Ultrasound Med. Biol.* 22:139–41
43. O'Brien WD Jr, Simpson DG, Frizzell LA, Zachary JF. 2001. Superthreshold behavior and threshold estimates of ultrasound-induced lung hemorrhage in adult rats: role of beamwidth. *IEEE Trans. Ultrasonics Ferroelectr. Freq. Control* 48:1695–705
44. O'Brien WD Jr, Simpson DG, Ho MH, Miller RJ, Frizzell LA, Zachary JF. 2003. Superthreshold behavior and threshold estimation of ultrasound-induced lung hemorrhage in pigs: role of age dependency. *IEEE Trans. Ultrasonics Ferroelectr. Freq. Control* 50:153–69
45. Raeman CH, Child SZ, Meltzer RS, Meltzer RS, Carstensen EL. 1997. Albunex® does not increase the sensitivity of the lung to pulsed ultrasound. *Echocardiography* 14:553–57
46. O'Brien WD Jr, Frizzell LA, Weigel RM, Zachary JF. 2000. Ultrasound-induced lung hemorrhage is not caused by inertial cavitation. *J. Acoust. Soc. Am.* 108:1290–97
47. Bailey MR, Dalecki D, Child SZ, Penney DP, Blackstock DT, Carstensen EL. 1996. Bioeffects of positive and negative acoustic pressures in vivo. *J. Acoust. Soc. Am.* 100:3941–46
48. Dalecki D, Child SZ, Raeman CH, Xing C, Gracewski S, Carstensen EL. 2000. Bioeffects of positive and negative acoustic pressures in mice infused with microbubbles. *Ultrasound Med. Biol.* 26:1327–32
49. Frizzell LA, Zachary JF, O'Brien WD Jr. 2003. Effect of pulse polarity and energy on ultrasound-induced lung hemorrhage in adult rats. *J. Acoust. Soc. Am.* 113:2912–18
50. Miller DL, Thomas RM. 1994. Heating as a mechanism for ultrasonically induced petechial hemorrhages in mouse intestine. *Ultrasound Med. Biol.* 20:493–503
51. Miller DL, Thomas RM. 1995. Thresholds for hemorrhages in mouse skin and intestine induced by lithotripter shockwaves. *Ultrasound Med. Biol.* 21:249–57
52. Dalecki D, Raeman CH, Child SZ, Carstensen EL. 1995. Thresholds for intestinal hemorrhage in mice exposed to a piezoelectric lithotripter. *Ultrasound Med. Biol.* 21:1239–46
53. Dalecki D, Raeman CH, Child SZ, Carstensen EL. 1995. Intestinal hemorrhage from exposure to pulsed ultrasound. *Ultrasound Med. Biol.* 21:1067–72
54. Raeman CH, Child SZ, Dalecki D, Mayer R, Parker KJ, Carstensen EL. 1994. Damage to murine kidney and intestine from exposure to the fields of a piezoelectric lithotripter. *Ultrasound Med. Biol.* 20:589–94
55. Miller DL, Gies RA. 1998. Gas-body-based contrast agent enhances vascular bioeffects of 1.09 MHz ultrasound on mouse intestine. *Ultrasound Med. Biol.* 24:201–8
56. Miller DL, Gies RA. 2000. The influence of ultrasound frequency and gas-body composition on the contrast agent-mediated enhancement of vascular bioeffect in mouse intestine. *Ultrasound Med. Biol.* 26:307–13
57. Dalecki D, Keller BB, Carstensen EL, Neel DS, Palladino JL, Noordergraaf A. 1991. Thresholds for premature ventricular contractions in frog hearts exposed to lithotripter fields. *Ultrasound Med. Biol.* 17:341–46

58. Delius M, Hoffman G, Steinbeck G, Conzen P. 1994. Biological effects of shock waves: induction of arrhythmia in piglet hearts. *Ultrasound Med. Biol.* 20:279–85
59. Dalecki D, Keller BB, Raeman CH, Carstensen EL. 1993. Effects of pulsed ultrasound on the frog heart: I. Thresholds for changes in cardiac rhythm and aortic pressure. *Ultrasound Med. Biol.* 19:385–90
60. MacRobbie AG, Raeman CH, Child SZ, Dalecki D. 1997. Thresholds for premature contractions in murine hearts exposed to pulsed ultrasound. *Ultrasound Med. Biol.* 23:761–65
61. Dalecki D, Child SZ, Raeman CH, Gildner CD. 2000. Premature cardiac contractions produced by ultrasound contrast agents. *J. Ultrasound Med.* 19:32
62. Li P, Cao L, Dou C, Armstrong WF, Miller D. 2003. Impact of myocardial contrast echocardiography on vascular permeability: an in vivo dose response study of delivery mode, pressure amplitude and contrast dose. *Ultrasound Med. Biol.* 9:1341–49
63. Zachary JF, Hartleban SA, Frizzell LA, O'Brien WD Jr. 2002. Arrhythmias in rat hearts exposed to pulsed ultrasound after intravenous injection of a contrast agent. *J. Ultrasound Med.* 21:1347–56
64. van der Wouw PA, Brauns AC, Bailey SE, Powers JE, Wilde AA. 2000. Premature ventricular contractions during triggered imaging with ultrasound contrast. *J. Am. Soc. Echocardiogr.* 13:288–94
65. Dalecki D, Raeman CH, Carstensen EL. 1993. Effects of pulsed ultrasound on the frog heart: II. An investigation of heating as a potential mechanism. *Ultrasound Med. Biol.* 19:391–98
66. Dalecki D, Raeman CH, Child SZ, Carstensen EL. 1997. Effects of pulsed ultrasound on the frog heart: III. The radiation force mechanism. *Ultrasound Med. Biol.* 23:275–85
67. Dalecki D, Raeman CH, Child SZ, Cox C, Francis CW, et al. 1997. Hemolysis in vivo from exposure to pulsed ultrasound. *Ultrasound Med. Biol.* 23:307–13
68. Killam AL, Greener Y, McFerran BA, Maniquis J, Bloom A, et al. 1998. Lack of bioeffects of ultrasound energy after intravenous administration of FS069 (Optison) in the anesthetized rabbit. *J. Ultrasound Med.* 17:349–56
69. Coleman AJ, Kodama T, Choi MJ, Adams T, Saunders JE. 1995. The cavitation threshold of human tissue exposed to 0.2 MHz pulsed ultrasound: preliminary measurements based on a study of clinical lithotripsy. *Ultrasound Med. Biol.* 21:405–17
70. Delius M, Jordan M, Liebich HG, Brendel W. 1990. Biological effects of shock waves: effect of shock waves on the liver and gallbladder wall of dogs—administration rate dependence. *Ultrasound Med. Biol.* 16:459–66
71. Delius M, Enders F, Xuan ZR, Liebich HG, Brendel W. 1988. Biological effects of shock waves: kidney damage by shock waves in dogs—dose dependence. *Ultrasound Med. Biol.* 14:117–22
72. Delius M, Jordan M, Eizenhoefer H, Marlinghaus E, Heine G, et al. 1988. Biological effects of shock waves: kidney hemorrhage by shock waves in dogs—administration rate dependence. *Ultrasound Med. Biol.* 14:689–94
73. Mayer R, Schenk E, Child SZ, Norton S, Cox C, et al. 1990. Pressure threshold for shock wave induced renal hemorrhage. *J. Urol.* 144:1505–9
74. Dalecki D, Raeman CH, Child SZ, Penney DP, Mayer R, Carstensen EL. 1997. The influence of contrast agents on hemorrhage produced by lithotripter fields. *Ultrasound Med. Biol.* 23:1435–39
75. Dalecki D, Raeman CH, Child SZ, Penney DP, Carstensen EL. 1997. Remnants of Albunex nucleate acoustic cavitation. *Ultrasound Med. Biol.* 23:1405–12
76. Miller DL, Gies RA. 1999. Consequences of lithotripter shockwave interaction with

gas body contrast agent in mouse intestine. *J. Urology* 162:606–9
77. Miller DL, Quddus J. 2000. Diagnostic ultrasound activation of contrast agent gas bodies induces capillary rupture in mice. *Proc. Natl. Acad. Sci. USA* 97:10179–84
78. Price RJ, Skyba DM, Kaul S, Skalak TC. 1998. Delivery of colloidal particles and red blood cells to tissue through microvessel ruptures created by targeted microbubble destruction with ultrasound. *Circulation* 98:1264–67
79. Wible JH Jr, Galen KP, Wojdyla JK, Hughes MS, Klibanov AL, Brandenburger GH. 2002. Microbubbles induce renal hemorrhage when exposed to diagnostic ultrasound in anesthetized rats. *Ultrasound Med. Biol.* 28:1535–46
80. Song J, Chappell JC, Qi M, VanGieson EJ, Kaul S, Price RJ. 2002. Influence of injection site, microvascular pressure and ultrasound variables on microbubble-mediated delivery of microspheres to muscle. *J. Am. Coll. Cardiol.* 39:726–31
81. Song J, Qi M, Kaul S, Price RJ. 2002. Stimulation of arteriogenesis in skeletal muscle by microbubble destruction with ultrasound. *Circulation* 106:1550–55
82. Simon RH, Ho SY, Lange SC, Uphoff DF, D'Arrigo JS. 1993. Applications of lipid-coated microbubble contrast to tumor therapy. *Ultrasound Med. Biol.* 19:123–25
83. Unger EC, Hersh E, Vannan M, Matsunaga TO, McCreery T. 2001. Local drug and gene delivery through microbubbles. *Prog. Cardio. Dis.* 44:45–54
84. Birnbaum Y, Luo H, Nagai T, Fishbein MC, Peterson TM, et al. 1998. Noninvasive in vivo clot dissolution without a thrombolytic drug: recanalization of thrombosed iliofemoral arteries with transcutaneous ultrasound combined with intravenous infusion of microbubbles. *Circulation* 97:130–34
85. Culp WC, Porter TR, Xie F, Goertzen TC, McCowan TC, et al. 2001. Microbubble potentiated ultrasound as a method of declotting thrombosed dialysis grafts: experimental study in dogs. *Cardiov. Intervent. Radiol.* 24:407–12
86. Unger EC, Hersh E, Vannan M, McCreery T. 2001. Gene delivery using ultrasound contrast agents. *Echocardiography* 18:355–61
87. Greenleaf WF, Bolander ME, Sarkar G, Goldring MB, Greenleaf JF. 1998. Artificial cavitation nuclei significantly enhance acoustically induced cell transfection. *Ultrasound Med. Biol.* 24:587–95
88. Tachibana K, Tachibana S. 1993. Use of ultrasound to enhance the local anesthetic effect of topically applied aqueous lidocaine. *Anesthesiology* 78:1091–96
89. Tachibana K. 1992. Transdermal delivery of insulin to alloxan-diabetic rabbits by ultrasound exposure. *Pharm. Res.* 9:952–54
90. Mitragotri S, Blankschtein D, Langer R. 1995. Ultrasound-mediated transdermal protein delivery. *Science* 269:850–52
91. Francis CW, Onundarson PT, Carstensen EL, Blinc A, Meltzer RS, et al. 1992. Enhancement of fibrinolysis in vitro by ultrasound. *J. Clin. Inv.* 90:2063–68
92. Tachibana K. 1992. Enhancement of fibrinolysis with ultrasound energy. *J. Vas. Interv. Rad.* 3:299–303
93. Tachibana K, Tachibana S. 1997. Prototype therapeutic ultrasound emitting catheter for accelerating thrombolysis. *J. Ultrasound Med.* 16:529–35
94. Nilsson AM, Odselius R, Roijer A. 1995. Pro- and antifibrinolytic effects of ultrasound on streptokinase-induced thrombolysis. *Ultrasound Med. Biol.* 21:833–40
95. Luo H, Nishioka T, Fishbein MC, Cercek B, Forrester JS, et al. 1996. Transcutaneous ultrasound augments lysis of arterial thrombi in vivo. *Circulation* 94:775–78
96. Suchkova V, Siddiqi FN, Carstensen EL, Dalecki D, Child S, Francis CW. 1998. Enhancement of fibrinolysis with 40-kHz ultrasound. *Circulation* 98:1030–35
97. Lanza GM, Wallace KD, Scott MJ,

Cacheris WP, Abendschein DR, et al. 1996. A novel site-targeted ultrasonic contrast agent with broad biomedical application. *Circulation* 94:3334–40
98. Dyson M, Brookes M. 1982. Stimulation of bone repair by ultrasound. *Ultrasound Med. Biol.* 8(Suppl. 1):50
99. Duarte LR. 1983. The stimulation of bone growth by ultrasound. *Arch. Ortho. Trauma Surg.* 101:153–59
100. Pilla AA, Mont MA, Nasser SA, Khan SA, Figueiredo M, et al. 1990. Non-invasive low-intensity pulsed ultrasound accelerates bone healing in the rabbit. *J. Orthop. Trauma* 4:246–53
101. Rubin C, Bolander M, Ryaby JP, Hadjiargyrou M. 2001. The use of low-intensity ultrasound to accelerate the healing of fractures. *J. Bone Joint Surg.* 83:259–70
102. Heckman JD, Ryaby JP, McCabe J, Frey JJ, Kilcoyne RF. 1994. Acceleration of tibial fracture healing by non-invasive, low-intensity pulsed ultrasound. *J. Bone Joint Surg. Am.* 76:26–34
103. Kristiansen TK, Ryaby JP, McCabe J, Frey JJ, Roe LR. 1997. Accelerated healing of distal radial fractures with the use of specific, low-intensity ultrasound. A multicenter, prospective, randomized, double-blind, placebo-controlled study. *J. Bone Joint Surg. Am.* 79:961–63
104. Dalecki D, Child SZ, Raeman CH, Penney DP, Mayer R, et al. 1997. Thresholds for fetal hemorrhages produced by a piezoelectric lithotripter. *Ultrasound Med. Biol.* 23:287–97
105. Dalecki D, Child SZ, Raeman CH, Cox C. 1999. Hemorrhage in murine fetuses exposed to pulsed ultrasound. *Ultrasound Med. Biol.* 25:1139–44
106. Foster KR, Wiederhold ML. 1978. Auditory responses in cats produced by pulsed ultrasound. *J. Acoust. Soc. Am.* 63:1199–205
107. Tsirulnikov EM, Vartanyan IA, Gersuni GV, Rosenblyum AS, Pudov VI, Gavrilov LR. 1988. Use of amplitude-modulated focused ultrasound for diagnosis of hearing disorders. *Ultrasound Med. Biol.* 14: 277–85
108. Dalecki D, Child SZ, Raeman CH, Carstensen EL. 1995. Tactile perception of ultrasound. *J. Acoust. Soc. Am.* 97:3165–70
109. Gavrilov LR. 1984. Use of focused ultrasound for stimulation of nerve structure. *Ultrasonics* 22:132–38
110. Gavrilov LR, Gershuni GV, Ilyinski OB, Tsirulnikov EM, Shchekanov EE. 1977. A study of reception with the use of focused ultrasound: I. Effects on the skin and deep receptor structures in man. *Brain Res.* 135:265–77
111. Gavrilov LR, Gershuni GV, Ilyinski OB, Tsirulnikov EM, Shchekanov EE. 1977. A study of reception with the use of focused ultrasound: II. Effects on the animal receptor structures. *Brain Res.* 135:279–85

Annu. Rev. Biomed. Eng. 2004. 6:249–73
doi: 10.1146/annurev.bioeng.6.040803.140055

First published online as a Review in Advance on February 6, 2004

# OCULAR BIOMECHANICS AND BIOTRANSPORT

C. Ross Ethier,[1] Mark Johnson,[2] and Jeff Ruberti[3]
*[1]Departments of Mechanical and Industrial Engineering, Ophthalmology, and Institute for Biomaterials and Biomedical Engineering, University of Toronto, Ontario, M5S 3G8, Canada; email: ethier@mie.utoronto.ca*
*[2]Department of Biomedical Engineering, Northwestern University, Evanston, Illinois 60208; email: m-johnson2@northwestern.edu*
*[3]Cambridge Polymer Group, Inc., Somerville, Massachusetts 02143, and Adjunct Assistant Scientist, Schepens Eye Research Institute, Boston, Massachusetts 02114-2500; email: jeff@campoly.com*

**Key Words** cornea, glaucoma, aqueous humor drainage, optic nerve head, Bruch's membrane

■ **Abstract** The eye transduces light, and we usually do not think of it as a biomechanical structure. Yet it is actually a pressurized, thick-walled shell that has an internal and external musculature, a remarkably complex internal vascular system, dedicated fluid production and drainage tissues, and a variety of specialized fluid and solute transport systems. Biomechanics is particularly involved in accommodation (focusing near and far), as well as in common disorders such as glaucoma, macular degeneration, myopia, and presbyopia. In this review, we give a (necessarily brief) overview of many of the interesting biomechanical aspects of the eye, concluding with a list of open problems.

CONTENTS

# INTRODUCTION

The eye is a remarkable organ, specialized for the conversion of photons into spatially organized and temporally resolved electrochemical signals. Biomechanics plays a major role in the normal and pathological function of the eye. We begin with a brief anatomical review of some of the biomechanically important parts of the eye.

## Overview of Ocular Anatomy

The outer envelope of the eye is formed by two connective tissues, the cornea and sclera (Figure 1, see color insert). Six extraocular muscles attach to the outer sclera, acting to rotate the eye in concert with a clever system of active pulleys (1). The corneoscleral envelope forms a closed shell, pierced at the back of the eye by the scleral canal and at other discrete locations by small vessels and nerves. The optic nerve, responsible for carrying information from the retina to the visual center in the brain, leaves the eye through the scleral canal. Light enters the eye by passing through the cornea, after which it traverses the anterior chamber, pupil, lens, and vitreous body before striking the retina. The lens is suspended by ligaments (the zonules) that attach to the inner fibers of the ciliary muscle; alterations in tone of these muscle fibers cause the zonules to tug on the lens, so that the lens changes shape to alter the focal length of the eye in a process known as accommodation.

The ciliary body consists of the ciliary muscle and a highly folded and vascularized inner layer known as the ciliary processes, which secrete a clear, colourless fluid called the aqueous humor. This fluid flows radially inward, bathing the lens, then flows anteriorly through the pupil to fill the anterior chamber and nourish the cornea, before draining out of the eye through specialized tissues in the angle formed by the iris and cornea. As we will see, this fluid flow is responsible for creating a positive pressure within the eye, the so-called intraocular pressure (IOP), which has many interesting biomechanical consequences. Additionally, the volume of vascular beds within the eye changes throughout the cardiac cycle, creating a time-varying component of the IOP in an effect known as the ocular pulse. The space behind the lens is filled with a relatively inert connective tissue called the vitreous body. It is quite porous and thus transmits the pressure from the anterior chamber throughout the interior of the eye.

# OCULAR BIOSOLID MECHANICS

The eye is subjected to a mean and time-varying internal pressure; furthermore, the ciliary muscle can create significant internal forces, whereas the extraocular muscles create external forces. Despite these forces, the eye must maintain the proper relative positions of all optical components so as to ensure high visual acuity. This leads to some interesting biosolid mechanics.

## Mechanics of the Sclera and Corneoscleral Envelope

The corneoscleral shell encloses the intraocular tissues and protects the eye from blunt injury. It is a surprisingly tough tissue that has a high elastic modulus and a very high rupture strength. Measurements on intact inflated human ocular globes have yielded average Young's moduli in the range of 5–13 MPa (3–5). The sclera is largely composed of circumferentially oriented types I and III collagen fibers and thus has a modulus in the circumferential direction much higher than in the radial (6).

Knowledge of the elastic properties of the sclera is important in several applications: improving the accuracy of methods to measure IOP and resistance to aqueous humor drainage, understanding the development of myopia (near-sightedness), and interpreting the magnitude of the ocular pulse. We first review the many studies done to measure mechanical properties of the sclera and to model the stress-strain behavior of the corneoscleral envelope. Then we examine the application of these findings.

Friedenwald (7) first proposed the "ocular rigidity function," describing the change in intraocular pressure, ($IOP$–$IOP_0$), with a change in ocular volume, $(V - V_0)$:

$$\ln\left[\frac{IOP}{IOP_0}\right] = K(V - V_0), \tag{1}$$

where $K$ is the coefficient of ocular rigidity. In humans, $K$ is approximately 0.05 $\mu l^{-1}$ (8), giving a compliance of the ocular envelope of roughly 1 $\mu$l/mmHg at a physiologic IOP of 15 mmHg; the bovine eye is considerably less stiff with an ocular rigidity that is roughly tenfold smaller.

Equation 1 is consistent with the mechanical properties of collagen, which is responsible for the high elastic modulus of the sclera. Specifically, collagen exhibits a stress ($\sigma$)/strain ($\varepsilon$) relationship of the form (9)

$$\sigma = A[e^{\alpha\varepsilon} - 1], \tag{2}$$

where A and $\alpha$ are material constants. Note that at low strains, A$\alpha$ is equivalent to the Young's modulus of the material.

The tangential (hoop) stress in the sclera can be related to the intraocular pressure using Laplace's relation: $\sigma = IOP\ R/(2h)$, where $R$ is the radius of the eye and $h$ is the thickness of the sclera. Considering small strains, such that $\varepsilon = (R - R_0)/R_0$ (but not so small that Equation 2 is linear), we let $V - V_0 = 4\pi\ R_0^2\ (R - R_0)$. Approximating Equation 2 as $\sigma = A \exp{(\alpha\ \varepsilon)}$, Equation 1 results. The approximation is reasonable when strains are large enough that the nonlinear term dominates Equation 2, which occurs for very small strains indeed because $\alpha$ is very large. Keeping the full form of Equation 2 leads to a modified form of the

Friedenwald equation (in the small strain limit):

$$\ln\left[\frac{IOP + \dfrac{2hA}{R}}{IOP_0 + \dfrac{2hA}{R}}\right] = \frac{\alpha}{V_0}(V - V_0). \tag{3}$$

McEwen & St. Helen (10) first introduced Equation 3, and Collins & Van der Werff (8) summarized their results for human eyes to obtain $\alpha/V_0 = 0.022\ \mu l^{-1}$ and $2hA/R = 9.5$ mmHg. If we let the typical radius and thickness of the human corneoscleral shell be 1.15 cm and 0.06 cm, respectively (8), then $\alpha = 140$ and the low strain modulus, $A\alpha$, is 1.7 MPa. Greene derives Equation 3 more rigorously and reviews the literature to give a range of values for $\alpha$, $A$, and the compliance of the eye (11).

Note that the ocular rigidity function really characterizes the properties of both the sclera and the cornea. Although the cornea is somewhat less stiff than the sclera (12–14), its elastic properties can also be described by a relationship analogous to Equation 2. Thus, Equation 3 actually describes the behavior of the corneoscleral envelope.

These formulations treat the sclera and cornea as elastic materials, but the ocular envelope also shows time-dependent deformations upon the application of stress. Viscoelastic models have been used to characterize this behavior (15–17), but, as in other tissues, a variety of time-constants are necessary to capture the behavior. This is likely due to the fact that the sclera is a biphasic material and thus better characterized by models that allow coupling of stresses with fluid motions in or out of the tissue (18, 19).

APPLICATIONS OF SCLERAL MECHANICS The most common use of the Friedenwald relationship is for tonometry (noninvasive measurement of IOP). There are different types of tonometers (20), the conceptually simplest of which is the Schiotz tonometer. This device measures the depth of indentation that occurs when a plunger of known weight is placed against the cornea. Gloster (21) summarized data for the relationship between intraocular pressure and the scale reading (for a given tonometer weight). However, this is the pressure in the eye with the tonometer distorting the eye. What is desired is the pressure of the undeformed eye. The indentation of the eye is equivalent to the injection of a fluid volume into the eye equal to the indentation volume. Gloster found a relationship between indentation depth and indentation volume of the tonometer. Then, using the Friedenwald relationship (Equation 1), the undeformed IOP can be found (22). This requires knowledge of the ocular rigidity, found either by using a population average or by using the Schiotz tonometer with two different plunger weights (22).

A related application of the Friedenwald relationship is in tonography in which a modified tonometer is used to estimate the aqueous humor drainage resistance in a live eye (23) (see also Aqueous Humor Dynamics, below). After the plunger increases the pressure in the eye, the pressure slowly decays as this indentation volume flows out via the aqueous humor drainage pathway. By measuring the change in pressure over a short period of time ($\Delta t$, usually 4 min.), Equation 1 can be used to calculate the volume decrease of the corneoscleral envelope during this period ($\Delta V_s$). Additionally, because the plunger indentation into the cornea increases as the pressure in the eye drops, this increased indentation volume ($\Delta V_c$) must be included in the estimate of the total volume that has passed out of the eye. Then, outflow facility, $C$, the inverse of aqueous drainage resistance, can be estimated as $C = (\Delta V_s + \Delta V_c)/(\Delta t\ \Delta P)$, where $\Delta P$ is the average increase in IOP that occurred during the tonography. Greene (11) emphasized that ocular rigidity should be determined for a given eye before performing tonography, as very different results are expected for eyes of differing volumes (compare Equations 1 and 3 to see that $K$ is inversely proportional to ocular volume). Note also that viscoelastic creep might confound the measurement of outflow facility by this method, but experimental studies indicate that this is not a serious error (24, 25).

Another important application of scleral mechanics is the understanding of myopia in which the axial length of the eye is too large to allow clear focussing of distant light rays on the retina. So far, we have considered the sclera to be a nonlinear elastic or viscoelastic material; however, the sclera has an elastic limit beyond which plastic deformation occurs (26, 27). Among the mechanical theories for explaining myopia, it has been postulated that these young eyes have (*a*) a genetically inherited decrease of this elastic limit, (*b*) higher than normal stresses on the sclera associated with accommodation and convergence that occur when reading (28), or (*c*) stretching caused by periodic increases in IOP owing to squinting or eye rubbing (27). It is possible that one or more of these mechanisms, combined with the physiological feedback loop responsible for growth of the eye (29–31), leads to the development of myopia.

## Corneal Biomechanics

The cornea is a multilaminate tissue, consisting of an anterior stratified squamous "tight" epithelium (~50 microns thick), a tough collagenous stroma, and a posterior "leaky" monolayer of actively pumping endothelial cells (~5 microns thick). Its combination of remarkable strength and transparency is due to the highly organized micro- and nanoscale structure of the stroma (32, 33). On the microscale, the stroma comprises a nematic stack of 250–400 lamellae (34) containing type I/V heterotypic collagen fibrils (35). These fibrils run preferentially in the meridonal, horizontal, and (in the periphery) circumferential directions (36), and together help bear the load imposed by the IOP (Figure 2). In fact, the load may be taken up in a complex manner both in the plane of the cornea and transversely (37–40). Remarkably, there is no consensus on how the cornea is loaded in vivo. On the nanoscale, hydrophilic proteoglycans surround the 35-nm monodisperse collagen fibrils and impose a relatively uniform spacing on the collagen. The cornea's transverse material properties are determined primarily by the 36–48 mM of fixed charge density associated with the presence of these organizing proteoglycans (41, 42).

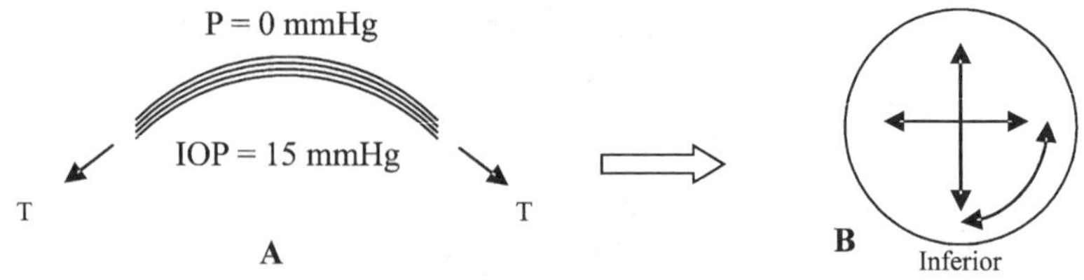


**Figure 2** Corneal tensile load bearing. (*A*) Transverse view of cornea. Conversion of the 15 mmHg pressure difference across the cornea results in a tangential tensile force that is carried by the stromal lamellae. (*B*) En face view of cornea. Lamellar fibrils are thought to be oriented in three preferential orientations, which explains the anisotropic nature of the measured tensile modulus in the stroma.

MATERIAL PROPERTIES To generate a nearly perfectly spherical, aberration-free surface, the cornea must distribute applied loads with remarkable precision. To effect predictable shape changes to correct refractive errors, the corneal response to tissue resection/ablation must be characterized. Thus, it is of interest to discern the material properties of the cornea, which are heterogeneous, highly anisotropic, nonlinear, and viscoelastic. For example, for meridonal loading at normal IOP, Young's secant modulus is largest in the central cornea (8.6 MPa), whereas for circumferential loading, the secant modulus is largest in the periphery (13.0 MPa) (5). Woo et al. (4) used finite element analysis to obtain a nonlinear effective stress-strain relationship for clamped inflated human corneas of the form of Equation 2 with $A = 5.4 \times 10^4$ dyne/cm$^2$ and $\alpha = 28.0$. A more recent study of 12 human corneas found $A = 1.75 \times 10^4$ dyne/cm$^2$ and $\alpha = 48.3$ (43). Stress relaxation curves demonstrating the viscoelastic nature of peripheral corneal strips were fit with the following empirical equation (44):

$$y = -0.0159 \ln(t) + 0.9785, \tag{4}$$

where $y$ is the normalized storage modulus at a fixed stretch ratio of 1.5 and $t$ is time in seconds.

SWELLING PRESSURE In the anterior-posterior direction, the mammalian corneal stroma lacks internal mechanical constraints. The stroma therefore has a tendency to imbibe water, which is quantified through its "swelling pressure" (45). To prevent swelling, which leads to opacity, the cornea is compressed by the combined action of its limiting membranes (46), as discussed in detail in Transport Within the Cornea, below. Therefore, it is of interest to understand the magnitude and nature of the swelling forces that must be controlled to preserve vision. Stromal swelling pressure depends strongly on hydration (Figure 3), and can be described by (47)

$$p = \gamma \exp(-\beta H), \tag{5}$$

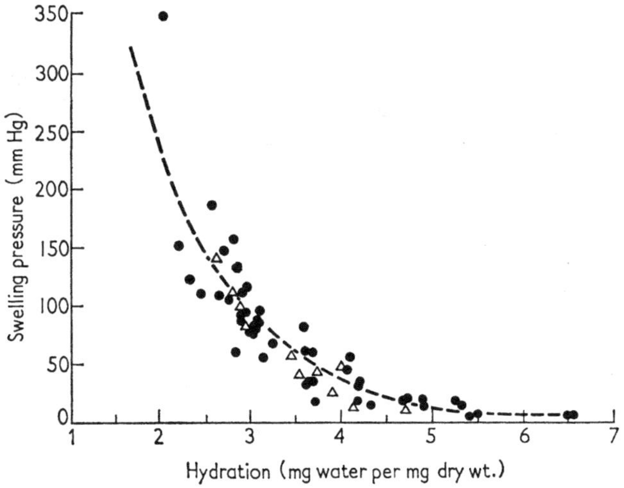


**Figure 3** Swelling pressure in rabbit (*filled circles*) and human (*open triangles*) corneal stroma versus stromal hydration (mass water/mass dry tissue). The broken curve represents steer swelling pressure. At normal hydration (3.2–3.4 mg $H_2O$/mg dry material), this stromal swelling pressure is approximately 60 mmHg (52). From Hedbys & Dohlman (53).

where $p$ is swelling pressure, $\gamma$ and $\beta$ are constants, and $H$ is the hydration of the stromal tissue. Equation 5 is a regression of experimental data and tells us little about the physics of stromal swelling forces. Taking a more fundamental physical approach, Eisenberg & Grodzinsky (48, 49) extended KLM (50, 51) biphasic theory to include the effects of ionic species, expressing the swelling stress in the stroma, $\sigma$, as a function of the strain, $\varepsilon$, and the concentration of ionic species, $c$:

$$\sigma(c, \varepsilon) = E_A(c)\varepsilon + \sigma_c(c), \tag{6}$$

where $E_A$ is the aggregate modulus [sum of the Lame's constants—2G(c) + λ(c)] and $\sigma_c$ is the chemical stress. Eisenberg & Grodzinsky were able to extract both $E_A$ and $\sigma_c$(c) as functions of $c$ and use Equation 6 to predict the free swelling of the corneal stroma with reasonable accuracy (48).

APPLICATION TO REFRACTIVE SURGERY An obvious application of corneal biomechanics is to predict the laser ablation profile that will optimize postoperative visual acuity in refractive corneal procedures. However, biomechanical modeling has not been particularly successful in this task. Instead, laser manufacturers depend on continually updated, proprietary empirical algorithms (54) based on direct shape-subtraction (55) formulas that have been modified and statistically optimized to the mean patient population postoperative response (54). This empirical approach has been quite successful with up to 97% of the subjects willing to recommend LASIK (Laser ASsisted In-situ Keratomileusis) to a friend (56). How, then, did the biomechanician fail, with the embarrassing result that human corneas became test cases for the development of a vast empirical database?

In spite of a sophisticated effort to model radial keratotomy (RK) refractive surgical outcomes during the late 1980s and early 1990s (57–61), the practical application of these models never really gained acceptance for four reasons: (*a*) Early RK models could not be validated (61); (*b*) the spatially variant mechanical properties of the stroma are not well defined on the relevant microscopic length scale (37); (*c*) the distribution of load in the stroma, which sets the local value of the nonlinear tensile modulus [to which refractive models are highly sensitive (43)] is not definitively known; and finally (*d*) the long-term stromal remodeling response is not addressed at all by mechanical models. These limitations, in combination with the undeniable effectiveness of the empirical approach, have virtually ensured that predictive biomechanical modeling of refractive procedures is not likely to enjoy resurgent popularity in the near future. In a further ironic twist, topographic corneal maps obtained following laser ablation surgeries are being used to "back out" information about stromal structure and material properties (54).

## Retina and Lamina Cribrosa Biomechanics

The retina is a remarkably fragile tissue, having a thickness of 250 $\mu$m (62) and a Young's modulus of only 20 kPa (63). It does not carry significant load, but it can tear, usually with drastic visual consequences. Retinal tears are often associated with age-related liquefaction and shrinkage of the vitreous body (64), but can also occur when the eye is subjected to large accelerations (65), such as in shaken baby syndrome (66).

The lamina cribrosa is one of the most biomechanically interesting tissues in the eye. It is a porous connective tissue that spans the scleral canal, mechanically supporting the retinal ganglion cells of the optic nerve as they pass through the scleral canal. The lamina cribrosa is very important in glaucoma, a group of diseases having a common clinical end point of visual field loss and characteristic changes to the optic nerve. Glaucoma is the second most common cause of blindness in western countries and afflicts approximately 65 to 70 million people worldwide (67). In the most common forms of glaucoma, IOP is elevated (to 21 mmHg or higher), and if this elevated IOP is sustained, retinal ganglion cell loss ensues and blindness eventually results. We do not yet completely understand the mechanism of ganglion cell loss, but studies have strongly suggested that the lamina cribrosa is the site of damage (68–70). This has led to the mechanical theory of glaucomatous optic neuropathy, which postulates that elevated mechanical stresses acting within the lamina cribrosa lead to nerve fiber damage, probably through activation of Type 1-$\beta$ astrocytes and/or other glial cells (71). Such mechanical effects may combine synergistically with altered vascular perfusion in the optic nerve head to damage retinal ganglion cells (see Blood Flow in the Eye, below).

In order to evaluate the possible role of mechanical stress in glaucoma, we must know something about the mechanical environment within the lamina cribrosa. Unfortunately, the lamina cribrosa is small, relatively inaccessible, soft, and surrounded by a much stiffer tissue (sclera). This makes experiments challenging, and most measurements have relied on post mortem histologic examination (72, 73), or other indirect measurements of deformation (74–76). Others have adopted a modeling approach, treating the lamina as a circular plate of finite thickness (77, 78). Unfortunately, the lamina is much more geometrically complex than such analytic treatments allow, and thus numerical modeling is an attractive option. Bellezza et al. (79) considered a simplified model of the lamina cribrosa consisting of regular networks of connective tissue "bridges" spanning an elliptical scleral canal. Their results showed remarkable stress elevations in the lamina cribrosa bridges, in some cases more than 100 times the applied IOP. Sigal et al. (80), also using a finite element approach, modeled the sclera, lamina cribrosa, and pre- and postlaminar nerve tissue, finding von Mises strains of up to 12% within the lamina at an IOP of 50 mmHg. Such models are relatively crude at present, assuming linear elasticity, tissue isotropy, and simplified geometries. Nonetheless, when supported by suitable experimental studies, they are a promising tool for unraveling the mysteries of lamina cribrosa biomechanics in glaucoma.

## Accommodation and Presbyopia

Although there are many changes that occur with aging, perhaps the most universal is the loss of the ability to accommodate, i.e., to change the focal length of the eye by changing lens shape. This condition is known as presbyopia, familiar to everyone who has purchased a pair of reading glasses, and typically begins during the fifth decade of life. Several hypotheses have been offered for the causes of presbyopia, including (*a*) a decreased elasticity of the lens, making it more resistant to deformation; (*b*) changes in the geometry of the anterior segment and the lens, resulting in a loss of mechanical effectiveness of zonular tightening; and (*c*) loss of ciliary muscle contractility.

There appears to be good evidence supporting all of these hypotheses. The lens definitely becomes stiffer with age (81–83). There are changes in the geometry of the anterior segment, including an anterior motion of the lens and of the ciliary muscle, an increased size and curvature of the lens, and a decreased anterior chamber depth (84). Other studies (85, 86) have shown that although the ciliary muscle loses its ability to contract in older individuals, the muscle itself is not weakened (87, 88) and remains sensitive to cholinergic agonists (89). Recent evidence indicates that changes in the connective tissues around the ciliary muscle may inhibit its ability to freely contract (90). Thus, the pathophysiology of presbyopia may be multifactorial.

# OCULAR BIOFLUID MECHANICS AND TRANSPORT

Blood flows through the eye, aqueous humor is produced within and drains from the eye, and interstitial fluid percolates through connective tissues within the eye. These myriad fluid pathways contain many fascinating and challenging biomechanical problems.

## Blood Flow in the Eye

All blood is supplied to the eye by the ophthalmic artery. The eye has two main vascular systems: the retinal and uveal. The retinal circulation is fed and drained by the central retinal artery and vein, both of which enter the eye through the scleral canal. The retinal circulation is responsible for supplying blood to the inner retina and is autoregulated (91, 92) so that it provides a nearly constant blood flow rate even as IOP increases up to 30 mmHg. Above this pressure, blood flow is reduced as IOP increases. As the blood flow to the inner aspects of the optic nerve head is also served by the retinal circulation (91), this may have some importance in glaucoma.

The uveal circulation can itself be divided into two parts. The anterior uveal circulation is responsible for supplying blood to vascular tissues of the anterior eye, in particular the iris and ciliary body, where it is involved in the formation of the aqueous humor (see Aqueous Humor Dynamics, below). The iridial circulation is autoregulated (91). The posterior uveal circulation feeds a specialized vascular bed known as the choroid, lying between the retina and sclera. The choroid supplies blood to the outer retina, which has a very high metabolic rate (93). In fact, the choroidal flow is the highest flow per perfused volume of any tissue in the body (8), with approximately 85% of total ocular blood flow passing through the choroid (91). Because the oxygen needs of even the retina are greatly exceeded by this supply (91), the reason for such a high perfusion rate is not known, although a number of creative hypotheses have been offered (94–97). The choroidal flow is thought not to be autoregulated (91), but there is some recent evidence to the contrary (98, 99). The uveal circulation is drained by a venous system consisting of two parts (100). Most blood drains through the vortex veins, four large veins (in the human) that exit the eye through the posterior sclera. The anterior ciliary veins drain part of the ciliary muscle.

The physiology of blood flow in the eye, particularly on the venous side, is strongly influenced by IOP. In most of the circulatory system, flow is determined by the difference between the arterial and venous pressures. However, in the eye, the perfusion pressure is the difference between the arterial pressure and IOP. This relates to the well-known problem of flow through collapsible tubes under the influence of an external pressure (101–103). When the external pressure surrounding a blood vessel is greater than the pressure within that vessel, the vessel collapses, initially at the distal end of the vessel, where the pressure is lowest. As this constriction is the location where most of the pressure drop occurs, upstream of this collapse region the pressure in the vessel is at least equal to the external pressure. Thus, while the arterial pressure in the eye is somewhat lower than in the rest of the body [in the uvea, 75 mmHg systolic and 35 mmHg diastolic (104)], venous pressure in the eye (other than in the sclera) is always above 15 mmHg. Pressures in the choriocapillaris are typically 5–10 mmHg higher than IOP (100).

The region of vessel collapse occurs in the veins as they pass from the vitreous chamber into the sclera. This collapse is necessary for the pressure in the vessel to drop from IOP to episcleral venous pressure [typically 8–10 mmHg in the eye (105,

106)]. The dramatic change in the vessel cross-section that occurs at this point is known as a vascular waterfall. It is a point of flow limitation, similar to what occurs at the nozzle throat in supersonic flow, or at a waterfall (102). In all of these flows, once the flow velocity has reached the wave speed at the point of flow limitation, the flow becomes insensitive to the downstream pressure. The consequence is that, as indicated above, ocular blood flow is very sensitive to the IOP. This is likely the reason why several of the circulations in the eye are autoregulated. It is also the basis for the theory that glaucomatous damage to the optic nerve is caused by reduced blood flow owing to the elevated IOP (107).

## Aqueous Humor Dynamics

For proper visual acuity the eye must be relatively rigid, yet the mammalian eye contains no bones. How then is rigidity maintained? Further, the lens and cornea must remain clear to allow light transmission, and therefore cannot be invested with a vasculature. How then are the cells nourished in these tissues? The eye has solved both problems with a common (and clever) mechanism: The corneoscleral shell is inflated by the production and drainage of the aqueous humor, which also serves to nourish the lens and cornea. The best analogy is a soccer ball with a slow leak whose air is constantly being replenished from a pump. The aqueous humor can also clear debris from within the eye, e.g., red cells from intraocular haemorrhage.

The aqueous humor is produced at $2.4 \pm 0.6$ $\mu$l/min (mean $\pm$ SD, daytime measurements in adults aged 20–83 years) (108). This corresponds to a turnover rate of 1% of the anterior chamber volume per minute, i.e., relatively slowly. Aqueous humor production varies diurnally: It is normally about 3.0 $\mu$l/min in the morning, 2.4 $\mu$l/min in the afternoon, and drops to 1.5 $\mu$l/min at night (108). It is produced primarily by active transport across epithelial cells lining the surface of the ciliary processes (109), and the rate of production is relatively independent of IOP.

The aqueous humor drains from the eye via two routes, the so-called conventional and uveo-scleral (or unconventional) routes. Uveo-scleral outflow normally carries only approximately 10% of total outflow (110, 111); we consider it again in Scleral Permeability and Drug Delivery to the Eye, below. Most aqueous humor instead drains via specialized tissues situated in the angle of the anterior chamber, located at the conjunction of the iris, cornea, and sclera. Beginning at the anterior chamber and moving exteriorly, these tissues are the trabecular meshwork, a porous connective tissue; Schlemm's canal, a collecting duct lined by a vascular-like endothelium; and the collector channels/aqueous veins. Direct pressure measurements (112, 113) and circumstantial evidence (114) indicate that most of the flow resistance in the normal nonglaucomatous eye is in the juxtacanalicular tissue (JCT) or the endothelial lining of Schlemm's canal. After leaving the aqueous veins, the aqueous humor mixes with blood in the episcleral veins, eventually draining back to the right heart (Figure 4, see color insert). The episcleral venous pressure is approximately 8–10 mmHg (105, 106), and the resistance of the conventional aqueous drainage tissues is approximately 3–4 mmHg/$\mu$l/min, resulting in an IOP of 15.5 $\pm$ 2.6 mmHg (mean $\pm$ SD) in the general population (115).

This would be an interesting curiosity if it were not for the problem of glaucoma. We know that elevated IOP is the main risk factor for glaucoma, and that lowering IOP helps preserve visual function (116). In the vast majority of glaucomas, the elevation in IOP is due to too much aqueous humor drainage resistance, and in the majority of these cases the elevated resistance is due to pathologic changes in the conventional drainage tissues. Despite years of intensive research, we understand little of how aqueous drainage resistance is controlled in normal and glaucomatous eyes.

One of the big questions in glaucoma research is: Where is the aqueous flow resistance? Models of Schlemm's canal as a compliant chamber with a porous, elastic wall suggest negligible flow resistance within the canal itself, except at extreme intraocular pressures (>50 mmHg) when the canal collapses (117). Known concentrations of proteoglycan-rich gels within the extracellular spaces of the juxtacanalicular tissue are consistent with the generation of significant flow resistance (118); recent data suggest that the turnover of this matrix is modulated by stretch-induced matrix metalloproteinases (MMP) activity within the trabecular meshwork (119–121). However, the evidence supporting a primary role for extracellular matrix is far from iron-clad (see review in 122), and researchers have looked elsewhere. The other "candidate" for generating flow resistance is the endothelial lining of Schlemm's canal. This cellular layer is unusual; for example, it has the highest permeability of any endothelium (123), with $L_p \geq 4 \times 10^{-8}$ cm$^2$ s/g, yet it is nonfenestrated (but see below). The cells are joined by tight junctions that become less tight as IOP increases (124) and are permeated by membrane-lined openings (pores) that, although poorly understood, are almost certainly involved in aqueous humor transport (125). The pores represent only approximately 0.1% of the total endothelial area and have a mean diameter just slightly over 1 $\mu$m (125). A model of the pores in the endothelial lining modulating the flow through a porous juxtacanalicular tissue (127) suggests that overall flow resistance may depend on an interaction between the endothelial pores and extracellular matrix.

The endothelial cells lining Schlemm's canal bulge prominently into the lumen of the canal, forming the so-called giant vacuoles. Evidence suggests these are passive structures that form in response to the "backward" basal-to-apical pressure gradient that is always present across the cells (128, 129). The extreme case is when you rub your eyes, instantaneously generating pressures as high as 80 mmHg (130)! These large IOPs form so many giant vacuoles that inner wall endothelial cells may stretch by as much as 50% (131), a harsh biomechanical environment indeed.

The biomechanics of aqueous humor flow within the anterior chamber are also interesting. Because the cornea is normally exposed to ambient air, the temperature at the posterior corneal surface is slightly less than body temperature, thus creating a temperature gradient across the anterior chamber. The resulting convection patterns (132, 133) tend to transport particles in vertical paths along the mid-peripheral

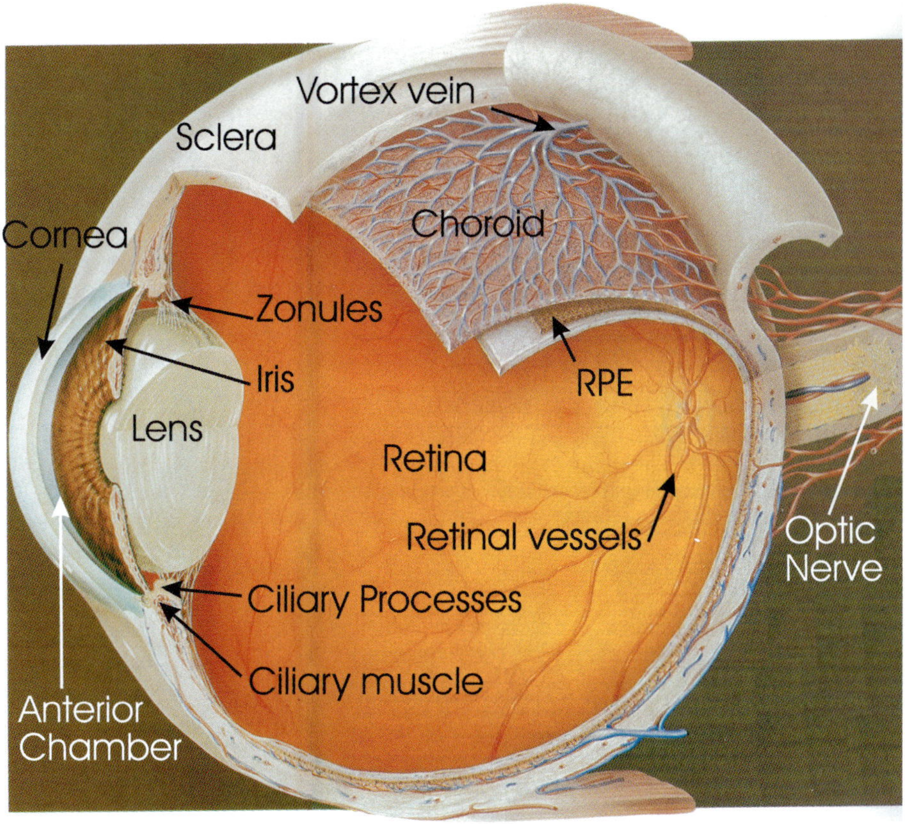


**Figure 1** Overview of ocular anatomy, with several key ocular components labelled. Modified from (2).

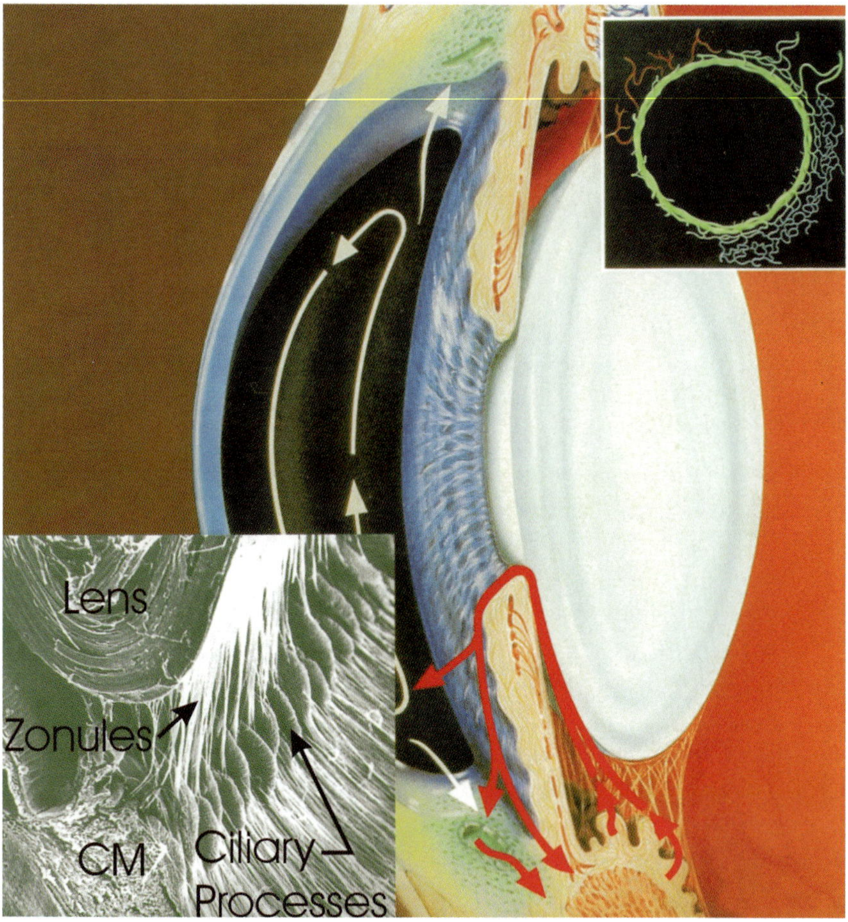


**Figure 4** View of anterior segment of eye, showing site of production of aqueous humor (ciliary processes) and drainage routes (*red arrows*). The white arrows in the anterior chamber show thermal convection patterns. The lower left inset is a scanning electron micrograph of the zonular apparatus (CM = ciliary muscle). The inset at upper right shows Schlemm's canal (*green*) as seen face-on. Green vessels anatomising with Schlemm's canal are collector channels; blue vessels are aqueous veins; red vessels are arterioles. Modified from (2).

cornea (Figure 4). The clinical correlate of this effect is pigment particles that are seen to accumulate along such paths in patients whose irises release abnormal amounts of pigments.

There is a form of glaucoma in which the elevated IOP is not due to changes in the drainage system of the eye per se. This is angle-closure glaucoma, when the iris pivots forward and blocks access to the drainage structures in the angle of the anterior chamber. There appears to be an anatomic predisposition to this situation. The iris is extremely pliable (134), and modeling has shown interesting interactions between iris deformation and aqueous flow through the pupil and between the lens and the iris, especially when the eye is perturbed by blinking (135, 136).

## Transport Within the Cornea

To maintain transparency, the corneal stroma must be prevented from swelling. The flows and forces that nourish and deturgesce the stroma are subtle and complex. Although there is some evidence for limbally derived lateral flow (137, 138) because of the 10:1 ratio of lateral to transverse diffusion distance, the corneal transport system is essentially one-dimensional in the AP (anterior-to-posterior) direction (Figure 5). To understand this AP transport, we must consider the role of the corneal membranes. The epithelium, with its complete tight junctions, primarily protects the stroma [although it does have some limited active pumping ability (139)], whereas the endothelium, with its incomplete tight junctions and its plethora of basolateral ATPases, removes fluid yet allows free diffusion of nutrients and cytokines from the aqueous humor (46). Globally, there is approximately a 20 micron/h net flow velocity out of the cornea to the tear film, driven by the transcorneal pressure gradient and by evaporation from the tear film (140). Intriguingly, however, the corneal endothelium can generate a fluid velocity of 40 microns/h in the opposite direction, effectively compressing the stroma (141).

Fluid transport through the cornea depends on the hydraulic permeabilities, $L_p$, of the endothelium, epithelium, and stroma. Isolating functioning membranes from

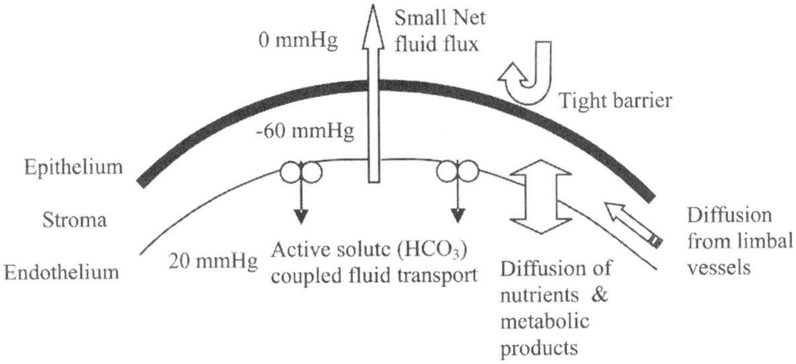


**Figure 5** Key elements of the corneal transport system.

the hydrophilic stroma to measure $L_p$ is not feasible. However, Klyce & Russell (142) were able to extract $L_p$ for both the endothelium ($42.0 \times 10^{-12}$ cm$^3$/dyne sec) and the epithelium ($6.1 \times 10^{-12}$ cm$^3$/dyne sec) by coupling thermodynamic representations of the membranes (143) to a dynamic stromal transport model (47) and fitting the model to the corneal response to osmotic challenges. As expected, the endothelium is more permeable to water than the epithelium (by a factor of seven). From the same series of experiments, the ratio of endothelial to epithelial NaCl permeability was much larger than one as well. To produce dynamic corneal transport models (e.g., 142), it is necessary to know the value of stromal hydraulic conductivity, $k/\eta$, as a function of tissue hydration. The elegant work of Hedbys & Mishima (144) relates the stromal hydraulic conductivity in both the in-plane and transverse direction to hydration (Figure 6).

Typically, stromal fluid transport and hydraulic conductivity have been measured on bulk tissue. Recently, however, Ruberti et al. (145) tracked microscale

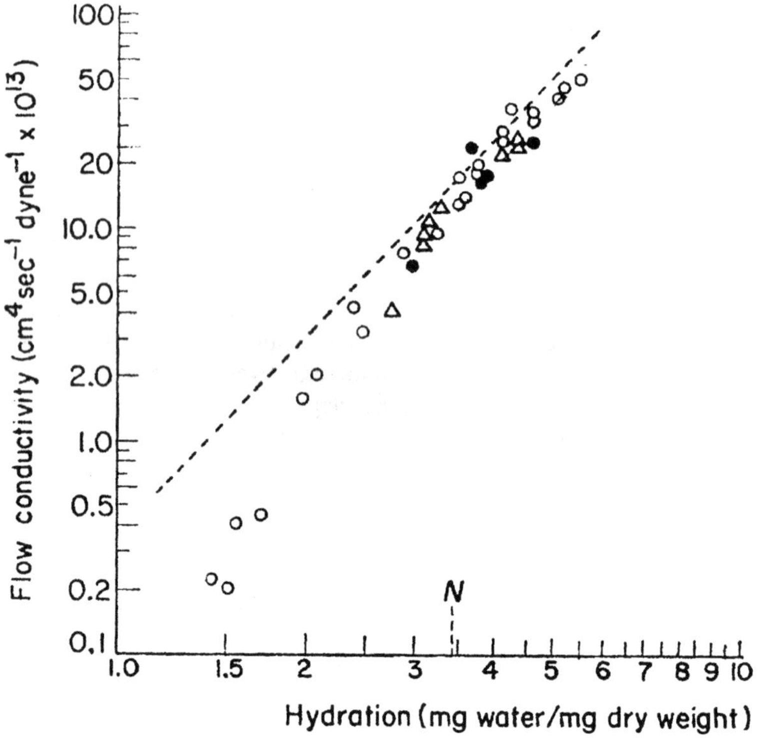


**Figure 6** Flow conductivity versus hydration across the cornea. The symbols refer to measurements taken with (*closed circles*) and without (*open circles*) Descemet's membrane in 0.9% NaCl, or without Descemet's membrane in distilled water (*triangles*). The broken line represents the flow conductivity versus hydration relationship for flow along the cornea. N is the normal corneal hydration. From Hedbys & Mishima (144).

intrastromal flows in response to corneal debridement, and Overby et al. (146) determined intrastromal specific hydraulic conductivity directly from structure-preserving micrographs. Such investigations promise to improve our understanding of microscale corneal transport dynamics.

## Transport Across Bruch's Membrane

In addition to the corneal endothelium, there are several sites of active transport in the eye, including the ciliary epithelium, responsible for production of aqueous humor, and the retinal pigment epithelium (RPE), which removes fluid from the retina and thus helps keep the retina attached (147–149).

The RPE rests on a basement membrane that is part of Bruch's membrane, a five-layer barrier structure that limits transport between the choroid and the outer retina. These five layers, beginning at the RPE and proceeding outward toward the choroid, are the basement membrane of the RPE, the inner collagenous layer, the elastin layer, the outer collagenous layer, and the basement membrane of the choriocapillaris (150). Oxygen, electrolytes, nutrients, and cytokines from the choroidal circulation must pass through this barrier to reach the retina, whereas waste products from the retina and water pumped by the RPE must pass back through this barrier to be eliminated into the blood stream.

Water transport through this membrane is the best studied of these transport processes. After the RPE pumps water from the retinal space into Bruch's membrane, the water moves under the influence of both hydrostatic and osmotic pressure gradients into the choroidal circulation (91, 151). The hydraulic resistance of Bruch's membrane increases with age (Figure 7). This increase has been hypothesized to contribute to the pathology of age-related macular degeneration (AMD) by inhibiting fluid transport by the RPE and consequently causing retinal detachment (152).

The age-related increase in the hydraulic resistance of Bruch's membrane is thought to be a consequence of lipid accumulation (153) because the age-related increase in resistance parallels the age-related accumulation of lipid in Bruch's membrane (Figure 7). These lipids may originate as waste products from the retina that are processed by the RPE (154).

It has been shown that there is a parallel age-related increase in the transport resistance of Bruch's membrane to protein transport (156), although that study may not have properly accounted for osmotic effects of the proteins examined. Little study has yet been done on the transport of other moieties across Bruch's membrane.

## Scleral Permeability and Drug Delivery to the Eye

Drug delivery to intraocular tissues is important in treating a variety of ocular diseases. Systemic administration of these agents is undesirable because it necessitates high plasma concentrations to achieve adequate intraocular dosing. Transcorneal delivery by passive diffusion is difficult because the drug needs to have

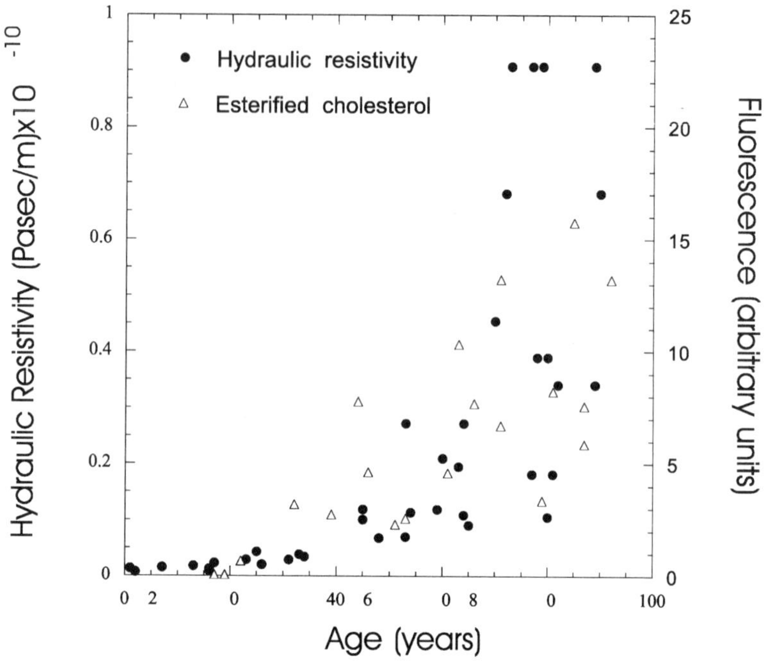


**Figure 7** Hydraulic resistivity (150) of excised Bruch's membrane/choroid (*closed symbols*) and fluorescence owing to histochemically detected esterified cholesterol in sections of normal Bruch's membrane (155) (*open symbols*) as a function of age.

hydrophobic characteristics to pass through the corneal epithelium and endothelium, and hydrophilic characteristics to pass through the corneal stroma. Furthermore, as soon as the agent enters the anterior chamber, it is carried out of the eye by the aqueous humor. Scleral delivery, especially for drugs destined for the retina (157), may be a more attractive route for drug administration (158), as the tight epithelial barriers of the cornea are not present on the sclera (159). However, the scleral stroma is still a significant barrier, and a number of studies have examined the permeability of this tissue.

As expected, scleral permeability to solute transport decreases with increasing solute molecular weight and increasing molecular radius, with the latter a better predictor of scleral permeability than the former (160). The posterior sclera is more permeable to solute transport than the anterior sclera, further supporting the sclera as an ideal route for drug delivery to the retina (161).

The specific hydraulic conductivity of the sclera is $2 \times 10^{-14}$ cm$^2$, typical of dense connective tissues (162). With a typical pressure difference across the sclera of 15 mmHg; a scleral thickness, $L$, of 0.6 mm (163); and a filtering area, $A$, of 11.5 cm$^2$ [the total scleral area (163)], we can use Darcy's law to estimate a maximum flow rate ($Q$) across the sclera of 0.3 $\mu$l/min. The flow rate can be used to examine several issues related to fluid flow though the scleral stroma.

The first question is the extent to which this flow impedes drug delivery across the sclera. The diffusional flux of a drug through a tissue can be estimated as

$$D_0(1 - \Phi)A\frac{\Delta C}{L}, \tag{7}$$

whereas the convective flux of a drug through that same tissue would be

$$QC(1 - \Phi). \tag{8}$$

Here $D_0$ is the diffusion coefficient of the tracer in free solution (for albumin $6 \times 10^{-7}$ cm$^2$/sec); $\Phi$ is the extent to which the tracer is retarded, relative to the fluid flow, from moving by the extracellular matrix (0 is unhindered, 1 completely hindered); and $\Delta C$ is the concentration difference across the sclera, which we assume is the same as the concentration of drug at the surface of the sclera. Using these formulas, the ratio of diffusional transport to convective transport is computed to be approximately 20 for molecules the size of albumin. In other words, for these parameters, diffusional transport of a drug across the sclera is more than an order-of-magnitude higher than transport of the drug by convection. Thus, bulk flow across the sclera should have minimal impact on drug delivery through the sclera.

We can also use the value of $Q$ to gain insight into the unconventional drainage pathway (Aqueous Humor Dynamics, above) that normally carries a small fraction of the aqueous humor from the eye. Aqueous humor draining via this pathway passes through the ciliary muscle, into the suprachoroidal space, and then passes (*a*) either through the sclera into the orbit or (*b*) through the sclera to the vortex veins and choroidal circulation, where it is absorbed. Arguments have been provided for each of these pathways (123, 164, 165). The value of $Q$ calculated above as 0.3 $\mu$l/min would appear to support the former pathway because this value is consistent with measured values of unconventional aqueous outflow rates (166). However, it is known that ciliary muscle contraction greatly affects the unconventional outflow (167), and that $PGF_{2\alpha}$ greatly increases unconventional outflow by decreasing the flow resistance of the interstitial spaces in the ciliary muscle (168, 169). This can only be the case if the flow resistance of the ciliary muscle is of the same order of magnitude or even larger than that of the sclera; otherwise, changes in the muscle would make little difference. But, in that case, the calculated flow rate of 0.3 $\mu$l/min must be an upper bound that does not consider the flow resistance of the ciliary muscle. A further argument against a trans-scleral flow is that unconventional outflow is not very pressure sensitive (170). Although this might be expected if the flow were primarily osmotically driven into the uveal vessels, this would not be the expected characteristic of a trans-scleral flow. Each of these considerations argue against trans-scleral flow, but are consistent with osmotic adsorption of the unconventional aqueous outflow by the choroidal circulation (123).

## SUMMARY AND OPEN PROBLEMS

From this brief summary it is clear that there is a great deal of interesting biomechanics in the eye. We are far from understanding all the relevant biomechanics in this understudied field, and hence we close with a list of open problems to tempt researchers.

- Why does presbyopia occur? There have been no biomechanical modeling studies that account for all of the physiological observations mentioned in Accommodation and Presbyopia (above) and attempt to comprehensively evaluate the mechanisms underlying presbyopia. More generally, fundamental studies about the biomechanics of accommodation are also needed.
- How is outflow resistance generated in the normal eye, and what goes wrong to increase this resistance in most forms of glaucoma?
- How does elevated IOP damage the optic nerve and lead to blindness in glaucoma?
- What are the biomechanics of myopia?
- How can we determine microscale material properties and corneal stress field noninvasively, in vivo? If this can be accomplished, then the biomechanicist might provide input for refractive corneal surgery on a case-by-case basis.
- How is the hydration of the cornea controlled? No control signal has been identified to date, yet corneas maintain their hydration in a relatively tight range. Recently, Ruberti & Klyce (171) demonstrated that 5% changes in NaCl concentration induced compensatory changes in endothelial pump rate, suggesting a possible homeostatic response triggered by NaCl.

## ACKNOWLEDGMENTS

Our work has benefited from ongoing grant support from the Canadian Institutes of Health Research (CRE), the Glaucoma Research Society of Canada (CRE), International Retinal Research Foundation (MJ), the American Health Assistance Foundation (MJ), and the National Institutes of Health (R01 EY014662; MJ).



## LITERATURE CITED

1. Demer JL. 2002. The orbital pulley system: a revolution in concepts of orbital anatomy. *Ann. NY Acad. Sci.* 956:17–32
2. Krey HF, Bräuer H. 1998. *Chibret Augenatlas: Eine Repetition für Ärtze mit Zeigetafeln für Patienten*. Munich: Chibret Med. Serv.
3. Jue B, Maurice DM. 1986. The mechanical properties of the rabbit and human cornea. *J. Biomech.* 19:847–53

4. Woo SL, Kobayashi AS, Schlegel WA, Lawrence C. 1972. Nonlinear material properties of intact cornea and sclera. *Exp. Eye Res.* 14:29–39
5. Hjortdal JO. 1996. Regional elastic performance of the human cornea. *J. Biomech.* 29:931–42
6. Battaglioli JL, Kamm RD. 1984. Measurements of the compressive properties of scleral tissue. *Invest. Ophthalmol. Vis. Sci.* 25:59–65
7. Friedenwald JS. 1937. Contribution to the theory and practice of tonometry. *Am. J. Ophthalmol.* 20:985–1024
8. Collins R, van der Werff TJ. 1980. Mathematical models of the dynamics of the human eye. In *Lecture Notes in Biomathematics*. Berlin: Springer-Verlag
9. Fung YC. 1967. Elasticity of soft tissues in simple elongation. *Am. J. Physiol.* 213:1532–44
10. McEwen WK, St Helen R. 1965. Rheology of the human sclera. Unifying formulation of ocular rigidity. *J. Biol. Chem.* 240:2003–10
11. Greene PR. 1985. Closed-form ametropic pressure-volume and ocular rigidity solutions. *Am. J. Optom. Physiol. Opt.* 62:870–78
12. Woo SL, Kobayashi AS, Schlegel WA, Lawrence C. 1972. Nonlinear material properties of intact cornea and sclera. *Exp. Eye Res.* 14:29–39
13. Woo SL-Y, Kobayashi AS, Lawrence C, Schlegel WA. 1972. Mathematical model of the corneo-scleral shell as applied to intraocular pressure-volume relations and applanation tonormetry. *Ann. Biomed. Eng.* 1:87–98
14. Nash IS, Greene PR, Foster CS. 1982. Comparison of mechanical properties of keratoconus and normal corneas. *Exp. Eye Res.* 35:413–24
15. Lyon C, McEwen WK, Shepherd MD. 1970. Ocular rigidity and decay curves analyzed by two nonlinear systems. *Invest. Ophthalmol. Vis. Sci.* 9:935–45
16. St. Helen R, McEwen WK. 1961. Rheology of the human sclera. I. Anelastic behavior. *Am. J. Ophthalmol.* 52:539
17. Downs JC, Suh JK, Thomas KA, Bellezza AJ, Burgoyne CF, Hart RT. 2003. Viscoelastic characterization of peripapillary sclera: material properties by quadrant in rabbit and monkey eyes. *J. Biomech. Eng.* 125:124–31
18. Mow VC, Holmes MH, Lai WM. 1984. Fluid transport and mechanical properties of articular cartilage: a review. *J. Biomech.* 17:377
19. Johnson M, Tarbell JM. 2001. A biphasic, anisotropic model of the aortic wall. *J. Biomech. Eng.* 123:52–57
20. McDermott JA. 1989. Tonography. See Ref. 172, pp. 293–99
21. Gloster J. 1965. Tonometry and tonography. *Int. Ophthalmol. Clin.* 5:911–1133
22. Fatt I. 1978. *Physiology of the Eye: An Introduction to the Vegetative Functions*. Boston, MA: Butterworth
23. Grant WM. 1950. Tonographic method for measuring the facility and rate of aqueous flow in human eyes. *Arch. Ophthalmol.* 44:204–14
24. Viernstein LJ, Kitazawa Y. 1970. Measurements of factors affecting the precision of tonometry and tonography. *Exp. Eye Res.* 9:91–97
25. Viernstein LJ, Cowan M. 1969. Static and dynamic measurements of the pressure-volume relationship in living and dead rabbit eyes. *Exp. Eye Res.* 8:183–92
26. Greene PR, McMahon TA. 1979. Scleral creep vs. temperature and pressure in vitro. *Exp. Eye Res.* 29:527–37
27. Ku DN, Greene PR. 1981. Scleral creep in vitro resulting from cyclic pressure pulses: applications to myopia. *Am. J. Optom. Physiol. Opt.* 58:528–35
28. Greene PR. 1980. Mechanical considerations in myopia: relative effects of accommodation, convergence, intraocular pressure, and the extraocular muscles. *Am. J. Optom. Physiol. Opt.* 57:902–14
29. Wiesel TN, Raviola E. 1977. Myopia and

eye enlargement after neonatal lid fusion in monkeys. *Nature* 266:66–68

30. Wallman J, Turkel J, Trachtman J. 1978. Extreme myopia produced by modest change in early visual experience. *Science* 201:1249–51
31. Goss DA, Wickham MG. 1995. Retinal-image mediated ocular growth as a mechanism for juvenile onset myopia and for emmetropization. A literature review. *Doc. Ophthalmol.* 90:341–75
32. Maurice D. 1957. The structure and transparency of the cornea. *J. Physiol.* 136:263–86
33. Goldman JN, Benedek GB. 1967. The relationship between morphology and transparency in the nonswelling corneal stroma of the shark. *Invest. Ophthalmol. Vis. Sci.* 6:574–600
34. Pouliquen Y. 1985. Fine structure of the corneal stroma. *Cornea* 3:168–77
35. Birk DE, Fitch JM, Babiarz JP, Linsenmayer TF. 1988. Collagen type I and type V are present in the same fibril in the avian corneal stroma. *J. Cell Biol.* 106:999–1008
36. Meek KM, Fullwood NJ. 2001. Corneal and scleral collagens—a microscopist's perspective. *Micron* 32:261–72
37. Shin TJ, Vito RP, Johnson LW, McCarey BE. 1997. The distribution of strain in the human cornea. *J. Biomech.* 30:497–503
38. Waring GO 3rd. 1999. A cautionary tale of innovation in refractive surgery. *Arch. Ophthalmol.* 117:1069–73
39. McPhee TJ, Bourne WM, Brubaker RF. 1985. Location of the stress-bearing layers of the cornea. *Invest. Ophthalmol. Vis. Sci.* 26:869–72
40. Hennighausen H, Feldman ST, Bille JF, McCulloch AD. 1998. Anterior-posterior strain variation in normally hydrated and swollen rabbit cornea. *Invest. Ophthalmol. Vis. Sci.* 39:253–62
41. Hodson S, O'Leary D, Watkins S. 1991. The measurement of ox corneal swelling pressure by osmometry. *J. Physiol.* 434:399–408
42. Otori T. 1967. Electrolyte content of the rabbit corneal stroma. *Exp. Eye Res.* 6:356–67
43. Bryant MR, McDonnell PJ. 1996. Constitutive laws for biomechanical modeling of refractive surgery. *J. Biomech. Eng.* 118:473–81
44. Zeng Y, Yang J, Huang K, Lee Z, Lee X. 2001. A comparison of biomechanical properties between human and porcine cornea. *J. Biomech.* 34:533–37
45. Flory PJ. 1953. *Principles of Polymer Chemistry*. Ithaca, NY: Cornell Univ. Press. 672 pp.
46. Maurice DM. 1984. The cornea and sclera. In *The Eye*, ed. H Davson. New York: Academic
47. Fatt I, Goldstick T. 1965. Dynamics of water transport in swelling membranes. *J. Colloid Sci.* 20:962–89
48. Eisenberg SR, Grodzinsky AJ. 1985. Swelling of articular cartilage and other connective tissues: electromechanochemical forces. *J. Orthop. Res.* 3:148–59
49. Eisenberg SR, Grodzinsky AJ. 1987. The kinetics of chemically induced nonequilibrium swelling of articular cartilage and corneal stroma. *J. Biomech. Eng.* 109:79–89
50. Myers ER, Lai WM, Mow VC. 1984. A continuum theory and an experiment for the ion-induced swelling behavior of articular cartilage. *J. Biomech. Eng.* 106:151–58
51. Mow VC, Kuei SC, Lai WM, Armstrong CG. 1980. Biphasic creep and stress relaxation of articular cartilage in compression? Theory and experiments. *J. Biomech. Eng.* 102:73–84
52. Hedbys B, Mishima S, Maurice D. 1963. The imbibition pressure of the corneal stroma. *Exp. Eye Res.* 2:99–111
53. Hedbys B, Dohlman C. 1963. A new method for the determination of the swelling pressure of the corneal stroma in vitro. *Exp. Eye Res.* 2:122–29
54. Roberts C. 2000. The cornea is not a piece of plastic. *J. Refract. Surg.* 16:407–13

55. Munnerlyn CR, Koons SJ, Marshall J. 1988. Photorefractive keratectomy: a technique for laser refractive surgery. *J. Cataract. Refract. Surg.* 14:46–52
56. Bailey MD, Mitchell GL, Dhaliwal DK, Boxer Wachler BS, Zadnik K. 2003. Patient satisfaction and visual symptoms after laser in situ keratomileusis. *Ophthalmology* 110:1371–78
57. Hanna KD, Jouve FE, Waring GO 3rd. 1989. Preliminary computer simulation of the effects of radial keratotomy. *Arch. Ophthalmol.* 107:911–18
58. Pinsky PM, Datye DV. 1991. A microstructurally-based finite element model of the incised human cornea. *J. Biomech.* 24:907–22
59. Velinsky SA, Bryant MR. 1992. On the computer-aided and optimal design of keratorefractive surgery. *Refract. Corneal. Surg.* 8:173–82
60. Vito RP, Shin TJ, McCarey BE. 1989. A mechanical model of the cornea: the effects of physiological and surgical factors on radial keratotomy surgery. *Refract. Corneal. Surg.* 5:82–88
61. Wray WO, Best ED, Cheng LY. 1994. A mechanical model for radial keratotomy: toward a predictive capability. *J. Biomech. Eng.* 116:56–61
62. Alamouti B, Funk J. 2003. Retinal thickness decreases with age: an OCT study. *Br. J. Ophthalmol.* 87:899–901
63. Jones IL, Warner M, Stevens JD. 1992. Mathematical modelling of the elastic properties of retina: a determination of Young's modulus. *Eye* 6(Pt. 6):556–59
64. Stevens JD, Jones IL, Warner M, Lavin MJ, Leaver PK. 1992. Mathematical modelling of retinal tear formation: implications for the use of heavy liquids. *Eye* 6(Pt. 1):69–74
65. David T, Smye S, Dabbs T, James T. 1998. A model for the fluid motion of vitreous humour of the human eye during saccadic movement. *Phys. Med. Biol.* 43:1385–99
66. Levin AV. 2002. Ophthalmology of shaken baby syndrome. *Neurosurg. Clin. N. Am.* 13:201–11, vi
67. Quigley HA. 1996. Number of people with glaucoma worldwide. *Br. J. Ophthalmol.* 80:389–93
68. Quigley HA, Addicks EM, Green WR, Maumenee AE. 1981. Optic nerve damage in human glaucoma; II: the site of injury and susceptibility to damage. *Arch. Ophthalmol.* 99:635
69. Quigley HA, Anderson DR. 1976. The dynamics and location of axonal transport blockade by acute intraocular pressure elevation in primate optic nerve. *Invest. Ophthalmol. Vis. Sci.* 15:606–16
70. Quigley HA, Flower RW, Addicks EM, McLeod DS. 1980. The mechanism of optic nerve damage in experimental acute intraocular pressure elevation. *Invest. Ophthalmol. Vis. Sci.* 19:505
71. Hernandez MR. 2000. The optic nerve head in glaucoma: role of astrocytes in tissue remodeling. *Prog. Retin. Eye Res.* 19:297–321
72. Yan DB, Metheetrairut A, Coloma FM, Trope GE, Heathcote JG, Ethier CR. 1994. Deformation of the lamina cribrosa by elevated intraocular pressure. *Br. J. Ophthalmol.* 78:643–48
73. Nesterov AP, Egoriv EA. 1986. Pathological physiology of primary open angle glaucoma. In *Glaucoma*, ed. J Cairns, pp. 382–96. Miami, FL: Grune Stratton
74. Yan DB, Flanagan JG, Farra T, Trope GE, Ethier CR. 1998. Study of regional deformation of the optic nerve head using scanning laser tomography. *Curr. Eye Res.* 17:903–16
75. Levy NS, Crapps EE. 1984. Displacement of optic nerve head in response to short-term intraocular pressure elevation in human eyes. *Arch. Ophthalmol.* 102:782–86
76. Levy NS, Crapps EE, Bonney RC. 1981. Displacement of the optic nerve head. Response to acute intraocular pressure elevation in primate eyes. *Arch. Ophthalmol.* 99:2166–74

77. He DQ, Ren ZQ. 1999. A biomathematical model for pressure-dependent lamina cribrosa behavior. *J. Biomech.* 32:579–84
78. Edwards ME, Good TA. 2001. Use of a mathematical model to estimate stress and strain during elevated pressure induced lamina cribrosa deformation. *Curr. Eye Res.* 23:215–25
79. Bellezza AJ, Hart RT, Burgoyne CF. 2000. The optic nerve head as a biomechanical structure: initial finite element modeling. *Invest. Ophthalmol. Vis. Sci.* 41:2991–3000
80. Sigal IA, Flanagan JG, Tertinegg I, Ethier CR. 2003. Investigation of the biomechanical environment within the optic nerve head by finite element modelling. In *Computational Fluid and Solid Mechanics 2003, Proc. Second MIT Conf.*, ed. KJ Bathe, pp. 1810–13. New York: Elsevier
81. Pau H, Kranz J. 1991. The increasing sclerosis of the lens and its relevance to accommodation and presbyopia. *Graefes Arch. Clin. Exp. Ophthalmol.* 229:294–96
82. Fisher R. 1971. The elastic constants of the human lens. *J. Physiol.* 212:147–80
83. Glasser A, Campbell M. 1998. Presbyopia and the optical changes in the human crystalline lens with age. *Vision Res.* 38:209–29
84. Koretz J, Cook C, Kaufman P. 1997. Accommodation and presbyopia in the human eye. Changes in the anterior segment and crystalline lens with focus. *Invest. Ophthalmol. Vis. Sci.* 38:569–78
85. Lütjen-Drecoll E, Tamm E, Kaufman P. 1988. Age-related loss of morphologic response to pilcarpine in rhesus monkey ciliary muscle. *Arch. Ophthalmol.* 106:1591
86. Neider M, Crawford K, Kaufman P, Bito L. 1990. In vivo videography of the rhesus monkey accommodative apparatus. Age-related loss of ciliary muscle response to central stimulation. *Arch. Ophthalmol.* 108:69
87. Fisher R. 1977. The force of contraction of human ciliary muscle during accommodation. *J. Physiol.* 270:51
88. Swegmark G. 1969. Studies with impedance cyclography on human ocular accommodation at diferent ages. *Acta Ophthalmol.* 47:1186
89. Pardue MT, Sivak JG. 2000. Age-related changes in human ciliary muscle. *Optom. Vis. Sci.* 77:204–10
90. Tamm E, Lutjen-Drecoll E, Jungkunz W, Rohen JW. 1991. Posterior attachment of ciliary muscle in young, accommodating old, presbyopic monkeys. *Invest. Ophthalmol. Vis. Sci.* 32:1678–92
91. Bill A. 1975. Blood circulation and fluid dynamics in the eye. *Physiol. Rev.* 55:383–416
92. Grunwald JE, Petrig BL, Robinson F. 1986. Retinal blood flow autoregulation in response to an acute increase in blood pressure. *Invest. Ophthalmol. Vis. Sci.* 27:1706–12
93. Wangsa-Wirawan ND, Linsenmeier RA. 2003. Retinal oxygen: fundamental and clinical aspects. *Arch. Ophthalmol.* 121:547–57
94. Parver LM, Auker C, Carpenter DO. 1980. Choroidal blood flow as a heat dissipating mechanism in the macula. *Am. J. Ophthalmol.* 89:641–46
95. Bill A. 1985. Some aspects of the ocular circulation. Friedenwald lecture. *Invest. Ophthalmol. Vis. Sci.* 26:410–24
96. Foulds W. 1990. The choroidal circulation and retinal metabolism: an overview. *Eye* 4:243–48
97. Linsenmeier RA, Padnick-Silver L. 2000. Metabolic dependence of photoreceptors on the choroid in the normal and detached retina. *Invest. Ophthalmol. Vis. Sci* 41:3117–23
98. Kiel JW, van Heuven WA. 1995. Ocular perfusion pressure and choroidal blood flow in the rabbit. *Exp. Eye Res.* 60:267–78
99. Kiel JW, Shepherd AP. 1992. Autoregulation of choroidal blood flow in the rabbit. *Invest. Ophthalmol. Vis. Sci.* 33:2399–410
100. Maepea O. 1992. Pressures in the anterior ciliary arteries, choroidal veins and

choriocapillaris. *Exp. Eye Res.* 54:731–36
101. Shapiro AH. 1977. Physiological and medical aspects of flow in collapsible tubes. *Proc. Can. Congr. Appl. Mech., 6th, Vancouver,* pp. 883–906
102. Shapiro AH. 1977. Steady flow in collapsible tubes. *J. Biomech. Eng.* 99:126–47
103. Kamm RD. 1987. Flow through collapsible tubes. In *Handbook of Bioengineering*, ed. R Skalak, S Chien. New York: McGraw-Hill
104. Cole D. 1966. Aqueous humor formation. *Doc. Ophthalmol.* 21:116–238
105. Phelps CD, Armaly MF. 1978. Measurement of episcleral venous pressure. *Am. J. Ophthalmol.* 85:35–42
106. Brubaker RF. 1967. Determination of episcleral venous pressure in the eye. A comparison of three methods. *Arch. Ophthalmol.* 77:110
107. Minckler DS, Spaeth GL. 1981. Optic nerve damage in glaucoma. *Surv. Ophthalmol.* 26:128–48
108. Brubaker RF. 1989. Measurement of aqueous flow by fluorophotometry. See Ref. 172, pp. 337–44
109. Bartels SP. 1989. Aqueous humor production. See Ref. 172, pp. 199
110. Becker B, Neufeld AH. 2002. Erratum. Pressure dependence of uveoscleral outflow. *J. Glaucoma* 11:545
111. Becker B, Neufeld AH. 2002. Pressure dependence of uveoscleral outflow. *J. Glaucoma* 11:464
112. Mäepea O, Bill A. 1989. The pressures in the episcleral veins, Schlemm's canal and the trabecular meshwork in monkeys: effects of changes in intraocular pressure. *Exp. Eye Res.* 49:645–63
113. Mäepea O, Bill A. 1992. Pressures in the juxtacanalicular tissue and Schlemm's canal in monkeys. *Exp. Eye Res.* 54:879–83
114. Ethier CR. 2002. The inner wall of Schlemm's canal. *Exp. Eye Res.* 74:161–72
115. Schottenstein EM. 1989. Intraocular pressure. See Ref. 172, pp. 301–17
116. Beck AD. 2003. Review of recent publications of the Advanced Glaucoma Intervention Study. *Curr. Opin. Ophthalmol.* 14:83–85
117. Johnson M, Kamm RD. 1983. The role of Schlemm's canal in aqueous outflow from the human eye. *Invest. Ophthalmol. Vis. Sci.* 24:320
118. Ethier CR, Kamm RD, Palaszewski BA, Johnson MC, Richardson TM. 1986. Calculation of flow resistance in the juxtacanalicular meshwork. *Invest. Ophthalmol. Vis. Sci.* 27:1741–50
119. Alexander JP, Samples JR, Acott TS. 1998. Growth factor and cytokine modulation of trabecular meshwork matrix metalloproteinase and TIMP expression. *Curr. Eye Res.* 17:276–85
120. Bradley JM, Vranka J, Colvis CM, Conger DM, Alexander JP, et al. 1998. Effect of matrix metalloproteinases activity on outflow in perfused human organ culture. *Invest. Ophthalmol. Vis. Sci.* 39:2649–58
121. Bradley JM, Kelley MJ, Zhu X, Anderssohn AM, Alexander JP, Acott TS. 2001. Effects of mechanical stretching on trabecular matrix metalloproteinases. *Invest. Ophthalmol. Vis. Sci.* 42:1505–13
122. Ethier CR. 2002. The inner wall of Schlemm's canal. *Exp. Eye Res.* 74:161–72
123. Johnson M, Erickson K. 2000. Mechanisms and routes of aqueous humor drainage. In *Principles and Practices of Ophthalmology*, ed. DM Albert, FA Jakobiec, pp. 2577–95. Philadelphia, PA: WB Saunders Co.
124. Ye W, Gong H, Sit A, Johnson M, Freddo TF. 1997. Interendothelial junctions in normal human Schlemm's canal respond to changes in pressure. *Invest. Ophthalmol. Vis. Sci.* 38:2460–68
125. Ethier CR. 2002. The inner wall of Schlemm's canal. *Exp. Eye Res.* 74:161–72
126. Deleted in proof

127. Johnson M, Shapiro A, Ethier CR, Kamm RD. 1992. The modulation of outflow resistance by the pores of the inner wall endothelium. *Invest. Ophthalmol. Vis. Sci.* 33:1670–75
128. Parc CE, Johnson DH, Brilakis HS. 2000. Giant vacuoles are found preferentially near collector channels. *Invest. Ophthalmol. Vis. Sci.* 41:2984–90
129. Grierson I, Lee WR. 1977. Light microscopic quantitation of the endothelial vacuoles in Schlemm's canal. *Am. J. Ophthalmol.* 84:234–46
130. Coleman DJ, Trokel S. 1969. Direct-recorded intraocular pressure variations in a human subject. *Arch. Ophthalmol.* 82:637–40
131. Ethier CR. 2002. The inner wall of Schlemm's canal. *Exp. Eye Res.* 74:161–72
132. Canning CR, Greaney MJ, Dewynne JN, Fitt AD. 2002. Fluid flow in the anterior chamber of a human eye. *IMA J. Math. Appl. Med. Biol.* 19:31–60
133. Heys JJ, Barocas VH. 2002. A boussinesq model of natural convection in the human eye and the formation of Krukenberg's spindle. *Ann. Biomed. Eng.* 30:392–401
134. Heys J, Barocas VH. 1999. Mechanical characterization of the bovine iris. *J. Biomech.* 32:999–1003
135. Heys JJ, Barocas VH. 2002. Computational evaluation of the role of accommodation in pigmentary glaucoma. *Invest. Ophthalmol. Vis. Sci.* 43:700–8
136. Heys JJ, Barocas VH, Taravella MJ. 2001. Modeling passive mechanical interaction between aqueous humor and iris. *J. Biomech. Eng.* 123:540–47
137. Green K, DeBarge LR, Cheeks L, Phillips CI. 1987. Centripetal movement of fluorescein dextrans in the cornea: relevance to arcus. *Acta Ophthalmol.* 65:538–44
138. Wiig H. 1990. Cornea fluid dynamics. II. Evidence for transport of radiolabelled albumin in rabbits by bulk flow. *Exp. Eye Res.* 50:261–67
139. Klyce SD. 1975. Transport of Na, Cl, and water by the rabbit corneal epithelium at resting potential. *Am. J. Physiol.* 228:1446–52
140. Mishima S, Maurice DM. 1961. The oily layer of the tear film and evaporation from the corneal surface. *Exp. Eye Res.* 1:39–45
141. Trenberth S, Mishima S. 1968. The effect of ouabain on the rabbit corneal endothelium. *Invest. Ophthalmol. Vis. Sci.* 7:44–52
142. Klyce S, Russell S. 1979. Numerical solution of coupled transport equations applied to corneal hydration dynamics. *J. Physiol.* 292:107–34
143. Kedem O, Katchalsky A. 1958. Thermodynamic analysis of the permeability of biological membranes to non-electrolytes. *Biochim. Biophys. Acta* 27:229–46
144. Hedbys B, Mishima S. 1962. Flow of water in the corneal stroma. *Exp. Eye Res.* 1:262–75
145. Ruberti JW, Klyce SD, Smolek MK, Karon MD. 2000. Anomalous acute inflammatory response in rabbit corneal stroma. *Invest. Ophthalmol. Vis. Sci.* 41:2523–30
146. Overby D, Ruberti J, Gong H, Freddo TF, Johnson M. 2001. Specific hydraulic conductivity of corneal stroma as seen by quick-freeze/deep-etch. *J. Biomech. Eng.* 123:154–61
147. Fatt I, Shantinath K. 1971. Flow conductivity of retina and its role in retinal adhesion. *Exp. Eye Res.* 12:218–26
148. Marmor MF, Abdul-Rahim AS, Cohen DS. 1980. The effect of metabolic inhibitors on retinal adhesion and subretinal fluid resorption. *Invest. Ophthalmol. Vis. Sci.* 19:893–903
149. Tsuboi S. 1987. Measurement of the volume flow and hydraulic conductivity across the isolated dog retinal pigment epithelium. *Invest. Ophthalmol. Vis. Sci.* 28:1776–82
150. Marshall J, Hussain AACS, Moore DJ, Patmore AL. 1998. Aging and Bruch's membrane. In *The Retinal Pigment*

*Epithelium: Function and Disease*, ed. MF Marmor, TJ Wolfensberger, pp. 669–92. New York: Oxford Univ. Press

151. Negi A, Marmor MF. 1983. The resorption of subretinal fluid after diffuse damage to the retinal pigment epithelium. *Invest. Ophthalmol. Vis. Sci.* 24:1475–79
152. Bird AC, Marshall J. 1986. Retinal pigment epithelial detachments in the elderly. *Trans. Ophthalmol. Soc. UK* 105:674–82
153. Ruberti JW, Curcio CA, Millican L, Menco BPhM, Huang J-D, Johnson M. 2003. Quick-freeze/deep-etch visualization of age-related lipid accumulation in Bruch's membrane. *Invest. Ophthalmol. Vis. Sci.* 44:1753–59
154. Malek G, Guidry C, Medeiros NE, Curcio CA. 2002. Localization of apolipoproteins and cholesterol in macular and peripheral Bruch's membrane, basal deposits (BD) and drusen of normal and age-related maculopathy eyes. *Invest. Ophthalmol. Vis. Sci.* 43:2789 (Abstr.) www.arvo.org
155. Curcio CA, Millican CL, Bailey T, Kruth HS. 2001. Accumulation of cholesterol with age in human Bruch's membrane. *Invest. Ophthalmol. Vis. Sci.* 42:265–74
156. Moore DJ, Clover GM. 2001. The effect of age on the macromolecular permeability of human Bruch's membrane. *Invest. Ophthalmol. Vis. Sci.* 42:2970–75
157. Ambati J, Gragoudas ES, Miller JW, You TT, Miyamoto K, et al. 2000. Transscleral delivery of bioactive protein to the choroid and retina. *Invest. Ophthalmol. Vis. Sci.* 41:1186–91
158. Geroski DH, Edelhauser HF. 2001. Transscleral drug delivery for posterior segment disease. *Adv. Drug Deliv. Rev.* 52:37–48
159. Hamalainen KM, Kananen K, Auriola S, Kontturi K, Urtti A. 1997. Characterization of paracellular and aqueous penetration routes in cornea, conjunctiva, and sclera. *Invest. Ophthalmol. Vis. Sci.* 38:627–34
160. Ambati J, Canakis CS, Miller JW, Gragoudas ES, Edwards A, et al. 2000. Diffusion of high molecular weight compounds through sclera. *Invest. Ophthalmol. Vis. Sci.* 41:1181–85
161. Boubriak OA, Urban JP, Bron AJ. 2003. Differential effects of aging on transport properties of anterior and posterior human sclera. *Exp. Eye Res.* 76:701–13
162. Levick JR. 1987. Flow through interstitium and other fibrous matrices. *Q. J. Exp. Physiol.* 72:409–37
163. Fatt I, Hedbys BO. 1970. Flow of water in the sclera. *Exp. Eye Res.* 10:243
164. Bill A. 1964. The drainage of albumin from the uvea. *Exp. Eye Res.* 3:179
165. Pederson JE, Gaasterland DE, MacLellan HM. 1977. Uveoscleral aqueous outflow in the rhesus monkey: importance of uveal reabsorption. *Invest. Ophthalmol. Vis. Sci.* 16:1008
166. Bill A, Phillips CI. 1971. Uveoscleral drainage of aqueous humor in human eyes. *Exp. Eye Res.* 12:275–81
167. Crawford K, Kaufman PL. 1987. Pilocarpine antagonizes prostaglandin F2 alpha-induced ocular hypotension in monkeys. Evidence for enhancement of Uveoscleral outflow by prostaglandin F2 alpha. *Arch. Ophthamol.* 105:1112–16
168. Lütjen-Drecoll E, Tamm E. 1988. Morphological study of the anterior segment of cynomolgus monkey eyes following treatment with prostaglandin $F_{2\alpha}$. *Exp. Eye Res.* 47:761–69
169. Gabelt B, Kaufman P. 1989. Prostaglandin F increases uveoscleral outflow in the cynomolgus monkey. *Exp. Eye Res.* 49: 389–402
170. Bill A. 1966. Conventional and uveoscleral drainage of aqueous humor in the cynomologous monkey (macaca irus) at normal and high intraocular pressures. *Exp. Eye Res.* 5:45
171. Ruberti JW, Klyce SD. 2003. NaCl osmotic perturbation can modulate hydration control in rabbit cornea. *Exp. Eye Res.* 76:349–59
172. Ritch R, Shields MB, Krupin T, eds. 1989. *The Glaucomas*. St. Louis, MO: C.V. Mosbey Co.

Annu. Rev. Biomed. Eng. 2004. 6:275–302
doi: 10.1146/annurev.bioeng.6.040803.140040

First published online as a Review in Advance on February 18, 2004

# MECHANOTRANSDUCTION AT CELL-MATRIX AND CELL-CELL CONTACTS

Christopher S. Chen,[1] John Tan,[1] and Joe Tien[2]
[1]*Department of Biomedical Engineering, Johns Hopkins School of Medicine, Baltimore, Maryland 21205; email: cchen@bme.jhu.edu*
[2]*Department of Biomedical Engineering, Boston University, Boston, Massachusetts 02215; email: jtien@bu.edu*

**Key Words** integrins, cadherins, focal adhesion, adherens junction, extracellular matrix, actin, myosin, cytoskeleton, mechanical force, tension

■ **Abstract** Mechanical forces play an important role in the organization, growth, maturation, and function of living tissues. At the cellular level, many of the biological responses to external forces originate at two types of specialized microscale structures: focal adhesions that link cells to their surrounding extracellular matrix and adherens junctions that link adjacent cells. Transmission of forces from outside the cell through cell-matrix and cell-cell contacts appears to control the maturation or disassembly of these adhesions and initiates intracellular signaling cascades that ultimately alter many cellular behaviors. In response to externally applied forces, cells actively rearrange the organization and contractile activity of the cytoskeleton and redistribute their intracellular forces. Recent studies suggest that the localized concentration of these cytoskeletal tensions at adhesions is also a major mediator of mechanical signaling. This review summarizes the role of mechanical forces in the formation, stabilization, and dissociation of focal adhesions and adherens junctions and outlines how integration of signals from these adhesions over the entire cell body affects how a cell responds to its mechanical environment. This review also describes advanced optical, lithographic, and computational techniques for the study of mechanotransduction.

CONTENTS

# INTRODUCTION

To perform as single integrated machines, multicellular organisms have evolved complex mechanisms to communicate signals throughout their bodies. One principal mechanism for this global coordination is the transmission of mechanical forces through viscoelastic tissues, cells, and fluids (1–3). Whether externally applied or internally generated, these forces play essential roles in the development of proper mammalian physiology and in the response of an organism to injury: Gravitational compressive forces control the deposition of bone; isotonic tension causes muscles to grow (2, 4). Normal hydrostatic pressure in blood vessels promotes the maturation of vascular smooth muscle, whereas hypertensive pressure causes the walls of arteries to thicken (5). Shear stresses that arise from the flow of blood help to prevent activation of coagulation cascades and maintain endothelium in an anti-inflammatory and antiatherogenic state (6, 7). Contractile forces generated by endothelial cells regulate vascular permeability; those generated by myofibroblasts in a wound reduce the area of granulation tissue over time (8–10).

Although it is clear that common physiological processes expose cells to a variety of mechanical stimuli, how cells sense and integrate these forces at the molecular level to produce coordinated behaviors is an open question. Cellular structures are subjected to stresses of 0.01–0.1 atm in vivo, equivalent to 1–10 nN per cell contact. Even small changes in the magnitudes or distribution of these forces may lead to compensatory remodeling of cell-matrix and cell-cell contacts and may initiate a variety of cell behaviors. For instance, a slight increase in time-averaged shear stress in an artery induces proliferation of vascular cells and widening of the artery until the shear stress renormalizes to (nearly) its initial value (11, 12).

Recently, it has become clear that cultured cells in vitro possess specific mechanisms to sense and generate mechanical forces and that mechanical signals provide a fundamental means for cells to respond to their microenvironment (13–23); whether the same mechanisms operate in vivo within multicellular organisms is currently under intense study (24, 25). Mechanotransduction, or the translation of mechanical signals into biochemical ones that affect cell function, appears to occur primarily at the surface of a cell in vitro (Figure 1, see color insert). In mesenchymal cells that are grown on two- or three-dimensional scaffolds of the extracellular matrix (ECM), mechanotransduction occurs at specialized structures that link cells to the ECM, such as the focal adhesions (FAs) that develop in cells cultured on a rigid substrate (13, 26). In epithelial cells, which are bound to the ECM basally and surrounded by neighboring cells laterally, mechanotransduction also occurs at cell-cell junctions called adherens junctions (AJs) (27–29). In both types of cells and in blood-borne cells, shear and hydrostatic stresses from surrounding fluid may provide yet another avenue for mechanical signaling (30–32).

Cells adhere to the ECM and to each other through specific classes of transmembrane adhesion receptors (33–35). These receptors bind to ligand extracellularly and provide an anchor to the intracellular cytoskeleton via cytoplasmic scaffolding proteins (29, 36). Linkages between external cellular contacts, adhesion receptors, and cytoskeleton provide a means for bidirectional communication between the inside and outside of a cell. Dynamic changes in adhesions and cytoskeletal systems may thus play a critical role in regulating mechanotransduction (37).

The cellular response to mechanical forces is inherently coupled to the internal organization of the cytoskeleton and to adhesion to surrounding cells and the ECM. Structural cues such as anisotropy or topography of the ECM or location of cell-cell contact can cause a cell to reorient its body, change its shape, or alter its functional state (38–40). Similarly, changes in the shape and internal organization of cells alter how cells adhere to their surroundings and affect their function (41–43). Application or removal of a gross external load from a cell causes the cell to actively adapt its adhesions and cytoskeleton and transduce the altered mechanical environment into biochemical signals (44).

This review focuses on the mechanical and biochemical properties of cell adhesions and how these adhesions might be involved in the ability of cells to transduce structural and mechanical signals into adaptive behaviors. First, we describe recent advances in techniques used for the study of mechanotransduction. Second, we examine the responses of single-cell-ECM and cell-cell adhesions to mechanical force, as well as the integration of mechanical signals over an entire cell, to produce observable behaviors. It is important to note, however, that not all forms of mechanotransduction take place at adhesions. For instance, shear stresses experienced by the endothelium are not only transmitted through cell bodies to basal adhesions but also appear to be directly transduced through receptors located within the apical membrane (31). In some cases, a single protein may act as a mechanosensor. For example, stretch-activated ion channels appear to change conductivity in response to stresses applied to the plasma membrane (45). For further details on non-adhesion-based mechanotransduction, we refer the reader to several recent reviews (31, 46, 47).

## TECHNIQUES TO STUDY MECHANOTRANSDUCTION

Studies of mechanotransduction examine how mechanical forces influence intracellular signaling and subsequent behaviors of cells. Typically, these studies perturb the mechanical state of a cell by varying the degree to which a cell is spread (48–52), the rigidity of the substrate to which a cell adheres (22, 53, 54), or the ability of a cell to generate intracellular forces (55). Measurements in these studies include observation of the assembly (or lack of assembly) of adhesions (19, 56, 57), biochemical analyses of proteins known to interact with adhesion complexes (58, 59), quantification of gross cell behaviors (proliferation, apoptosis, migration, or differentiation) (41, 60–62), and measurements of forces exerted by cells (15, 18, 19, 63).

Early experiments exposed cells to spatially uniform mechanical environments and measured the averaged response of cells to these stimuli. To control the degree of cell spreading, cells were cultured on substrates coated with different densities of ECM proteins (49); the denser the adsorbed layer, the better the cell spread. To control the rigidity of the substrate, cells were cultured on thin flexible sheets of polymer, or in three-dimensional gels of ECM (usually collagen) that were cross-linked for different times (53, 54, 64). To control the ability of a cell to generate contractile forces, cells were cultured in the presence of agents that destabilized or enhanced cytoskeletal filaments throughout the entire cell (55). Analyses of cell adhesions and downstream signaling relied on several standard biological techniques, including immunofluorescence, Western blotting, and assays for proliferation and apoptosis.

Although the results of these experiments demonstrated a strong correlation between mechanical forces and changes in cell behaviors, these experiments could not prove a causal relationship between the two. The realization that cell-matrix and cell-cell contacts may be the primary sites of mechanotransduction has motivated the development of techniques to control or record the mechanical state of a cell with the spatial resolution of a single cell contact ($\sim$1 $\mu$m). These techniques—coupled with advanced optical methods for probing a cell, such as the use of fluorescent fusion proteins that target to adhesions (56) and the use of correlational microscopy to determine how adhesions evolve over time (56, 57)—have begun to elucidate the causal relationships between mechanical forces and intracellular signaling. Three recent developments have proven to be invaluable in the study of mechanotransduction: (*a*) measurements of the distribution of mechanical stresses exerted by a cell with subcellular resolution, (*b*) application of force locally to only a portion of the cell membrane, and (*c*) confinement of the areas at which a cell can exert mechanical force.

## Measurement of Forces Exerted by Cells

Cells exert nanonewton-scale contractile forces against adhesive structures that couple the cell to its external environment (20). In vitro studies of these minute forces have relied on the culture of cells on soft materials such as uniformly cross-linked hydrogels or flexible rubber membranes, where the degree of cross-linking controls mechanical compliance (Figure 2*A*, see color insert) (14, 22, 53, 65–67). Initial experiments with thin membranes demonstrated conclusively that cells exerted contractile forces (also referred to as tension or traction forces). Contractile forces generated by cells deformed rubber membranes to form microscopic wrinkles that were easily observed by phase-contrast microscopy (53). Subsequent studies have focused on dynamic changes in the magnitude and direction of forces exerted by cells and how these forces correlate with the shapes of cells during cytokinesis and cell migration (65, 66).

Quantitation of force exerted by cells on thin membranes consisted of counting the number of wrinkles near cell bodies, measuring the lengths of these wrinkles, and using these values to calculate the total force exerted on the membrane (66). Because membranes deformed grossly in these studies, it was difficult, if not impossible, to calculate the force exerted locally by cells with subcellular resolution. Improvements on this setup led to the development of a method called traction force microscopy to quantify force exerted by cell (Figure 2*B*) (68). Here, cells are plated onto a membrane that is pre-stressed to prevent wrinkling of its surface. Force that is generated by the cells deforms the membrane only slightly; fiduciary markers, such as spherical beads embedded within the membrane, aid in measurement of local displacements. Because the substrate deforms only within a plane, is basically incompressible (i.e., has a Poisson's ratio of 0.5) and is linearly elastic, the stress field $\mathbf{F}(\mathbf{r})$ and displacement field $\mathbf{u}(\mathbf{r}')$ are related by a Fredholm integral equation of the first kind:

$$u_i(r) = \int dr' G_{ij}(r - r')F_j(r'), \tag{1}$$

where $\mathbf{G}(\mathbf{r} - \mathbf{r}')$ is the tensorial Green's function of the elastic isotropic halfspace and represents the displacement at $\mathbf{r}$ that results from the application of a point force at $\mathbf{r}'$. For instance, the displacement at $\mathbf{r}$ that results from a single point force at $\mathbf{r}'$ is given by Equations 2 and 3:

$$u_x(r) = G_{xx}(r - r')F_x(r') + G_{xy}(r - r')F_y(r') \tag{2}$$

$$u_y(r) = G_{yx}(r - r')F_x(r') + G_{yy}(r - r')F_y(r') \tag{3}$$

Given a displacement field $\mathbf{u}$ measured from the movement of embedded beads, the challenge in traction force microscopy is to invert Equation 1 to obtain the stress field $\mathbf{F}$. Because the integral operation is a smoothing operation, inversion does not always lead to a unique solution (71). As with any inversion operation, regularization schemes are often used to provide additional information to restrict the set of possible solutions (72); examples of commonly used guides include the assumption that force can be exerted only at focal adhesions and that only the least complex solution is used (68). The complete description of computational methods to calculate force and the derivation of the Green's function have been well described (73).

The recent use of microfabricated regular arrays of fluorescent particles as markers has allowed better tracking of the deformation field (Figure 2*C*) (15); algorithms for inversion of Equation 1 have also improved and no longer require the continual use of supercomputers. The computation is still sufficiently intensive, which makes the analysis of forces exerted by large populations of cells impractical. Moreover, because the displacement of discrete markers cannot fully describe the deformation of a continuous surface, finding a unique solution of force can be achieved only by placing constraints on the deformation field, on the nature of the cellular forces, or on the location of adhesions (67).

These limitations are inherent to the use of flat, continuous substrates where a deformation at one location can propagate to another part. Alternatives to these substrates for measurement of force initially used a microfabricated device containing a horizontally mounted cantilever that deflected along one axis as individual cells migrated across it (Figure 2*D*) (18). Because the moveable unit in these devices (the cantilever) is mechanically decoupled from its surroundings, lateral deflections of the cantilever result only from local forces exerted on it; measurements of these deflections give a direct value for the local force generated at the cell surface. As originally designed, however, the geometry of the cantilever (with the flexible arm in the same plane as the displacement) restricted the measurement of force to one axis and a few locations (18).

We anticipated that, by altering the design of the device so that the arm of the cantilever did not reside in the same plane as the displacement, it would be possible to place multiple cantilevers in a single device and thus to measure local forces across the entire body of a cell (Figure 2*E*). In practice, we used lithographic techniques to mold arrays of closely spaced vertical cantilevers (i.e., microneedles or posts) in a silicone elastomer; cells attached and spread across the tips of multiple posts and bent the posts as the cells probed the tips (63). For small deflections, the posts behave like simple springs so that their deflections are directly proportional to the local forces applied by the attached cell. This behavior is described for beams composed of linearly elastic material under pure bending by Equation 4,

$$F = \left(\frac{3EI}{L^3}\right)\delta, \tag{4}$$

where F, E, I, L, and $\delta$ are the bending force, Young's modulus, moment of inertia, length, and resulting deflection of the post, respectively (74). Because each post moves independently of its neighbors, its deflection directly reports the direction and magnitude of the local cell-generated force without the need for a priori assumptions.

## Application of Localized Forces to Cells

In the previously described methods, the substrate passively responds to forces exerted by the cultured cell. Often, however, it is useful to be able to deliberately expose a cell to external mechanical force and then observe its response (Figure 3). The first studies in this area used stretchable membranes to impart a uniform strain (and, by extrapolation, a uniform stress) to cells (75). As with techniques for the measurement of force, methods for the application of force have gradually evolved beyond the use of spatially homogeneous substrates; recent advances have enabled the exposure of selected portions of a cell to a controlled stress.

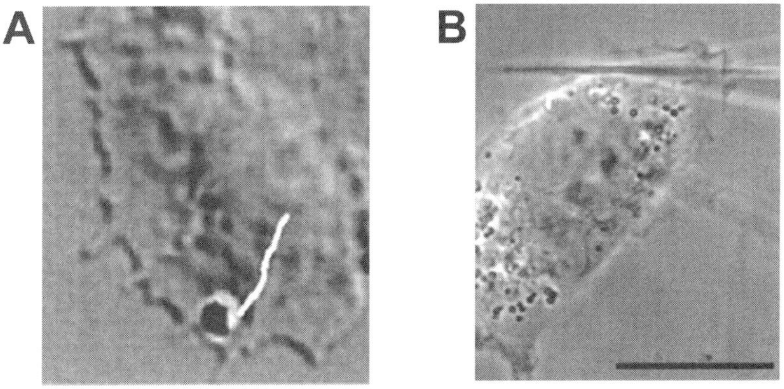


**Figure 3** Techniques to apply external forces to cells: (*A*) Movement of optically trapped microbeads on the cell surface measures both the externally imposed force and the reaction generated by the cell. Reproduced with permission from Reference 20. (*B*) Deformation of the cell membrane by a micropipette imparts a gross force to the area of contact. Reproduced with permission from Reference 16.

Many of these advances rely on the use of micrometer-sized beads that can be manipulated by an external electromagnetic field (Figure 3*A*) (20, 21, 76). In these studies, beads are coated with ECM proteins and are allowed to passively settle onto cells or are placed directly on the cell membrane. Application of a magnetic field to an attached paramagnetic bead forces the bead to align in the direction of the magnetic field; this technique generates a twisting stress that rotates the cell membrane (21). Application of a non-uniform electromagnetic field, such as that resulting from focusing light through an optical lens, to an attached bead whose index of refraction differs from that of its surroundings attracts the bead to the regions of highest light intensity; this technique (known as optical tweezers) generates a lateral stress that pulls and pushes the cell membrane (77). Equations to describe the force exerted on a bead in these magnetic setups or optical tweezers are well known and lead to straightforward calculations of force exerted on attached beads. Because these techniques are compatible with optical microscopy, it is possible to simultaneously exert force on the bead and observe whether the bead can escape from its magnetic alignment or optical trap. The degrees to which beads resist their applied forces can thus give a direct measurement of the force exerted by the cell on the beads in response to the force exerted on the cell by the beads.

Other techniques to impart a localized force to cells use the controlled movement of an attached micropipette across the surface of a cell (Figure 3*B*) (16, 78). These techniques may consist of (*a*) translating a rigid tip a defined distance and using simplifying assumptions of the mechanical properties of the cell to calculate the applied force (16), (*b*) translating a flexible cantilever across the cell and calculating the applied force from Equation 4, and (*c*) translating a rigid tip against the underlying substrate of a cell to increase or decrease the local stiffness of a gel or membrane (78). Here, the determination of exerted force is not as exact as with magnetic or optical forces, but these tip-based methods are often favored because they are easily implemented with nothing more than a translation stage and optical microscope.

## Confinement of Cell-Matrix and Cell-Cell Contacts

A complementary set of techniques controls where cells can exert force with subcellular resolution (Figure 4). These techniques all rely on the use of nonadhesive surfaces to restrict the regions to which a cell can adhere and exert force (79). In early studies, cells were cultured on thin films of palladium that were patterned by evaporation through a fine metal mask (mesh size ~100 $\mu$m) on a nonadhesive substrate (51, 52). Cells were restricted to the islands of metal and adjusted their shapes to the shapes of the islands. Subsequently, many strategies to create more complex patterns by using lithographic printing techniques have been developed (79a, 79b), one of which involves contact printing of small organothiols onto a thin film of gold defines adhesive and nonadhesive regions (Figure 4*A*) (41, 80–82). Micro-contact printing of these features is not limited to discrete adhesive islands (in contrast to surfaces made by evaporation through a mask) and can be readily applied to non-planar substrates (81). Cells cultured on these patterned surfaces adhere selectively to the adhesive regions; because the stamp used for printing is made by microlithography, the definition of adhesive surfaces takes place with sub 100-nm

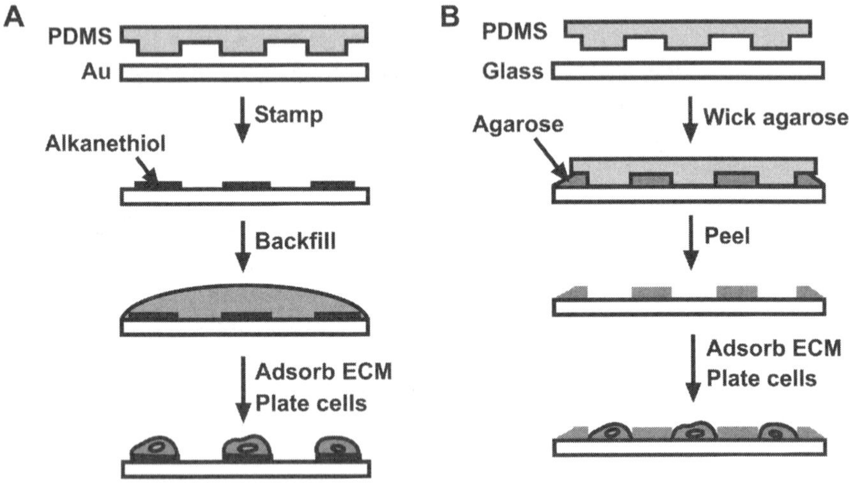


**Figure 4** Techniques to confine the locations of cell-matrix and cell-cell contacts: (*A*) Micro-contact printing of adhesive and nonadhesive regions on a flat surface controls the locations of cell-matrix contacts. (*B*) Micromolding of a nonadhesive gel further confines the locations of cell-cell contacts. The gel in (*B*), which is several micrometers thick, physically restricts the formation of cell-cell contacts, whereas the nanometer-thick printed regions in (*A*) do not.

resolution and allows a single cell to attach to multiple, discrete micrometer-scale patches.

To control where cells can contact neighboring cells, we have also used lithographic techniques to mold thin nonadhesive gels of agarose into microscale meshes (Figure 4*B*) (60, 83). The molded agarose forms walls that block cells from making contact with their neighbors. Cells cultured through a suitably patterned mesh thus can adhere to the ECM and other cells in defined locations.

The development of techniques to measure force exerted by cells, to expose cells to defined forces, and to localize where cells exert force, all with subcellular resolution, has led to recent breakthroughs in the study of mechanotransduction at cell-ECM and cell-cell contacts. We anticipate that the development of techniques with even finer (nm scale) spatial resolution and techniques that allow rapid dynamic changes in the forces exerted at an adhesion will uncover new insights into mechanical signaling in cells.

# MECHANOTRANSDUCTION AT CELL-MATRIX CONTACTS

## Structure of Cell-Matrix Adhesions

Recent studies have shown that many distinct types of adhesions exist between cells and the ECM; these adhesions differ in size, shape, and biochemical composition and probably differ in function as well (84). The best-characterized and largest of these structures is the focal adhesion (FA; also known as a focal contact) (13). These adhesions are transient in nature, and form in many types of cells that are cultured on a substrate coated with ECM. All adherent cells bind to the ECM through integrins—transmembrane receptors that bind to specific motifs on numerous ECM proteins (85). The binding of integrins to the ECM causes them to cluster and leads to the recruitment of a battery of cytoplasmic signaling and structural proteins to form FAs at the site of integrin clustering (13, 86, 87). Numerous structural proteins (e.g., vinculin, talin, $\alpha$-actinin, and paxillin) act as scaffolding proteins that strengthen cell adhesion by anchoring FAs to the actin cytoskeleton (13, 86). It is thought that these proteins are able to provide this anchoring function because some of these proteins bind actin filaments directly, whereas others contain domains that can bind to actin-binding proteins. When these proteins coalesce with clusters of integrins, they likely bind to each other through a multitude of interactions to link the integrins to the actin cytoskeleton. Other types of cell-matrix adhesions that have recently been identified—focal complexes, fibrillar adhesions and three-dimensional matrix adhesions—are structurally similar to FAs but differ subtly in composition and morphology (24, 56, 88).

## Forces that Regulate Assembly of Focal Adhesions

The distinguishing features of the four different cell-matrix adhesions (FAs, focal complexes, fibrillar adhesions, and three-dimensional matrix adhesions) suggest a central role for mechanical forces in their development. Focal complexes are found within minutes after suspended cells are placed in contact with an ECM-coated surface (88). These complexes are small, punctate, and exist primarily at the periphery of a spreading cell or at the leading edge of a migrating one (88, 89). Slightly proximal to these focal complexes are the larger FAs. Observations made with time-lapse fluorescence microscopy suggest that focal complexes are one of the precursors of FAs. In cells that express genetically engineered FA proteins linked to green fluorescent protein, focal complexes gradually move centripetally inward from the boundary of a cell, elongate, and evolve into FAs as more adhesion proteins and actin are recruited to the adhesion (56).

The maturation of these complexes into FAs appears to require the application of mechanical stress to the adhesions (15, 90). Early studies demonstrated that altering the activity of several biochemical signaling pathways, particularly those that involve myosin light chain kinase (MLCK) and the small GTPase Rho, regulated both the contractility of the actin cytoskeleton and the formation of FAs (14, 90). Specifically, the number of FAs present in a cell correlated strongly with the contractility of the cytoskeleton. However, these studies did not determine whether it was the biochemical activity of these signals, or the resultant mechanical stresses, that caused FAs to form.

Two different approaches that do not require tampering with endogenous signaling pathways also suggest that mechanical forces have a direct role in the formation of FAs. In the first approach, investigators used flexible substrates that deform when attached cells contract to measure the local distribution of forces that are generated by cells at their adhesions (Figure 3*A*) (15, 63, 67). Studies using this approach have demonstrated that the size of individual focal adhesions (as determined by fluorescence microscopy) correlates loosely with the measured local forces. [Intriguingly, at a subset of smaller adhesions ($<1\ \mu m^2$ in area), cells exerted significant traction force that does not correlate with adhesion size.] This study also provided strong evidence that forces and focal adhesions correlate in un-manipulated cells, whose signaling pathways remain intact; nevertheless, cause and effect were not distinguished.

In the second approach, investigators applied external forces directly to adhesions (Figure 3*B*) (16, 19, 20, 91). Applying force to FAs from externally bound beads or pipettes led to assembly of components into FAs (16). This force-dependent assembly of FAs resulted in increased strength of adhesion; the strength of adhesion increased with the amount of force applied (20). Taken together, these studies suggest that intracellular tension against initial cell-ECM contacts is necessary for these contacts to develop into FAs. These studies have clearly shown that the application of force causes FAs to increase in size, to stabilize, and to strengthen their coupling to the cell (presumably through the actin cytoskeleton). Externally applied mechanical forces can replace the activation of Rho-associated kinase (ROCK), a downstream effector of Rho that regulates cell contractility, but cannot replace the function of mDia1, an effector of Rho that allows actin to polymerize (16).

These findings collectively suggest that maturation of FAs requires either tensile forces generated by actin-myosin contraction of the anchoring actin filaments

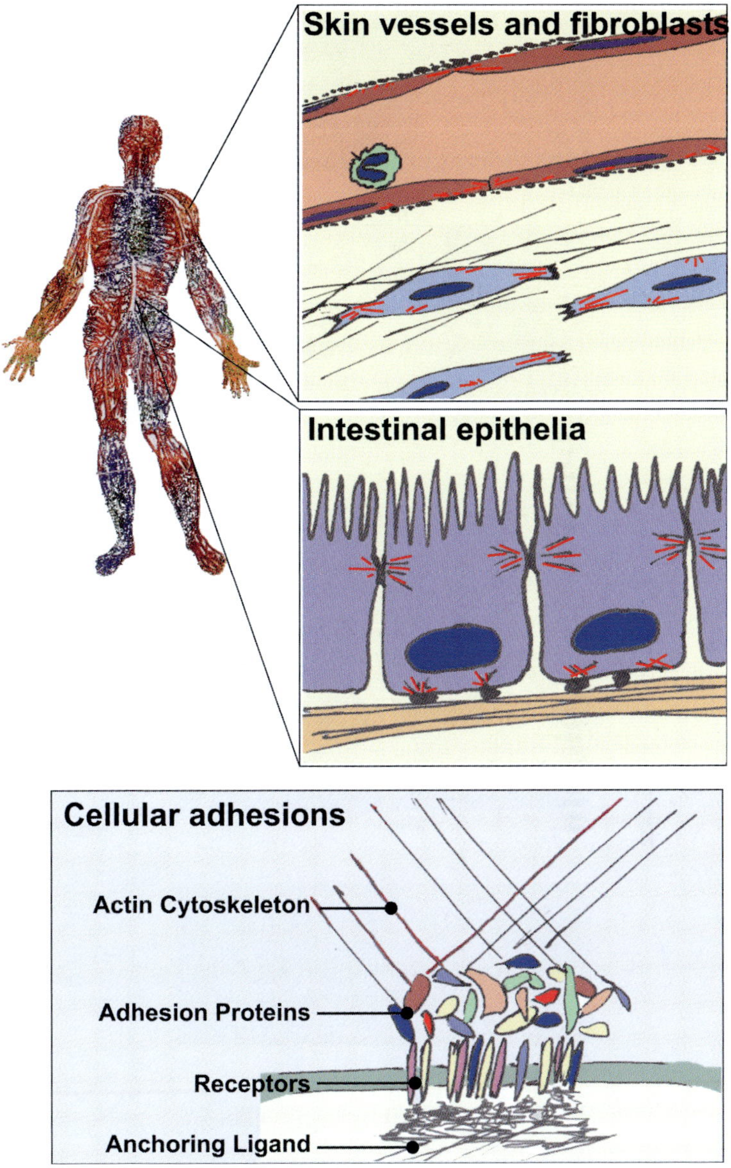


**Figure 1** Transmission of mechanical forces to a cell may occur at cell-matrix and cell-cell adhesions. Mechanotransduction at mesenchymal cells relies primarily on cell-matrix contacts, whereas that in epithelial cells makes use of both cell-matrix and cell-cell contacts. All cells may be exposed to shear and hydrostatic stresses from surrounding fluid.

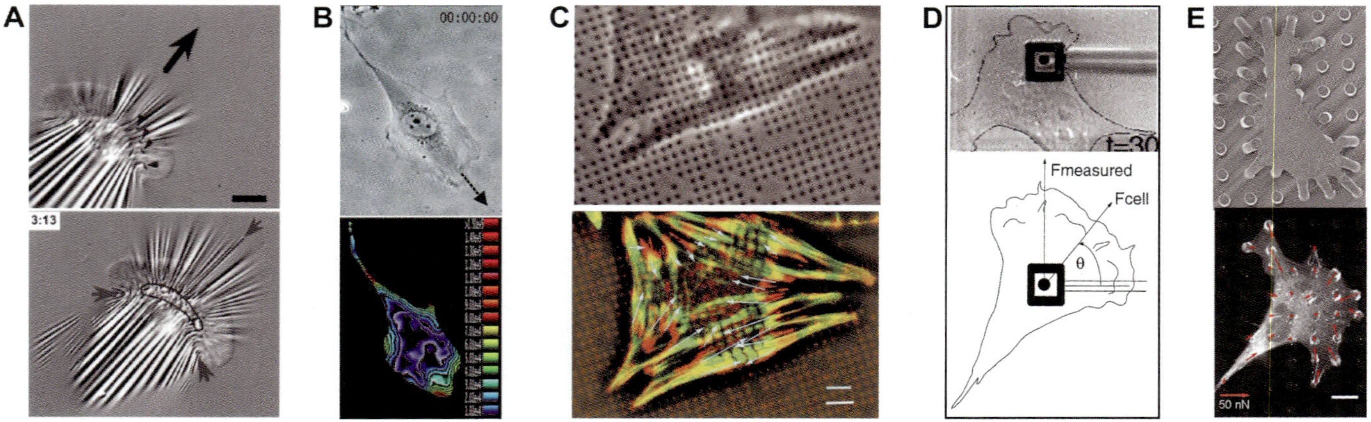


**Figure 2** Techniques for the measurement of forces exerted by cells: (*A*) Contraction of a thin membrane by cells generates microscopic wrinkles in the membrane. Reproduced with permission from Reference 69. (*B*, *C*) Translation of beads or patterned markers embedded in an elastic surface yields a stress map of the entire cell body. Reproduced with permission from References 17 and 70. (*D*) Bending of a cantilever measures the force generated at a single area under a cell. Reproduced with permission from Reference 18. (*E*) Bending of an array of posts measures force generated at multiple locations across the cell body. Reproduced with permission from Reference 63.

or external loading of the bound ECM. In addition, these findings outline a three-stage process for the formation of FAs in cultured cells: Occupation of integrins by ligand initiates condensation of FA proteins, clustering of integrins by multivalent ECM recruits further components of FAs, and exertion of tensile forces through integrins to the ECM provides a signal to mature the adhesions.

Fibrillar adhesions appear to be a separate form of FAs and manifest as streaks that lie centripetal to FAs (56, 57). Time-lapse recordings have shown that fibrillar adhesions quickly slide centripetally from FAs to the central region beneath the cell; these adhesions appear to originate from the proximal ends of FAs (56). Fibrillar adhesions appear to track along actin stress fibers that anchor into the originating FA and move at speeds comparable to the treadmilling rate of actin. These adhesions contain slightly different mixtures of components and integrin subtypes than do FAs and are enriched in fibronectin and $\alpha_5\beta_1$ integrin (57). Culture of cells on ECM that is chemically cross-linked onto a rigid substrate greatly reduces the formation of fibrillar adhesions and favors the formation of FAs instead. These results suggest that FAs form when the cell can exert large stresses against an ECM, whereas fibrillar adhesions form when the ECM can support only smaller contractile forces. Whether this hypothesis is correct awaits the use of optical tweezers or compliant substrates to determine the effect of force on the formation of fibrillar adhesions.

Adhesions to a three-dimensional matrix appear to be a distinct class of structures that form only when cells are cultured on naturally assembled ECM fibrils (versus a flat adsorbed layer of ECM). This three-dimensional ECM typically consists of a fibrous composite of collagen, proteoglycans, elastin, and adhesive glycoproteins (92). It is usually oriented, highly porous, and heavily cross-linked. The three-dimensional matrix adhesions appear to have a composition distinct from FAs, fibrillar adhesions, and focal complexes; in particular, they lack phosphorylated focal adhesion kinase (24). What remains unclear is whether these matrix adhesions form as a result of the difference in matrix architecture, mechanical compliance, or ligand presentation, such as might result from the hydration state of the matrix. When the compliant three-dimensional ECM is either compressed into a sheet or chemically cross-linked to produce a rigid three-dimensional ECM, the distribution of adhesion proteins changes. These results suggest that mechanical forces again may play a key role in the formation of these adhesions; they also suggest that the architecture of the ECM—whether flat or a porous volume—may control the localization of proteins to these adhesions.

Several aspects of the cell-matrix adhesions that are likely relevant for cell mechanics remain unresolved. First, it is not clear how the compositions of adhesions differ between cells or between adhesions in a single cell, and how a particular composition determines downstream signaling. No stoichiometric relationships have been determined in defining the composition of these adhesions, and, given the numerous proteins that are involved, it is uncertain whether specific stoichiometries should even exist in these structures. In fact, a wide range of compositions may provide similar functions to the different types of matrix adhesions (84). In vitro several of these FA proteins appear to be redundant for normal cell adhesion and function. In vivo, however, deletion of any of these proteins in mice is lethal, suggesting that at different times during development there are periods where each of these scaffolding proteins is critical for adhesive function (93).

The composition of these adhesions has been determined predominantly by two distinct approaches: (*a*) the cells can be labeled with immunofluorescent probes and fluorescence microscopy used to detect the distribution of specific proteins in the adhesions, or (*b*) the adherent cells can be permeabilized to remove most cellular proteins and the remaining adhesions solubilized for electrophoretic separation and detection by Western blot. With immunostaining, the distinctions between different classes of adhesions have been made by the presence or absence of specific integrins or FA proteins within the structures and by the morphology of these adhesions. These methods have not yet determined whether these adhesions are indeed distinct subtypes or, instead, vary along a continuum in adhesion composition and properties. However, the complexity and compaction of proteins in these adhesions raise the possibility that fluorescent markers may not be able to penetrate adhesions to label targeted proteins adequately. Methods to selectively collect a particular class of adhesions for biochemical analysis would greatly aid in resolving these issues.

Second, it is not yet clear if there is a particular organization to these adhesive structures. Apart from knowing that integrins exist at the plasma membrane and that actin is linked to the cytoplasmic domains of FAs, the internal structure of these adhesions is basically unknown. From a comprehensive list of positive protein-protein interactions and a list of proteins present at an adhesion, it may be possible to guess the three-dimensional arrangement present at the adhesion. The use of fluorescence resonance energy transfer (FRET) techniques to determine the spacings between proteins may prove useful here (94).

Third, the mechanical properties of these adhesions remain unclear. Given the large number of interconnected protein-protein interactions that arise during adhesion formation, one expects that much of the mechanical stability arises from binding energies between these scaffolding proteins. Because many of the binding energies between proteins have not yet been determined, it is difficult to estimate the theoretical strength of these adhesion sites, let alone the relative contribution of each protein-protein interaction to the strength of these adhesions.

Fourth, it is not clear how the different compositions or mechanical properties of cell adhesions lead to changes in biochemical signaling. Because the molecular definition of these adhesions remains vague, it has been difficult to uncover how specific signaling events arise.

## Forces that Regulate Signaling at Focal Adhesions

In all adherent cells, adhesion is needed for proper metabolism, protein synthesis, and survival (95, 96). Although it is well-known that signaling through integrins regulates the formation of FAs (13), only recently has it become evident that the mechanical and structural changes associated with maturation of adhesions in turn affect signaling (58, 97). Thus cell-matrix adhesions not only play a physical role in organizing cells into tissues but also provide an important biochemical role in the regulation of many cellular processes.

Many signaling proteins (e.g., src, FAK, Ras) localize within cell-matrix adhesions (84, 87). Because these signaling proteins function in cascades initiated by growth factors, their concentration at adhesions suggests that adhesions may act to coordinate integrin and growth factor signaling (96). For example, it is known that most adherent cells will undergo apoptosis quickly in the absence of either adhesion or soluble growth factors and will proliferate only in the presence of both signals (98). In fact, growth factor receptors themselves are thought to localize to FAs. Because specific integrins within these adhesions appear to interact with specific growth factor receptors (99, 100), these adhesions may enable cells to generate unique responses when exposed to particular combinations of ECM and growth factors. For example, signaling through basic fibroblast growth factor receptor in endothelial cells requires ligation of the integrin $\alpha_v\beta_3$, whereas signaling through vascular endothelial growth factor receptor uses $\alpha_v\beta_5$; because $\alpha_v\beta_3$ and $\alpha_v\beta_5$ bind to different classes of ECM proteins, the response of endothelial cells to a given growth factor depends on its underlying ECM (101, 102). Thus adhesions provide a physical structure that allows many important biochemical signals to initiate fundamental changes in cell behavior. Because these adhesions continually remodel in response to changes in the composition, architecture, and mechanical properties of the cell-matrix interface, they appear to be a central mechanism by which cells can change behavior in response to structural and mechanical cues.

Increasing mechanical stress at FAs by increasing intracellular tension or applying extracellular forces leads to important changes in signaling at FAs through focal adhesion kinase (FAK) and its downstream partners (17, 97). FAK appears to be the earliest marker of FA signaling whose activity changes with tension. Recent studies show that applying mechanical stretch can increase FAK phosphorylation, sustain the activation of the mitogen-activated protein kinase ERK, and cause cells to proliferate (103, 104). The activation of FAK by autophosphorylation of tyrosine397 is required for ERK activation and cyclin-dependent progression through $G_1$ (105). Kinase-dead mutations in FAK appear to abrogate ERK activation and cell proliferation caused by mechanical forces (106, 107); expression of constitutively active FAK, on the other hand, can transform cells so that they proliferate in suspension (108). These findings imply that increases in cytoskeletal tension may be transduced into a proliferative signal in FAs, possibly through changes in FAK activity and that this signal represents a crucial component of adhesion-dependent growth in cells. The hypothesized link between tension and proliferation might explain why agonists that increase cytoskeletal tension, such as thrombin or angiotensin II, cause smooth muscle cells to proliferate (109–111).

Because FAs do not form without the generation of intracellular tension, it has been difficult to determine whether the pro-proliferative effects of tension are mediated by the presence of FAs or whether tension has additional direct effects on the activity of signaling proteins. Recent results have provided tantalizing evidence that tension may modulate the activity of proteins in a recruitment-independent manner. Application of mechanical stretch to permeabilized cells, i.e., depleted of additional cytoplasmic proteins that can localize to FAs, can itself result in phosphorylation of paxillin, FAK, and Cas (17). This result implies that stretch may possibly alter the conformation and thus the activity of molecules that have already been recruited to FAs. Changes in activity that result from changes in conformation are well known for the FA proteins vinculin and src (112); although tension-generated changes in cell signaling have previously been ascribed to binding of soluble factors to FA proteins, the demonstration that some of these changes can take place in the absence of soluble factors suggests that additional mechanisms for altering biochemical activity operate in adherent cells.

## Integrated Forces Alter Cell Behavior

The response of a cell to changes in its mechanical environment depends on the integration of signals transduced at numerous distinct FAs; in vitro a cell typically forms numerous adhesions to surrounding ECM. How these signals from each adhesion are coordinated over the entire cell to drive cell behavior collectively must be considered in the context in which mechanical tension is generated throughout the cell. The ability of a cell to generate tension depends partly on the architecture of its anchoring cytoskeleton; cytoskeletal structure, in turn, varies with the global placement of adhesions. This interplay has led to the hypothesis that cell shape—as controlled by the location of cell-matrix adhesions—may regulate cell behavior through changes in intracellular tension and downstream signaling at FAs (37).

It has been known for some time that ligation of integrins alone is insufficient to support cell proliferation. Folkman & Moscona (48) first observed that cells proliferated only when allowed to spread and flatten against a solid substrate, suggesting that cell morphology may provide a regulatory signal for cell function. Studies later showed that the projected area of the cell (cell spreading) can be directly controlled by the density of immobilized ECM; increased cell spreading led to increased proliferation (113). Because ECM coating density not only affects cell spreading but also integrin activation, it remained controversial whether the effects of increased cell area merely reflected increased integrin activation or were separate from it (114–116).

To generate substrates that could decouple cell spreading from ECM coating density, we developed a micropatterning technique to synthesize surfaces that contained micrometer-scale ECM-coated islands surrounded by nonadhesive regions (Figure 4*A*). Cells cultured on these substrates attached and spread to fill the patterned islands (41). Cells that were plated on smaller islands coated with saturating densities of the ECM protein fibronectin were smaller in size and proliferated less (41, 117). Similar studies have shown that changes in cell spreading can also affect the differentiated function of cells (43, 118). Thus it appears that cell spreading independently regulates cells through a mechanism that is distinct from direct integrin ligation (117). Given that cell shape and cytoskeletal architecture are linked and that cytoskeletal architecture in part drives the organization of FAs, these studies strongly suggest that signaling through matrix adhesions transduces the effects of changes in cell shape.

Cell spreading appears to modulate proliferation by regulating levels of tension within the actin cytoskeleton. Blocking actomyosin tension production in spread cells by inhibiting MLCK or by disrupting the actin cytoskeleton arrests cell cycle progression in late $G_1$, as if cells were not spread (119). Direct measurements of the traction forces exerted by cells have shown that increased cell spreading increases the magnitude of tensile forces that cells exert against their adhesions (21, 63). These forces appear to be regulated in part by the Rho signaling pathway, which plays a major role in the generation of stress fibers and intracellular tension in adherent cells (90, 120).

Spreading-induced changes in cytoskeletal tension may regulate cell proliferation through changes in signaling through Rho. Microinjection of constitutively activated RhoA promotes DNA synthesis, whereas C3 exoenzyme, which ADP ribosylates and inactivates Rho, blocks DNA synthesis (121, 122). One Rho effector, Rho kinase (ROCK), is involved in the generation of cytoskeletal tension. Inhibition of ROCK with the compound Y-27632 or with expression of dominant-negative ROCK suppresses the mitogen-induced DNA synthesis of vascular cells in vitro and in vivo (123–125). ROCK directly phosphorylates both smooth muscle and nonmuscle myosin II regulatory light chain (MLC) and MLC phosphatase to synergistically increase MLC phosphorylation and myosin II contractility (126–128). Blocking Rho, ROCK, MLCK, or myosin activity leads to the same phenotype of cell cycle arrest; because MLCK acts to increase cell tension, it is thought that Rho acts through tension as well to exert its effect on cell proliferation (129).

Changes in cytoskeletal tension may be translated into appropriate proliferative signals by the interplay between cell shape, Rho, and FAs. First, inhibition of Rho greatly reduces the formation of FAs (14, 90). Second, cell spreading increases the total area of FAs quantity in a tension-dependent manner (130). Third, the activation of FAK reduces the activation of Rho (58). Because cells in culture are constantly exposed to agonists, such as lysophosphatidic acid (LPA), that activate Rho, cell shape may act in culture as a master switch to control the area of FAs, activation of Rho, generation of tension, and progression through the cell cycle.

A similar model may apply to the control of cell migration, this time through a different Rho family GTPase, Rac. Here, the data are less conclusive than for the role of Rho and tension in proliferation. Cells migrate, in part, by polarizing the distribution of force that they exert against their adhesions (131). Activation of Rac leads to the formation of lamellipodia, which are commonly observed at the leading edge of migrating cells and appear essential for migration (88). Moreover, activated Rac leads to the formation of focal complexes between cells and their substrate, which further recruit and activate Rac at the membrane. Cortically oriented tension (i.e., parallel to the cell periphery) decreases the activation of Rac and reduces the extension of lamellipodia, whereas radial tension has the opposite effect (132, 133). Taken together, these findings support a model in which the coordinated directions of mechanical tension—which is needed for persistent migration—control the local activation of Rac through focal complexes. This activation may result in extension or retraction of lamellipodia, which leads to further formation of adhesions and redirection of contractile forces.

In contrast to cell proliferation, cell migration appears to be favored at intermediate levels of spreading. In fact, the speed of migration exhibits a unimodal dependence on the degree of cell-ECM contact (134). This variation can be mimicked by culturing cells on substrates of varying stiffnesses. Cells migrate most on substrates of intermediate stiffness and may be induced to migrate in a specific direction by local stiffening of the substrate with a rigid tip (62). These effects may be regulated through FAK because FAK-null cells do not respond to local variations in the rigidity of the substrate and migrate less than do cells with wild-type FAK (78). How signals from FAK regulate the activation of Rac is unclear, although the inhibition of Rho by active FAK suggests that FAK may enhance signaling through Rac by inhibiting Rho and thus changing the magnitudes or directions of cell tension. Mechanical forces may thus provide a link between cell proliferation and migration through the assembly of FAs and focal complexes and through regulation of FAK and Rho family GTPases.

# MECHANOTRANSDUCTION AT CELL-CELL CONTACTS

Cell-cell adhesions, similar to cell-matrix adhesions, are emerging as important players in mechanotransduction. Distinct types of cell-cell adhesions include AJs, tight junctions, and gap junctions, which are mediated by cadherins, occludins, and connexins, respectively (135–137). In some cases, especially with blood-borne cells, intercellular adhesions may be mediated by integrins (138). Among these different cell-cell adhesions, the AJ is perhaps one of the most important for transmitting mechanical signals directly to the actin cytoskeleton. The homotypic engagement of cadherins, a family of transmembrane $Ca^{2+}$-dependent adhesion molecules, initiates the formation of AJs and recruits scaffolding proteins that anchor the actin cytoskeleton (139).

## Similarities Between Focal Adhesions and Adherens Junctions

Focal adhesions and AJs exhibit many striking similarities (Figure 1). First, both consist of dense clusters of transmembrane receptors that attach the cell to the external environment. Second, both provide a highly dynamic and responsive mechanical link to the actin cytoskeleton. Third, the architecture of both FAs and AJs consists of a large number of signaling and structural molecules that cluster at the junction through multiple, redundant protein-protein interactions. Several of these components, including $\alpha$-actinin, Arp2/3, zyxin, moesin, and vinculin, are shared by both types of adhesions (140).

These similarities have motivated the idea that, as in FAs, mechanical force regulates the formation of AJs and their downstream signaling. In contrast to FAs, however, where the role of cytoskeletal tension in regulating adhesion formation is clear, the response of AJs to tension remains controversial. For instance, increasing Rho GTPase RhoA-mediated cytoskeletal tension can change the morphology of AJs and increase the permeability of cell-cell junctions (141, 142), whereas increasing sphingosine-1-phosphate-mediated cytoskeletal tension appears to stabilize AJs and decrease permeability (143). Similarly, it has been reported that disruption of the cytoskeleton can disturb AJs, leading to loss of cadherins from cell-cell junctions (144); however, we have found that pharmacologically disrupting the cytoskeleton may have no effect on the localization of cadherin (60). Some of these differences may be attributed to differences in experimental conditions and in the particular cell types studied, but no consistent picture of the interaction between mechanical forces and AJs has emerged. Not surprisingly, experiments to determine the effect of tension on AJs often lead to simultaneous changes at FAs that complicate interpretation of data.

## Does Force Regulate Assembly and Signaling at Adherens Junctions?

The ability to quantitatively measure force at cell-cell junctions may help reconcile some of the findings and shed light on the role of tension at cell-cell junctions. Although the existence of endogenous tension at cell-cell contacts has not been demonstrated, cadherin-based adhesions are clearly capable of supporting large forces. Suspended cells expressing E-cadherin will adhere to each other and require >100 nN of force to separate them (W.A. Thomas, personal communication). Likewise, the compaction of epithelial layers during morphogenesis generates substantial compressive force (145, 146).

The localization of components to AJs may be driven by tension. One of these components, vinculin, binds various cytoskeletal proteins, including actin, $\alpha$-actinin, talin, paxillin, VASP, and protein kinase C (147). Vinculin plays a key role in coupling FAs to the cytoskeleton, and the amount of vinculin localized to FAs correlates with the amount of local tension (15, 63). Whether vinculin in AJs plays a similar role, however, is unknown. Another component of cell-cell junctions is $\beta$-catenin, which binds along with several adaptor proteins to the cytoplasmic domains of cadherins (148). When localized to AJs, $\beta$-catenin plays a structural role in linking cadherin to the actin cytoskeleton. When phosphorylated on tyrosine, however, $\beta$-catenin can dissociate from AJs and translocate to the nucleus, where it interacts with the TCF/LEF family of transcription factors to regulate the expression of genes such as *cyclin D* and c-*myc* that regulate cell cycle progression (149–151). Tension at cell-cell junctions may play a role in stabilizing AJs and controlling downstream proliferative signaling pathways by regulating the fraction of $\beta$-catenin that is bound to AJs or freely diffusing in the cytoplasm.

Although direct evidence for the effects of mechanical force on AJs remains elusive, evidence for the effects of cadherin engagement on cytoskeletal organization and cell function is accumulating. Perhaps the clearest indication of the regulation of cell structure by cadherins lies in the requirement for expression of cadherins to define apical and basolateral domains in the formation of differentiated epithelial monolayers (27, 152). It has also been shown that cadherin-mediated cell-cell contact decreases cell-ECM adhesion. For example, increasing the density of cells on a substrate leads to increased intercellular contact and decreased cell spreading on the substrate, a phenomenon described as contact inhibition of cell spreading (60, 83, 153). Many studies have also suggested that cadherin engagement inhibits proliferation or contact inhibition of proliferation: For example, exogenous expression of VE-cadherin in Chinese hampster ovary cells results in decreased growth rates, whereas blocking the function of VE-cadherin leads to increased proliferation (154). Similarly, transformed cells that lack a variety of components of AJs exhibit higher rates of proliferation than when they are transfected with N- or E-cadherin (155, 156). Recent evidence suggests that the engagement of cadherins blocks proliferation by increasing p27kip1 levels and inhibiting cell cycle progression into S-phase (157).

We have used a lithographic method to demonstrate that, when preventing contact inhibition of cell spreading by holding cell-matrix contact constant, cadherin-mediated cell-cell contact no longer inhibits proliferation but instead acts as a stimulatory signal for cell proliferation in vascular cells (60, 83). Moreover, this signal requires intact signaling through MLCK, the Rho pathway, and PI3-kinase. In cells that are allowed to spread freely in this system, cadherin-mediated inhibition of cell spreading is restored and proliferation is arrested. These results imply that AJs can generate two opposing signals that affect cell proliferation: an inhibitory signal involving effects on cell spreading and a stimulatory signal through cell-cell contact-mediated increases in intracellular tension. In most previous experiments with mass cultures, the antiproliferative effects of reduced cell spreading (and reduced tension at FAs) presumably overrode the effects of additional tension generated at AJs and resulted in lower proliferative rates. When cell spreading is held constant, however, the effect of AJ-mediated tension is to increase proliferation.

Recent studies indirectly suggest that cadherins can stimulate such tension by increasing Rho activity. Cadherin engagement appears to sequester a Rho inhibitor, p120 catenin (158, 159). Cadherin engagement also initiates signaling of Rac, a Rho GTPase that causes membrane ruffling (160). In all, while little data exist to provide a clear model of how mechanical forces might alter the structure or signaling of AJs, the engagement of cadherins appears to have dramatic effects on cytoskeletal organization and tension. Thus AJs are at least indirectly involved in modulating mechanotransduction, if not direct sites for such mechanochemical signaling.

## Crosstalk Between Focal Adhesions and Adherens Junctions

Our results and those of others have consistently emphasized a link between signaling at FAs and AJs in controlling cell behavior. An emerging principle is that the formation of FAs and AJs results in antagonistic behaviors. For instance, increasing cell-cell adhesion mechanically competes with and hence decreases cell-substrate adhesion (161, 162). Also, adhesion of ECM- or cadherin-coated beads to the cell surface leads to selective reinforcement of FAs and AJs, respectively (163). Thus the extent to which this interplay results from the redistribution of cytoskeletal tension to FAs and AJs or from the release or sequestration of soluble factors that interact with both types of adhesions is unknown.

## FUTURE DIRECTIONS

Much work still needs to be undertaken to create a coherent consistent theory of mechanotransduction at cell-matrix and cell-cell contacts. Unsolved questions include the following: First, and most importantly, what is the nature of the mechanosensor in cells? Is it a stretch-sensitive protein (or group of proteins) that can signal only when its conformation changes? Is it the lateral clustering of membrane proteins at adhesions that occurs when these proteins experience a force parallel to the cell membrane? We believe that multiple proteins are responsible for mechanosensing in a cell. For example, stretch of a chain of proteins may alter all of their conformations and thereby alter their ability to bind, recruit, or modify other cytoplasmic proteins.

Second, how is the shape of a cell determined? In our experiments with culturing cells on microscale islands, we have consistently observed that cells will spread to fill an island if the island is small, but will not if the island is too large. Does the stiffness of the substrate determine when the cell "knows" to stop spreading? Does a cell keep spreading until its adhesions can no longer support the contractile forces exerted on them? Previous results have suggested that whether a cell is under isometric or isotonic tension plays a role in determining if it can spread farther (164). The inhibitory effect of FAK on Rho implies that there is a negative feedback loop that acts to stabilize intracellular tension. Might a cell spread only until the "correct" tension is reached? The majority of our experience with cell shape involves culture on a flat surface; how do we investigate these effects when cells are embedded in three-dimensional scaffolds?

Third, how do the different types of FAs, AJs, ECM, integrins, and cell-cell adhesion molecules interact? In addition, how do these different combinations manifest in different types of cells (transformed versus normal, human versus nonhuman)? Variations in results owing to the use of different cells or differently prepared substrates have rarely been addressed and are often rationalized as investigator-specific anomalies. Whereas the effects of different types of ECM on cell behavior are well known, other types of differences may play a larger role than previously suspected: Swiss 3T3 mouse fibroblasts, a cell type commonly used in studies of mechanotransduction, are favored because they form particularly large FAs. Removing serum from the culture media of these cells causes FAs to disassemble quickly, but this effect is not seen for some other cell types. To what extent, then, are data specific to a particular type of cell? Likewise, differences in how ECM proteins are adsorbed may lead to unexpected changes in the conformation of adsorbed proteins that can influence the clustering of cell adhesion molecules (165). For instance, adsorbed cadherin fusion proteins do not elicit the same behaviors as native cadherins embedded in a fluid lipid membrane (C.M. Nelson, J. Tien & C.S. Chen, unpublished results).

Fourth, is the only purpose of cytoskeletal tension to drive the maturation of adhesions and to enhance adhesion-based signaling? The force generated by cells can not only alter intracellular structures but also had been shown to alter the structure and organization of the extracellular matrix (166, 167). Although we and others have focused nearly exclusively on examining the effects of tension generated by the actin-myosin cytoskeleton, other cytoskeletal systems such as microtubules and intermediate filaments play a part in determining the mechanical properties of a cell (1). It seems reasonable to expect that these less-studied systems may also affect mechanical signaling in cells (albeit indirectly, because complexes do not appear to mechanically couple these other filaments to adhesions). One hypothesis claims that microtubules act as elements to resist compressive forces in cells; depolymerization of microtubules should thus increase cytoskeletal tension, and mimic the effect of enhancing cell contractility, as suggested by some recent studies (168, 169). Transmission of mechanical force may also alter the shape of the cell nucleus and thereby regulate the nuclear import of transcription factors (170, 171). These forces may even direct the organization of chromatin and physically alter the accessibility of genes to transcriptional complexes (172). However, attempts to test these hypotheses have been limited by the lack of direct methods to measure intracellular forces.

In all, there are numerous opportunities for researchers to advance the study of mechanotransduction. Given that many breakthroughs have occurred hand-in-hand with the development of new tools to observe or to perturb cells, we expect that new methods to analyze cells in three dimensions with submicrometer resolution and over fine timescales should open new avenues of investigation in this area.

**The *Annual Review of Biomedical Engineering* is online at http://bioeng.annualreviews.org**

## LITERATURE CITED

1. Ingber DE. 1998. The architecture of life. *Sci. Am.* 278:48–57
2. Thompson DA. 1961. *On Growth and Form*. Cambridge, UK: Cambridge Univ. Press. 346 pp.
3. Fung YC. 1993. *Biomechanics: Mechanical Properties of Living Tissues*. New York: Springer-Verlag. 568 pp.
4. Guyton AC. 1991. *Textbook of Medical Physiology*. Philadelphia, PA: Saunders. 1014 pp.
5. Folkow B. 1982. Physiological aspects of primary hypertension. *Physiol. Rev.* 62: 347–504
6. Cines DB, Pollak ES, Buck CA, Loscalzo J, Zimmerman GA, et al. 1998. Endothelial cells in physiology and in the pathophysiology of vascular disorders. *Blood* 91:3527–61
7. Gimbrone MA Jr. 1999. Vascular endothelium, hemodynamic forces, and atherogenesis. *Am. J. Pathol.* 155:1–5

8. Shepro D, D'Amore P. 1984. Physiology and biochemistry of the vascular wall endothelium. In *Microcirculation*, ed. EM Renkin, CC Michel, pp. 103–64. Bethesda, MD: Am. Physiol. Soc.
9. Dunphy JE. 1963. The fibroblast—a ubiquitous ally for the surgeon. *N. Engl. J. Med.* 268:1367–77
10. Singer AJ, Clark RA. 1999. Cutaneous wound healing. *N. Engl. J. Med.* 341:738–46
11. Cowan DB, Langille BL. 1996. Cellular and molecular biology of vascular remodeling. *Curr. Opin. Lipidol.* 7:94–100
12. Langille BL. 1995. Blood flow-induced remodeling of the artery wall. In *Flow-Dependent Regulation of Vascular Function*, ed. JA Bevan, G Kaley, GM Rubanyi, pp. 277–99. New York: Am. Physiol. Soc.
13. Burridge K, Fath K, Kelly T, Nuckolls G, Turner C. 1988. Focal adhesions: transmembrane junctions between the extracellular matrix and the cytoskeleton. *Annu. Rev. Cell Biol.* 4:487–525
14. Chrzanowska-Wodnicka M, Burridge K. 1996. Rho-stimulated contractility drives the formation of stress fibers and focal adhesions. *J. Cell Biol.* 133:1403–15
15. Balaban NQ, Schwarz US, Riveline D, Goichberg P, Tzur G, et al. 2001. Force and focal adhesion assembly: a close relationship studied using elastic micropatterned substrates. *Nat. Cell Biol.* 3:466–72
16. Riveline D, Zamir E, Balaban NQ, Schwarz US, Ishizaki T, et al. 2001. Focal contacts as mechanosensors: externally applied local mechanical force induces growth of focal contacts by an mDia1-dependent and ROCK-independent mechanism. *J. Cell Biol.* 153:1175–86
17. Sawada Y, Sheetz MP. 2002. Force transduction by Triton cytoskeletons. *J. Cell Biol.* 156:609–15
18. Galbraith CG, Sheetz MP. 1997. A micromachined device provides a new bend on fibroblast traction forces. *Proc. Natl. Acad. Sci. USA* 94:9114–18
19. Galbraith CG, Yamada KM, Sheetz MP. 2002. The relationship between force and focal complex development. *J. Cell Biol.* 159:695–705
20. Choquet D, Felsenfeld DP, Sheetz MP. 1997. Extracellular matrix rigidity causes strengthening of integrin-cytoskeleton linkages. *Cell* 88:39–48
21. Wang N, Butler JP, Ingber DE. 1993. Mechanotransduction across the cell surface and through the cytoskeleton. *Science* 260:1124–27
22. Pelham RJJ, Wang Y-L. 1997. Cell locomotion and focal adhesions are regulated by substrate flexibility. *Proc. Natl. Acad. Sci. USA* 94:13661–65
23. Burridge K, Chrzanowska-Wodnicka M. 1996. Focal adhesions, contractility, and signaling. *Annu. Rev. Cell Dev. Biol.* 12: 463–518
24. Cukierman E, Pankov R, Stevens DR, Yamada KM. 2001. Taking cell-matrix adhesions to the third dimension. *Science* 294:1708–12
25. Kano Y, Katoh K, Fujiwara K. 2000. Lateral zone of cell-cell adhesion as the major fluid shear stress-related signal transduction site. *Circ. Res.* 86:425–33
26. Izzard CS, Lochner LR. 1976. Cell-to-substrate contacts in living fibroblasts: an interference reflexion study with an evaluation of the technique. *J. Cell Sci.* 21:129–59
27. Rodriguez-Boulan E, Nelson WJ. 1989. Morphogenesis of the polarized epithelial cell phenotype. *Science* 245:718–25
28. Bissell MJ, Nelson WJ. 1999. Cell-to-cell contact and extracellular matrix. Integration of form and function: the central role of adhesion molecules. *Curr. Opin. Cell Biol.* 11:537–39
29. Gumbiner BM. 1996. Cell adhesion: the molecular basis of tissue architecture and morphogenesis. *Cell* 84:345–57
30. Davies PF. 1995. Flow-mediated endothelial mechanotransduction. *Physiol. Rev.* 75:519–60
31. Shyy JY, Chien S. 1997. Role of integrins in cellular responses to mechanical

stress and adhesion. *Curr. Opin. Cell Biol.* 9:707–13
32. Acevedo AD, Bowser SS, Gerritsen ME, Bizios R. 1993. Morphological and proliferative responses of endothelial cells to hydrostatic pressure: role of fibroblast growth factor. *J. Cell. Physiol.* 157:603–14
33. Takeichi M. 1991. Cadherin cell adhesion receptors as a morphogenetic regulator. *Science* 251:1451–55
34. Juliano RL, Haskill S. 1993. Signal transduction from the extracellular matrix. *J. Cell Biol.* 120:577–85
35. Schwartz MA, Schaller MD, Ginsberg MH. 1995. Integrins: emerging paradigms of signal transduction. *Annu. Rev. Cell Dev. Biol.* 11:549–99
36. Jockusch BM, Bubeck P, Giehl K, Kroemker M, Moschner J, et al. 1995. The molecular architecture of focal adhesions. *Annu. Rev. Cell Dev. Biol.* 11:379–416
37. Chicurel ME, Chen CS, Ingber DE. 1997. Cellular control lies in the balance of forces. *Curr. Opin. Cell Biol.* 10:232–39
38. Dunn GA, Brown AF. 1986. Alignment of fibroblasts on grooved surfaces described by a simple geometric transformation. *J. Cell Sci.* 83:313–40
39. Brunette DM, Chehroudi B. 1999. The effects of the surface topography of micromachined titanium substrata on cell behavior in vitro and in vivo. *J. Biomech. Eng.* 121:49–57
40. Bissell MJ, Weaver VM, Lelievre SA, Wang F, Petersen OW, Schmeichel KL. 1999. Tissue structure, nuclear organization, and gene expression in normal and malignant breast. *Cancer Res.* 59:1757s–63
41. Chen CS, Mrksich M, Huang S, Whitesides GM, Ingber DE. 1997. Geometric control of cell life and death. *Science* 276:1425–28
42. Watt FM, Jordan PW, O'Neill CH. 1988. Cell shape controls terminal differentiation of human epidermal keratinocytes. *Proc. Natl. Acad. Sci. USA* 85:5576–80
43. Thomas CH, Collier JH, Sfeir CS, Healy KE. 2002. Engineering gene expression and protein synthesis by modulation of nuclear shape. *Proc. Natl. Acad. Sci. USA* 99:1972–77
44. Boonstra J. 1999. Growth factor-induced signal transduction in adherent mammalian cells is sensitive to gravity. *FASEB J.* 13:S35–42
45. Guharay F, Sachs F. 1984. Stretch-activated single ion channel currents in tissue-cultured embryonic chick skeletal muscle. *J. Physiol.* 352:685–701
46. Hamill OP, Martinac B. 2001. Molecular basis of mechanotransduction in living cells. *Physiol. Rev.* 81:685–740
47. Ghazi A, Berrier C, Ajouz B, Besnard M. 1998. Mechanosensitive ion channels and their mode of activation. *Biochimie* 80:357–62
48. Folkman J, Moscona A. 1978. Role of cell shape in growth control. *Nature* 273:345–49
49. Ingber DE, Folkman J. 1989. Mechanochemical switching between growth and differentiation during fibroblast growth factor-stimulated angiogenesis in vitro: role of extracellular matrix. *J. Cell Biol.* 109:317–30
50. Ingber DE, Madri JA, Folkman J. 1987. Endothelial growth factors and extracellular matrix regulate DNA synthesis through modulation of cell and nuclear expansion. *In Vitro Cell. Dev. Biol.* 23:387–94
51. Ireland GW, Dopping-Hepenstal P, Jordan P, O'Neill C. 1987. Effect of patterned surfaces of adhesive islands on the shape, cytoskeleton, adhesion and behaviour of Swiss mouse 3T3 fibroblasts. *J. Cell Sci. Suppl.* 8:19–33
52. O'Neill C, Jordan P, Ireland G. 1986. Evidence for two distinct mechanisms of anchorage stimulation in freshly explanted and 3T3 Swiss mouse fibroblasts. *Cell* 44:489–96
53. Harris AK, Wild P, Stopak D. 1980. Silicone rubber substrata: a new wrinkle

in the study of cell locomotion. *Science* 208:177–80

54. Harris AK, Stopak D, Wild P. 1981. Fibroblast traction as a mechanism for collagen morphogenesis. *Nature* 290:249–51
55. Flusberg DA, Numaguchi Y, Ingber DE. 2001. Cooperative control of Akt phosphorylation, bcl-2 expression, and apoptosis by cytoskeletal microfilaments and microtubules in capillary endothelial cells. *Mol. Biol. Cell* 12:3087–94
56. Zamir E, Katz M, Posen Y, Erez N, Yamada KM, et al. 2000. Dynamics and segregation of cell-matrix adhesions in cultured fibroblasts. *Nat. Cell Biol.* 2:191–96
57. Katz BZ, Zamir E, Bershadsky A, Kam Z, Yamada KM, Geiger B. 2000. Physical state of the extracellular matrix regulates the structure and molecular composition of cell-matrix adhesions. *Mol. Biol. Cell* 11:1047–60
58. Ren XD, Kiosses WB, Sieg DJ, Otey CA, Schlaepfer DD, Schwartz MA. 2000. Focal adhesion kinase suppresses Rho activity to promote focal adhesion turnover. *J. Cell Sci.* 113:3673–78
59. Chen Q, Kinch MS, Lin TH, Burridge K, Juliano RL. 1994. Integrin-mediated cell adhesion activates mitogen-activated protein kinases. *J. Biol. Chem.* 269:26602–5
60. Nelson CM, Chen CS. 2003. VE-cadherin simultaneously stimulates and inhibits cell proliferation by altering cytoskeletal structure and tension. *J. Cell Sci.* 116: 3571–81
61. Dike LE, Chen CS, Mrksich M, Tien J, Whitesides GM, Ingber DE. 1999. Geometric control of switching between growth, apoptosis, and differentiation during angiogenesis using micropatterned substrates. *In Vitro Cell. Dev. Biol. Anim.* 35:441–48
62. Lo CM, Wang HB, Dembo M, Wang YL. 2000. Cell movement is guided by the rigidity of the substrate. *Biophys. J.* 79: 144–52
63. Tan JL, Tien J, Pirone DM, Gray DS, Bhadriraju K, Chen CS. 2003. Cells lying on a bed of microneedles: an approach to isolate mechanical force. *Proc. Natl. Acad. Sci. USA* 100:1484–89
64. Nakagawa S, Pawelek P, Grinnell F. 1989. Long-term culture of fibroblasts in contracted collagen gels: effects on cell growth and biosynthetic activity. *J. Invest. Dermatol.* 93:792–98
65. Lee J, Leonard M, Oliver T, Ishihara A, Jacobson K. 1994. Traction forces generated by locomoting keratocytes. *J. Cell Biol.* 127:1957–64
66. Burton K, Taylor DL. 1997. Traction forces of cytokinesis measured with optically modified elastic substrata. *Nature* 385:450–54
67. Beningo KA, Wang YL. 2002. Flexible substrata for the detection of cellular traction forces. *Trends Cell Biol.* 12:79–84
68. Dembo M, Oliver T, Ishihara A, Jacobson K. 1996. Imaging the traction stresses exerted by locomoting cells with the elastic substratum method. *Biophys. J.* 70:2008–22
69. Burton K, Park JH, Taylor DL. 1999. Keratocytes generate traction forces in two phases. *Mol. Biol. Cell* 10:3745–69
70. Munevar S, Wang YL, Dembo M. 2001. Distinct roles of frontal and rear cell-substrate adhesions in fibroblast migration. *Mol. Biol. Cell* 12:3947–54
71. Arfken GB. 1985. *Mathematical Methods for Physicists*. Orlando, FL: Academic. 985 pp.
72. Wallace W, Schaefer LH, Swedlow JR. 2001. A workingperson's guide to deconvolution in light microscopy. *Biotechniques* 31:1076–97
73. Landau LD, Lifshitz EM. 1986. *Theory of Elasticity*. Oxford, UK: Pergamon. 187 pp.
74. Archer RR, Lardner TJ. 1978. *An Introduction to the Mechanics of Solids*. New York: McGraw-Hill. 628 pp.
75. Sadoshima J, Takahashi T, Jahn L, Izumo S. 1992. Roles of mechano-sensitive ion channels, cytoskeleton, and contractile activity in stretch-induced immediate-early

gene expression and hypertrophy of cardiac myocytes. *Proc. Natl. Acad. Sci. USA* 89:9905–9
76. Maksym GN, Fabry B, Butler JP, Navajas D, Tschumperlin DJ, et al. 2000. Mechanical properties of cultured human airway smooth muscle cells from 0.05 to 0.4 Hz. *J. Appl. Physiol.* 89:1619–32
77. Kuo SC, Sheetz MP. 1992. Optical tweezers in cell biology. *Trends Cell Biol.* 2: 116–18
78. Wang HB, Dembo M, Hanks SK, Wang Y. 2001. Focal adhesion kinase is involved in mechanosensing during fibroblast migration. *Proc. Natl. Acad. Sci. USA* 98:11295–300
79. Tien J, Chen CS. 2002. Patterning the cellular microenvironment. *IEEE Eng. Med. Biol.* 21:95–98
79a. Folch A, Toner M. 2000. Microengineering of cellular interactions. *Annu. Rev. Biomed. Eng.* 2:227–56
79b. Whitesides GM, Ostuni E. Takayama S, Jiang X, Ingber DE. 2001. Soft lithography in biology and biochemistry. *Annu. Rev. Biomed. Eng.* 3:335–73
80. Singhvi R, Kumar A, Lopez G, Stephanopoulos GN, Wang DIC, Whitesides GM. 1994. Engineering cell shape and function. *Science* 264:696–98
81. Mrksich M, Chen CS, Xia Y, Dike LE, Ingber DE, Whitesides GM. 1996. Controlling cell attachment on contoured surfaces with self-assembled monolayers of alkanethiolates on gold. *Proc. Natl. Acad. Sci. USA* 93:10775–78
82. Mrksich M, Dike LE, Tien J, Ingber DE, Whitesides GM. 1997. Using microcontact printing to pattern the attachment of mammalian cells to self-assembled monolayers of alkanethiolates on transparent films of gold and silver. *Exp. Cell Res.* 235:305–13
83. Nelson CM, Chen CS. 2002. Cell-cell signaling by direct contact increases cell proliferation via a PI3K-dependent signal. *FEBS Lett.* 514:238–42
84. Zamir E, Geiger B. 2001. Molecular complexity and dynamics of cell-matrix adhesions. *J. Cell Sci.* 114:3583–90
85. Ruoslahti E. 1996. RGD and other recognition sequences for integrins. *Annu. Rev. Cell Dev. Biol.* 12:697–715
86. Miyamoto S, Akiyama SK, Yamada KM. 1995. Synergistic roles for receptor occupancy and aggregation in integrin transmembrane function. *Science* 267:883–85
87. Plopper G, Ingber DE. 1993. Rapid induction and isolation of focal adhesion complexes. *Biochem. Biophys. Res. Commun.* 193:571–78
88. Nobes CD, Hall A. 1995. Rho, rac, and cdc42 GTPases regulate the assembly of multimolecular focal complexes associated with actin stress fibers, lamellipodia, and filopodia. *Cell* 81:53–62
89. Kiosses WB, Shattil SJ, Pampori N, Schwartz MA. 2001. Rac recruits high-affinity integrin $\alpha_v\beta_3$ to lamellipodia in endothelial cell migration. *Nat. Cell Biol.* 3:316–20
90. Ridley AJ, Hall A. 1992. The small GTP-binding protein rho regulates the assembly of focal adhesions and actin stress fibers in response to growth factors. *Cell* 70:389–99
91. Felsenfeld DP, Schwartzberg PL, Venegas A, Tse R, Sheetz MP. 1999. Selective regulation of integrin–cytoskeleton interactions by the tyrosine kinase Src. *Nat. Cell Biol.* 1:200–6
92. Hay ED. 1991. Collagen and other matrix glycoproteins in embryogenesis. In *Cell Biology of Extracellular Matrix*, ed. ED Hay, pp. 419–62. New York: Plenum
93. Ilic D, Furuta Y, Kanazawa S, Takeda N, Sobue K, et al. 1995. Reduced cell motility and enhanced focal adhesion contact formation in cells from FAK-deficient mice. *Nature* 377:539–44
94. Miyawaki A, Llopis J, Heim R, McCaffery JM, Adams JA, et al. 1997. Fluorescent indicators for $Ca^{2+}$ based on green fluorescent proteins and calmodulin. *Nature* 388:882–87

95. Stoker M, O'Neill C, Berryman S, Waxman V. 1968. Anchorage and growth regulation in normal and virus-transformed cells. *Int. J. Cancer* 3:683–93
96. Schwartz MA. 1997. Integrins, oncogenes, and anchorage independence. *J. Cell Biol.* 139:575–78
97. Leopoldt D, Yee HF Jr, Rozengurt E. 2001. Calyculin-A induces focal adhesion assembly and tyrosine phosphorylation of $p125^{Fak}$, $p130^{Cas}$, and paxillin in Swiss 3T3 cells. *J. Cell. Physiol.* 188:106–19
98. Frisch SM, Francis H. 1994. Disruption of epithelial cell-matrix interactions induces apoptosis. *J. Cell Biol.* 124:619–26
99. Mettouchi A, Klein S, Guo W, Lopez-Lago M, Lemichez E, et al. 2001. Integrin-specific activation of Rac controls progression through the $G_1$ phase of the cell cycle. *Mol. Cell* 8:115–27
100. Schneller M, Vuori K, Ruoslahti E. 1997. $\alpha_v\beta_3$ integrin associates with activated insulin and PDGF$\beta$ receptors and potentiates the biological activity of PDGF. *EMBO J.* 16:5600–7
101. Friedlander M, Brooks PC, Shaffer RW, Kincaid CM, Varner JA, Cheresh DA. 1995. Definition of two angiogenic pathways by distinct $\alpha_v$ integrins. *Science* 270:1500–2
102. Alavi A, Hood JD, Frausto R, Stupack DG, Cheresh DA. 2003. Role of Raf in vascular protection from distinct apoptotic stimuli. *Science* 301:94–96
103. Numaguchi K, Eguchi S, Yamakawa T, Motley ED, Inagami T. 1999. Mechanotransduction of rat aortic vascular smooth muscle cells requires RhoA and intact actin filaments. *Circ. Res.* 85:5–11
104. Domingos PP, Fonseca PM, Nadruz W Jr, Franchini KG. 2002. Load-induced focal adhesion kinase activation in the myocardium: role of stretch and contractile activity. *Am. J. Physiol. Heart Circ. Physiol.* 282:H556–64
105. Renshaw MW, Price LS, Schwartz MA. 1999. Focal adhesion kinase mediates the integrin signaling requirement for growth factor activation of MAP kinase. *J. Cell Biol.* 147:611–18
106. Li W, Duzgun A, Sumpio BE, Basson MD. 2001. Integrin and FAK-mediated MAPK activation is required for cyclic strain mitogenic effects in Caco-2 cells. *Am. J. Physiol. Gastrointest. Liver Physiol.* 280:G75–87
107. Li S, Kim M, Hu YL, Jalali S, Schlaepfer DD, et al. 1997. Fluid shear stress activation of focal adhesion kinase. Linking to mitogen-activated protein kinases. *J. Biol. Chem.* 272:30455–62
108. Frisch SM, Vuori K, Ruoslahti E, Chan-Hui PY. 1996. Control of adhesion-dependent cell survival by focal adhesion kinase. *J. Cell Biol.* 134:793–99
109. Seasholtz TM, Zhang T, Morissette MR, Howes AL, Yang AH, Brown JH. 2001. Increased expression and activity of RhoA are associated with increased DNA synthesis and reduced $p27^{Kip1}$ expression in the vasculature of hypertensive rats. *Circ. Res.* 89:488–95
110. Stouffer GA, Sarembock IJ, McNamara CA, Gimple LW, Owens GK. 1993. Thrombin-induced mitogenesis of vascular SMC is partially mediated by autocrine production of PDGF-AA. *Am. J. Physiol. Cell Physiol.* 265:C806–11
111. Hahn AW, Resink TJ, Kern F, Buhler FR. 1993. Peptide vasoconstrictors, vessel structure, and vascular smooth-muscle proliferation. *J. Cardiovasc. Pharmacol.* 22:S37–43
112. Johnson RP, Craig SW. 1995. F-actin binding site masked by the intramolecular association of vinculin head and tail domains. *Nature* 373:261–64
113. Ingber DE. 1990. Fibronectin controls capillary endothelial cell growth by modulating cell shape. *Proc. Natl. Acad. Sci. USA* 87:3579–83
114. Clark EA, Brugge JS. 1995. Integrins and signal transduction pathways: the road taken. *Science* 268:233–39
115. Hynes RO. 1992. Integrins: versatility,

modulation, and signaling in cell adhesion. *Cell* 69:11–25
116. Tamkun JW, deSimone DW, Fonda D, Patel RS, Buck C, et al. 1986. Structure of integrin, a glycoprotein involved in the transmembrane linkage between fibronectin and actin. *Cell* 46:271–82
117. Chen CS, Mrksich M, Huang S, Whitesides GM. 1998. Micropatterned surfaces for control of cell shape, position and function. *Biotechnol. Progr.* 14:356–63
118. Moiseeva EP. 2001. Adhesion receptors of vascular smooth muscle cells and their functions. *Cardiovasc. Res.* 52:372–86
119. Huang S, Chen CS, Ingber DE. 1998. Control of cyclin D1, p27Kip1 and cell cycle progression in human capillary endothelial cells by cell shape and cytoskeletal tension. *Mol. Biol. Cell* 9:3179–93
120. Hall A. 1998. Rho GTPases and the actin cytoskeleton. *Science* 279:509–14
121. Yamamoto M, Marui N, Sakai T, Morii N, Kozaki S, et al. 1993. ADP-ribosylation of the rhoA gene product by botulinum C3 exoenzyme causes Swiss 3T3 cells to accumulate in the G1 phase of the cell cycle. *Oncogene* 8:1449–55
122. Olson MF, Ashworth A, Hall A. 1995. An essential role for Rho, Rac, and Cdc42 GTPases in cell cycle progression through G1. *Science* 269:1270–72
123. Sawada N, Itoh H, Ueyama K, Yamashita J, Doi K, et al. 2000. Inhibition of rho-associated kinase results in suppression of neointimal formation of balloon-injured arteries. *Circulation* 101:2030–33
124. Uchida S, Watanabe G, Shimada Y, Maeda M, Kawabe A, et al. 2000. The suppression of small GTPase rho signal transduction pathway inhibits angiogenesis in vitro and in vivo. *Biochem. Biophys. Res. Commun.* 269:633–40
125. Uehata M, Ishizaki T, Satoh H, Ono T, Kawahara T, et al. 1997. Calcium sensitization of smooth muscle mediated by a Rho-associated protein kinase in hypertension. *Nature* 389:990–94
126. Kimura K, Ito M, Amano M, Chihara K, Fukata Y, et al. 1996. Regulation of myosin phosphatase by Rho and Rho-associated kinase (Rho-kinase). *Science* 273:245–48
127. Amano M, Ito M, Kimura K, Fukata Y, Chihara K, et al. 1996. Phosphorylation and activation of myosin by Rho-associated kinase (Rho-kinase). *J. Biol. Chem.* 271:20246–49
128. Ishizaki T, Maekawa M, Fujisawa K, Okawa K, Iwamatsu A, et al. 1996. The small GTP-binding protein Rho binds to and activates a 160 kDa Ser/Thr protein kinase homologous to myotonic dystrophy kinase. *EMBO J.* 15:1885–93
129. Geiger B, Bershadsky A. 2001. Assembly and mechanosensory function of focal contacts. *Curr. Opin. Cell Biol.* 13:584–92
130. Chen CS, Alonso JL, Ostuni E, Whitesides GM, Ingber DE. 2003. Cell shape provides global control of focal adhesion assembly. *Biochem. Biophys. Res. Commun.* 307:355–61
131. Lauffenburger DA, Horwitz AF. 1996. Cell migration: a physically integrated molecular process. *Cell* 84:359–69
132. Katsumi A, Milanini J, Kiosses WB, del Pozo MA, Kaunas R, et al. 2002. Effects of cell tension on the small GTPase Rac. *J. Cell Biol.* 158:153–64
133. Parker KK, Brock AL, Brangwynne C, Mannix RJ, Wang N, et al. 2002. Directional control of lamellipodia extension by constraining cell shape and orienting cell tractional forces. *FASEB J.* 16:1195–204
134. Palecek SP, Loftus JC, Ginsberg MH, Lauffenburger DA, Horwitz AF. 1997. Integrin-ligand binding properties govern cell migration speed through cell-substratum adhesiveness. *Nature* 385: 537–40
135. Vasioukhin V, Fuchs E. 2001. Actin dynamics and cell-cell adhesion in epithelia. *Curr. Opin. Cell Biol.* 13:76–84
136. Balda MS, Matter K. 1998. Tight junctions. *J. Cell Sci.* 111:541–47
137. Kumar NM, Gilula NB. 1996. The gap

junction communication channel. *Cell* 84:381–88
138. Hynes RO, Lander AD. 1992. Contact and adhesive specificities in the associations, migrations, and targeting of cells and axons. *Cell* 68:303–22
139. McNeill H, Ryan TA, Smith SJ, Nelson WJ. 1993. Spatial and temporal dissection of immediate and early events following cadherin-mediated epithelial cell adhesion. *J. Cell Biol.* 120:1217–26
140. Nagafuchi A. 2001. Molecular architecture of adherens junctions. *Curr. Opin. Cell Biol.* 13:600–3
141. Wojciak-Stothard B, Potempa S, Eichholtz T, Ridley AJ. 2001. Rho and Rac but not Cdc42 regulate endothelial cell permeability. *J. Cell Sci.* 114:1343–55
142. Dudek SM, Garcia JG. 2001. Cytoskeletal regulation of pulmonary vascular permeability. *J. Appl. Physiol.* 91:1487–500
143. Garcia JG, Liu F, Verin AD, Birukova A, Dechert MA, et al. 2001. Sphingosine 1-phosphate promotes endothelial cell barrier integrity by Edg-dependent cytoskeletal rearrangement. *J. Clin. Invest.* 108:689–701
144. Hordijk PL, Anthony E, Mul FP, Rientsma R, Oomen LC, Roos D. 1999. Vascular-endothelial-cadherin modulates endothelial monolayer permeability. *J. Cell Sci.* 112:1915–23
145. Hutson MS, Tokutake Y, Chang MS, Bloor JW, Venakides S, et al. 2003. Forces for morphogenesis investigated with laser microsurgery and quantitative modeling. *Science* 300:145–49
146. Foty RA, Pfleger CM, Forgacs G, Steinberg MS. 1996. Surface tensions of embryonic tissues predict their mutual envelopment behavior. *Development* 122: 1611–20
147. Critchley DR. 2000. Focal adhesions—the cytoskeletal connection. *Curr. Opin. Cell Biol.* 12:133–39
148. Gumbiner BM. 1995. Signal transduction of beta-catenin. *Curr. Opin. Cell Biol.* 7:634–40
149. Piedra J, Martinez D, Castano J, Miravet S, Dunach M, de Herreros AG. 2001. Regulation of $\beta$-catenin structure and activity by tyrosine phosphorylation. *J. Biol. Chem.* 276:20436–43
150. Hecht A, Kemler R. 2000. Curbing the nuclear activities of $\beta$-catenin. Control over Wnt target gene expression. *EMBO Rep.* 1:24–28
151. Tetsu O, McCormick F. 1999. $\beta$-catenin regulates expression of cyclin D1 in colon carcinoma cells. *Nature* 398:422–26
152. Drubin DG, Nelson WJ. 1996. Origins of cell polarity. *Cell* 84:335–44
153. Fagotto F, Gumbiner BM. 1996. Cell contact-dependent signaling. *Dev. Biol.* 180:445–54
154. Caveda L, Martin-Padura I, Navarro P, Breviario F, Corada M, et al. 1996. Inhibition of cultured cell growth by vascular endothelial cadherin (cadherin-5/VE-cadherin). *J. Clin. Invest.* 98:886–93
155. Levenberg S, Yarden A, Kam Z, Geiger B. 1999. p27 is involved in N-cadherin-mediated contact inhibition of cell growth and S-phase entry. *Oncogene* 18:869–76
156. Stockinger A, Eger A, Wolf J, Beug H, Foisner R. 2001. E-cadherin regulates cell growth by modulating proliferation-dependent $\beta$-catenin transcriptional activity. *J. Cell Biol.* 154:1185–96
157. St Croix B, Sheehan C, Rak JW, Florenes VA, Slingerland JM, Kerbel RS. 1998. E-cadherin-dependent growth suppression is mediated by the cyclin-dependent kinase inhibitor $p27^{KIP1}$. *J. Cell Biol.* 142:557–71
158. Grosheva I, Shtutman M, Elbaum M, Bershadsky AD. 2001. p120 catenin affects cell motility via modulation of activity of Rho-family GTPases: a link between cell-cell contact formation and regulation of cell locomotion. *J. Cell Sci.* 114:695–707
159. Anastasiadis PZ, Moon SY, Thoreson MA, Mariner DJ, Crawford HC, et al. 2000. Inhibition of RhoA by p120 catenin. *Nat. Cell Biol.* 2:637–44

160. Noren NK, Niessen CM, Gumbiner BM, Burridge K. 2001. Cadherin engagement regulates Rho family GTPases. *J. Biol. Chem.* 276:33305–8
161. Lauffenburger DA, Griffith LG. 2001. Who's got pull around here? Cell organization in development and tissue engineering. *Proc. Natl. Acad. Sci. USA* 98:4282–84
162. Ryan PL, Foty RA, Kohn J, Steinberg MS. 2001. Tissue spreading on implantable substrates is a competitive outcome of cell-cell vs. cell-substratum adhesivity. *Proc. Natl. Acad. Sci. USA* 98:4323–27
163. Levenberg S, Katz BZ, Yamada KM, Geiger B. 1998. Long-range and selective autoregulation of cell-cell or cell-matrix adhesions by cadherin or integrin ligands. *J. Cell Sci.* 111:347–57
164. Grinnell F. 2003. Fibroblast biology in three-dimensional collagen matrices. *Trends Cell Biol.* 13:264–69
165. Garcia AJ, Vega MD, Boettiger D. 1999. Modulation of cell proliferation and differentiation through substrate-dependent changes in fibronectin conformation. *Mol. Biol. Cell* 10:785–98
166. Baneyx G, Baugh L, Vogel V. 2002. Fibronectin extension and unfolding within cell matrix fibrils controlled by cytoskeletal tension. *Proc. Natl. Acad. Sci. USA* 99:5139–43
167. Ohashi T, Kiehart DP, Erickson HP. 1999. Dynamics and elasticity of the fibronectin matrix in living cell culture visualized by fibronectin-green fluorescent protein. *Proc. Natl. Acad. Sci. USA* 96:2153–58
168. Bershadsky A, Chausovsky A, Becker E, Lyubimova A, Geiger B. 1996. Involvement of microtubules in the control of adhesion-dependent signal transduction. *Curr. Biol.* 6:1279–89
169. Liu BP, Chrzanowska-Wodnicka M, Burridge K. 1998. Microtubule depolymerization induces stress fibers, focal adhesions, and DNA synthesis via the GTP-binding protein Rho. *Cell Adhes. Commun.* 5:249–55
170. Feldherr CM, Akin D. 1993. Regulation of nuclear transport in proliferating and quiescent cells. *Exp. Cell Res.* 205:179–86
171. Yen A, Pardee AB. 1979. Role of nuclear size in cell growth initiation. *Science* 204:1315–17
172. Pienta KJ, Coffey DS. 1992. Nuclear-cytoskeletal interactions: evidence for physical connections between the nucleus and cell periphery and their alteration by transformation. *J. Cell. Biochem.* 49:357–65

Annu. Rev. Biomed. Eng. 2004. 6:303–29
doi: 10.1146/annurev.bioeng.6.040803.140240

First published online as a Review in Advance on February 18, 2004

# FUNCTIONAL EFFICACY OF TENDON REPAIR PROCESSES

David L. Butler, Natalia Juncosa, and Matthew R. Dressler
*Department of Biomedical Engineering, Noyes-Giannestras Biomechanics Laboratory, University of Cincinnati, Cincinnati, Ohio 45221-0048; email: david.butler@uc.edu, juncosln@email.uc.edu, matthew.dressler@uc.edu*

**Key Words** functional tissue engineering, evaluation, injury, design parameters, biomechanics

■ **Abstract** Despite various attempts to repair and replace injured tendon, an understanding of the repair processes and a systematic approach to achieving functional efficacy remain elusive. In this review the epidemiology of tendon injury and repair is first examined. Using a traditional paradigm for repair assessment, the biology and biomechanics of normal tendon, natural healing, and repair are then explored. New treatment strategies such as functional tissue engineering are discussed, including a functional approach to treatment that involves the development of in vivo functional design parameters to judge the acceptability of a repair outcome. The paper concludes with future directions.

CONTENTS



1523-9829/04/0815-0303$14.00

# INTRODUCTION

Soft tissue injuries and repairs are quite common. Tendon, ligament, and joint capsular injuries represent 45% of the 32 million musculoskeletal injuries each year in the United States (1, 2). Tendon injuries are especially common, requiring surgical repair to replace the shoulder's rotator cuff tendons (51,000 per year), the Achilles tendon (44,000 per year), and the patellar tendon (42,000 per year) (1–14). The frequency of these injuries is expected to rise as the population ages and remains active (1, 2, 15–17). Although some surgical procedures are successful, many must be revised, in part owing to the large unknown forces sustained by the tendon repair during activities of daily living.

This review describes normal tendon biology and biomechanics and tendon repair processes using a general paradigm (Figure 1). Following a tendon injury, a treatment is prescribed and the tissue is permitted to either heal naturally or receive surgical repair. The success of the repair is judged by contrasting specific response measures against normal properties. The circular and iterative nature of this process is discussed. The relevance of these comparisons is then explored before concluding with future directions.

## Biology and Biomechanics of Normal Tendon

To evaluate injured and repaired tissues, physicians and engineers have traditionally used normal tissue as a benchmark. Having knowledge of normal allows determination of differences between normal and injured states and guidance in devising repair strategies. Therefore, this review of tendon repair processes begins by providing a brief characterization of normal tissue and also discusses the assays

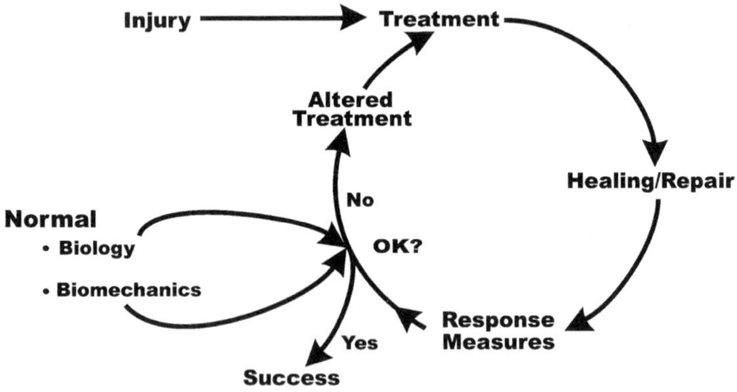


**Figure 1** Traditional paradigm of tendon repair. Following an injury, a treatment is tried, healing or repair permitted, and specific response measures compared with values for normal tissue. If unacceptable, the process is repeated until repair measures compare favorably with normal values.

and measurements that are used to compare normal tendon to injured and repaired tendon.

BIOLOGY OF CELLS AND EXTRACELLULAR MATRIX Spanning between skeletal muscle and bone, tendon transmits muscle force to bone attachments to effect movement of lower limbs during gait, and motion of the thorax, upper extremities, and head during activities of daily living. As such, tendon plays critical biological and biomechanical roles in the homeostasis of the organism. These roles are played out through a reciprocal relationship between the tendon's cellular and extracellular compartments.

Spindle-shaped tendon cells or tenocytes are the primary cell type found in normal uninjured tendon (18). An intricate microvascular supply nourishes these tenocytes, permitting them to maintain their local extracellular environment (18). Spatial variations exist in cell phenotype with the appearance of more rounded than spindle-shaped cells near the attachment sites into bone (19–21). Rounded cells are also prevalent in the fibrocartilage-rich contact zone where the tendon wraps around bone (19–27).

Tenocytes synthesize a wide array of extracellular matrix (ECM) proteins in a well-ordered structure. Among the most prolific of these proteins is collagen, which is organized in a parallel arrangement. At the macrostructural level, tendon collagen consists of parallel and crimped primary and secondary fiber bundles (fascicles), the periodicity of which dramatically decreases close to the tendon insertion into bone (28–30). Each bundle contains fibers visible at the light microscope level. Under scanning and transmission electron microscopy, the fibers are composed of fibrils (100–500 nm in diameter), the fundamental building blocks of tendon, which in turn contain microfibrils (diameter 3.6 nm). At the molecular level (detected by X-ray diffraction), aligned and staggered tropocollagen molecules (length 280 nm; diameter 1.5 nm) are bound through transient and permanent (pyridinium) cross-links that permit force transmission along the entire tendon structure (31, 32).

The biochemistry of tendon extracellular matrix reveals primarily type I collagen along with glycoproteins. Type I collagen represents approximately 95% of all collagen present and 65–80% of the dry mass in tendon (18, 33). Other collagens are less prevalent but play an important role. For example, type V collagen copolymerizes with type I collagen to regulate tendon fibril diameter during fibrillogenesis (34) and aging (35). Type III collagen synthesis increases during early repair but is believed to then decrease as new type I collagen is synthesized and organized (36–39). Other glycoproteins such as decorin (located in the tropocollagen interstices) are also believed to regulate fibril diameter and to provide fibril-to-fibril and fibril-to-proteoglycan binding (40, 41).

FAILURE AND SUBFAILURE BIOMECHANICS To judge the fate of tendon healing and repair, the biomechanical properties of the normal tendon are usually determined and then used as a benchmark for comparison. Traditionally, uninjured normal

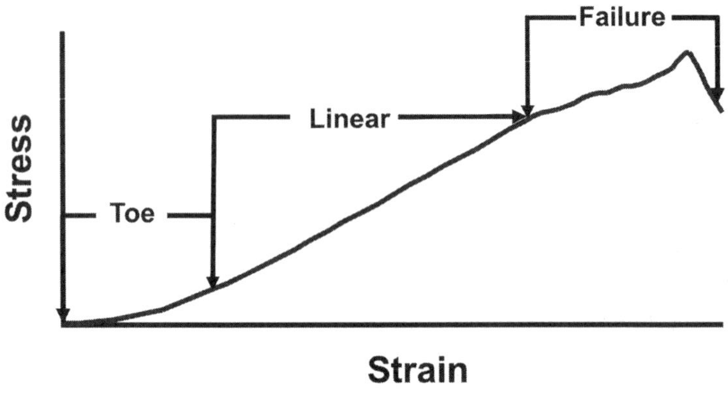


**Figure 2** Stress-strain curve showing the initial nonlinear toe region followed by a linear region up to a failure region. Serial and progressive drops occur in the curve during the failure process.

tendons are failed in tension to determine their ultimate or failure properties. The bone is gripped at one end and the tendon at the other (except in cases like the patellar tendon that has a sesamoid bone that permits gripping at both ends) (36–39). After aligning the centerline axis of the tendon with the loading axis to more uniformly distribute forces across the fibers, the tissue is rapidly failed in tension while force and displacement are recorded. To permit comparisons among tissues with different dimensions, the force is usually normalized by the tissue's initial cross-sectional area (tensile stress) and the displacement is normalized by the initial tissue length (tensile strain). Plotting the two parameters against each other up to failure results in a nonlinear stress-strain response (Figure 2) composed of three regions. In the toe region, the curve is concave upward, and the modulus or slope continually increases. In the linear region, the modulus becomes nearly constant. This is followed by the failure region, where small reductions in stress occur with progressive decreases in slope up to maximum stress and then rapid or progressive return to zero stress, depending on tissue organization. Linear modulus and maximum stress can range from 500 to 1000 MPa and 60 to 100 MPa, respectively, depending on fiber bundle organization, anatomical location, and species (35, 42–45). Corresponding strains to maximum stress can range from 13% to 22% when measured between grips and even lower (~5% to 8%) if strains are measured optically in the tendon midsubstance (13, 35, 43). Linear moduli nearly double using optically based strain measurements (1400 to 1700 MPa) (35, 42, 43).

More relevant, however, may be a tendon's subfailure properties because normal and repair tissues do not routinely fail in vivo. The subfailure response of tendon is typically characterized by controlling load and measuring increasing tensile deformation (static or cyclic creep), controlling deformation and measuring decreasing load (static or cyclic stress relaxation), and/or monitoring changes in loading and unloading behavior (hysteresis). Although these tests are straightforward to perform, setting the testing conditions (e.g., peak stresses in creep and peak strains in relaxation) are more difficult if the operator is trying to simulate the in vivo setting (see Functional Approach to Treatment, below). Simulation also requires knowledge of in vivo temporal events (such as rates of loading and duty cycles), which are not typically done during creep or relaxation testing.

TENDON ANATOMY, BIOCHEMISTRY, AND BIOMECHANICS Whereas the structural hierarchy of collagen and the biomechanical properties are reasonably well accepted, the mechanisms of force transmission through this hierarchy are not as clear. As a result, investigators continue to seek correlates of normal tendon anatomy, chemistry, and mechanical properties (46, 47). Examples include correlation of force with fibril diameter (35, 48, 49), cross-link density (50–52), and collagen composition (40, 53–55).

Understanding the dynamic and complex interplay of a tendon's constituents is critical to formalizing structure-function relationships and to effectively repairing a damaged tissue. Fibril diameter, for example, is influenced not only by type V collagen but also by type III collagen and decorin. (*a*) As a fibrillar collagen, type V can form homotypic fibrils composed of a single collagen type, but they more often coassemble into heterotypic fibrils with type I collagen (56). Its inhibitory effect on fibril diameter [e.g., in the cornea (34, 54)] presumably arises at the molecule's N terminus, where its hinged configuration protrudes radially outward and perpendicular to the long axis of the fibril (34). The hinged region controls fibril diameter through steric and static inhibitions (53). (*b*) Type III collagen, present during development and after injury, also may control fibril diameter through its N terminus, as does type V, but it does so closer to the surface of the type I collagen fibrils (57). (*c*) Decorin, a small proteoglycan, has also been implicated in controlling fibril diameter, where it interacts directly with specific regions on the collagen fibril. Although decorin's action is not thoroughly understood, mouse knockout studies and antisense treatments point to its involvement in controlling fibril diameter (40). Such studies in normal tendon are critical when attempting to repair or regenerate the injured tendon microstructure to improve force transmission.

## Modes of Injury

Acute and chronic tendon injuries differ in their modes and treatments. Acute injuries typically arise from trauma, whereas chronic injuries often occur after repetitive subfailure mechanical events followed by inflammation (58, 59). Acute extensor tendon injuries (e.g., closed tendon injuries of the hand and wrist) can be treated with nonoperative management (59, 60), but acute closed flexor tendon injuries usually require operative intervention. Chronic injuries can be associated with inflammation (tendonitis), without inflammation (tendinosis), or involve the surrounding tissue (peritendinitis). Delayed diagnosis may result in less successful operative intervention and even produce permanent disability regardless of treatment. Surprisingly, athletes often return quickly to their preinjury level of participation regardless of treatment (59, 60); however, they then remain at higher risk for future injury and degeneration.

An example of overuse injury is found in the rotator cuff tendons, which do not spontaneously heal, in part due to the complex anatomy and extended range of motion of the shoulder joint, as well as to the relative weakening and hypovascularization of the cuff tendons (5). Acute tears commonly occur in athletes participating in overhead sports (61), whereas chronic degeneration and tearing tend to occur in older more sedentary subjects (6). Chronic degeneration increases both the frequency and size of the tears with aging and is considered the primary contributing factor in tendon pathogenesis (5, 7, 62). Untreated partial defects of the rotator cuff, whether traumatic or degenerative in origin, can sometimes progress toward massive connective tissue tears (5, 61, 63). As degenerative weakening of the rotator cuff progresses, the stability and mechanics of the shoulder joint are greatly compromised.

The Achilles tendon is often injured traumatically, but it is also frequently involved in chronic injuries. Acute Achilles tendon injury and pain usually occur in active individuals, when the tendon is subjected to high or unusual loads. Surgical repair after rupture is encouraged in patients seeking to continue sports participation, as the rerupture rate in those treated conservatively has been shown to be significantly higher than those treated surgically (4). If the tendon remains intact, the long-term outcomes in those managed conservatively has been reported to be similar to those treated operatively (4, 64, 65). In contrast to acute injuries, Achilles tendinopathies are caused by repeated microinjuries coupled with a degenerative or failed healing response. Although the process of tendon disruption that leads to microinjury is unknown, it may fail to stimulate an adequate inflammatory response to begin the reparative cycle (66). Whereas acute tendon injuries heal with a standard triphasic response (see Healing Process, below) and return slowly to a structure that resembles normal tendon organization (40), it is unclear why overuse tendinopathies do not similarly respond with this triphasic response. Tendinopathy is noninflammatory and can be resistant to treatment, as symptoms may persist despite both conservative and surgical intervention (64, 67, 68).

## BIOLOGY AND BIOMECHANICS OF NATURAL HEALING

Although surgical repair is frequently performed, one option is to allow the tendon to heal naturally, without any intervention. We first discuss this healing process or cascade. Several issues related to natural healing are then reviewed, providing operative controls or baseline healing data against which various surgical treatment options can be compared. As such, these data provide benchmark biomechanics for newly synthesized tissue, important data for establishing structure-function relationships for scar tissue, and for contrasting basic healing with healing induced through primary surgical repair and tissue engineering approaches.

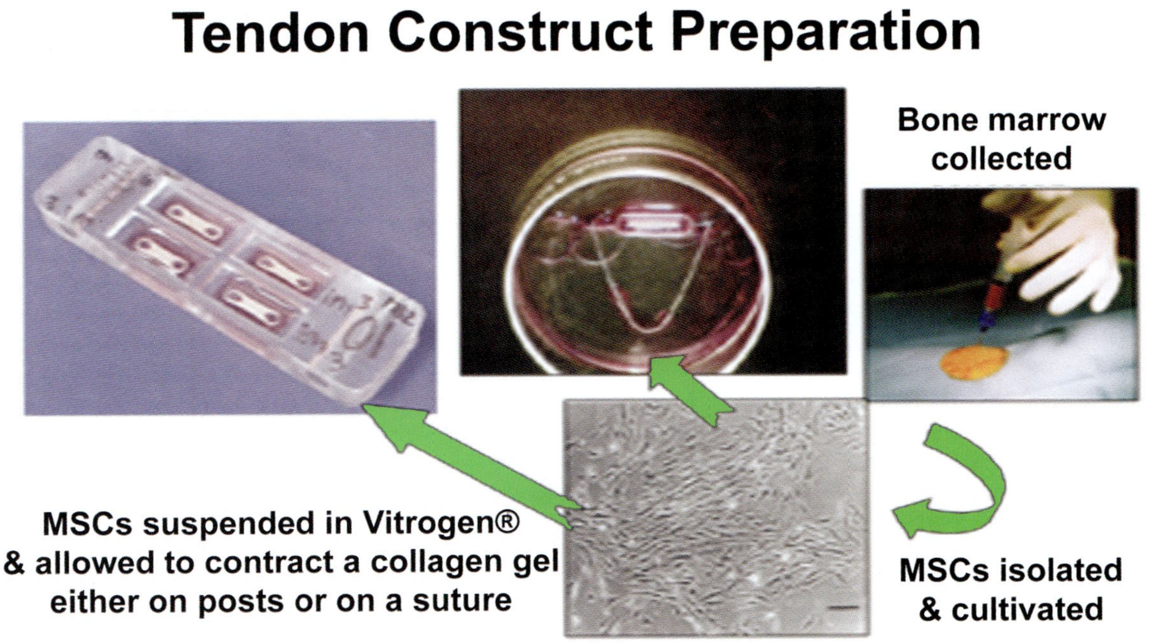


**Figure 3** A tissue-engineered approach to create tendon repairs. Mesenchymal stem cells (MSCs) are isolated from bone marrow, cultivated and proliferated in culture, and delivered either to a glass boat containing a tensioned suture or to a silicone dish containing four wells with posts protruding from the base of each well.

## Healing Process

The wound healing cascade is well known, generally shared among soft connective tissues, and only briefly reviewed in this section. More detailed discussions exist in the literature (40, 69–72).

Inflammation after injury protects the body by eliminating and diluting harmful agents, preventing further injury, supplying large quantities of oxygen and nutrients needed for repair, and allowing the entry of clotting agents. Inflammation is triggered by several chemical mediators, (e.g., histamines, kinins, prostaglandins, complement, lymphokines) (40). During histogenesis, the clot formed during inflammation is transformed into granulation tissue, so called for its visually granular appearance caused by the capillaries that permeate the clot. Macrophages digest and remove the clot while providing a continuing source of growth factors. As fibroblasts infiltrate the wound, blood vessels form to carry oxygen and nutrients to the developing tissue. Finally, during remodeling, granulation tissue is supplanted by new collagen synthesis and deposition and by remodeling myofibroblasts that contract the matrix along the axis of the tendon. Wound healing cells and their matrix exist in a dynamic reciprocity whereby cells deposit new matrix and the matrix modulates gene expression and cell-matrix receptors (69). Through cell-cell and cell-matrix interactions, collagen fibrils align with fibroblasts and join end-to-end with other fibrils in the wound and at the margin via covalent cross-links (69). Most fibroblasts then enter apoptosis (programmed cell death), thereby transitioning from a highly cellular granulation tissue to a less densely populated scar tissue.

## Issues with Natural Healing

There are four important issues to consider in natural healing: (*a*) the source of cells (intrinsic and/or extrinsic), (*b*) the source of nutrition (vascular or synovial), (*c*) the consequences of a gap in the muscle-tendon complex, and (*d*) whether a conservative treatment actually heals a tendon wound sufficiently. (*a*) Intrinsic repair relies solely on the tissue's own cells to effect healing, whereas extrinsic repair relies on cellular infiltration from external tissue sources including the synovial sheath. Typically, both modes are involved, the extrinsic being involved early and the intrinsic at later intervals. One consequence of extrinsic repair is the appearance of adhesions as surrounding tissues incorporate into the scar. This process, which is extremely common in flexor tendons, often results in impaired range of motion. (*b*)Vascularity is key in this healing process in most regions of the tendon, except in the so-called pulley regions that rely on synovial diffusion. (*c*) When the gap from a retracted tendon is not restored, the range of motion and strength generated by affected muscle diminishes greatly. Gap dimensions (length, width, and thickness), gap shape, and the extent of disruption are all expected to affect the outcome. As might be expected, the rate and extent of natural healing slow as the gap dimensions increase (73). Fewer cells are required to fill a smaller gap with scar tissue than to fill a larger gap, and the presence of some intact tissue in a partial thickness injury can maintain gap length during the healing process. Of course, scalpel incisions introduced at surgery to control gap dimensions do not reflect the actual type of injury that occurs in vivo and hence represent a "best care scenario" of healing rate and magnitude. (*d*) During natural healing, forces from the in-series muscle would seem capable of retracting the failed ends and leaving a large gap to fill. In one study involving transection and partial resection of the Achilles tendon in the sheep model, the wound site appeared to heal spontaneously without postoperative immobilization and resulted in sufficient stability within 12 months without surgical readaptation (74). All sheep regained partial weight-bearing capacity after at least 6 weeks and showed no limping or gait restrictions after at least 8 weeks (74). However, the wound site was still weak (low failure force) compared with normal tissue, possibly a result of the forces generated by the soleus and gastrocnemius muscles to create ankle plantar flexion. In a second report, unsutured and sutured central-third repairs were compared in the rabbit patellar tendon model (75). Several measures (failure load, ultimate stress, and stiffness) showed significant initial declines but gradually returned to normal 9 months after the injury. No significant differences were reported between the two groups for collagen content, failure load, ultimate stress, and stiffness (75). Although these results suggest that conservative treatment is no better than operative repair, the level of activity in the rabbits may not have challenged either scar tissue. Because these values were not compared with normal values, neither may have achieved acceptable values.

Some tissues heal well without surgical repair, depending on the specific tissue, the extent of the injury, and the postinjury rehabilitation regime (4, 10, 74). Not surprisingly, tendon ends in apposition achieve a better biomechanical outcome than those where a gap must be filled with scar tissue (73, 76). Partial tendon tears may function sufficiently well without any treatment (77, 78). Complete Achilles tendon tears appear to heal better when the ankle is maintained in plantar flexion. However, flexor tendon injuries in the hand often require surgery to re-establish contact between the tendon ends, and rotator cuff injuries heal incompletely after 12 weeks (79).

## Biomechanics of Natural Healing

Whereas healing tendons can withstand nearly half of normal failure force over time, the temporal changes in repair strength are nonlinear and exhibit a rapid early increase in strength followed by slower improvements. The tendons often do not achieve normal tendon failure force in the long-term. For example, only 1.5 months after creating a defect injury in the patellar tendon, the repair tissue achieves 7–9% of normal failure force (42). By 3 and 6 months after injury, however, repair tissue failure force has modestly changed to only 11% and 8% of normal, respectively. A patellar tendon defect in the goat knee generates a higher relative failure force than in the rabbit model, but even 21 months after surgery, the repair tissue filling the injury achieves only 49% of normal failure force values (80). Similarly, Achilles tendon scars reached 48% of normal failure force after 0.5 months (81). Even rotator cuff tears tolerate 42% of failure load after 3 months in spite of the fact that they still possess open voids in the scar tissue (79).

Whether these healing percentages are satisfactory depends on several factors including the expected tissue loads transmitted by the in-series muscle in vivo (see Functional Approach to Treatment, below) and changes that occur in the quality of the tissue scar over time. Repair quality often remains inferior because of the creation of a large collagen callus at the wound site consisting of small, poorly organized collagen fibrils (42, 74, 80) and increased cellularity and vascularity (neither of which contributes to load-bearing capabilities) (80). Although the cross-sectional area of this large callus tissue decreases over time (42, 79, 80), the area still has larger than normal values at later repair intervals (79). Two material parameters, maximum stress and linear modulus, are generally low in the scar compared with normal values. For example, maximum stress values in the patellar tendon scar are about 19% of normal values at 6 months (42) and 35% of normal after 21 months (80). Achilles tendon maximum stress values are 10% of normal at 2 weeks (81) and 57% of normal after 12 months (74).

# BIOLOGY AND BIOMECHANICS OF SURGICAL REPAIR

## Clinical Outcomes Following Surgical Repair

Clinically, surgeons repair tendons that do not heal well on their own using a variety of traditional and innovative methods that vary with tendon location. Conventional treatments seek to increase repair strength by increasing the number of core sutures or by using a wire loop to pretension the core suture (82–87). Others use internal stainless steel tendon anchors (88). (*a*) Flexor tendon—flexor tendon repair remains a significant challenge (89). Multi-strand, multi-grasp suture techniques are typically used (85, 90–92). Three methods [Tajima, Savage, and eight-strand repair (92a)] significantly improve gliding function compared with those that feature external knots (Kessler and Tsuge) and those that tend to bunch at the repair site (double-loop locking suture) (90). Eight-strand repair shows the greatest initial failure force of all tested methods (90). (*b*) Achilles tendon—repairing ruptured Achilles tendon has been difficult because the repair is often not strong enough to allow early active range of motion exercises of the foot and ankle and early weight-bearing (93–95). Kirschmayer core suture and cross-stitch epitenon suture (96) appear to have stronger initial mechanical properties (97) than previous methods of Achilles tendon repair. Open repair using a Kessler-type suture and apposition sutures (95), combined with accelerated rehabilitation, appears to improve recovery of foot function, mobility, and strength. (*c*) Rotator cuff tendons—surgeons advocate early primary anatomic repair of rotator cuff tears followed by careful rehabilitation (61). Chronic degenerative injuries, however, often generate excessive tension following primary repair and may fail (98). In fact, primary repairs of larger chronic tears can fail up to 38% of the time owing to tendon weakening and muscle atrophy (7, 99). Extensive tendon mobilization has been advocated to treat large cuff defects to reduce tissue tension, improve repair strength, and restore joint stability (100, 101). Even with these techniques, however, failure rates can reach 40% due to muscle contraction, decreased range of joint motion, neurovascular damage, or postoperative alteration of normal shoulder mechanics (100, 101). Arthroscopic rotator cuff repair is another means of treatment. This technique can achieve good to excellent results in a large percentage of patients, independent of tear size (102–105). Repairing u-shaped tears by converging the margins produces results comparable to those of crescent-shaped tears repaired directly by a tendon-to-bone technique (102). There is a rapid return to full overhead function after arthroscopic rotator cuff repair (average, 4 months for all tear sizes) (102, 103, 105, 106).

## Biology of Primary Repair

When injuries are repaired with suture, the biological response is similar to that outlined above. The addition of the suture, however, can engender an additional foreign body reaction. The extent of the reaction depends on the suture material and its biodegradability. Nonabsorbable materials will become enveloped by fibrous capsule, whereas absorbable materials, on the other hand, illicit a migration of giant cells and other phagocytes into the wound site (107). Increased inflammation (108) causes a more diffuse repair of lower repair quality and risks adhesion formation that can limit gliding and range of motion (109).

## Biomechanics of Primary Repair

Various techniques have been used to repair tendons in animal studies (86, 87, 89, 110–112). Conventional treatments seek to increase repair strength by increasing the number of core sutures (86, 87, 89, 110). A four- or eight-strand suture technique in the canine model was employed to repair the flexor digitorum profundus (86). The eight-strand suture technique did not result in increased stiffness or strength compared with a four-strand technique, and the ultimate force did not increase with time (86). These lower failure forces were consistent with reduced collagen content. In the pig model (89), a four-strand adaptation of the Kessler technique was found to be significantly stronger than the modified Kessler technique (89) and easier to perform than other multi-strand suture techniques. Partial lacerations in the canine flexor tendon (110) have also been repaired using Lee, modified four-strand Savage, Kessler, modified Kessler, and augmented Becker core suture techniques. The modified Kessler and modified Savage repair techniques were shown to be significantly stronger than the Lee suture method. However, all these repair techniques were weaker than unrepaired tendons (110). Based on these results, it would be appropriate to pursue other innovative approaches to improve repair strength. The persistent question, however, is how good is good enough?

# NEW TREATMENT STRATEGIES

## Tissue Engineering

New approaches are being developed to treat tendon injuries including the use of tissue engineering (TE), which combines principles of engineering and biology to fabricate new generations of reparative tissue constructs (113, 114). The process usually involves the creation of constructs for surgery that contain cells alone, scaffold alone, or cells and scaffolds combined (113–115). Those constructs that include cells typically require the manipulation of the cells in culture (in vitro phase) prior to their implantation at surgery (in vivo phase). Differentiated tenocytes can be handled in culture, as well as undifferentiated mesenchymal stem cells. The in vitro phase often requires cell proliferation to increase the number of cells and differentiation to control cell phenotype, which then must be maintained after introducing a delivery vehicle or scaffold (Figure 3, see color insert).

IN VITRO TISSUE ENGINEERING STUDIES In many in vitro tissue engineering studies, cells are delivered on two-dimensional substrates or in three-dimensional constructs. These studies are usually performed in bioreactors designed to apply physical stimuli (e.g., strain or stress) to the cell-based structures as they mature. Delivering these stimuli to control cell phenotype and matrix expression seems warranted on the basis of the pioneering studies of Yasuda et al. and Hayashi et al. showing the rapid and large reductions in material properties after stress shielding the patellar tendon in vivo (116, 117, 119). It is now well known that cells attached to deforming two-dimensional substrates can modify their orientation and cytoskeleton (120–123), their proliferation rates (121, 124–127), and their protein transcription (mRNA) or synthesis (127–130). Similar effects occur using tendon cells on substrates, including increased DNA synthesis (124) and the expression of novel genes (130).

Understanding the mechanisms by which cells that are attached to substrates sense mechanical stimuli and alter gene expression and protein synthesis is important to engineering an appropriate construct. Two leading mediators of this signal transduction are the integrin family of membrane-bound ECM receptors and stretch-activated ion channels. Cytoskeletal tension is known to regulate cell and nuclear shape (131, 132). Integrins bind matrix molecules on the cell surface, and the cytoplasmic tail binds to the cytoskeleton via $\alpha$-actinin or talin (133–135). These bound integrin subunits then cluster to form focal adhesions. In the case of stretch-activated ion channels, cell deformation (by plasma membrane indentation, tension, or shear stress) induces rapid internal calcium transients (136–140). The stretch-activated channel is linked to the cytoskeleton that, in turn, affects cell behavior (141). These responses to mechanical stimulation, regardless of the initial mechanism, activate a kinase cascade (e.g., ERK, FAK) that then modulates gene expression. Replicating normal cell-cell and cell-ECM events in culture would seem advantageous.

Whereas in vitro studies examining the effects of mechanical stimulation of cells on two-dimensional monolayers are valuable, studies in three dimensions more accurately model cell-ECM interactions (142). Novel bioreactors for three-dimensional culture have been developed to fabricate and condition constructs for tendon and ligament repair in a stable environment (37°C, 95% relative humidity, 5% $CO_2$). Many of these reactors utilize cells seeded in collagen gels for examination under static (42, 108, 143–145) and dynamic conditions (146–148). Under static conditions, the cells can contract a gel around a tensioned suture (42, 108, 143) or around a pair of posts (144, 145) in a manner dependent on cell and collagen densities (cell-to-collagen ratio) and time. Nuclei align more rapidly with the suture axis and elongate more fully at higher cell-to-collagen ratios (143). Typically, the construct is fabricated, gripped, and stretched cyclically using a linear motor (146), stepper motor, and pulley system (147), or a stepper and gear system (148). The tissue-engineered constructs can be maintained in culture for several weeks with several media exchanges and then removed for evaluation. Some of the bioreactors have load cells that can monitor the development of the tissue in real time (146, 147).

Although several methods of mechanical stimulation of tendon or ligament have been reported, one study to tissue engineer the anterior cruciate ligament is noteworthy. In order to direct differentiation of MSCs via mechanical stimulation, Altman et al. (127, 148) developed a unique bioreactor similar to those described above, but capable of delivering translational and rotational strains (10% strain and 90° rotation at one cycle per minute) to account for the helical orientation of the collagen fibers and the complex loading experienced by the tissue. After 21 days of stimulation, MSCs expressed mRNA for types I and III collagen and tenascin-C, all of which are indicators of a fibroblast phenotype, but there was no upregulation of osteo- or chondro-specific markers. Histologically the cells appeared elongated and in parallel with the helically oriented collagen fibers. Unfortunately, no mechanical tests were performed to evaluate the quality of the resulting tissue-engineered ligament.

IN VIVO REPAIR (SURGICAL EVALUATION) STUDIES AND BIOMECHANICS Many of the recent tissue engineering studies designed to accelerate tendon repair have compared results for undifferentiated MSC repair with those for natural repair and sham control (42, 108, 149–151). MSCs are typically mixed with type I collagen gels and implanted in window and central full-length defects in the rabbit patellar tendon (42, 149) and in gap defects in the Achilles tendon (108, 150, 151). Compared with repairs containing only collagen gels, MSC-gel composites introduced in window defects result in modest 18% to 33% improvements in the material properties of the repair tissue (149). However, when the MSC-gel construct is first organized in culture (permitted to contract around sutures) before being implanted in gap defect wounds in the Achilles tendon, the resulting repair biomechanics are vastly improved compared with natural healing (108). In fact, the structural properties for the MSC-seeded repairs are twice those for natural healing as early as 4 weeks after the procedure, suggesting the potential for more rapid return to normal function. Maximum force and stiffness generated by the repairs achieve 66% and 54% of normal values, respectively, values that would appear to be satisfactory but not really established. When these cell-gel-suture composites are then seeded at three different MSC concentrations (1, 4, and 8 million cells per ml) for repair of central patellar tendon defects in the rabbit (42, 149), the cell-seed repairs are 50% greater in maximum force and stiffness at 12 weeks compared with values for natural repair tissues. At 12 weeks after surgery, maximum stress and modulus of the grafted repairs are 37% and 94%, respectively, greater than for natural repair tissues (42). However, no significant differences were found in repair outcome among the three cell density conditions (42). Using a poly-lactide-co-glycolide acid (PLGA) scaffold instead of collagen gel with suture, MSCs were found to produce denser matrix than scaffold alone, and an apparent crimp pattern was evident at 4 weeks (150). At 12 weeks, the stiffness of the repair tissue treated by PLGA with MSCs reached 87% compared with 56% in repairs using PLGA alone. The addition of the MSCs resulted in a 55% improvement in stiffness over the scaffold alone (151); however, there was only a small but insignificant difference in the modulus.

Autologous tenocytes have also been used in different configurations and animal models to improve tendon repair outcome. Tenocytes have been mixed with unwoven polyglycolic acid (PGA) fibers and wrapped with intestinal submucosa to form a cell-scaffold construct for the hen flexor digitorum profundus (FDP) (152). The engineered tendons resemble natural tendons not only in gross appearance and histologic structure but also in biomechanical properties. Biomechanical analysis in the hen FDP (152) demonstrates increased maximum stress for the engineered tendons with time, which reached 83% of normal tendon strength at 14 weeks. However, the maximum stress of the scaffold material (PGA) accounts for only 9% of normal tendon strength, indicating poor tissue quality. Porcine small intestinal submucosa has also been used to replace a completely resected infraspinatus tendon in the dog model (61). The gross appearance, histologic continuity, and failure mode of the constructs mimic the results for sham-operated and native infraspinatus tendons. Although the ultimate strength of the small intestinal submucosa repairs was significantly less than that of native infraspinatus tendons, it was similar to that of reimplanted tendons at 3 and 6 months (61). The results of these studies (42, 61, 108, 149, 151, 152) indicate that tendon tissue could be engineered in vivo to bridge a tendon defect.

## Functional Approach to Treatment

The past and current approaches that have been used to evaluate and direct tendon repair therapies (Figure 1) have contributed greatly to the treatment of injuries. To further advance tendon repair, we propose a shift in approach from making comparisons under idealized in vitro conditions that may not capture the true in vivo operating conditions. Instead, we propose an alternative approach based

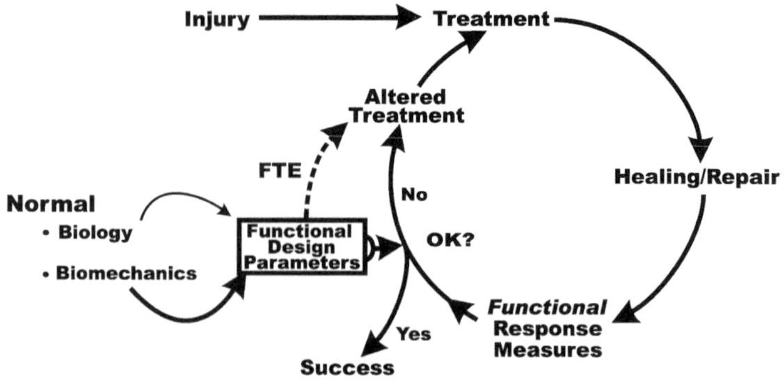


**Figure 4** Functional design parameters incorporated in an alternative paradigm for tendon repair treatment. These design parameters are selected after establishing the in vivo environment that acts on the normal tissue and recognizing that the repairs might also experience these in vivo signals. It is hoped that the iterative process of improving repair outcome measures is shortened. These measures might also be used in functional tissue engineering (FTE) to stimulate the tissue-engineered constructs to accelerate this iterative process.

on functional tissue engineering (113, 114, 153) that seeks to regain functional efficacy by restoring both the in vivo joint kinematics as well as the regional tissue properties.

NEED FOR INCORPORATING FUNCTIONALITY IN REPAIR ASSESSMENT AND TISSUE ENGINEERING The unpredictable nature of tendon repair suggests that an alternative approach be taken. A revised paradigm, shown in Figure 4, provides functional design parameters that are based on in vivo function rather than on a comparison of repair parameters with standard biomechanical parameters for normal tissue such as stiffness and maximum force. In so doing, this approach seeks to better meet the expected need for the repairing tissue in vivo. These functional design parameters also serve as stimulation inputs for a tissue-engineered construct before surgery using principles of functional tissue engineering (FTE ) (113, 114, 153). This approach, which utilizes a FTE road map, is depicted in Figure 5. Following an injury, a differentiated or undifferentiated cell source must be selected, isolated, and propagated. After introducing biopolymers and then permitting morphogenesis, growth factors and mechanical signals can be timed in culture to optimize the resulting tissue substitute. After surgical implantation, wound healing, and histogenesis, the tissue either undergoes regeneration to a normal tissue or more likely undergoes repair. The question remains, have we achieved functional efficacy? If the answer is yes then we can move into product development; if not, the problem needs to be identified and the construct re-engineered. To illustrate the approach shown in Figure 4, we now revisit the behavior of normal tissue but focus on in vivo function rather than failure biomechanics. Functional design parameters are

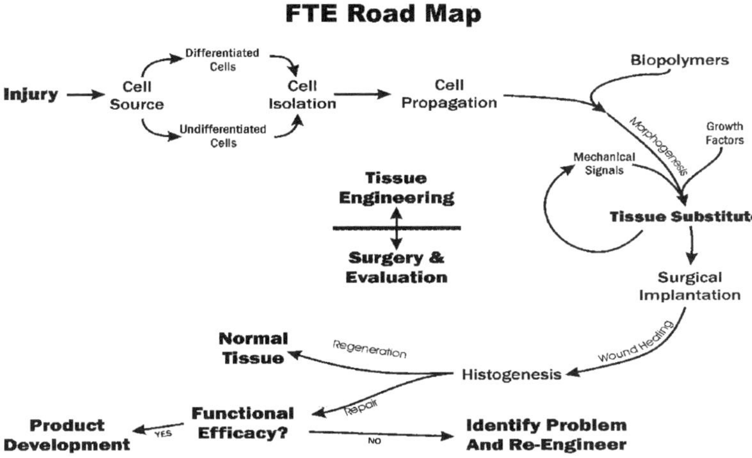


**Figure 5** Functional tissue engineering road map consisting of a tissue engineering phase (in culture) and a surgery and evaluation phase (in vivo). After injury, either differentiated or undifferentiated cells are isolated, propagated, mixed with biopolymers, permitted to undergo morphogenesis, and possibly exposed to mechanical signals and/or growth factors. The resulting tissue-engineered substitute is ready for surgical implantation, wound healing, and histogenesis. Ideally, there is true regeneration to normal tissue, which is a rare event, or else an inferior repair. This repair must be judged as to its functional efficacy. If efficacious, product development can proceed; if not, we must identify the problem and re-engineer. Comparison with normal in vivo behavior is essential.

determined after which this functional approach is applied to our tendon tissue engineered repair data (Applying a Functional Approach to Tissue Engineering, below).

ESTABLISHING IN VIVO FUNCTION, IN VIVO FORCES, AND STRAINS Tendons rapidly transmit large in-series muscle forces to produce joint movement. These transmitted forces are difficult to measure and may reach many times body weight, much larger than forces transmitted by ligaments that connect bone to bone at a joint. Numerous investigators (154–159) have measured these in vivo tendon and ligament forces using buckle E-type gauges (160), implantable force transducers (154, 155, 158, 159), modified pressure transducers (154), and devices involving fiber optical technology (161). In vivo muscle filament strains have also been measured using laser diffraction techniques and correlated with tendon strains (162). Typically, force-time patterns are parameterized by measuring peak and minimum forces and rates of change in force (154, 155, 159) (Figure 6). Peak tendon forces and the rates of rise and fall in in vivo force increase with increasing levels of activity (154, 155, 159). Actual peak force values vary with anatomical location

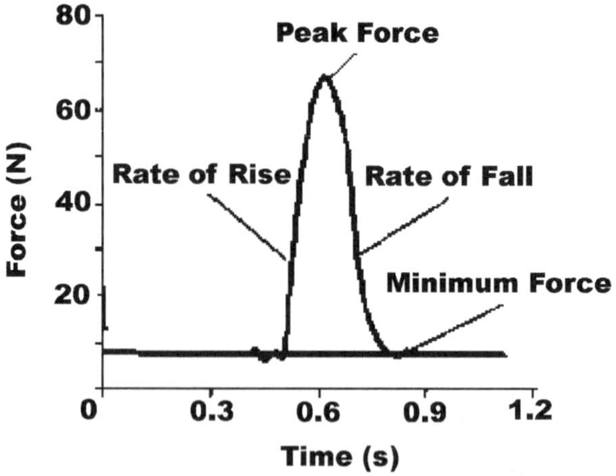


**Figure 6** In vivo force signal for the rabbit patellar tendon. Four parameters are shown for one hop in vivo. They include the peak force, the minimum force, and the rates of rise and fall in force. These parameters can be used to establish functional design parameters for tendon repair.

and species, reaching 100 N in the rabbit patellar tendon and Achilles tendon and approximately 1000 N in the goat patellar tendon (154, 155, 159). Minimum tendon force during quiet standing remains nearly constant in the patellar, Achilles, and flexor digitorum profundus tendons (154, 155, 159). In vivo strains for these tendons have been calculated from these in vivo forces for rabbit patellar tendon and oscillate between 1% and 4% (159). These results can then be used to set functional design parameters.

SETTING FUNCTIONAL DESIGN PARAMETERS Ideally, we seek to design a repair that matches the failure properties of specific tendon models (42, 108, 149). Although this outcome may be achieved in some repair scenarios, this is often at the expense of much larger elongations and strains than experienced by the normal tendon. More often, the repairs are only fractions of normal tissue failure force or stiffness. Developing a common set of functional design parameters is useful.

One way to develop such a common set is to determine how the recorded in vivo forces compare with the failure properties for the normal tissue. Revisiting the in vivo forces measured in the previous section for the rabbit FDP (155) and goat patellar tendon (154), forces and stresses approach 30% to 40% of their failure forces during the most vigorous activities, whereas rabbit patellar and Achilles tendon (159) forces achieve only about 10% and 20% of failure forces, respectively. To design tendon repairs that meet and actually exceed in vivo functional demands, (154, 155, 159, 161, 162), in vivo forces and strains as described above should be recorded for each specific tendon model. After obtaining these in vivo data, researchers should add an extra buffer or safety factor for each parameter (maximum force, stiffness, energy, etc.) and then consider comparing each value with the corresponding failure property and thus generate a set of relevant functional design parameters for specific tendon models.

It is also important to recognize that these thresholds for in vivo force are activity-level dependent and can be used to set design parameters for different repair approaches. Using the conventional force-displacement and stress-strain curves for normal tendon, the associated in vivo displacements and strains can be calculated (159). With this information, the in vivo stiffness and strain energy ranges can be established. The functional design parameters can be selected on the basis of these in vivo force and displacement thresholds (Figure 6). The selection of the parameters will depend on whether the tendon repair needs to match the in vivo forces (stresses) or displacements (strains) for a low, intermediate, or high level of activity.

For example, our group has used actual in vivo forces and displacements to mechanically stimulate tendon tissue–engineered constructs in culture. Because these constructs are initially compliant and weak, we impose minimum (1%) and maximum or peak strains (3%–4%) rather than in vivo forces during construct maturation. These minimum and peak forces are converted to strains using constitutive (stress-strain) relationships from the contralateral normal tendon. We then impose these strains in custom-designed bioreactors early after construct creation. This approach of delivering simulated in vivo signals will hopefully improve the mechanical properties of the constructs before surgery and lead to functionally efficaceous repair biomechanics after surgery.

The essential issue is that design parameters do not need to be chosen at random. These parameters should instead take into consideration the in vivo environment and the in vivo functional demands that likely vary with anatomical location and species. The functional design parameters will serve as landmarks to compare with the response outcome of each tendon repair and establish whether good is good enough.

APPLYING A FUNCTIONAL APPROACH TO TISSUE ENGINEERING Revisiting our tendon repair data, these functional design parameters can help us assess whether the repair is acceptable or whether new treatments and iterations are required (Figure 4). For the tissue-engineered repairs for rabbit patellar tendon (42, 149), the window defect and full-length central repairs are 9% to 11% of failure force, comparable to the 11% peak force measured in vivo (159) but thus not acceptable for the levels of activity imposed. By contrast, the failure forces for the rabbit Achilles tendon are 66% of normal failure force and thus well above the 20% of failure force from in vivo force measurements.

However, these repairs may still not be acceptable if the repair tissues do not meet other criteria. For example, if the forces in the repair achieve the threshold of in vivo force (IVF), but do so at a large additional repair displacement (ARD) (Figure 7), then the repair may not be functioning as needed. Thus it is also important to compare these displacements at a common IVF, as well as compare the

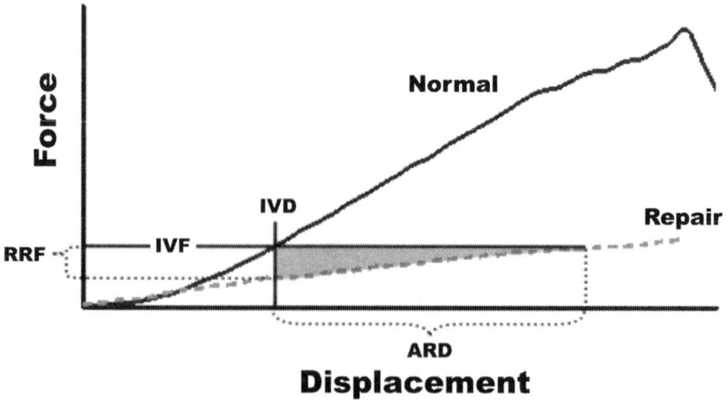


**Figure 7** Force displacement curve for normal and repair tendons. Based on in vivo measurements, thresholds of in vivo force (IVF) and in vivo displacement (IVD) can be established for a specific activity. Note the additional repair displacement (ARD) when comparing repair tissue with normal tissue at a common IVF threshold. Similarly, for a common IVD threshold, note the reduced repair force (RRF) generated by the healing tissue. The relative sizes of ARD and RRF dictate how successful the repair is compared with normal tissue under common force and displacement conditions, respectively.

repair and normal stiffness at this threshold. Alternatively, if the tissue is expected to be functioning more in a displacement-controlled setting (i.e., thresholds of in vivo displacement or IVD), then the associated reduced repair force (RRF) should be determined for each activity level.

## FUTURE DIRECTIONS: FACTORS IN TENDON REPAIR BIOLOGY AND BIOMECHANICS

In spite of the long and sustained progress made by countless investigators in trying to understand and evaluate repair processes after tendon injury, much remains to be accomplished. Most notably, we must focus on identifying and quantifying various factors affecting the biology and biomechanics of tendon repair as well as their interaction. At present, our understanding of tendon biology is quite descriptive, including the various phases of repair (inflammation, histogenesis, and remodeling) and their time course. Tendon biomechanical parameters appear to better quantify the state of the repair tissue over time, but even these measures can be simply convenient to record in the laboratory rather than a more realistic assessment of in vivo events. Agreeing on what measures should be utilized and actually performing these studies remain major challenges for the orthopedic science community. However, once these experiments are identified and agreed to, they may form the basis for assessment of the repair state of other soft and hard tissues in the body. In so doing, we should be better able to chart how best to proceed with new and innovative repair technologies and thereby effect more rapid return of the patient to preinjury status.

Armed with a set of more realistic biological and biomechanical assessment tools, investigators can then begin to judge the effects of other factors on tendon repair. The roles of aging, immobility, exercise, and gender on natural tendon repair processes require closer scrutiny as they form the foundation for judging repair events. Other cell and gene therapies can then be carefully screened in light of these natural repair outcomes. The effects of new surgical techniques, such as tissue shrinkage methods and local drug delivery, can then be quantified. And as new and exciting technologies are uncovered, the field retains a basis for judging both their safety and efficacy. Rapid assessment will also lead to lower development costs as less successful methods are discarded and more promising techniques are pursued using a rational treatment paradigm.

## ACKNOWLEDGMENTS

Portions of the research presented in this review were supported by a grant from the National Institutes of Health (AR 46574) given to the University of Cincinnati, NIH SBIR grant (AR42618), by Cincinnati Sports Medicine Research and Education Foundation, and VA Merit review grant (Gregory Boivin). The authors thank Gregory Boivin, Hani Awad, Randy Young, Stephen Gordon, David Fink, John West, Matthew Harris, and Shun Yoshida for much of our work presented in this review, and Kyle Adkins for his assistance in the creation of the figures.

**The *Annual Review of Biomedical Engineering* is online at http://bioeng.annualreviews.org**

## LITERATURE CITED

1. Praemer A, Furner S, Rice D. 1992. *Musculoskeletal Condition in the United States*. Parke Ridge, IL: Am. Acad. Orthop. Surg. 199 pp.
2. Praemer AF, Furner S, Rice DP. 1999. *Musculoskeletal Condition in the United States*. Parke Ridge, IL: Am. Acad. Orthop. Surg. 182 pp.
3. Wong J, Barrass V, Maffulli N. 2002. Quantitative review of operative and nonoperative management of Achilles tendon ruptures. *Am. J. Sports Med.* 30:565–75
4. Kocher MS, Bishop J, Marshall R, Briggs KK, Hawkins RJ. 2002. Operative versus nonoperative management of acute Achilles tendon rupture: expected-value decision analysis. *Am. J. Sports Med.* 30: 783–90
5. Soslowsky LJ, Thomopoulos S, Tun S, Flanagan CL, Keefer CC, et al. 2000. Neer Award 1999. Overuse activity injures the supraspinatus tendon in an animal model: a histologic and biomechanical study. *J. Shoulder Elbow Surg.* 9:79–84
6. Cofield RH, Parvizi J, Hoffmeyer PJ, Lanzer WL, Ilstrup DM, Rowland CM. 2001. Surgical repair of chronic rotator cuff tears. A prospective long-term study. *J. Bone Joint Surg. Am.* 83-A:71–77
7. Romeo AA, Hang DW, Bach BR Jr, Shott

S. 1999. Repair of full thickness rotator cuff tears. Gender, age, and other factors affecting outcome. *Clin. Orthop.* 367:243–55

8. Yamaguchi K, Levine WN, Marra G, Galatz LM, Klepps S, Flatow EL. 2003. Transitioning to arthroscopic rotator cuff repair: the pros and cons. *Instr. Course Lect.* 52:81–92
9. Liu SH, Nguyen TM. 1999. Ankle sprains and other soft tissue injuries. *Curr. Opin. Rheumatol.* 11:132–37
10. Huang HH, Qureshi AA, Biundo JJ Jr. 2000. Sports and other soft tissue injuries, tendinitis, bursitis, and occupation-related syndromes. *Curr. Opin. Rheumatol.* 12:150–54
11. Butler D. 1989. Kappa Delta Award paper. Anterior cruciate ligament: its normal response and replacement. *J. Orthop. Res.* 7:910–21
12. Noyes FR, Barber-Westin SD. 1997. A comparison of results in acute and chronic anterior cruciate ligament ruptures of arthroscopically assisted autogenous patellar tendon reconstruction. *Am. J. Sports Med.* 25:460–71
13. Woo S, Chan S, Yamaji T. 1997. Biomechanics of knee ligament healing, repair and reconstruction. *J. Biomech.* 30:431–39
14. Ruotolo C, Nottage WM. 2002. Surgical and nonsurgical management of rotator cuff tears. *Arthroscopy* 18:527
15. Buckwalter JA, Lane NE. 1997. Athletics and osteoarthritis. *Am. J. Sports Med.* 25:873–81
16. Buckwalter J, Woo S, Goldberg V, Hadley E, Booth F, et al. 1993. Soft-tissue aging and musculoskeletal function. *J.Bone Joint Surg. Am.* 75:1533–48
17. Horan MA, Little RA, eds. 1998. *Injury in the Aging*. Cambridge/New York: Cambridge Univ. Press. 365 pp.
18. Amiel D, Frank C, Harwood F, Fronek J, Akeson W. 1984. Tendons and ligaments: a morphological and biochemical comparison. *J. Orthop. Res.* 1:257–65
19. Benjamin M, Ralphs JR. 1998. Fibrocartilage in tendons and ligaments—an adaptation to compressive load. *J. Anat.* 193:481–94
20. Rufai A, Ralphs JR, Benjamin M. 1995. Structure and histopathology of the insertional region of the human Achilles tendon. *J. Orthop. Res.* 13:585–93
21. Evans EJ, Benjamin M, Pemberton DJ. 1990. Fibrocartilage in the attachment zones of the quadriceps tendon and patellar ligament of man. *J. Anat.* 171:155–62
22. Almekinders L, Baynes A, Bracey L. 1995. An in vitro investigation into the effects of repetitive motion and nonsteroidal antiinflammatory medication on human tendon fibroblasts. *Am. J. Sports Med.* 23:119–23
23. Gillard GC, Birnbaum P, Reilly HC, Merrilees MJ, Flint MH. 1979. The effect of charged synthetic polymers on proteoglycan synthesis and sequestration in chick embryo fibroblast cultures. *Biochim. Biophys. Acta* 584:520–28
24. Gillard GC, Reilly HC, Bell-Booth PG, Flint MH. 1979. The influence of mechanical forces on the glycosaminoglycan content of the rabbit flexor digitorum profundus tendon. *Connective Tissue Res.* 7:37–46
25. Vogel KG, Ordog A, Pogany G, Olah J. 1993. Proteoglycans in the compressed region of human tibialis posterior tendon and in ligaments. *J. Orthop. Res.* 11:68–77
26. Fallon J, Blevins FT, Vogel K, Trotter J. 2002. Functional morphology of the supraspinatus tendon. *J. Orthop. Res.* 20:920–26
27. Giori NJ, Beaupre GS, Carter DR. 1993. Cellular shape and pressure may mediate mechanical control of tissue composition in tendons. *J. Orthop. Res.* 11:581–91
28. Butler DL, Sheh MY, Stouffer DC, Samaranayake VA, Levy MS. 1990. Surface strain variation in human patellar tendon and knee cruciate ligaments. *J. Biomech. Eng.* 112:38–45

29. Kastelic J, Galeski A, Baer E. 1978. The multicomposite structure of tendon. *Connective Tissue Res.* 6:11–23
30. Butler DL, Grood ES, Noyes FR, Zernicke RF, Brackett K. 1984. Effects of structure and strain measurement technique on the material properties of young human tendons and fascia. *J. Biomech.* 17:579–96
31. Bailey A, Paul R, Knott L. 1998. Mechanisms of maturation and ageing of collagen. *Mech. Ageing Dev.* 106:1–56
32. Kuhn K. 1987. The classical collagens: Types I, II, and III. In *Structure and Function of Collagen Types*. pp. 1–42. San Diego: Academic
33. Kannus P. 2000. Structure of the tendon connective tissue. *Scand J. Med. Sci. Sports* 10:312–20
34. Linsenmayer T, Gibney E, Igoe F, Gordon M, Fitch J, et al. 1993. Type V collagen: molecular structure and fibrillar organization of the chicken alpha 1(V) $NH_2$-terminal domain, a putative regulator of corneal fibrillogenesis. *J. Cell Biol.* 121:1181–89
35. Dressler MR, Butler DL, Wenstrup R, Awad HA, Smith F, Boivin GP. 2002. A potential mechanism for age-related declines in patellar tendon biomechanics. *J. Orthop. Res.* 20:1315–22
36. Liu SH, Yang RS, al-Shaikh R, Lane JM. 1995. Collagen in tendon, ligament, and bone healing. A current review. *Clin. Orthop.* 318:265–78
37. Riley GP, Harrall RL, Constant CR, Chard MD, Cawston TE, Hazleman BL. 1994. Tendon degeneration and chronic shoulder pain: changes in the collagen composition of the human rotator cuff tendons in rotator cuff tendinitis. *Ann. Rheum Dis.* 53:359–66
38. Holz U. 1980. Achilles tendon rupture and achillodynia. The importance of tissue regeneration. *Fortschr. Med.* 98:1517–20
39. Niyibizi C, Kavalkovich K, Yamaji T, Woo SL. 2000. Type V collagen is increased during rabbit medial collateral ligament healing. *Knee Surg. Sports Traumatol. Arthrosc.* 8:281–85
40. Frank C, Shrive N, Hiraoka H, Nakamura N, Kaneda Y, Hart D. 1999. Optimisation of the biology of soft tissue repair. *J. Sci. Med. Sport* 2:190–210
41. Derwin KA, Soslowsky LJ, Kimura JH, Plaas AH. 2001. Proteoglycans and glycosaminoglycan fine structure in the mouse tail tendon fascicle. *J. Orthop. Res.* 19:269–77
42. Awad HA, Boivin GP, Dressler MR, Smith FN, Young RG, Butler DL. 2003. Repair of patellar tendon injuries using a cell-collagen composite. *J. Orthop. Res.* 21:420–31
43. Tohyama H, Yasuda K. 2000. Extrinsic cell infiltration and revascularization accelerate mechanical deterioration of the patellar tendon after fibroblast necrosis. *J. Biomech. Eng.* 122:594–99
44. Lewis G, Shaw KM. 1997. Tensile properties of human tendon Achilles: effect of donor age and strain rate. *J. Foot Ankle Surg.* 36:435–45
45. Wren TA, Yerby SA, Beaupre GS, Carter DR. 2001. Mechanical properties of the human Achilles tendon. *Clin. Biomech.* 16:245–51
46. Derwin KA, Soslowsky LJ. 1999. A quantitative investigation of structure-function relationships in a tendon fascicle model. *J. Biomech. Eng.* 121:598–604
47. Wren TA, Yerby SA, Beaupre GS, Carter DR. 2001. Influence of bone mineral density, age, and strain rate on the failure mode of human Achilles tendons. *Clin. Biomech.* 16:529–34
48. Parry D, Barnes G, Craig A. 1978. A comparison of the size distribution of collagen fibrils in connective tissues as a function of age and a possible relation between fibril size distribution and mechanical properties. *Proc. R. Soc. London Ser. B* 203:305–21
49. Parry DA. 1988. The molecular and fibrillar structure of collagen and its relationship to the mechanical properties of

connective tissue. *Biophys. Chem.* 29: 195–209

50. Frank C, McDonald D, Wilson J, Eyre D, Shrive N. 1995. Rabbit medial collateral ligament scar weakness is associated with decreased collagen pyridinoline crosslink density. *J. Orthop. Res.* 13:157–65
51. Vogel HG. 1980. Influence of maturation and aging on mechanical and biochemical properties of connective tissue in rats. *Mech. Ageing Dev.* 14:283
52. Amiel D, Kuiper SD, Wallace CD, Harwood FL, VandeBerg JS. 1991. Age-related properties of medial collateral ligament and anterior cruciate ligament: a morphologic and collagen maturation study in the rabbit. *J. Gerontol.* 46:B159
53. Yurchenco PD, Birk DE, Mecham RP, eds. 1994. *Extracellular Matrix Assembly and Structure*. San Diego: Academic. 468 pp.
54. White J, Werkmeister J, Ramshaw J, Birk D. 1997. Organization of fibrillar collagen in the human and bovine cornea: collagen types V and III. *Connective Tissue Res.* 36:165–74
55. Birk D, Mayne R. 1997. Localization of collagen types I, III and V during tendon development. Changes in collagen types I and III are correlated with changes in fibril diameter. *Eur. J. Cell Biol.* 72:352–61
56. Birk D, Fitch J, Babiarz J, Doane K, Linsenmayer T. 1990. Collagen fibrillogenesis in vitro: interaction of types I and V collagen regulates fibril diameter. *J. Cell Sci.* 95:649–57
57. Kadler K, Holmes D, Trotter J, Chapman J. 1996. Collagen fibril formation. *Biochem. J.* 316:1–11
58. Almekinders LC. 1998. Tendinitis and other chronic tendinopathies. *J. Am. Acad. Orthop. Surg.* 6:157–64
59. Rockwell WB, Butler PN, Byrne BA. 2000. Extensor tendon: anatomy, injury, and reconstruction. *Plast. Reconstr. Surg.* 106:1592–603
60. Stamos BD, Leddy JP. 2000. Closed flexor tendon disruption in athletes. *Hand Clin.* 16:359–65
61. Dejardin LM, Arnoczky SP, Ewers BJ, Haut RC, Clarke RB. 2001. Tissue-engineered rotator cuff tendon using porcine small intestine submucosa. Histologic and mechanical evaluation in dogs. *Am. J. Sports Med.* 29:175–84
62. Soslowsky LJ, Thomopoulos S, Esmail A, Flanagan CL, Iannotti JP, et al. 2002. Rotator cuff tendinosis in an animal model: role of extrinsic and overuse factors. *Ann. Biomed. Eng.* 30:1057–63
63. Iannotti JP, Norris TR. 2003. Influence of preoperative factors on outcome of shoulder arthroplasty for glenohumeral osteoarthritis. *J. Bone Joint Surg. Am.* 85-A:251–58
64. Bressel E, McNair PJ. 2001. Biomechanical behavior of the plantar flexor muscle-tendon unit after an Achilles tendon rupture. *Am. J. Sports Med.* 29:321–26
65. Davis JJ, Mason KT, Clark DA. 1999. Achilles tendon ruptures stratified by age, race, and cause of injury among active duty U.S. military members. *Mil. Med.* 164:872–73
66. Marsolais D, Cote CH, Frenette J. 2001. Neutrophils and macrophages accumulate sequentially following Achilles tendon injury. *J. Orthop. Res.* 19:1203–9
67. Cook JL, Khan KM, Purdam C. 2002. Achilles tendinopathy. *Man. Ther.* 7:121–30
68. Mazzone MF, McCue T. 2002. Common conditions of the Achilles tendon. *Am. Fam. Physician* 65:1805–10
69. Clark R, Singer AJ. 2000. Wound repair: basic biology to tissue engineering. In *Principles of Tissue Engineering*, ed. RP Lanza, RS Langer, J Vacanti, pp. 857–78. San Diego: Academic
70. Beredjiklian PK. 2003. Biologic aspects of flexor tendon laceration and repair. *J. Bone Joint Surg. Am.* 85-A:539
71. Swift ME, Burns AL, Gray KL, DiPietro LA. 2001. Age-related alterations in the inflammatory response to dermal injury. *J. Invest. Dermatol.* 117:1027

72. Mast BA. 1997. Healing in other tissues. *Surg. Clin. N. Am.* 77:529
73. Gelberman RH, Boyer MI, Brodt MD, Winters SC, Silva MJ. 1999. The effect of gap formation at the repair site on the strength and excursion of intrasynovial flexor tendons. An experimental study on the early stages of tendon healing in dogs. *J. Bone Joint Surg. Am.* 81:975–82
74. Bruns J, Kampen J, Kahrs J, Plitz W. 2000. Achilles tendon rupture: experimental results on spontaneous repair in a sheep model. *Knee Surg. Sports Traumatol. Arthrosc.* 8:364–69
75. Li CK, Maffulli N, Lee K, Chan KM. 1998. A prospective randomized trial of suture of the patellar tendon defect after harvesting. *Arthroscopy* 14:682–89
76. Boyer MI, Gelberman RH, Burns ME, Dinopoulos H, Hofem R, Silva MJ. 2001. Intrasynovial flexor tendon repair. an experimental study comparing low and high levels of in vivo force during rehabilitation in canines. *J. Bone Joint Surg. Am.* 83-A:891–99
77. Erhard L, Zobitz ME, Zhao C, Amadio PC, An K-N. 2002. Treatment of partial lacerations in flexor tendons by trimming. A biomechanical in vitro study. *J. Bone Joint Surg. Am.* 84-A:1006
78. McCarthy DM, Tramaglini DM, Chan SS, Schmidt CC, Sotereanos DG, Herndon JH. 1995. Effect of partial laceration on the structural properties of the canine FDP tendon: an in vitro study. *J. Hand Surg.* 20:795–800
79. Carpenter J, Thomopoulos S, Flanagan C, DeBano C, Soslowsky L. 1998. Rotator cuff defect healing: a biomechanical and histologic analysis in an animal model. *J. Shoulder Elbow Surg.* 7:599–605
80. Proctor C, Jackson D, Simon T. 1997. Characterization of the repair tissue after removal of the central one-third of the patellar ligament. An experimental study in a goat model. *J. Bone Joint Surg. Am.* 79:997–1006
81. Reddy GK, Stehno-Bittel L, Enwemeka CS. 1999. Matrix remodeling in healing rabbit Achilles tendon. *Wound Repair Regen.* 7:518–27
82. Zatiti SC, Mazzer N, Barbieri CH. 1998. Mechanical strengths of tendon sutures. An in vitro comparative study of six techniques. *J. Hand Surg.* 23:228–33
83. Xie RG, Zhang S, Tang JB, Chen F. 2002. Biomechanical studies of 3 different 6-strand flexor tendon repair techniques. *J. Hand Surg.* 27:621–27
84. Tang JB, Wang B, Chen F, Pan CZ, Xie RG. 2001. Biomechanical evaluation of flexor tendon repair techniques. *Clin. Orthop.* 386:252–59
85. Veitch A, Firoozbakhsh K, Pribyl CR, McNally T. 2000. In vitro biomechanical evaluation of the double loop suture for flexor tendon repair. *Clin. Orthop.* 377:228–34
86. Silva MJ, Boyer MI, Ditsios K, Burns ME, Harwood FL, et al. 2002. The insertion site of the canine flexor digitorum profundus tendon heals slowly following injury and suture repair. *J. Orthop. Res.* 20:447–53
87. Zhao C, Amadio PC, Momose T, Couvreur P, Zobitz ME, An KN. 2001. The effect of suture technique on adhesion formation after flexor tendon repair for partial lacerations in a canine model. *J. Trauma* 51:917–21
88. Gordon L, Tolar M, Rao KT, Ritchie RO, Rabinowitz S, Lamb RP. 1998. Flexor tendon repair using a stainless steel internal anchor. Biomechanical study on human cadaver tendons. *J. Hand Surg.* 23:37–40
89. Smith AM, Evans DM. 2001. Biomechanical assessment of a new type of flexor tendon repair. *J. Hand Surg.* 26:217–19
90. Winters SC, Seiler JG III, Woo SL, Gelberman RH. 1997. Suture methods for flexor tendon repair. A biomechanical analysis during the first six weeks following repair. *Ann. Chir. Main Memb. Super.* 16:229–34
91. Raposio E, Cella A, Barabino P, Santi P. 1999. Two modified techniques for

flexor tendon repair. *Plast. Reconstr. Surg.* 103:1691–95

92. Gill RS, Lim BH, Shatford RA, Toth E, Voor MJ, Tsai TM. 1999. A comparative analysis of the six-strand double-loop flexor tendon repair and three other techniques: a human cadaveric study. *J. Hand Surg. Am.* 24:1315–22

92a. Winters SC, Gelberman RH, Woo SL, Chan SS, Grewal R, Seiler JG III. 1998. The effects of multiple-strand suture methods on the strength and excursion of repaired intrasynovial flexor tendons: a biomechanical study in dogs. *J. Hand Surg.* 23:97–104

93. Fernandez-Fairen M, Gimeno C. 1997. Augmented repair of Achilles tendon ruptures. *Am. J. Sports Med.* 25:177–81

94. Jaakkola JI, Hutton WC, Beskin JL, Lee GP. 2000. Achilles tendon rupture repair: biomechanical comparison of the triple bundle technique versus the Krakow locking loop technique. *Foot Ankle Int.* 21:14–7

95. Speck M, Klaue K. 1998. Early full weightbearing and functional treatment after surgical repair of acute Achilles tendon rupture. *Am. J. Sports Med.* 26:789–93

96. Aoki M, Ogiwara N, Ohta T, Nabeta Y. 1998. Early active motion and weightbearing after cross-stitch Achilles tendon repair. *Am. J. Sports Med.* 26:794–800

97. Kim PT, Aoki M, Tokita F, Ishii S. 1996. Tensile strength of cross-stitch epitenon suture. *J. Hand Surg.* 21:821–23

98. Gerber C, Schneeberger AG, Perren SM, Nyffeler RW. 1999. Experimental rotator cuff repair. A preliminary study. *J. Bone Joint Surg. Am.* 81:1281–90

99. Rokito AS, Cuomo F, Gallagher MA, Zuckerman JD. 1999. Long-term functional outcome of repair of large and massive chronic tears of the rotator cuff. *J. Bone Joint Surg. Am.* 81:991–7

100. Miniaci A, MacLeod M. 1999. Transfer of the latissimus dorsi muscle after failed repair of a massive tear of the rotator cuff. A two to five-year review. *J. Bone Joint Surg. Am.* 81:1120–27

101. Celli L, Rovesta C, Marongiu MC, Manzieri S. 1998. Transplantation of teres major muscle for infraspinatus muscle in irreparable rotator cuff tears. *J. Shoulder Elbow Surg.* 7:485–90

102. Burkhart SS, Danaceau SM, Pearce CE Jr. 2001. Arthroscopic rotator cuff repair: analysis of results by tear size and by repair technique: margin convergence versus direct tendon-to-bone repair. *Arthroscopy* 17:905–12

103. Bennett WF. 2003. Arthroscopic repair of massive rotator cuff tears: a prospective cohort with 2- to 4-year follow-up. *Arthroscopy* 19:380–90

104. Gartsman GM, Khan M, Hammerman SM. 1998. Arthroscopic repair of full-thickness tears of the rotator cuff. *J. Bone Joint Surg. Am.* 80:832–40

105. Bennett WF. 2003. Arthroscopic repair of anterosuperior (supraspinatus/subscapularis) rotator cuff tears: a prospective cohort with 2- to 4-year follow-up. Classification of biceps subluxation/instability. *Arthroscopy* 19:21–33

106. Norberg FB, Field LD, Savoie FH III. 2000. Repair of the rotator cuff. Mini-open and arthroscopic repairs. *Clin. Sports Med.* 19:77–99

107. Setzen G, Williams EF III. 1997. Tissue response to suture materials implanted subcutaneously in a rabbit model. *Plast. Reconstr. Surg.* 100:1788–95

108. Young RG, Butler DL, Weber W, Caplan AI, Gordon SL, Fink DJ. 1998. Use of mesenchymal stem cells in a collagen matrix for Achilles tendon repair. *J. Orthop. Res.* 16:406–13

109. Gelberman RH, Manske PR, Akeson WH, Woo SL, Lundborg G, Amiel D. 1986. Flexor tendon repair. *J. Orthop. Res.* 4:119–28

110. Zobitz ME, Zhao C, Amadio PC, An KN. 2000. Comparison of mechanical properties of various suture repair techniques in

a partially lacerated tendon. *J. Biomech. Eng.* 122:604–7
111. Tang JB, Pan CZ, Xie RG, Chen F. 1999. A biomechanical study of Tang's multiple locking techniques for flexor tendon repair. *Chir. Main* 18:254–60
112. Wada A, Kubota H, Taketa M, Miuri H, Iwamoto Y. 2002. Comparison of the mechanical properties of polyglycolide-trimethylene carbonate (Maxon) and polydioxanone sutures (PDS2) used for flexor tendon repair and active mobilization. *J. Hand Surg.* 27:329–32
113. Butler D, Goldstein S, Guilak F. 2000. Functional tissue engineering: the role of biomechanics. *J. Biomech. Eng.* 122:570–75
114. Guilak F, Butler DL, Goldstein SA, Mooney D, eds. 2003. *Functional Tissue Engineering.* New York: Springer-Verlag. 480 pp.
115. Lanza RP, Langer RS, Vacanti J, eds. 2000. *Principles of Tissue Engineering.* San Diego: Academic. 995 pp.
116. Ohno K, Yasuda K, Yamamoto N, Kaneda K, Hayashi K. 1993. Effects of complete stress-shielding on the mechanical properties and histology of in situ frozen patellar tendon. *J. Orthop. Res.* 11:592–602
117. Yamamoto N, Ohno K, Hayashi K, Kuriyama H, Yasuda K, Kaneda K. 1993. Effects of stress shielding on the mechanical properties of rabbit patellar tendon. *J. Biomech. Eng.* 115:23–28
118. Deleted in proof
119. Yamato M, Adachi E, Yamamoto K, Hayashi T. 1995. Condensation of collagen fibrils to the direct vicinity of fibroblasts as a cause of gel contraction. *J. Biochem.* 117:940–46
120. Buck RC. 1980. Reorientation response of cells to repeated stretch and recoil of the substratum. *Exp. Cell Res.* 127:470–74
121. Buckley MJ, Banes AJ, Levin LG, Sumpio BE, Sato M, et al. 1988. Osteoblasts increase their rate of division and align in response to cyclic, mechanical tension in vitro. *Bone Miner. Res.* 4:225–36
122. Dartsch PC, Hammerle H, Betz E. 1986. Orientation of cultured arterial smooth muscle cells growing on cyclically stretched substrates. *Acta Anat.* 125:108–13
123. Neidlinger-Wilke C, Grood E, Wang J-C, Brand R, Claes L. 2001. Cell alignment is induced by cyclic changes in cell length: studies of cells grown in cyclically stretched substrates. *J. Orthop. Res.* 19:286
124. Zeichen J, van Griensven M, Bosch U. 2000. The proliferative response of isolated human tendon fibroblasts to cyclic biaxial mechanical strain. *Am. J. Sports Med.* 28:888–92
125. Banes AJ, Gilbert J, Taylor D, Monbureau O. 1985. A new vacuum-operated stress-providing instrument that applies static or variable duration cyclic tension or compression to cells in vitro. *J. Cell Sci.* 75:35–42
126. Brighton CT, Strafford B, Gross SB, Leatherwood DF, Williams JL, Pollack SR. 1991. The proliferative and synthetic response of isolated calvarial bone cells of rats to cyclic biaxial mechanical strain. *J. Bone Joint Surg. Am.* 73:320–31
127. Altman GH, Horan RL, Martin I, Farhadi J, Stark PR, et al. 2002. Cell differentiation by mechanical stress. *FASEB J.* 16:270–72
128. Skutek M, van Griensven M, Zeichen J, Brauer N, Bosch U. 2001. Cyclic mechanical stretching modulates secretion pattern of growth factors in human tendon fibroblasts. *Eur. J. Appl. Physiol.* 86:48–52
129. Carver W, Nagpal ML, Nachtigal M, Borg TK, Terracio L. 1991. Collagen expression in mechanically stimulated cardiac fibroblasts. *Circ. Res.* 69:116–22
130. Banes AJ, Horesovsky G, Larson C, Tsuzaki M, Judex S, et al. 1999. Mechanical load stimulates expression of novel genes in vivo and in vitro in avian flexor tendon cells. *Osteoarthritis Cartilage* 7:141
131. Ingber DE, Dike L, Hansen L, Karp S,

Liley H, et al. 1994. Cellular tensegrity: exploring how mechanical changes in the cytoskeleton regulate cell growth, migration, and tissue pattern during morphogenesis. *Int. Rev. Cytol.* 150:173–224
132. Ingber DE. 1997. Tensegrity: the architectural basis of cellular mechanotransduction. *Annu. Rev. Physiol.* 59:575–99
133. Bockholt SM, Burridge K. 1993. Cell spreading on extracellular matrix proteins induces tyrosine phosphorylation of tensin. *J. Biol. Chem.* 268:14565–67
134. Nuckolls GH, Romer LH, Burridge K. 1992. Microinjection of antibodies against talin inhibits the spreading and migration of fibroblasts. *J. Cell Sci.* 102: 753–62
135. Clark EA, Brugge JS. 1995. Integrins and signal transduction pathways: the road taken. *Science* 268:233–39
136. Sanderson MJ, Charles AC, Dirksen ER. 1990. Mechanical stimulation and intercellular communication increases intracellular $Ca^{2+}$ in epithelial cells. *Cell Regul.* 1:585–96
137. Goligorsky MS. 1988. Mechanical stimulation induces $Ca^{2+}{}_i$ transients and membrane depolarization in cultured endothelial cells. Effects on $Ca^{2+}{}_i$ in co-perfused smooth muscle cells. *FEBS Lett.* 240:59–64
138. Davies PF, Tripathi SC. 1993. Mechanical stress mechanisms and the cell. An endothelial paradigm. *Circ. Res.* 72:239–45
139. Fleischer S, Inui M. 1989. Biochemistry and biophysics of excitation-contraction coupling. *Annu. Rev. Biophys. Biophys. Chem.* 18:333–64
140. Geiger RV, Berk BC, Alexander RW, Nerem RM. 1992. Flow-induced calcium transients in single endothelial cells: spatial and temporal analysis. *Am. J. Physiol. Cell Physiol.* 262:C1411–17
141. Guharay F, Sachs F. 1984. Stretch-activated single ion channel currents in tissue-cultured embryonic chick skeletal muscle. *J. Physiol.* 352:685–701
142. Grinnell F. 2003. Fibroblast biology in three-dimensional collagen matrices. *Trends Cell Biol.* 13:264–69
143. Awad H, Butler D, Harris M, Ibrahim R, Wu Y, et al. 2000. In vitro characterization of mesenchymal stem cell-seeded collagen scaffolds for tendon repair: effects of initial seeding density on contraction kinetics. *J. Biomed. Mater. Res.* 51:233–40
144. Bell E, Ivarsson B, Merrill C. 1979. Production of a tissue-like structure by contraction of collagen lattices by human fibroblasts of different proliferative potential in vitro. *Proc. Natl. Acad. Sci. USA* 76:1274–78
145. Huang D, Chang T, Aggarwal A, Lee R, Ehrlich H. 1993. Mechanisms and dynamics of mechanical strengthening in ligament-equivalent fibroblast-populated collagen matrices. *Ann. Biomed. Eng.* 21:289–305
146. Cacou C, Palmer D, Lee DA, Bader DL, Shelton JC. 2000. A system for monitoring the response of uniaxial strain on cell seeded collagen gels. *Med. Eng. Phys.* 22:327–33
147. Langelier E, Rancourt D, Bouchard S, Lord C, Stevens P, et al. 1999. Cyclic traction machine for long-term culture of fibroblast-populated collagen gels. *Ann. Biomed. Eng.* 27:67–72
148. Altman GH, Lu HH, Horan RL, Calabro T, Ryder D, et al. 2002. Advanced bioreactor with controlled application of multidimensional strain for tissue engineering. *J. Biomech. Eng.* 124:742–49
149. Awad HA, Butler DL, Boivin GP, Smith FN, Malaviya P, et al. 1999. Autologous mesenchymal stem cell-mediated repair of tendon. *Tissue Eng.* 5:267–77
150. Ouyang HW, Goh JC, Mo XM, Teoh SH, Lee EH. 2002. The efficacy of bone marrow stromal cell-seeded knitted PLGA fiber scaffold for Achilles tendon repair. *Ann. NY Acad. Sci.* 961:126–29
151. Ouyang HW, Goh JC, Thambyah A, Teoh SH, Lee EH. 2003. Knitted poly-lactide-co-glycolide scaffold loaded with bone

marrow stromal cells in repair and regeneration of rabbit Achilles tendon. *Tissue Eng.* 9:431–39
152. Cao Y, Liu Y, Liu W, Shan Q, Buonocore SD, Cui L. 2002. Bridging tendon defects using autologous tenocyte engineered tendon in a hen model. *Plast. Reconstr. Surg.* 110:1280–89
153. Guilak F. 2002. Functional tissue engineering—the role of biomechanics in reparative medicine. *Ann. NY Acad. Sci.* 961:193–95
154. Korvick D, Cummings J, Grood E, Holden J, Feder S, Butler D. 1996. The use of an implantable force transducer to measure patellar tendon forces in goats *J. Biomech.* 29:557–61
155. Malaviya P, Butler D, Korvick D, Proch F. 1998. In vivo tendon forces correlate with activity level and remain bounded: evidence in a rabbit flexor tendon model. *J. Biomech.* 31:1043–49
156. Hasler EM, Herzog W. 1998. Quantification of in vivo patellofemoral contact forces before and after ACL transection. *J. Biomech.* 31:37–44
157. Herzog W, Leonard TR. 1996. Soleus forces and soleus force potential during unrestrained cat locomotion. *J. Biomech.* 29:271–79
158. Herzog W, Archambault JM, Leonard TR, Nguyen HK. 1996. Evaluation of the implantable force transducer for chronic tendon-force recordings. *J. Biomech.* 29:103–9
159. Juncosa N, West JR, Galloway MT, Boivin GP, Butler DL. 2003. In vivo forces used to develop design parameters for tissue engineered implants for rabbit patellar tendon repair. *J. Biomech.* 36:483–88
160. Komi PV, Fukashiro S, Jarvinen M. 1992. Biomechanical loading of Achilles tendon during normal locomotion. *Clin. Sports Med.* 11:521–31
161. Finni T, Komi PV, Lukkariniemi J. 1998. Achilles tendon loading during walking: application of a novel optic fiber technique. *Eur. J. Appl. Physiol. Occup. Physiol.* 77:289–91
162. Lieber RL, Loren GJ, Friden J. 1994. In vivo measurement of human wrist extensor muscle sarcomere length changes. *J. Neurophysiol.* 71:874–81

Annu. Rev. Biomed. Eng. 2004. 6:331–62
doi: 10.1146/annurev.bioeng.6.040803.140111

First published online as a Review in Advance on April 2, 2004

# FLUID MECHANICS OF HEART VALVES

Ajit P. Yoganathan, Zhaoming He, and S. Casey Jones
*Wallace H. Coulter Department of Biomedical Engineering, Georgia Institute of Technology, Atlanta, Georgia 30332-0535; email: ajit.yoganathan@bme.gatech.edu*

**Key Words** mechanical heart valves, bioprosthetic valves, computational fluid dynamics, laser Doppler velocimetry, native heart valves

■ **Abstract** Valvular heart disease is a life-threatening disease that afflicts millions of people worldwide and leads to approximately 250,000 valve repairs and/or replacements each year. Malfunction of a native valve impairs its efficient fluid mechanic/hemodynamic performance. Artificial heart valves have been used since 1960 to replace diseased native valves and have saved millions of lives. Unfortunately, despite four decades of use, these devices are less than ideal and lead to many complications. Many of these complications/problems are directly related to the fluid mechanics associated with the various mechanical and bioprosthetic valve designs. This review focuses on the state-of-the-art experimental and computational fluid mechanics of native and prosthetic heart valves in current clinical use. The fluid dynamic performance characteristics of caged-ball, tilting-disc, bileaflet mechanical valves and porcine and pericardial stented and nonstented bioprostheic valves are reviewed. Other issues related to heart valve performance, such as biomaterials, solid mechanics, tissue mechanics, and durability, are not addressed in this review.

CONTENTS

# INTRODUCTION

The human heart is a pump that sends oxygenated blood and nutrients to various organs in the body. It consists of four chambers and four valves. During the average human lifespan, the heart beats approximately three billion times. Heart disease is currently the major cause of death in the world, with heart valve disease being one of the main afflictions of the cardiovascular system. The most commonly affected valves are the mitral, aortic, and tricuspid valves. Valve malfunction affects hemodynamic performance in two primary ways in terms of forward and reverse flow, respectively:

- Stenosis: A narrowing of the valve, which increases the resistance to blood flow and therefore generates a larger pressure drop across the valve
- Incompetence: The failure of the valve leaflets to close completely resulting in retrograde blood flow (regurgitation) when the valve should be shut

Both of these pathological conditions reduce the efficiency of the heart and place additional stress and strain upon it. Surgical repair or replacement of the diseased valve with a heart valve prosthesis is necessary to restore valve function. Presently, approximately 180,000 prosthetic valves are implanted each year throughout the world.

The first clinical use of a cardiac valve prosthesis took place in 1952, when Dr. Charles Hufnagel implanted an artificial caged-ball valve in the descending aorta to compensate for aortic insufficiency. Since then, the achievements in valve design and the success of artificial heart valves as replacements have been remarkable (1). More than 50 different cardiac valve prostheses, listed in Tables 1 and 2, have been introduced over the past 40 years (2). Unfortunately, even

**TABLE 1** Mechanical prostheses (revised from 2)

| | |
|---|---|
| Monoleaflet | Bjork-Shiley monostrut mechanical prosthesis |
| | Sorin Monoleaflet allcarbon mechanical prosthesis |
| | Medtronic-Hall mechanical prosthesis |
| | Omnicarbon mechanical prosthesis |
| | Ultracor mechanical prosthesis |
| Bileaflet | St. Jude Medical Standard mechanical prosthesis |
| | St. Jude Medical Hemodynamic Plus mechanical prosthesis |
| | St. Jude Medical Regent mechanical prosthesis |
| | CarboMedics mechanical prosthesis |
| | Edwards Tekna mechanical prosthesis |
| | Sorin Bicarbon mechanical prosthesis |
| | ATS mechanical prosthesis |
| | ON-X mechanical prosthesis |
| | Medtronic Advantage mechanical prosthesis |
| | Medtronic Parallel mechanical prosthesis |
| | Edwards MIRA mechanical prosthesis |

**TABLE 2** Bioprostheses (revised from 2)

| | |
|---|---|
| Stented porcine | Hancock standard porcine bioprosthesis |
| | Carpentier-Edwards standard porcine bioprosthesis |
| | Carpentier-Edwards Supra-A |
| | Hancock II porcine bioprosthesis |
| | Hancock Modified Office porcine bioprosthesis |
| | St. Jude Medical-Biocor porcine bioprosthesis |
| | St. Jude Medical-Bioplant porcine bioprosthesis |
| | Medtronic Mosaic porcine bioprosthesis |
| | Aortech Aspire porcine bioprosthesis |
| | Labcor porcine bioprosthesis |
| | St. Jude Medical Epic porcine bioprosthesis |
| | CarboMedics Synergy St porcine bioprosthesis |
| Stented pericardial | Carpentier-Edwards Perimount pericardial bioprosthesis |
| | Mitroflow Synergy PC pericardial bioprosthesis |
| | St. Jude Medical Biocor pericardial bioprosthesis |
| | Sorin Pericarbon More pericardial bioprosthesis |
| | Labcor pericardial bioprosthesis |
| Stentless porcine and pericardial | St. Jude Medical-Toronto SPV stentless porcine bioprosthesis |
| | Medtronic Freestyle stentless porcine bioprosthesis |
| | Cryolife-O'Brien stentless porcine bioprosthesis |
| | Cryolife-Ross stentless porcine pulmonary bioprosthesis |
| | Edwards Prima Plus stentless porcine bioprosthesis |
| | Sorin PericarbonTM Freedom stentless pericardial bioprosthesis |
| | Aortech Aspire stentless porcine bioprosthesis |
| | St. Jude Medical Biocor stentless porcine bioprosthesis |
| | Labcor Stentless Porcine Bioprosthesis |
| | St. Jude Medical QuattroTM stentless mitral bioprosthesis |
| | Shelhigh skeletorized super-stentless aortic porcine bioprosthisis |
| | Shelhigh porcine pulmonic valve conduit |
| | Medtronic-Venpro Contegra pulmonary valved conduit |
| Allografts | Cryo Valve aortic valve with/without conduit |
| | Cryo Valve mitral valve |
| | Cryo Syner graft valve |
| Autografts | Pulmonary autografts for aortic root |
| | Autologous pericardial aortic valve |

after many years of experience, problems associated with heart valve prostheses have not been eliminated, demonstrating that none of these valves are ideal for valve replacement. New designs continue to be developed. To date, the most serious problems and complications with current prosthetic valves are the following (1, 3–5):

- Thrombosis and thromboembolism
- Anticoagulant-related hemorrhage

- Tissue overgrowth
- Infection
- Paravalvular leaks owing to healing defects
- Valve failure owing to material fatigue or chemical change.

These incidences may be caused by either mechanical or biological events. Both mechanical and biological valve designs have their own advantages and disadvantages. Of the current prosthetic valves, the four most commonly used types are (*a*) caged ball, (*b*) tilting disc, (*c*) bileaflet, and (*d*) bioprostheses (tissue or biological valve).

Many of the above-mentioned complications are directly related to the fluid mechanics associated with the various mechanical and bioprosthetic valve designs. This review focuses on the state-of-the-art experimental and computational fluid mechanics of native and prosthetic heart valves in current clinical use. Other issues related to heart valve performance, such as biomaterials, solid mechanics, tissue mechanics, and durability, are not addressed here.

## NATIVE HEART VALVE FUNCTION

The tricuspid and pulmonic valves on the right side of the heart regulate the flow of blood that is returned from the body to the lungs for oxygenation, whereas the mitral and aortic valves on the left side of the heart control the flow of oxygenated blood to the body. The aortic and pulmonic valves allow blood to be pumped from the ventricles into the arteries on the left and right sides of the heart, respectively. Similarly, the mitral and tricuspid valves regulate blood flow between the atria and ventricles of the left and right sides of the heart, respectively. The aortic and pulmonic valves open during systole when the ventricles are contracting and close during diastole when the ventricles are filling through the open mitral and tricuspid valves. During isovolumic contraction and relaxation, all four valves are closed.

When closed, the pulmonic and tricuspid valves must withstand a pressure of approximately 30 mm Hg. In contrast, the aortic valve withstands a pressure of approximately 100 mm Hg, whereas the mitral valve closes against pressures up to 150 mm Hg. Because of this extreme cyclic loading, the valves on the left side of the heart are particularly predisposed to disease. Hemodynamics may play a critical role in valve pathology. This section focuses on the aortic and mitral valves, and, where necessary, pertinent references are made to the pulmonic and tricuspid valves.

### Valve Anatomy

The aortic valve is composed of three semilunar cusps, or leaflets, contained within a connective tissue sleeve. Attachment of the leaflets forms the annular ring of the aortic valve and separates the aorta from the left ventricle. Superior to this ring is a structure called the aortic sinus, which comprises three bulges at the root of the aorta. The anatomy of the pulmonic valve is similar to that of the aortic valve, but the valve annulus is slightly larger than that of the aortic valve.

The mitral and tricuspid valves are similar in structure. Both valves are composed of four primary elements: (*a*) the valve annulus, (*b*) the valve leaflets, (*c*) the papillary muscles, and (*d*) the chordae tendineae. The base of the mitral leaflets forms the mitral annulus, which attaches to the atrial and ventricular walls and the aortic root. Two semicircular leaflets extend from the ventricular side of the annulus. At the free edges of the leaflets, the chordae tendineae insert at multiple locations and extend to the tips of the papillary muscles.

The mitral annulus is an elliptical, or D-shaped, ring. It undergoes dynamic changes during the cardiac cycle by changing in size and by moving three-dimensionally. Recent studies involving the measurement of annular shape have shown that the mitral annulus is not planar, but instead forms a three-dimensional saddle shape (6–9). Two main leaflets, called anterior and posterior leaflets, cover most of the valve orifice area during valve closure. The two small scallops between the leaflets, called commissure leaflets, provide coaptation compensation in case of disease (10, 11). The papillary muscles attach to the wall of the ventricle and tether the mitral valve in place via the chordae tendineae. This tethering prevents the mitral valve from prolapsing into the atrium during ventricular ejection.

Unlike the mitral valve, the tricuspid valve has three leaflets: (*a*) the anterior leaflet, (*b*) the posterior leaflet with a variable number of scallops, and (*c*) the septal leaflet. The tricuspid valve is larger and structurally more complicated than the mitral valve. From each papillary muscle, several chordae tendineae originate and branch into several insertion areas on the leaflets. The chordae, which attach to the tip of the free leaflet edge, are called marginal chordae and are usually thinner, whereas the basal chordae, which insert into the basal region and close to the annulus, are usually thicker. The marginal chordae tendineae function to keep the leaflets stationary, whereas the basal chordae seem to act more as supports (12).

## Valve Dynamics

The aortic valve opens at the beginning of systole as the left ventricle contracts and closes before the start of diastole as the ventricle relaxes and fills from the atrium. Systole lasts about one third of the cardiac cycle and begins when the aortic valve opens, which typically takes only 20 to 30 ms (13). Blood rapidly accelerates through the valve and reaches a peak velocity after the leaflets have fully opened. Peak velocity is reached during the first third of systole after which time the flow begins to decelerate rapidly, albeit not as fast as its initial acceleration. The adverse pressure gradient that is developed affects the low momentum fluid near the wall of the aorta more than that at the center, causing reverse flow in the sinus region (14). As shown in Figure 1 (15), during systole the pressure difference required to drive the blood through the aortic valve is on the order of only a few millimeters of mercury; however, the diastolic pressure difference reaches 80 mm Hg in normal individuals. The valve closes near the end of the deceleration phase of systole with

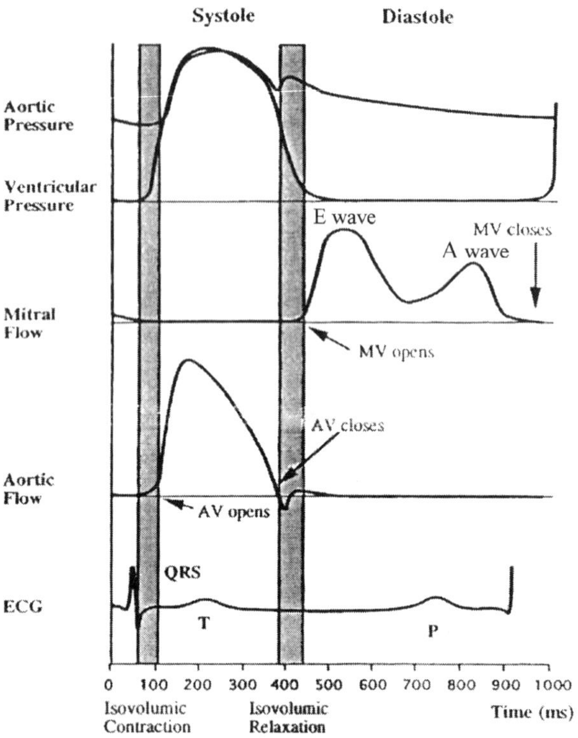


**Figure 1** Typical pressure and flow curves for the aortic and mitral valves (15).

very little reverse flow through the valve. All cardiac valves are closed during both isovolumic contraction and isovolumic relaxation.

The aortic valve varies in size and also translates, mainly along the axis of the aorta, during the cardiac cycle as the heart contracts and dilates. The perimeter of the annulus reaches a minimum at the end of systole and a maximum at the end of diastole. Studies in canines have shown that there is a 20% perimeter change for an aortic pressure variation of 120/80 mm Hg (16). During systole, vortices develop in all three sinuses behind the leaflets of the aortic valve. These vortices help to close the aortic valve quickly so that an efficient and fast closure is obtained. The closing volume, or backflow during closure, has been estimated to be less than 5% of the forward flow (17). In healthy individuals, blood flows through the aortic valve at the beginning of systole owing to the transvalvular pressure and rapidly accelerates to its peak value of 1.35 ± 0.35 m/s (18). This value for children is slightly higher at 1.5 ± 0.3 m/s (19). At the end of systole, there is a short period of reverse flow that can be measured with Doppler ultrasound. This reverse flow is probably due to either a small closing volume or the velocity of the valve leaflets as they move toward their closed position. The velocity profile on the valve orifice plane is almost flat, with the flow skewed slightly toward the septal wall (18, 20). Highly skewed velocity profiles and corresponding helical flow patterns have been observed in the human aortic arch using magnetic resonance phase velocity mapping (20).

Pulmonic valve flow behaves similarly to that of the aortic valve, but the magnitude of the velocity is not as great. Typical peak velocities for healthy adults are $0.75 \pm 0.15$ m/s; again these values are slightly higher for children at $0.9 \pm 0.2$ m/s (21). A rotation of the peak velocity can be observed in the velocity profiles downstream of the pulmonary artery. During acceleration the peak velocity in the pulmonary artery rotates counterclockwise (22).

The mitral valve leaflets, chordae tendineae, and papillary muscles all participate to ensure normal functioning of the valve. The blood flow through the mitral valve is biphasic during diastole. The first peak, called the E-wave, is due to ventricular relaxation, whereas the second peak, called the A-wave, is caused by contraction of the left atrium. During isovolumic relaxation the pressure in the left atrium exceeds that in the left ventricle, causing the mitral valve cusps to open. Blood flows through the open valve from the left atrium to the left ventricle during diastole. The velocity profiles at both the annulus and the mitral valve tips are skewed during the filling phase (23). The initial filling is enhanced by the active relaxation of the ventricle. The E-wave in the mitral flow curve occurs during the early ventricular filling phase. The peak velocities in the normal E-wave in healthy individuals range from 0.5 to 0.8 m/s (24, 25). Following active ventricular relaxation, the fluid begins to decelerate and the mitral valve undergoes partial closure. The atrium then contracts and the blood accelerates through the valve again to the secondary peak of the A-wave. In healthy individuals, the velocity during the A-wave is typically lower than during the E-wave. Thus, normal diastolic filling of the left ventricle shows two distinct peaks in the mitral flow curve, with no flow leaking back through the valve during systole.

A primary focus in explaining the fluid mechanics of mitral valve function has been to understand the closing mechanism of the valve. Bellhouse (26) first proposed that the vortices generated by ventricular filling were important for the partial closure of the mitral valve following early diastole. In vitro experiments suggest that without the strong outflow tract vortices, the mitral valve would remain open at the onset of ventricular contraction, thus resulting in more regurgitation than with the ventricular vortices. Later in vitro experiments by Reul et al. (27) suggest that an adverse pressure differential during mid-diastole could explain both the flow deceleration and the partial valve closure. Thus, they proposed that vortices might provide additional closing effects at the initial stage. Yellin et al. (28) put forth that chordal tension, flow deceleration, and ventricular vortices were important in valve closure, with chordal tension being a necessary condition for the other two. Studies using magnetic resonance imaging to visualize the three-dimensional flow field in the left ventricle have shown that in normal individuals a large anterior vortex is present at the initial partial closure of the valve as well as following atrial contraction (29).

The motion of the mitral valve complex has been a focus of many studies. The mitral apparatus moves and changes shape during the cardiac cycle. Studies have shown that the mitral annulus is a three-dimensional shape instead of a flat shape (6–9). According to these studies, during systole the annular circumference decreases from the diastolic value owing to the contraction of the ventricle, and this reduction in area ranges from 10% to 25%. Animal studies (30) have demonstrated that there is a 36% reduction in mitral area from the peak diastolic area. This reduction enables the leaflets to cover the smaller orifice. Not only does the annulus change size, it also translates during the cardiac cycle. The movement of the annulus toward the atrium suggests an increase in the efficiency of blood flow into the ventricle because the distance between the annulus and the apex of the ventricle is shortened during contraction (31).

The movement of the papillary muscles is also important in maintaining proper mitral valve function. Papillary muscles hold the mitral valve in position and prevent it from prolapsing during ventricular contraction. Even though the papillary muscles move with the heart and contract, the distance between the papillary muscle tips and the annulus measured in normal individual during systole was found to remain constant (32). However, in patients with mitral valve prolapse, this distance decreases, and in patients with ventricular dilation, this distance increases, which leads to mitral regurgitation (33).

The normal function of the mitral valve requires balanced interplay between the components of the mitral valve apparatus. Engineering studies involving mitral valve function have provided some insight into its mechanical properties and function. Further fundamental and detailed studies are needed to aid surgeons in repairing the diseased mitral valve and in understanding the changes in function owing to mitral valve pathologies. These studies are crucial for improving the design of prosthetic valves that more closely replicate native valve function.

The tricuspid flow profile is similar to that of the mitral valve; however, the velocities in the tricuspid valve are lower because it has a larger valve orifice. In addition, the tricuspid valve opens earlier and closes later than the mitral valve (21).

# IN VITRO FLUID MECHANICS OF PROSTHETIC HEART VALVES

## Engineering Concerns and Hemodynamic Assessment of Prosthetic Heart Valves

The basic engineering concerns for heart valve design are hemodynamics, durability, and the biological response to the prosthetic implant. From an engineering perspective, the ideal heart valve design should

- Produce minimal pressure drops
- Yield relatively small regurgitation volumes

- Minimize production of turbulence
- Not induce regions of high shear stresses
- Not create stagnation or flow separation regions in the flow fields in its immediate vicinity or within its superstructure.

PRESSURE DROP A pressure drop is a measure of flow potential energy losses that occur when viscous blood flows through the heart valve. It is an indication of heart valve efficiency. A large pressure drop across a prosthetic aortic valve requires a larger systolic pressure in the left ventricle to drive flow through the circulation. The pressure drop should be minimized when dealing with prosthetic valves because left ventricular pressure is the primary determinant of myocardial oxygen consumption (34). A well-designed valve will not significantly impede the blood flow, thus creating a small pressure drop across the valve.

EFFECTIVE ORIFICE AREA AND PERFORMANCE INDEX Effective orifice area (EOA) is an index of how well a valve design utilizes its primary or internal stent orifice area. It is defined as (35)

$$EOA(\text{cm}^2) = \frac{Q_{rms}}{51.6\sqrt{\Delta p}}, \tag{1}$$

where $Q_{rms}$ is the root mean square systolic/diastolic flow rate (cm$^3$/s) and $\Delta p$ is the mean systolic/diastolic pressure drop (mm Hg). EOA is related to the degree to which the prosthesis obstructs the flow of blood. A larger EOA corresponds to a smaller pressure drop and, therefore, a smaller energy loss. However, EOA is also a function of the valve size. Another measure of a valve's resistance to forward flow is the performance index (PI), which is the ratio of the EOA to the valve sewing ring area. The PI normalizes EOA by valve size and shows how well a valve design utilizes its total mounting area. Thus, it provides a measure of the valve's resistance characteristics independent of the size.

REGURGITATION Regurgitation results from reverse flow during valve closure and leakage. Typically, it is measured by percentage of stroke volume. Regurgitant volume is the total volume of fluid through the valve per beat owing to the retrograde flow. It is equal to the sum of the closing volume and leakage volume. The closing volume is the volume of retrograde flow through the valve during valve closure. Any fluid volume accumulation after valve closure is due to leakage and is referred to as the leakage volume. Figure 2 illustrates in vitro regurgitant volumes (closing and leakage). Regurgitation is dependent on valve type and size and increases with increasing valve diameter. Typically, the regurgitant volume is higher for mechanical valves than for bioprosthetic valves.

FLOW PATTERNS AND TURBULENT SHEAR STRESSES The velocity and turbulent shear stress patterns in the immediate vicinity of and within a prosthetic heart

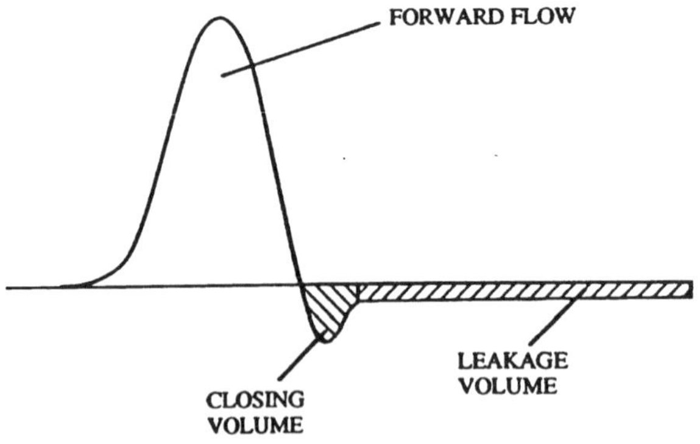


**Figure 2** Flow cycle divided into forward flow, closing volume, and leakage volume (38).

valve determine its long-term clinical performance. Flow velocity and shear stress patterns can be significantly different for various prosthetic heart valve designs. Regions of stagnation and flow separation adjacent to a prosthetic heart valve can lead to thrombus formation, tissue overgrowth, and/or calcification. Elevated levels of shear stress lead to sublethal and/or lethal damage to blood cells, such as hemolysis, as well as platelet activation. The hemolysis threshold for Reynolds shear stress can be as low as 400 $Nm^{-2}$ (36), and in three-dimensional stress analysis this threshold is considered to be at least 600 $Nm^{-2}$ (37). This lethal stress level is also affected by the residence time of the cell in the damaging fluid environment, which further complicates the damage mechanism. The peak turbulent shear stresses are higher when the valves are used in the aortic position than when they are used in the mitral position.

## Mechanical Heart Valves

There are three major mechanical heart valve (MHV) designs based on the occluder structure: caged-ball, tilting disc, and bileaflet valve. The fluid characteristics of these three types of valve are discussed below based on in vitro measurements conducted with 27 mm aortic valves, except where noted. The velocities and turbulent shear stresses were obtained at peak systole at a cardiac output of 6.0 L per minute and a heart rate of 70 beats per minute. All downstream distances are measured from the valve sewing ring.

CAGED-BALL VALVE The Starr-Edwards caged-ball valve, the only one currently in clinical use, has good reliability but poor hemodynamic performance. The flow goes through the annulus and around the ball forming a circumferential jet that separates from the ball as shown in Figure 3 (38). The jet flow has high velocities in the annular region, with a maximum velocity of 2.2 m/s at peak systole. A region of low velocity reverse flow in the wake distal to the ball is formed at peak systole and

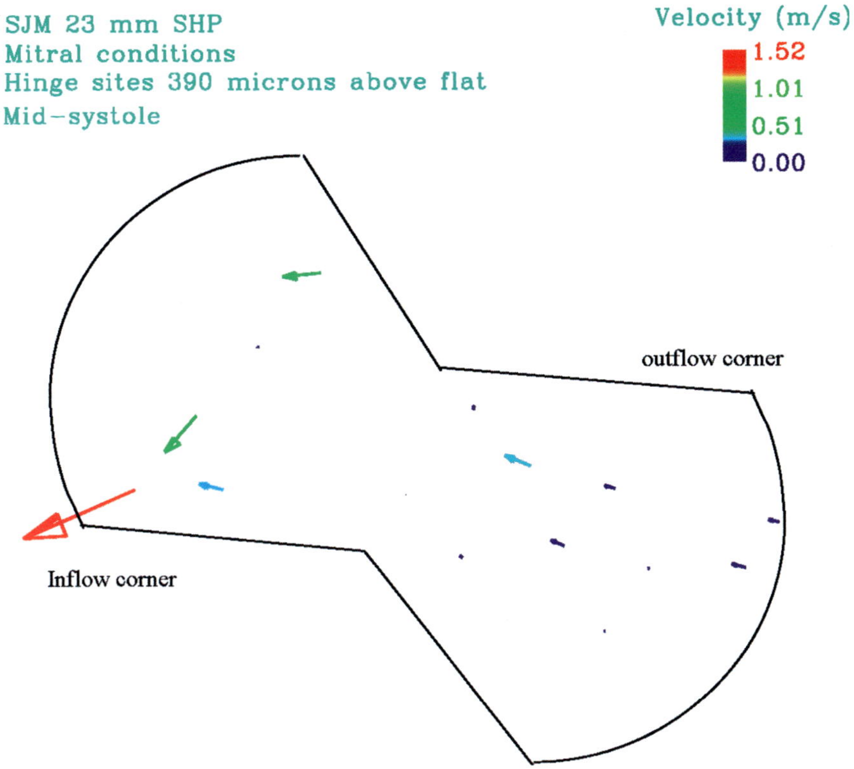


**Figure 6** St. Jude Medical Regent mitral valve (23 mm) hinge flow field at mid-diastole, 390 μm above flat (41).

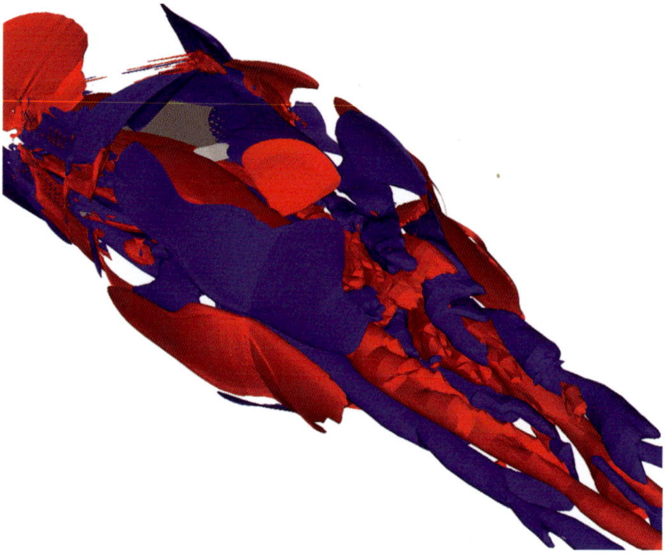

**Figure 9** CFD prediction of the complex three-dimensional flow distal to a model bileaflet MHV at Re = 1200 (89). The figure shows positive (*red*) and negative (*blue*) isosurfaces of streamwise vorticity. The direction of flow is out of the page.

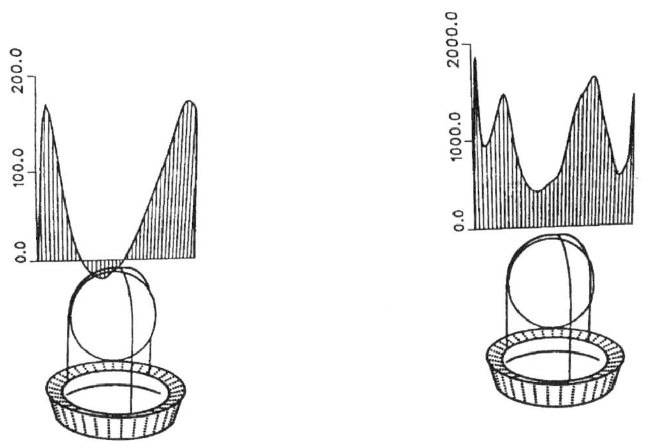


(a) Numbers are velocity in cm/s

(b) Numbers are turbulent shear stresses in dynes/cm$^2$

**Figure 3** (*a*) Velocity profile 30 mm downstream on the centerline for the Starr-Edwards ball valve at peak systole; (*b*) turbulent shear stress profile 30 mm downstream on the centerline for the Starr-Edwards ball valve at peak systole (38).

during the deceleration phase. The velocity in the central part of the flow channel is low during the deceleration phase. The ball generates a large wake in the central part of the flow field that begins in early systole and grows into a region of reverse flow lasting from peak to end systole. Peak reverse velocities in the wake region can be as high as 0.25 m/s. The flow field in the mitral position is similar to that in the aortic position. These vortex regions are responsible for the thrombogenicity of the valve. The caged-ball valve has a larger pressure drop than the tilting disc and bileaflet designs owing to its larger wake region. The performance index ranges from 0.30 to 0.36.

The regurgitant flow of the valve is mainly due to closing volume because the valve seals well with almost no leakage flow. Typical values for the regurgitant volume are approximately 5 ml/beat. These data are listed in Tables 3 and 4.

High turbulent shear stresses of 1850 dynes/cm$^2$ are generated at the edges of the annular jet, and the turbulence intensity during peak systole does not decay very rapidly downstream of the valve. Turbulent shear stresses as high as 3500 dynes/cm$^2$ have been estimated immediately adjacent to the flow channel wall and the ball occluder.

TILTING DISC VALVE The most commonly used tilting disc valve, the Medtronic-Hall mechanical valve, has major and minor orifices divided by a tilting disc. Two high-velocity jets flow from both the major and minor orifice outflow regions during systole. The flow on each side of the strut is nearly symmetric with similar

**TABLE 3** In vitro hemodynamic data for common aortic valve prostheses[a] (61)

| Valve type | Valve | Size | Regurgitant volume (ml/beat) | EOA[b] ($cm^2$) | PI |
|---|---|---|---|---|---|
| Caged ball | Starr-Edwards 1260 | 27 | 5.5 | 1.75 | 0.30 |
| | | 25 | 4.3 | 1.62 | 0.33 |
| | | 21 | 2.5 | 1.23 | 0.36 |
| Tilting disc | Björk-Shiley Convexo-Concave | 27 | 8.5 | 2.59 | 0.45 |
| | | 25 | 7.3 | 2.37 | 0.48 |
| | | 21 | 5.5 | 1.54 | 0.45 |
| | Björk-Shiley Monostrut | 27 | 9.2 | 3.34 | 0.58 |
| | | 25 | 7.6 | 2.62 | 0.53 |
| | | 23 | 6.9 | 2.00 | 0.48 |
| | | 21 | 5.9 | 1.45 | 0.42 |
| | | 19 | 5.5 | 1.07 | 0.38 |
| | Medtronic-Hall | 27 | 9.6 | 3.64 | 0.64 |
| | | 25 | 8.4 | 3.07 | 0.62 |
| | | 23 | 7.3 | 2.26 | 0.54 |
| | | 20 | 6.2 | 1.74 | 0.51 |
| Bileaflet | St. Jude Medical Standard | 27 | 10.8 | 4.09 | 0.71 |
| | | 25 | 9.9 | 3.23 | 0.66 |
| | | 23 | 8.3 | 2.24 | 0.54 |
| | | 21 | 6.8 | 1.81 | 0.52 |
| | | 19 | 6.8 | 1.21 | 0.43 |
| | St. Jude Medical Regent | 29 | 13.5 | 4.98 | 0.75 |
| | | 27 | 12.3 | 4.40 | 0.77 |
| | | 25 | 11.2 | 3.97 | 0.81 |
| | | 23 | 10.3 | 3.47 | 0.83 |
| | | 21 | 9.0 | 2.81 | 0.81 |
| | | 19 | 7.6 | 2.06 | 0.73 |
| | | 17 | 6.3 | 1.56 | 0.69 |
| | CarboMedics | 27 | 7.5 | 3.75 | 0.65 |
| | | 25 | 6.1 | 3.14 | 0.64 |
| | | 23 | 6.51 | 2.28 | 0.55 |
| | | 21 | 3.4 | 1.66 | 0.48 |
| | | 19 | 3.0 | 1.12 | 0.40 |
| | Sorin Bicarbon[c] | 27 | | 3.06 | 0.71 |
| | | 25 | | 2.39 | 0.69 |
| | | 23 | | 2.07 | 0.73 |
| | | 21 | | 1.54 | 0.67 |
| | | 19 | | 0.97 | 0.55 |
| Stented bioprosthesis | Carpentier-Edwards Porcine 2625 | 27 | <3 | 1.95 | 0.34 |
| | | 25 | <2 | 1.52 | 0.31 |
| | | 21 | <2 | 1.28 | 0.37 |

(*Continued*)

TABLE 3 (*Continued*)

| Valve type | Valve | Size | Regurgitant volume (ml/beat) | EOA[b] ($cm^2$) | PI |
|---|---|---|---|---|---|
| | Carpentier-Edwards Porcine 2650 | 27 | <2 | 2.74 | 0.48 |
| | | 25 | <2 | 2.36 | 0.48 |
| | | 21 | <2 | 1.38 | 0.40 |
| | | 19 | <2 | 1.17 | 0.41 |
| | Carpentier-Edwards Pericardial 2900 | 27 | <3 | 3.70 | 0.64 |
| | | 25 | <2 | 3.25 | 0.66 |
| | | 21 | <2 | 1.88 | 0.54 |
| | | 19 | <2 | 1.56 | 0.55 |
| | Hancock Porcine 242 | 27 | <3 | 2.14 | 0.37 |
| | | 25 | <2 | 1.93 | 0.39 |
| | | 23 | <2 | 1.73 | 0.42 |
| | | 21 | <2 | 1.31 | 0.38 |
| | | 19 | <2 | 1.15 | 0.41 |
| | Hancock MO Porcine 250 | 25 | <2 | 2.16 | 0.44 |
| | | 23 | <2 | 1.94 | 0.47 |
| | | 21 | <2 | 1.43 | 0.41 |
| | | 19 | <2 | 1.22 | 0.43 |
| | Hancock II Porcine 410 | 27 | <2 | 2.36 | 0.41 |
| | | 25 | <2 | 2.10 | 0.43 |
| | | 23 | <2 | 1.81 | 0.44 |
| | | 21 | <2 | 1.48 | 0.43 |
| | Ionescu-Shiley Standard Pericardial | 27 | <3 | 2.35 | 0.41 |
| | Mosaic Porcine | 29 | <3 | 3.15 | 0.48 |
| | | 27 | <2 | 2.81 | 0.49 |
| | | 25 | <2 | 2.11 | 0.43 |
| | | 23 | <2 | 1.74 | 0.42 |
| | | 21 | <1 | 1.54 | 0.44 |
| | Mitroflow Pericardial | 29 | <4 | 3.71 | 0.56 |
| | | 23 | <3 | 2.12 | 0.51 |
| | | 19 | <2 | 1.34 | 0.47 |
| Nonstented bioprosthesis | Medtronic Freestyle Porcine | 27 | <4 | 3.75 | 0.65 |
| | | 25 | <4 | 3.41 | 0.69 |
| | | 23 | <3 | 2.69 | 0.65 |
| | | 21 | <2 | 2.17 | 0.63 |
| | | 19 | <2 | 1.84 | 0.65 |

[a]HR = 70 bpm; CO = 5 L/min typical; 120/80 mm Hg aortic pressure.

[b]EOA computed from Equation 1.

[c]Values obtained from (63).

EOA = effective orifice area; PI = performance index.

**TABLE 4** In vitro hemodynamic data for common mitral valve prostheses[a] (61)

| Valve type | Valve | Size | Regurgitant volume (ml/beat) | EOA[b] ($cm^2$) | PI |
|---|---|---|---|---|---|
| Caged ball | Starr-Edwards 1260 | 30 | | 1.99 | 0.28 |
| | | 28 | | 1.66 | 0.27 |
| | | 26 | | 1.56 | 0.29 |
| Tilting disc | Björk-Shiley Standard | 31 | | 3.40 | 0.45 |
| | | 29 | 6.7 | 2.79 | 0.42 |
| | | 25 | | 2.15 | 0.44 |
| | Björk-Shiley Convexo-concave | 29 | 10.1 | 2.96 | 0.45 |
| | | 27 | 8.3 | 2.28 | 0.40 |
| | | 25 | | 2.03 | 0.41 |
| | Medtronic-Hall | 31 | 10.0 | 3.53 | 0.47 |
| | | 29 | 10.0 | 3.53 | 0.53 |
| | | 27 | 8.9 | 2.73 | 0.47 |
| | | 25 | 7.2 | 2.23 | 0.45 |
| Bileaflet | St. Jude Medical Standard | 31 | 13.1 | 3.67 | 0.48 |
| | | 29 | 10.9 | 3.40 | 0.51 |
| | | 27 | 9.7 | 2.81 | 0.49 |
| Stented bioprosthesis | Hancock Porcine 342 | 35 | <4 | 2.72 | 0.28 |
| | | 33 | <4 | 2.54 | 0.30 |
| | | 31 | <4 | 2.36 | 0.31 |
| | | 29 | <4 | 2.11 | 0.32 |
| | | 27 | <2 | 1.77 | 0.31 |
| | | 25 | <2 | 1.63 | 0.33 |
| | Hancock II Porcine | 33 | <4 | 2.66 | 0.31 |
| | | 31 | <3 | 2.29 | 0.30 |
| | | 29 | <3 | 2.05 | 0.31 |
| | | 27 | <2 | 1.78 | 0.31 |
| | | 25 | <2 | 1.59 | 0.32 |
| | Carpentier-Edwards Porcine 6650 | 27 | <2 | 2.03 | 0.35 |
| | Carpentier-Edwards Porcine 6900 | 27 | <2 | 2.68 | 0.47 |
| | Carpentier-Edwards Porcine 6625 | 31 | <4 | 2.58 | 0.39 |
| | Ionescu-Shiley Standard Pericardial | 31 | <5 | 3.00 | 0.40 |
| | | 27 | <2 | 1.77 | 0.31 |
| | | 25 | <2 | 1.61 | 0.33 |
| | Mosaic Porcine | 33 | <4 | 2.38 | 0.28 |
| | | 31 | <3 | 2.26 | 0.30 |
| | | 29 | <3 | 2.02 | 0.31 |
| | | 27 | <2 | 1.71 | 0.30 |
| | | 25 | <2 | 1.55 | 0.32 |
| Nonstented bioprosthesis | Mitral Valve Allograft[c] | 25 | | 3.38 | 0.69 |
| | | 23 | | 1.80 | 0.43 |

[a]HR = 70 bpm; CO = 5 liters/min typical.

[b]EOA computed from Equation 1.

[c]In vitro measurements at 5 L/min.

spatial structure and velocity magnitude. However, the major orifice jet is larger and has a slightly higher velocity than the minor orifice jet. The peak velocities measured 7 mm downstream of the valve are 2.1 m/s and 2 m/s in the major and minor orifice regions, respectively, as shown in Figure 4 (38). A region of reverse flow adjacent to the wall in the minor orifice region at peak systole extends 2 mm from the wall, with a maximum reverse velocity of 0.25 m/s. The size of this region increases during the deceleration phase to 8 mm from the wall. A small region of flow separation is adjacent to the wall in the major orifice region as illustrated by Figure 4. In the minor orifice region, a profound velocity defect forms 7 mm and persists 11 mm distal to the minor orifice strut. Furthermore, the region adjacent to the wall immediately downstream from the minor orifice is stagnant during the acceleration and deceleration phases and has very low velocities ($<0.15$ m/s) during peak systole.

The tilting disc design has slightly lower regurgitant volumes than the bileaflet design. It has a regurgitant volume of approximately 9 ml/beat for a 27 mm valve size, and smaller valves have lower regurgitant volumes. Tilting disc valves typically have PIs ranging from 0.40 to 0.65 (Tables 3 and 4). Leakage flow through the gap between the disc and housing can form jets, and these jets are advantageous owing to the potential washing of the gap region. However, the velocities of these regurgitant jets range from 2 to 5 m/s, and turbulent stresses are several times greater than in the forward flow field.

In the major orifice region, high turbulent shear stresses are confined to narrow regions at the edges of the major orifice jet. The peak turbulent shear stress at peak systole increases from 1200 to 1500 dynes/cm$^2$, 7 to 13 mm downstream of the valve, respectively. During the acceleration and deceleration phases, the turbulent shear stresses are relatively low, and high turbulent shear stresses are more dispersed in the minor orifice region. The turbulent shear stress profiles across the major and minor orifices 15 mm downstream of the valve show peak turbulent shear stresses at the lower edges of the orifice jets.

BILEAFLET VALVE The most commonly used bileaflet valve, the St. Jude Medical (SJM) mechanical valve, has two semicircular leaflets that divide the area available for forward flow into three regions: two lateral orifices and a central orifice. The major part of the forward flow emerges from the two lateral orifices. A triple jet pattern, shown in Figure 5, characterizes the forward flow (38). The lateral and central orifice jets reach maximum velocities of 2.2 m/s and 2 m/s, respectively, along the centerline plane 8 mm downstream of the valve at peak systole. The velocities of the jets are maintained as the flow travels from 8 to 13 mm downstream. After traveling 20 or 30 mm, the three jets merge into a central flow region. The velocity profile shows two defects that correspond to the wakes of the two leaflets. The flow is more evenly distributed across the flow chamber during the deceleration than during the acceleration phase, and more flow emerges from central orifice during the deceleration phase than during the acceleration phase. Regions of flow separation lie around the jets adjacent to the flow channel wall as the flow separates

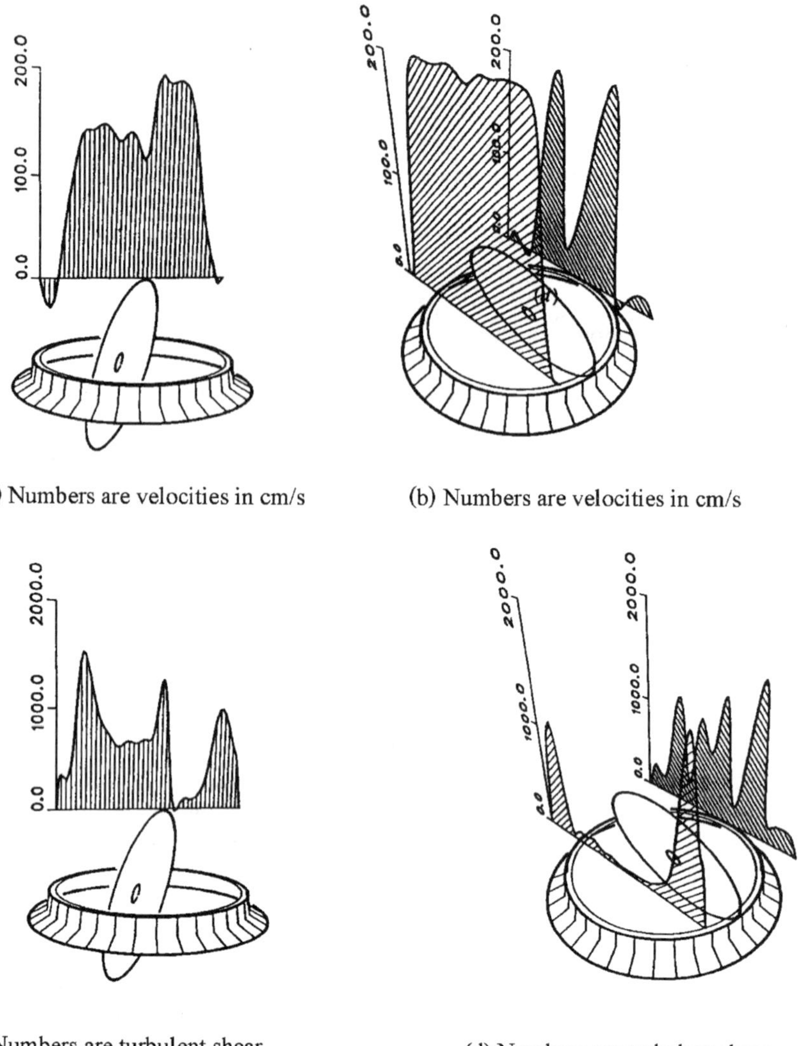


(a) Numbers are velocities in cm/s

(b) Numbers are velocities in cm/s

(c) Numbers are turbulent shear stresses in dynes/cm$^2$

(d) Numbers are turbulent shear stresses in dynes/cm$^2$

**Figure 4** (*a*) Velocity profile 15 mm downstream on the centerline across the major and minor orifices of the Medtronic-Hall tilting disc valve (major orifice to the *right*) at peak systole; (*b*) velocity profiles 13 mm downstream in the major and minor orifices of the Medtronic-Hall tilting disc valve at peak systole; (*c*) turbulent shear stress profile 15 mm downstream on the centerline across the major and minor orifices of the Medtronic-Hall tilting disc valve (major orifice to the *right*) at peak systole; (*d*) turbulent shear stress profiles 13 mm downstream in the major and minor orifices of the Medtronic-Hall tilting disc valve at peak systole (38).

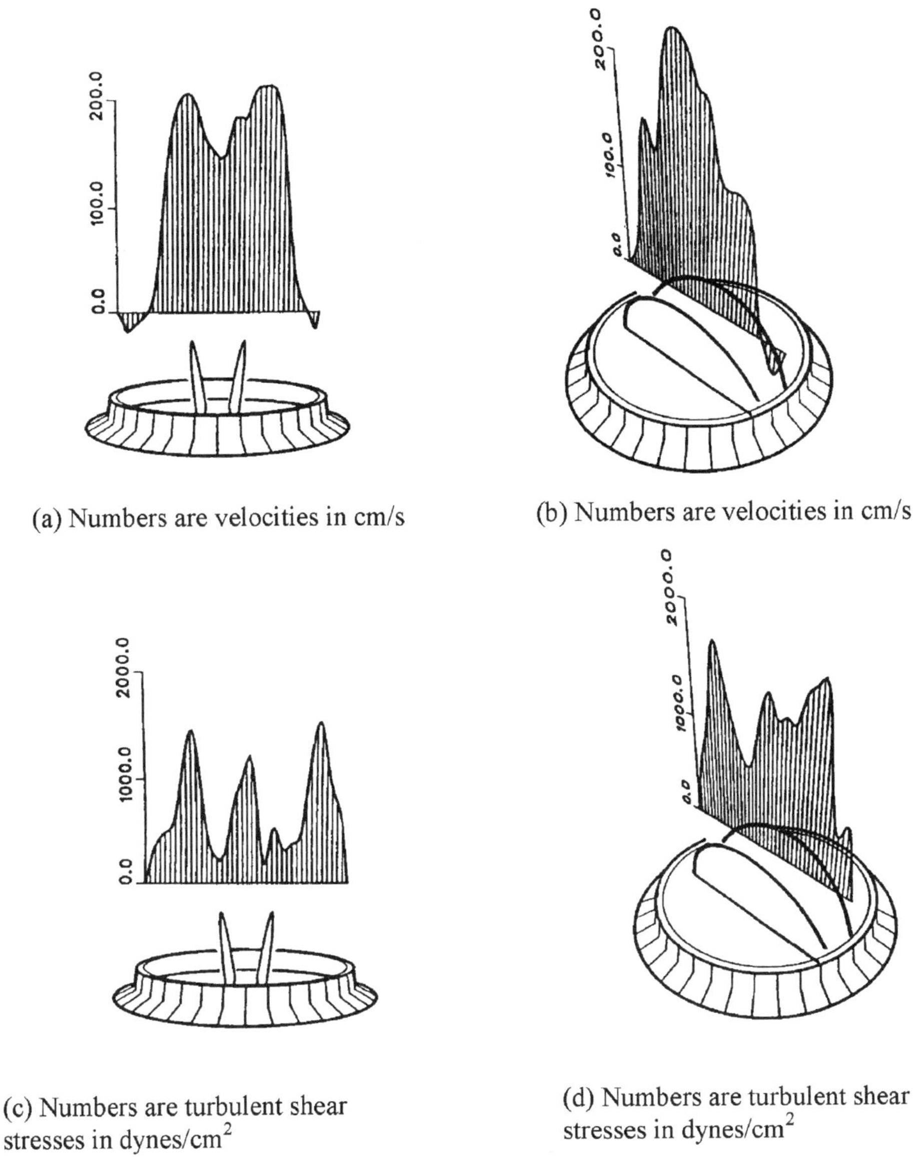


**Figure 5** (*a*) Velocity profile 13 mm downstream on the centerline for the St. Jude Medical bileaflet valve at peak systole; (*b*) velocity profile 13 mm downstream across the central orifice for the St. Jude Medical bileaflet valve at peak systole; (*c*) turbulent shear stress profile 13 mm downstream of the centerline orifice for the St. Jude Medical bileaflet valve at peak systole; (*d*) turbulent shear stress profile 13 mm downstream across the central orifice for the St. Jude Medical bileaflet valve at peak systole (38).

from the orifice ring, and small regions of low-velocity reverse flow are adjacent to the pivot/hinge mechanism of the valve.

Regurgitant flow characteristics of the bileaflet design are similar to those for the tilting disc design, but the bileaflet valve has slightly larger regurgitant volumes than the tilting disc valve. Regurgitant volumes are summarized in Tables 3 and 4. Leakage flow through the bileaflet valve occurs primarily through the pivots as well as through peripheral gap between the leaflets and the housing. The mean velocity in the leakage jet 1 mm upstream of the valve is approximately 2–3 m/s with turbulent shear stress levels exceeding 3000 dynes/$cm^2$. The bileaflet design in general has lower pressure drops than the caged-ball and tilting disc mechanical valve designs, and these data are listed in Tables 3 and 4.

High turbulent shear stresses occur at locations of high-velocity gradients immediately distal to the valve leaflets, as shown in Figure 5. The peak turbulent shear stresses along the centerline plane at peak systole are 1150 and 1500 dynes/$cm^2$ at planes 8 and 13 mm downstream of the valve, respectively. The profiles across the central orifice show that the flow is very disturbed in this region. The maximum turbulent shear stress in the central orifice region is 1700 dynes/$cm^2$ during peak systole 11 mm downstream of the valve. It is probable that even higher turbulent shear stresses occur closer to the valve.

HINGE FLOW STUDIES The hinge region is considered to be one of the most critical components of a bileaflet MHV because it directly affects valve durability, local fluid dynamics, functionality, and thrombus formation. The geometry of the hinge is normally a butterfly shape when viewed from the side, which matches the semicircular or square ear projections of the leaflets. More attention has been given to the hinge region of bileaflet valves in terms of hemodynamics as well as durability because the Medtronic Parallel valve was found to have a high incidence of thrombus formation within its hinge region. Laser Doppler velocimetry (LDV) and computational fluid dynamics (CFD) were used to investigate the flow characteristics within the hinge regions (39–43).

The hinge regions are washed twice during each cardiac cycle, once during the forward flow phase when the valve is open and again during the leakage phase when the valve is closed. The forward flow velocities within the hinge region are lower than the leakage flow velocities. Figure 6 (see color insert) shows the velocity map in the hinge region of the SJM Regent mitral valve during the leakage phase. High velocities occur in the inflow or outflow corners of the hinge region. The maximum velocity always occurs in the inflow corner during the leakage phase. The hinge flow depends very much upon the geometry of the hinge. The SJM Regent valve has a semicircular projection on the leaflet, which mates to a similarly shaped recess in the valve housing. The streamlined geometry of the hinge provides a smooth hinge flow, effectively minimizing the formation of unwanted vortex structures and complex flow seen in the Medtronic Parallel valve. The geometry of the Medtronic Parallel hinge recess is characterized by sudden expansion and contraction zones, which give rise to unsteady flow, vortex structures, and stagnation zones. The

**TABLE 5** Peak phase-averaged velocities and turbulent shear stresses measured within the hinge region of different bileaflet valve designs (41–43)

| Manufacture | Model | Size (mm) | Peak leakage velocity (m/s) | Peak turbulent shear stress (dyne/cm$^2$) |
|---|---|---|---|---|
| St. Jude Medical | Standard | 25 | 3.50 | 7200 |
| St. Jude Medical | Hemodynamic Plus | 17 | 1.3 | 2900 |
| St. Jude Medical | Regent | 23 | 1.50 | 2600 |
| St. Jude Medical | Regent | 17 | 0.75 | 2000 |
| CarboMedics | | 23 | 3.17 | 5640 |
| Medtronic | Parallel | 27 | 4.00 | 8000 |

turbulent shear stress has been measured at levels up to 2600 dyne/cm$^2$ (42). These flow features may be due to the contracting geometry of the corner site or to a narrow gap between the leaflet pivot and housing wall. In general, the streamlined hinge design of the SJM Regent valve has lower peak velocities, turbulent shear stresses, and a more favorable flow pattern. Table 5 lists the peak velocities and turbulent shear stresses in the hinge regions of different bileaflet valve designs in the mitral position.

CAVITATION IN MECHANICAL HEART VALVES Cavitation is the rapid formation and collapse of vapor-filled bubbles caused by a transient reduction in local pressure below the liquid vapor pressure (44). There are many micro bubbles in the liquid, which are called nuclei. The nuclei dilate rapidly into bubbles at a given temperature when the ambient pressure decreases to a critical pressure. The bubbles will collapse if the ambient pressure increases from this critical pressure. The violent collapse of cavitation bubbles generates intense shock waves and high-speed reentrant jets causing damage to the nearby material, which is called cavitation damage. The typical pattern of cavitation damage is pitting on the structure near the cavitation site. Pitting and erosion on some clinically explanted MHVs suggest that cavitation occurs under normal physiological conditions in the human body (45, 46). Pitting has only been reported on mechanical valves used in the mitral position. No pitting has been found on bioprosthetic heart valves.

Cavitation occurs on the inflow side of the mitral valve occluder surface at the instant when the occluder impacts the housing. The cavitation duration includes bubble incipience, development, and collapse. Its magnitude is on the order of a few hundred microseconds. The bubble collapse produces unique pressure characteristics, such as high-pressure oscillation, which is often used to detect cavitation (47, 48). Cavitation is more involved with local fluid dynamics and is therefore structure dependent. There are several factors that influence cavitation in MHVs: occluder closing velocity (49, 50), ventricular loading rate (51, 52), squeeze flow (53, 54), valve mounting (55), and occluder material properties (56, 57). In general, five major fluid mechanics causes of cavitation have been documented: (*a*) pressure oscillations, (*b*) flow deceleration, (*c*) tip vortices (58), (*d*) streamline contraction, and (*e*) squeeze jets (53). Recent evidence shows that the squeeze jets contribute more to cavitation than any other factor. During the formation of these jets, the fluid trapped between the occluder and housing is squeezed out of the gap during valve closure to form a high-speed jet. This jet mixes with fluid outside the gap and forms a strong shear layer in which vortices are so intense that pressure in the cores is low enough to lead to cavitation. These jets can be subdivided into squeeze jets and transvalvular jets (59), which can both cause jet vortex cavitation in the valve. This theory is supported by cavitation damage observed in the housing ring close to the leaflet contact site. Computational fluid dynamics has been utilized to show that the squeeze jet velocity can be as high as 14 m/s (53). Tip vortices are also considered to be an important cause of cavitation.

## Bioprosthetic Valves

Bioprosthetic valves, or tissue valves, are composed of three biological leaflets derived from porcine aortic valve leaflets or bovine pericardium, which are treated/fixed in a gluteraldehyde solution. They are geometrically similar to the natural aortic valve. The annular ring is cloth-covered and molded to function similarly to the aortic annulus. Metal or polymeric stents provide support to the leaflets at their commissures in stented bioprosthetic designs, whereas the leaflet commissures in nonstented aortic valve design must be attached to the native aorta for support. All trileaflet bioprosthetic designs have an orifice located in the center of the annulus. Bioprosthetic valves exhibit higher pressure drops than most mechanical valves, particularly in the small sizes, which have stenotic characteristics. The pressure drop increases when the tissue is calcified. The fluid characteristics of these bioprosthetic valves are discussed below based on in vitro measurements conducted using 27 mm aortic valve designs. The velocities and turbulent shear stresses were obtained at peak systole at a cardiac output of 6.0 L per minute and a heart rate of 70 beats per minute.

STENTED VALVES Bioprosthetic valves do not have an occluder in the central orifice when the valve is open. These valves tend to produce a high-velocity jet-like forward flow with a slightly laterally directed motion, as shown in Figure 7. The flow is much more evenly distributed along the outflow channel than that of mechanical valves. When the jet-like flow leaves the bioprosthetic valve, it dissipates very rapidly as it flows downstream. The peak aortic velocities in the Carpentier-Edwards porcine valve range from 2 to 3 m/s at peak systole. Usually, regions of flow separation are not generated throughout the systolic period inside the valve orifice outflow region. However, the annular region between the outflow surfaces of the leaflets and the flow chamber wall is stagnant throughout systole. The flow exiting the valve tends to accelerate toward the center of the flow channel then decelerate. All stented porcine tissue valves are mildly stenotic compared to the

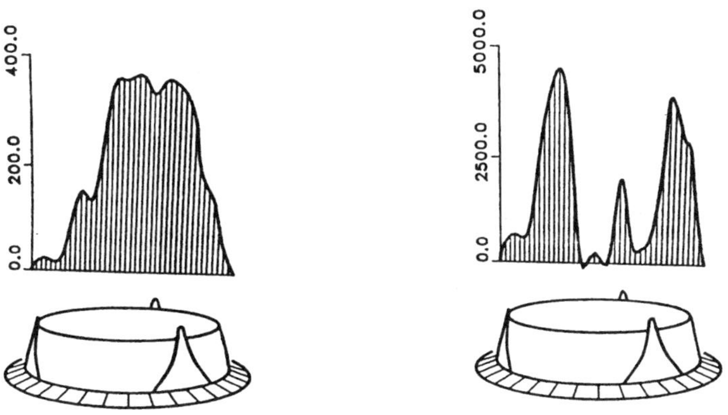


(a) Numbers are velocities in cm/s

(b) Numbers are turbulent shear stresses in dynes/cm$^2$

**Figure 7** (*a*) Velocity profile 15 mm downstream on the centerline for the Carpentier-Edwards 2625 porcine valve at peak systole; (*b*) turbulent shear stress profile 15 mm downstream on the centerline for the Carpentier-Edwards 2625 porcine valve at peak systole (38).

natural valve. As a result, performance indices of common stented porcine tissue valves range from 0.3 to 0.4. This stenotic behavior is due to stent restriction to leaflet opening, construction of the leaflets, stiffness of the fixed tissue, and man-made commissures. Typical EOAs range from 1.3 to 2.5 cm$^2$ for 21 mm to 27 mm porcine aortic valves, respectively (60). The EOA and PI values for several bioprosthetic valves are listed in Tables 3 and 4. All bioprosthetic valves exhibit some degree of regurgitant flow in the closing volume. Leakage volume is essentially zero in properly functioning native valves, and regurgitant volumes are less than 2 ml/beat for most tissue valves. The closing volumes are generally lower than those in mechanical prostheses.

High turbulent shear stresses occur at the edge of the central jet through the Carpentier-Edwards porcine valve (Figure 7). The maximum turbulent shear stresses range from 1000 to 4500 dynes/cm$^2$. The turbulent shear stresses at the edge of the jet increase as the flow travels downstream.

Another commonly used stented bioprosthesis is the Carpentier-Edwards pericardial valve. Its flow patterns in the aortic position are superior to that of the porcine valve. It has a larger EOA of 3.70 cm$^2$ and a maximum velocity of 1.80 m/s 17 mm downstream of the valve, as shown in Figure 8. The jet flow field downstream of the pericardial valve is more evenly distributed and closer to that of a nonstented porcine aortic valve. The high turbulent shear stresses at peak systole are confined to a narrow region, with a maximum value of 850 dynes/cm$^2$ (38).

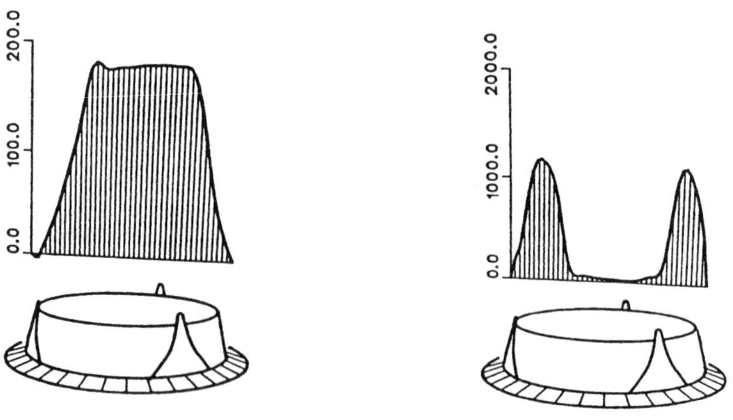


(a) Numbers are velocities in cm/s

(b) Numbers are turbulent shear stresses in dynes/cm$^2$

**Figure 8** (*a*) Velocity profile 17 mm downstream on the centerline for the Carpentier-Edwards pericardial valve at peak systole; (*b*) turbulent shear stress profile 17 mm downstream on the centerline for the Carpentier-Edwards pericardial valve at peak systole (38).

NONSTENTED VALVES Nonstented prosthetic valves are comprised of a natural porcine valve or part of an intact aorta. The original right and left coronary arteries are ligated with short remnants. Most of these nonstented valves are used in the aortic position. For aortic valves, the flow accelerates uniformly through the valve with an apparent uniform and flat profile downstream of the valve. The peak velocity at the leaflet tip is approximately 1.25 to 2.00 m/s, and unlike the stented bioprostheses, there is no jet with steep velocity gradients. Usually, nonstented valves exhibit large EOAs and low regurgitation with good leaflet coaptation. The removal of the stent results in less forward flow obstruction and significantly improves the hemodynamic performance. Tables 3 and 4 show EOAs for some nonstented valves. Nonstented valve function depends largely upon whether the valve geometry matches the specific patient. Additionally, total root or an inclusion cylinder valve geometry technique yields better EOA results than partially or fully scalloped valve configurations (61).

Mitral valve heterografts are considered to be nonstented bioprostheses. The flow data for these mitral heterografts are limited owing to difficulty in valve development. Fixation of mitral heterografts in gluteraldehyde can reduce the orifice area and increase regurgitation (62). The function of mitral heterografts is strongly dependent upon the implantation technique owing to the complex structure of the mitral valve apparatus.

Homograft valves are cryopreserved human valves and can be categorized as nonstented valves. They are similar to the natural valves in geometry except that the leaflets become stiff and the annulus shrinks slightly after cryopreservation. They exhibit small closing volumes and modest leakage. They have low pressure drops with large EOAs as compared with mechanical valves and stented bioprotheses. Typical values of EOAs and PIs for homograft valves are listed in Tables 3 and 4.

## COMPUTATIONAL MODELING OF NATIVE AND PROSTHETIC VALVES

The development of computational models of the fluid mechanics in heart valves is motivated by medical and economic concerns as well as efficiency. First, sufficiently accurate and descriptive computational models would serve as an excellent tool for scientific and medical research. Second, computational models would provide valve developers with a means of validating and predicting valve performance to improve the product development process and make it more cost effective. Third, fast and accurate computational models could be used in clinical settings if combined with medical imaging and other cardiovascular diagnostic techniques to provide real-time information to improve patient care.

Developing computational models of heart valves to meet these goals is challenging for the current generation of CFD software and computer hardware. This difficulty stems from the fact that the fluid mechanics of heart valves includes several phenomena that are difficult problems in their own right, such as fluid-structure interaction in which the motion of the valve leaflets drive most of the fluid motion and the wide disparity in length scales from the large-scale motions with length scales in the valve orifice (~25 mm) to the flow in the hinge regions of mechanical valves (~100 $\mu$m). Moreover, the flow is pulsatile owing to the heart cycle and possibly unsteady owing to vortex shedding from the leaflets and other parts of the valve structure. The flow can become turbulent at peak flow through the valve, and such turbulence is thought to play an important role in clinical phenomena, such as platelet activation and thrombosis formation and embolization. The important timescales of the flow also vary widely from more than one heart cycle for the effects of fluid stresses on blood cells to milliseconds when the valve closes where cavitation is an issue. Developing a comprehensive CFD model that can address even a few of these issues within the same computational model is a formidable task that has not yet been achieved. However, such a coupled model is necessary if the goals mentioned above are to be reached, namely producing a computational model that can aid in the scientific discovery of the role that fluid mechanics plays in heart valve function and disease and as a product-development tool to improve existing valve designs and create new prosthetic heart valves whether mechanical or biological.

In the past several decades, development of CFD models for heart valves has focused primarily on predicting the large-scale flow features in MHVs. Much of this research has focused on evaluating the effectiveness of different numerical methods or on validation—comparing the results of in vitro fluid mechanics experiments with model results. Most recent work of this type has been largely successful on a qualitative basis, but it is mainly limited to predicting the steady, forward flow in the valve. More recently, research has attempted to extend the numerical methods to coupling the motion of the valve leaflets with motion of the fluid to have a truly predictive model. Other recent research has reexamined the assumptions used in earlier forward-flow only work and extended the models to include important local flow features, such as cavitation and unsteadiness.

In what follows, the development and use of CFD for predicting the flow in heart valves is traced. This discussion begins with two-dimensional models that were developed in the 1970s and continues with the development of three-dimensional fluid-only models that are being used today. Other numerical issues that are particularly important for typical heart valve geometries, namely symmetry and grid resolution, are also discussed. Finally, the future of CFD for heart valve modeling is discussed, along with some considerations that should guide future work.

## Two-Dimensional Models

Two-dimensional models of the flow through heart valves were developed in the 1970s using the vorticity-stream function formulation of the Navier–Stokes equation, which is convenient and efficient in two dimensions but unwieldy in three dimensions. In these studies, the geometry of the native and prosthetic heart valves was greatly simplified because the numerical methods were limited to simple Cartesian grids (64, 65). However, even at this early stage, Hung & Schuessler (64) were able to include leaflet motion in the simulation by manipulating the boundary conditions on the leaflet surface. Au & Greenfield (66) predicted the steady flow through a tilting disk valve. Their work tried to infer thrombosis formation from laminar flow predictions at Re = 100, a volumetric flow much below physiological values. Using a similar CFD model, separation behind the valve leaflets was predicted by Underwood & Mueller (67, 68) for Re = 500. Idelsohn et al. (69) performed a comparative study of the caged-disk, tilting-disk, and caged-ball prosthetic valves using a finite-element CFD method with Re of 900 to 2000 for the various valves. This method avoided some of the difficulty encountered in previous studies that used regular computational grids. Stevenson et al. (70, 71) used a curvilinear formulation of the vorticity-stream-function form of the Navier-Stokes equations to circumvent the problem with Cartesian grids. Their work also accounted for turbulence effects using the $k$-$\varepsilon$ turbulence model. Nonetheless, all of the above methods were limited to two-dimensional or axisymmetric flow.

More recently Huang et al. (72) performed time-accurate two-dimensional simulations of a tilting disk heart valve using a grid resolution of over 90,000 nodes, much larger than any previous heart valve simulation, for Re between 10 and 1000. King et al. (73) performed a steady two-dimensional finite element simulation of a bileaflet heart valve at Re = 3000.

To predict two-dimensional fluid-structure interactions, Peskin (74) developed an immersed boundary method to couple the blood flow to the structure of the heart and its valves. He used the method to predict the flow through a mitral valve mounted in a straight tube and in the left heart (75). He also used it to predict the flow through prosthetic valves (76). The early version of the immersed boundary method was limited to very low Re. Peskin & McQueen (77) extended the method to larger Re, and the results showed no qualitative differences between the flow at Re = 20 and Re = 200. More recently, de Hart et al. (78) developed a two-dimensional fictitious domain finite element code to predict the unsteady flow in the aortic valve.

## Three-Dimensional Models

In the mid-to-late 1990s, the computer resources available to heart valve researchers increased to the point at which three-dimensional simulations of MHVs could be performed. Shim & Chang (79) performed a three-dimensional analysis of a tilting disk valve at Re = 210 and Re = 450 under steady flow conditions. They assumed the flow to be symmetric with respect to vertical plane of symmetry and discretized one half of the valve geometry using a grid with approximately 32,000 nodes. Their results suggested the presence of longitudinal vortices downstream of the leaflet. King et al. (80, 81) extended their two-dimensional simulations to three dimensions by using one quarter of the valve geometry. These simulations used a sinusoidally varying inlet velocity to mimic the acceleration phase of systole with a peak Re = 3000. Kiris et al. (82) used a multiblock method with approximately 22,000 nodes to predict the three-dimensional flow in a fixed tilting-disk valve. They used the full three-dimensional geometry for steady flow and varied the Re from 2000 to 6000. Krafczyk et al. (83) used a lattice-Boltzmann method with over 5 million particles to predict the flow in a full three-dimensional model of a fixed bileaflet valve using a time-varying inflow with a peak Re = 1800.

To achieve three-dimensional predictions of fluid-structure interaction, Peskin & McQueen (84, 85) extended their immersed boundary method to three dimensions and successfully computed the flow in the whole heart, albeit at a Re much below the physiological range. Their three-dimensional method was also applied to heart valves (86); however, difficulties still exist with extending their method to predict the turbulent flow that often occurs in diseased or MHVs. de Hart et al. (87, 88) extended their fictitious domain fluid-structure interaction code to predict the flow and motion of fiber-reinforced stentless bioprosthetic and native aortic valves. Because of the cost of their numerical method, their work was limited to predicting only one sixth of the valve with a limited spatial resolution of the fluid and valve leaflets using only 26,500 degrees of freedom.

## Issues for Future Modeling

Ge et al. (89) performed simulations to evaluate several numerical issues related to modeling the large-scale flow in MHVs. In particular, they focused on the complex three-dimensionality of the flow (see Figure 9, see color insert) and the role that grid resolution plays in the predicted flow field. Using a bileaflet heart valve within a simplified aortic sinus as a model, they studied the role of symmetry in predicting the onset of unsteadiness in the MHV with increasing Re. They found that the flow just distal to the leaflets is extremely sensitive to the cross-sectional grid resolution. Less than adequate grid resolution caused the flow in these regions to become unnaturally unsteady. Ge et al. (89) suggested that a grid resolution on the order of 1–2 million will be needed for grid-independent solutions in MHVs. Moreover, Ge et al. (89) showed that the flow for relatively low Re (Re = 1200) was fully three dimensional, thus calling into question some of the previous work at higher Re that assumed that the flow was symmetric about either the horizontal or both the horizontal and vertical symmetry planes of the valve.

It is also important to realize that many of the phenomena that researchers, engineers, and clinicians want to predict using numerical models, namely thrombosis formation and fate of emboli, probably require even more detailed grid resolution than that suggested by Ge et al. (89). Prakash & Ethier (90) found that CFD-based predictions of wall shear stress in the human right coronary artery were particularly sensitive to mesh refinement and required many more grid nodes to achieve grid-independence than the velocity field alone. The clinical issues that are of interest in MHV and native heart valves are at least as stringent.

Rosenfield et al. (93) studied the different unsteady forcings that occur in MHV flows, namely the unsteadiness owing to pulsatilty, vortex shedding, and the closing of the valve. Their results suggest that to get a true picture of the performance of the valve, one must predict the flow through the entire heart cycle. Even though their work was limited to two dimensions, they readily acknowledged that the flow in MHV is fully three dimensional and suggested in line with Ge et al. (89) that the grid refinement necessary for accurate predictions was much larger than is currently being used.

Aluri & Chandran (91) and Lai et al. (92) numerically studied the affect of valve closure on the potential for cavitation formation for MHVs. Because of the complexity of the phenomena and the desire to focus on the detailed flow patterns near the tips of the leaflets, they were also restricted to two-dimensional models. Laminarization and turbulence are important phenomena in prosthetic heart valves but have not yet been modeled together. Numerical methods capable of allowing laminar and turbulent flow to coexist in the same domain are needed. At present, variants of large-eddy simulation techniques appear to be the most promising for predicting the turbulence and relaminarization that occur during the cardiac cycle.

## IMPLICATIONS FOR THROMBUS FORMATION

In the vicinity of mechanical aortic heart valves, where peak turbulent shear stresses can easily exceed 1500 dyne/cm$^2$ and mean turbulent shear stresses are frequently in the range of 200–600 dyne/cm$^2$, and platelet activation and aggregation may readily occur. Data indicating that shear-induced platelet damage is cumulative are particularly relevant to heart valves. During an individual excursion through the replacement valve, the combination of shear magnitude and exposure time may not induce platelet aggregation. However, as a result of multiple journeys though the artificial valve, shear-induced damage may accumulate to a degree sufficient to promote thrombosis and subsequent embolization.

All of the aortic and mitral valve designs (mechanical and tissue) studied to date create mean turbulent shear stress in excess of 20 $N/m^2$ during the major portion of systole and diastole, which could lead to blood element damage. In the case of mechanical prostheses, owing to the presence of foreign surfaces, the chances for blood cell damage are increased. Furthermore, the regions of flow stagnation and/or flow separation that occur adjacent to the superstructures of these valve designs could promote the deposition of damaged blood elements, leading to thrombus formation on the prosthesis.

The clinical performance of the Medtronic Parallel valve is an example of the effects of these flow patterns on the likelihood of thromboembolic complications. This valve showed superior forward flow hemodynamics in an in vivo porcine model, suggesting a good clinical performance. However, the Medtronic Parallel valve performed very poorly in clinical trials, with approximately 20% of the patients in these trials developing thrombosis. Patient and material factors were statistically eliminated as potential reasons for the poor performance. Subsequent in vitro analysis of flow through the valve pivot revealed regions of highly disturbed vortical flow within this area during the leakage phase. Thrombi from explant valves were localized within the pivots to these disturbed flow regions.

## CONCLUSIONS

Direct comparison of the "total" performance of artificial heart valves is difficult, if not impossible. The precise definition of the criteria used to benchmark valve performance varies from study to study. To investigate long-term performance, large numbers of patients and lengthy observation periods are required. During these periods there may be an evolution in valve materials or design and in the medical treatment of patients with prosthetic heart valves. The age of the patient at implant and the underlying valvular heart disease(s) are extremely important factors in valve choice and longevity as well. Additionally, a valve design suited for the aortic position may be inappropriate for the mitral position. Consequently, it is not possible to categorize a particular valve as the best. All valves currently in use, mechanical and bioprosthetic, produce relatively large turbulent stresses, which can cause lethal and or sublethal damage to red cells and platelets, and also produce larger pressure gradients and regurgitant volumes than normal heart valves.

There are three promising directions for further advances in heart valves (and therefore three challenges for engineers designing new heart valves):

- Improved hemodynamic characteristics, especially reduction and/or elimination of low-flow regions (stagnation, flow separation) within and/or adjacent to the prosthetic heart valve and vessel surfaces, and high turbulent shear stresses along the edges of jets produced by valve outflow and/or leakage flow

- Improved thromboresistance with new and better artificial materials
- Improved durability of new tissue valves through the use of nonstented tissue valves, new anticalcification treatments, and better fixation treatments.

Although the current prosthetic heart valves in clinical use leave room for further improvements, the superior prognosis for the patient with a replacement heart valve is dramatic and convincing.

## ACKNOWLEDGMENTS

The authors acknowledge the support from the National Heart Lung and Blood Institute (grants HL-070262, HL-52009). We also acknowledge the editorial assistance of Anna Fallon and Jennifer Ritchie.

**The *Annual Review of Biomedical Engineering* is online at http://bioeng.annualreviews.org**

## LITERATURE CITED

1. Roberts WC. 1976. Choosing a substitute cardiac valve; type, size, surgeon. *Am. J. Cardiol.* 38:633–44
2. Jamieson WR. 2002. Current and advanced prostheses for cardiac valvular replacement and reconstruction surgery. *Surg. Technol. Int.* 10:121–49
3. Bodnar E, Frater R. 1991. *Replacement Cardiac Valves*. New York: Pergamon
4. Butchart EG, Bodnar E. 1992. *Thrombosis, Embolism and Bleeding*. London: ICR Publ.
5. Giddens DP, Yoganathan AP, Schoen FJ. 1993. Prosthetic cardiac valves. *Cardiovasc. Pathol.* 2(3)(Suppl.):167S–77
6. Ormiston JA, Shah PM, Tei C, Wong M. 1981. Size and motion of the mitral valve annulus in man: a two-dimensional echocardiographic method and findings in normal subjects. *Circulation* 64:113–20
7. Levine RA, Handshumacher MD, Sanfilippo AJ, Hagege AA, Harrigan P, et al. 1989. Three-dimensional echocardiographic reconstruction of the mitral valve, with implications for the diagnosis of mitral valve prolapse. *Circulation* 80:589–98
8. Gorman JH, Gupta KB, Streicher JT, Gorman RC, Jackson BM, et al. 1996. Dynamic three-dimensional imaging of the mitral valve and left ventricle by rapid sonomicrometry array localization. *J. Thorac. Cardiovasc. Surg.* 112:712–26
9. Karlsson MO, Glasson JR, Bolger AF, Daughters GT, Komeda M, et al. 1998. Mitral valve opening in the ovine heart. *Am. J. Physiol.Heart Circ. Physiol.* 274:H552–63
10. He S, Fontaine AA, Schwammenthal E, Yoganathan AP, Levine RA. 1997. Integrated mechanism for functional mitral regurgitation: leaflet elongation versus coapting force: in vitro study. *Circulation* 96:1826–34
11. He S, Lemmon JD, Weston MW, Jensen MAO, Levine RA, et al. 1999. Mitral valve compensation for annular dilatation: in vitro study into the mechanisms of functional mitral regurgitation with an adjustable annulus model. *J. Heart Valve Dis.* 8:294–302

12. Kunzelman KS, Cochran RP, Murphree SS, Ring WS, Verrier ED, Eberhart RC. 1993. Differential collagen distribution in the mitral valve and its influence on biomechanical behaviour. *J. Heart Valve Dis.* 2:236–44
13. Bellhouse BJ. 1969. Velocity and pressure distributions in the aortic valve. *J. Fluid Mech.* 37:587–600
14. Reul H, Talukdar N. 1979. Heart valve mechanics. In *Quantitative Cardiovascular Studies Clinical and Research Applications of Engineering Principles*, ed. NHC Hwang, DR Gross, DJ Patel, pp. 527–64. Baltimore, MD: Univ. Park Press
15. Yoganathan AP, Hopmeyer J, Heinrich R. 1995. Mechanics of heart valve. See Ref. 94, chapter 13, pp. 440–53
16. Thrbrikar M, Heckman JL, Nolan SP. 1993. High speed cine-radiographic study of aortic valve leaflet motion. *J. Heart Valve Dis.* 2:653–61
17. Bellhouse BJ, Bellhouse E. 1969. Fluid mechanics of model normal and stenosed aortic valve. *Circ. Res.* 25:693–704
18. Rossvoll O, Samstad S, Torp HG, Linker DT, Skjaerpe T, et al. 1991. The velocity distributation in the aortic annulus in normal subjects: a quantitative analysis of two-dimensional Doppler flow maps. *J. Am. Soc. Echocardiogr.* 4:367–78
19. Hatle L, Angelsen B. 1985. *Doppler Ultrasound in Cardiology Physical Principles and Clinical Applications*. Philadelphia, PA: Lea & Febiger
20. Kilner PJ, Yang GZ, Mohiaddin RH, Firmin DN, Longmore DB. 1993. Helical and retrograde secondary flow patterns in the aortic arch studied by three-dimensional magnetic resonance velocity mapping. *Circulation.* 88(Pt. I):2235–47
21. Weyman AE. 1994. *Principles and Practices of Echocardiography*. Philadelphia, PA: Lea & Febiger
22. Sloth E, Houlind KC, Oyre S, Kim WY, Pedersen EM, et al. 1994. Three-dimensional visualization of velocity profiles in the human main pulmonary artery with magnetic resonance phase-velocity mapping. *Am. Heart J.* 128:1130–38
23. Kim W, Bisgaard T, Nielsen SL, Poulsen JK, Pedersen EM, et al. 1994. Two-dimensional mitral flow velocity profiles in pig models using epicardial Doppler echocardiography. *J. Am. Coll. Cardiol.* 24: 532–45
24. Samstad SO, Torp HG, Linker DT, Rossvoll O, Skjaerpe T, et al. 1989. Cross sectional early mitral flow velocity profiles from colour Doppler. *Br. Heart J.* 62:177–84
25. Oh JK, Appleton CP, Hatle LK, Nishimura RA, Seward JB, et al. 1997. The noninvasive assessment of left ventricular diastolic function with two-dimensional and Doppler echocardiography. *J. Am. Soc. Echocardiogr.* 10:246–70
26. Bellhouse BJ. 1972. The fluid mechanics of a model mitral valve and left ventricle. *Cardiovasc. Res.* 6:199–210
27. Reul J, Talukder N, Muller E. 1981. Fluid mechanics of the natural mitral valve. *J. Biomech.* 14:361–72
28. Yellin EL, Peskin C, Yoran C, Koenigsberg M, Matsumoto M, et al. 1981. Mechanisms of mitral valve motion during diastole. *Am. J. Physiol. Heart Circ. Physiol.* 241:H389–400
29. Kim WY, Walker PG, Pederson EM, Poulsen JK, Houlind KC, et al. 1995. Mitral ammular function assessed by 3D imaging for mitral valve surgery. *J. Heart Valve Dis.* 3:483–90
30. Tsakiris AG, von Bernuth G, Rastelli GC, Bourgeois MJ, Titus JL, et al. 1971. Size and motion of the mitral valve annulus in anesthetized intact dogs. *J. Appl. Physiol.* 30:611–18
31. Simonson JS, Schiller NB. 1989. Descent of the base of the left ventricle: an echocardiographic index of left ventricular function. *J. Am. Soc. Echocardiogr.* 2:25–35
32. Sanfilippo AJ, Harrigan P, Popovic AD, Weyman AE, Levine RA. 1992. Papillary muscle traction in mitral valve prolapse: quantitation by two-dimensional echocardiography. *J. Am. Coll. Cardiol.* 19:564–71

33. Otsuji Y, Handshumacher MD, Schwammenthal E, Jiang L, Song JK, et al. 1997. Insights from three-dimensional echocardiography into the mechanism of functional mitral regurgitation: direct in vivo demonstration of altered leaflet tethering geometry. *Circulation* 96:1999–2008
34. Sarnoff S, Braunwald E, Welch GH, Case RB, Stainsby WN, et al. 1958. Hemodynamic determinants of oxygen consumption of the heart with special reference to the tension-time index. *Am. J. Physiol.* 192:141–47
35. Yoganathan AP, Chaux A, Gray R, Woo YR, DeRobertis M, et al. 1984. Bileaflet, tilting disc and porcine aortic valve substitutes: in vitro hydrodynamic characteristics. *J. Am. Coll. Cardiol.* 3:313–20
36. Sallam AM, Hwang NHC. 1984. Human red blood cell hemolysis in a turbulent shear flow: contribution of Reynolds shear stress. *Biorheology* 21:783–97
37. Grigioni M, Daniele C, D'Avenio G, Barbaro V. 1999. A discussion on the threshold limit for hemolysis related to Reynolds shear stress. *J. Biomech.* 32:1107–12
38. Yoganathan AP. 1995. 123 cardiac valve prostheses. See Ref. 94, pp. 1847–70
39. Gross J, Shu M, Dai F, Ellis J, Yoganathan A. 1996. A microstructural flow analysis within a bileaflet mechanical heart valve hinge. *J. Heart Valve Dis.* 596:581–90
40. Ellis J, Healy T, Fontaine A, Saxena R, Yoganathan A. 1996. Velocity measurements and flow patterns within the hinge region of a Medtronic parallel bileaflet mechanical valve with clear housing. *J. Heart Valve Dis.* 5(6):591–99
41. Ellis JT, Travis BR, Yoganathan AP. 2000. An in vitro study of the hinge and near-field forward flow dynamics of the St. Jude Medical Regent bileaflet mechanical heart valve. *Ann. Biomed. Eng.* 28:524–32
42. Ellis JT, Yoganathan AP. 2000. A comparison of the hinge and near-hinge flow fields of the St. Jude Medical Hemodynamic Plus and Regent bileaflet mechanical heart valves. *J. Thorac. Cardiovasc. Surg.* 119:83–93
43. Leo HL, He ZM, Ellis J, Yoganathan A. 2002. Micro flow fields in the hinge region of Carbomedics bileaflet mechanical valve design. *J. Thorac. Cardiovasc. Surg.* 124: 561–74
44. Knapp RJ, Daily JW, Hammitt FG. 1970. *Cavitation.* New York: McGraw-Hill Int. Book Co.
45. Kafesjian R, Wieting DW, Ely J, Chahine GL, Frederick GS, Watson RE. 1989. Characterization of cavitation potential of pyrolitic carbon. *Proc. Int. Symp. Heart Valve Dis.*, London, pp. 12–16
46. Klepetko W. 1989. Leaflet fracture in Edwards-Duromedics bileaflet valves. *J. Thorac. Cardiovasc. Surg.* 97:90–94
47. Chahine GL 1996. Scaling of mechanical heart valves for cavitation inception: observation and acoustic detection. *J. Heart Valve Dis.* 5(2):207–15
48. Zapanta CM, Stinebring DR, Sneckenberger DS, Deutsch S, Geselowitz DB, et al. 1996. In vivo observation of cavitation on prosthetic heart valves. *ASAIO J.* 42:M550–55
49. Richard G, Beavan A, Strzepa P. 1994. Cavitation threshold ranking and erosion characteristics of bileaflet heart valve prosthesis. *J. Heart Valve Dis.* 3(Suppl.1):S94–101
50. Lee CS, Chandran KB, Chen LD. 1996. Cavitation dynamics of Medtronic Hall mechanical heart valve prosthesis: fluid squeezing effect. *J. Biomech. Eng.* 118:97–105
51. Graf T, Fisher H, Reul H, Rau G. 1991. Cavitation potential of mechanical heart valve prostheses. *Int. J. Artif. Organs* 14:169–74
52. Graf T, Reul H, Dietz W, Wilmes R, Rau G. 1992. Cavitation of mechanical heart valves under physiological conditions. *J. Heart Valve Dis.* 1:131–41
53. Makhijani, VB, Yang HQ, Singhal, AK, Hwang NHC. 1994. An experimental computational analysis of MHV cavitation: effects of leaflet squeezing and rebound. *J. Heart Valve Dis.* 3(Suppl.1):235–48

54. Bluestein D, Einav S, Hwang NHC. 1994. A squeeze flow phenomenon at the closing of a bileaflet mechanical heart valve prosthesis. *J. Biomech.* 27:1369–78
55. Wu ZJ, Gao BZ, Hwang NHC. 1995. Transient pressure at closing of a monoleaflet mechanical heart valve prosthesis: mounting compliance effect. *J. Heart Valve Dis.* 4:553–67
56. Lee CS, Aluri S, Chandran KB. 1996. Effect of valve holder flexibility on cavitation initiation with mechanical heart valve prostheses: an in vitro study. *J. Heart Valve Dis.* 5:104–13
57. Sneckenberger DS, Stinebring DR, Deutsch S, Geselowitz DB, Tarbell JM, et al. 1996. Mitral heart valve cavitation in an artificial heart environment. *J. Heart Valve Dis.* 5(2):216–27
58. Lamson TC, Stinebring DR, Deutsch S, Rosenberg G, Tarbell JM. 1991. Real-time in vitro observation of cavitation in a prosthetic heart valve. *ASAIO Trans.* 37:M351–53
59. He Z, Xi B, Zhu K, Hwang NHC. 2001. Mechanisms of mechanical heart valve cavitation: investigation using a tilting disk valve model. *J. Heart Valve Dis.* 10:666–74
60. Yoganathan AP, Woo YR, Williams FP. 1983. In *Advances in Cardiac Valves*, ed. ME Debakey, pp. 229–46. New York: Dun-Donnelley Publ. Corp.
61. Yoganathan AP, Travis BR. 2000. Fluid dynamics of prosthetic valves. In. *The Practice of Clinical Echocardiography,* ed. CM Otto. Philedelphia, PA: WB Saunders. 2nd ed.
62. Jensen M, Lemmon J, Gessaghi VC, Conrad C, Levine RA, Yoganathan AP. 2001. Harvested porcine mitral xenograft fixation: impact on fluid dynamic performance. *J. Heart Valve Dis.* 10:111–24
63. Badano L, Mocchegiani R, Bertoli G, DeGaetano G, Carratino L, et al. 1997. Normal echocardiographic characteristics of the Sorin bicarbon bileaflet prosthetic heart valve in the mitral and aortic positions. *J. Am. Soc. Echocardiogr.* 10:632–43
64. Hung TK, Schuessler GB. 1971. Computational analysis as an aid to the design of heart valves. *Chem. Eng. Prog. Symp. Ser.* 67:8–17
65. Au AD, Greenfield HS. 1975. Computer graphics analysis of stresses in blood flow through a prosthetic heart valve. *Comput. Biol. Med.* 4:279–91
66. Au AD, Greenfield HS. 1977. Computer prediction of thrombogenic sites for a tilting-disc prosthetic heart valve. *Comput. Biomed. Res.* 10:165–82
67. Underwood FN, Mueller TJ. 1977. Numerical study of the steady axisymmetric flow through a disk-type prosthetic heart valve in a constant diameter chamber. *J. Biomech. Eng.* 99:91–97
68. Underwood FN, Mueller TJ 1979. Numerical study of the steady axisymmetric flow through a disk-type prosthetic heart valve in an aortic-shaped chamber. *J. Biomech. Eng.* 101:198–204
69. Idelsohn SR, Costa LE, Ponso R. 1985. A comparative computational study of blood flow through prosthetic heart valves using the finite element method. *J. Biomech.* 18:97–115
70. Stevenson DM, Yoganathan, AP. 1985. Numerical simulation of steady turbulent flow through trileaflet aortic heart valves—I. computational scheme and methodology. *J. Biomech.* 18:899–907
71. Stevenson DM, Yoganathan AP, Williams FP. 1985. Numerical simulation of steady turbulent flow through trileaflet aortic heart valves—II. results on five models. *J. Biomech.* 18:909–26
72. Huang ZJ, Merkle CL, Abdallah S, Tarbell JM. 1994. Numerical simulation of unsteady laminar flow through a tilting disk heart valve: prediction of vortex shedding. *J. Biomech.* 27:391–402
73. King MJ, David T, Fisher J. 1994. An initial parametric study on fluid flow through bileaflet mechanical heart valves using

computational fluid dynamics. *J. Eng. Med.* 208:63–72
74. Peskin CS. 1972. Flow patterns around heart valves: a numerical method. *J. Comput. Phys.* 10:252–71
75. Peskin CS. 1977. Numerical analysis of blood flow in the heart. *J. Comput. Phys.* 25: 220–52
76. McCracken MF, Peskin CS. 1980. A vortex method for blood flow through heart valves. *J. Comput. Phys.* 35:183–205
77. Peskin CS, McQueen DM. 1980. Modeling prosthetic heart valves for numerical analysis of blood flow through the heart. *J. Comput. Phys.* 37:113–32
78. de Hart J, Peters GWM, Schreurs PJG, Baaijens FPT. 2000. A two-dimensional fluid-structure interaction model of the aortic valve. *J. Biomech.* 33:1079–88
79. Shim EB, Chang KS. 1997. Numerical analysis of three-dimensional Björk-Shiley valvular flow in an aorta. *J. Biomech. Eng.* 119:45–51
80. King MJ, Corden J, David T, Fisher J. 1996. A three-dimensional, time-dependent analysis of flow through a bileaflet mechanical heart valve: comparison of experimental and numerical results. *J. Biomech.* 29:609–18
81. King MJ, David T, Fisher J. 1997. Three-dimensional study of the effect of two leaflet opening angles on the time-dependent flow through a bileaflet mechanical heart valve. *Med. Eng. Phys.* 19:235–41
82. Kiris C, Kwak D, Rogers SE, Chang ID. 1997. Computatinoal approach for probing the flow through artificial heart devices. *J. Biomech. Eng.* 119:452–60
83. Krafczyk M, Cerrolaza M, Schulz M, Rank E. 1998. Analysis of 3D transient blood flow passing through an artificial aortic valve by lattice–Boltzmann methods. *J. Biomech.* 31:453–62
84. Peskin CS, McQueen DM. 1989. A three-dimensional computational method for blood flow in the heart. I. immersed elastic fibers in a viscous incompressible fluid. *J. Comput. Phys.* 81:372–405
85. Peskin CS, McQueen DM. 1989. A three-dimensional computational method for blood flow in the heart. II. Contractile fibers. *J. Comput. Phys.* 82:289–97
86. Peskin CS, McQueen DM. 1997. Fluid dynamics of the heart and its valves. In *Case Studies in Mathematical Modeling—Ecology, Physiology, and Cell Biology*, ed. HG Othmer, FR Adler, MA Lewis, JC Dallon, pp. 410, Upper Saddle River, NJ: Prentice Hall
87. de Hart J, Peters GWM, Schreurs PJG, Baaijens FPT. 2003. A computational fluid-structure interaction analysis of a fiber-reinforced stentless aortic valve. *J. Biomech.* 36:699–712
88. de Hart J, Peters GWM, Schreurs PJG, Baaijens FPT. 2003. A computational fluid-structure interaction analysis in the aortic valve. *J. Biomech.* 36:103–12
89. Ge L, Jones SC, Sotiropoulos F, Healy TM, Yoganathan AP. 2003. Numerical simulation of flow in mechanical heart valves: grid resolution and the assumption of flow symmetry. *J. Biomech. Eng.* 125:709–18
90. Prakash S, Ethier CR. 2001. Requirements for mesh resolution in 3D computational hemodynamics. *J. Biomech. Eng.* 123:134–44
91. Aluri S, Chandran KB. 2001. Numerical simulation of mechanical mitral heart valve closure. *Ann. Biomed. Eng.* 29:665–76
92. Lai YG, Chandran KB, Lemmon J. 2002. A numerical simulation of mechanical heart valve closure fluid dynamics. *J. Biomech.* 35:881–92
93. Rosenfeld M, Avrahami I, Einav S. 2002. Unsteady effects on the flow across tilting disk valves. *J. Biomech. Eng.* 124:21–29
94. Bronzino JD, ed. 1995. *The Biomedical Engineering Handbook*. Boca Raton: CRC Press. 2nd ed.

Annu. Rev. Biomed. Eng. 2004. 6:363–95
doi: 10.1146/annurev.bioeng.6.040803.140143


# MOLECULAR MACHINES

C. Mavroidis,[1] A. Dubey,[2] and M.L. Yarmush[3]

[1]*Department of Mechanical and Industrial Engineering, Northeastern University, Boston, Massachusetts 02115; email: mavro@coe.neu.edu*

[2]*Department of Mechanical and Aerospace Engineering, Rutgers University, Piscataway, New Jersey 08854; email: dubey@rci.rutgers.edu*

[3]*Department of Biomedical Engineering, Rutgers University, Piscataway, New Jersey 08854; email: ireis@sbi.org*

**Key Words** molecular motors, nanomachines, nanodevices, nanomotors, bionanotechnology

■ **Abstract** Molecular machines are tiny energy conversion devices on the molecular-size scale. Whether naturally occurring or synthetic, these machines are generally more efficient than their macroscale counterparts. They have their own mechanochemistry, dynamics, workspace, and usability and are composed of nature's building blocks: namely proteins, DNA, and other compounds, built atom by atom. With modern scientific capabilities it has become possible to create synthetic molecular devices and interface them with each other. Countless such machines exist in nature, and it is possible to build artificial ones by mimicking nature. Here we review some of the known molecular machines, their structures, features, and characteristics. We also look at certain devices in their early development stages, as well as their future applications and challenges.

CONTENTS

# INTRODUCTION

Molecular machines can be defined as devices that can produce useful work through the interaction of individual molecules at the molecular scale of length. A convenient unit of measurement at the molecular scale would be a nanometer. Hence, molecular machines also fall into the category of nanomachines. Molecular machines depend on inter- and intramolecular interactions for their function. These interactions include forces such as the ionic and Van der Waal's forces and are a function of the geometry of the individual molecules. The interaction between two given molecules can be well understood by a set of laws governing them, which brings in a definite level of predictability and controllability of the underlying mechanics. Mother Nature has her own set of molecular machines that have been working for centuries and have become optimized for performance and design over the ages. As our knowledge and understanding of these numerous machines continues to increase, we now see a possibility of using the natural machines, or creating synthetic ones from scratch, by mimicking nature. In this review, we try to understand the principles, theory, and utility of the known molecular machines and look into the design and control issues for creation and modification of such machines. A majority of natural molecular machines are protein based, whereas the DNA-based molecular machines are mostly synthetic. Nature deploys proteins to perform various cellular tasks, from moving cargo to catalyzing reactions, whereas DNA has been retained as an information carrier. Hence, it is understandable that most of the natural machinery is built from proteins. With the powerful crystallographic techniques now available, protein structures are clearer than ever. The ever-increasing computing power makes it possible to dynamically model protein folding processes and predict the conformations and structure of lesser known proteins. These findings help unravel the mysteries associated with the molecular machinery and pave the way for the production and application of these miniature machines in various fields, including medicine, space exploration, electronics and military. We divide the molecular machines into three broad categories—protein based, DNA-based, and chemical molecular motors.

# ATP-BASED PROTEIN MOLECULAR MACHINES

Three naturally existing rotary motors have been identified and studied in detail so far. Two form the $F_0F_1$-ATP synthase, and the third one is the bacterial flagellar motor. The protein-based molecular motors rely on an energy-rich molecule known as adenosine triphosphate (ATP), which is basically a nucleotide having three phosphate molecules that play a vital role in its energetics, and make it an indispensable commodity of life. The machines described in this section, the $F_0F_1$-ATPase, the kinesin, myosin, and dynein superfamily of protein molecular machines, and bacteria flagellar motors all depend, directly or indirectly, on ATP for their input energy. These machines, which have been carrying out vital life functions both inside and outside cells for millions of years, have now been segregated out of their natural environment and are seen as energy conversion devices to obtain forces, torques, and motion. One disadvantage associated with ATP dependence is that the ATP creation machinery itself could be many times heavier and bulkier than the motors, thereby making the assembly more complex. These machines perform best in their natural environment, and in the near future it may not be possible to have them as a part of feasible biomimetic molecular machinery.

## The $F_0F_1$-ATP Synthase Motors

ATP is regarded as the energy currency of biological systems (1). The ATP molecule owes much of its energy to the terminal three phosphate ions attached to an adenosine base (2). In 1941 the role of ATP in the energy conversion process in living beings was recognized (3). However, the mode of transfer and structure of the enzyme was unknown. When this currency is utilized (i.e., the energy of the molecule that is used to drive a biological process), the terminal anhydride bond in the ATP molecule has to be split. This leaves adenosine diphosphate (ADP) and a phosphate ion (Pi) as the products, which are recombined to form ATP by a super efficient (4) enzyme motor assembly called the $F_0F_1$-ATP synthase ($F_0F_1$-ATPase). ATP synthase is present inside the mitochondria of animal cells, in plant chloroplasts, in bacteria, and some other organisms. ATP synthase was first seen in 1962 in an electron microscopy experiment on bovine heart mitochondria, as 10 nm diameter knobs (5). Their importance in energy conversion was realized, but their functioning was still unknown. In 1966 the relation of the thus far unknown knobs to the production of ATP was established (6), which provided one of the first structures of the enzyme.

The ATP synthase is actually a combination of two motors functioning together, the hydrophobic transmembrane $F_0$-ATPase motor and the globular $F_1$-ATPase motor (7). Both motors have distinct structures and functions. There are different abbreviations used for the $F_1$-ATPase based on their sources; the heart mitochondrial motors are called $mF_1$, chloroplast motors are $cF_1$, those obtained from *Escherichia coli* are termed $EcF_1$, and the ones from Kagawa's thermophilic bacterium are known as $TF_1$ (2). The $F_0$ motor has organism-dependant structural variations. In addition, the regulation of catalysis in ATP synthase depends on the organism's source (1). In animal mitochondria, this motor is embedded in the inner mitochondrial membrane and uses an ion-motive force for its function. Initially, however, it was believed that the force was proton-motive (8) only until it was shown that, in some cases, $Na^+$ ions induce the motive force for the $F_0$ motor (9); hence the term ion-motive force. The proton-motive force can be defined as the work per unit charge that a proton traveling through a membrane can perform.

STRUCTURE: $F_1$-ATPase MOTOR The $F_1$ motor, powered by hydrolysis of ATP, is composed of a central protein stalk, called the $\gamma$-subunit, surrounded by three copies each of $\alpha$- and $\beta$-subunits. The $\alpha$- and $\beta$-subunits are arranged

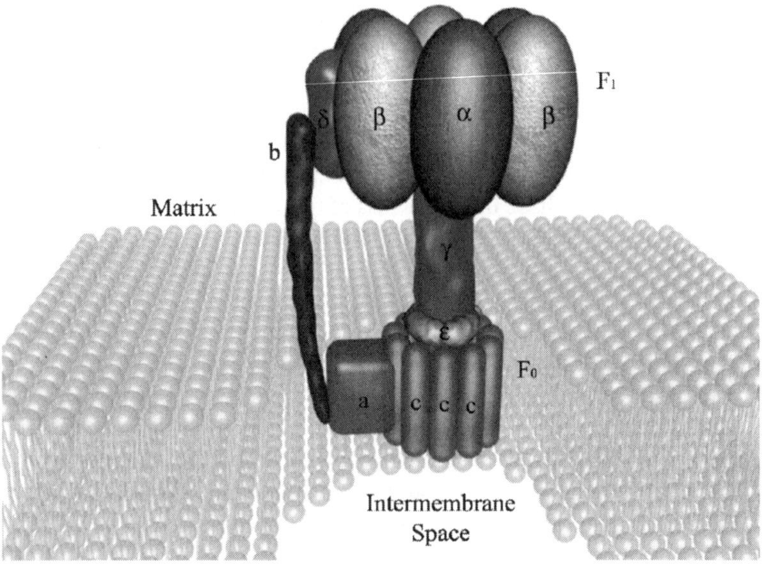


**Figure 1** The $F_0F_1$-ATPase motors. The $F_0$ motor is embedded in the inner mitochondrial membrane of the mitochondria. $F_0$ is typically composed of *a*, *b*, and *c* subunits as shown. The $F_1$ motor is the soluble region composed of three $\alpha$-, three $\beta$-, one each of $\gamma$-, $\delta$- and $\varepsilon$-subunits.

alternately so that they make a symmetric circular pattern when viewed from the top. There are $\delta$-subunits attached to the periphery of the $\alpha$-$\beta$ cylinder and the $\varepsilon$-subunits are present at the base of the $\gamma$-subunits, as shown in Figure 1. Hence, the $F_1$ motor is composed of nine polypeptides (10). The $\alpha$- and the $\beta$-subunits contain nucleotide-binding sites that bind ATP/ADP molecules. The nucleotide-binding sites in the $\alpha$-subunits simply bind the nucleotide, whereas those in the $\beta$-subunit actually perform the catalysis. The *a*, *b*, and the *c* subunits shown in Figure 1 are a part of the $F_0$ motor discussed below.

FUNCTION: $F_1$-ATPase MOTOR The binding-change mechanism to explain the function of $F_1$-ATPase was proposed in 1973 (11). The mechanism, as known today, shows that each of the $\beta$-subunits take three forms: O (open), L (loose), and T (tight) binding site. When the subunit is in the O form, it is catalytically inactive and has very low affinity to bind substrates. In the L form, the subunit loosely binds substrates (ADP and Pi), although it is catalytically inactive. In the T form, the ADP and Pi are converted into a tightly bound ATP until a conformational change converts the T-site into an O-site, thereby allowing the release of the newly formed ATP (12). The mechanism is shown in Figure 2.

The conformational change in the $\beta$-subunits is triggered by the rotation of the 4.5 nm long $\gamma$-subunit, which acts as a link connecting the $F_1$-ATPase to the

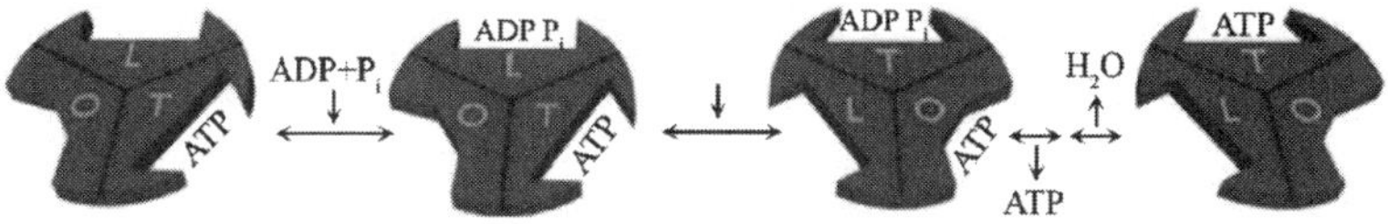


**Figure 2** The binding-change mechanism of $F_1$-ATPase. The three catalytic sites bind ADP/ATP alternately in L (loose), T (tight) and O (open) fashion. ADP and Pi are initially loosely bound, then the binding becomes tight, with the conversion of ADP + Pi into ATP, which is finally released when the open conformation is achieved.

$F_0$-ATPase. This was shown experimentally in 1997 (13). In this experiment, the $F_1$-ATPase was attached to a nickel-coated glass surface; a 1–3 $\mu$m long fluorescently labeled actin filament was attached to the other end of the $\gamma$-subunit. The rotation could then be observed through a fluorescence microscope, which was extremely interesting because the motor has a diameter of about 10 nm, whereas it could support and rotate a structure about one hundred times larger! However, the rate of rotation was reduced by 50 times to 1 rotation per second. The experimental setup is shown in Figure 3. $F_1$-ATPase can produce 80–100 pN-nm of rotary torque (4).

STRUCTURE: $F_0$-ATPase MOTOR Since the rotation of the $\gamma$-subunit has been shown to play the essential role in ATP creation, it is now imperative to see what causes the

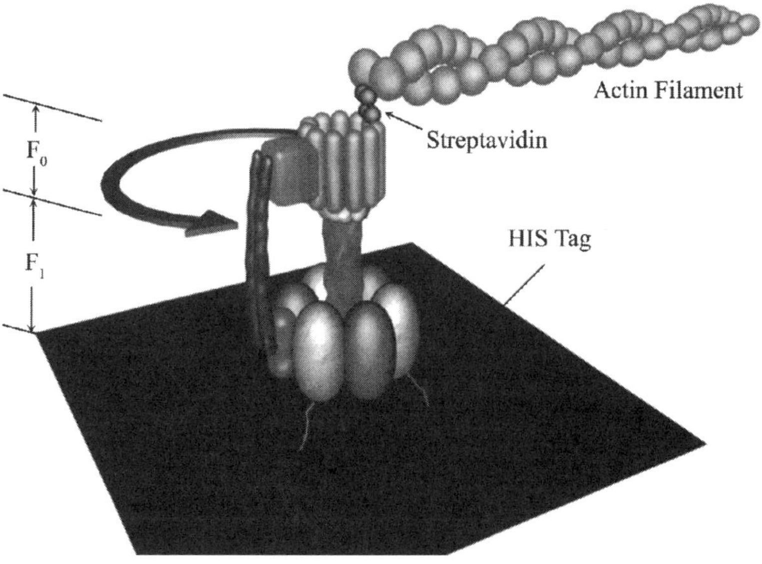


**Figure 3** Rotation of the ATPase motor as shown experimentally in (13). A 1–4 $\mu$m long fluorescently tagged actin filament was attached to the $F_0$-ATPase using streptavidin to observe the rotation of the ATP synthase motor.

$\gamma$-subunit to rotate. The answer lies in the functioning of the $F_0$-ATPase motor. Although the structure of the $F_0$-ATPase is not as well known as that of the $F_1$-ATPase, findings indicate that its structure depends on its source. The $F_0$ domain from the eubacterial enzymes, exemplified by *E. coli.* (14), has three types of subunits termed *a*, *b*, and *c* with 1 unit of *a*, 2 units of *b*, and 9 to 12 (15) units of *c* subunits (16, 17). Hence the subunit *a*, the two *b*, and the twelve *c* subunits in Figure 1 belong to the $F_0$-ATPase motor. In yeast, the $F_0$ has only 10 *c* subunits (18). The $F_0$ "turbine" from plant chloroplasts was found to have 14 *c* subunits (19), whereas a $Na^+$-driven specimen from bacteria was found to have 14 such subunits (20).

FUNCTION: $F_0$-ATPase MOTOR A flow of ions through the membrane propels the observed reversible (21) rotation of $F_0$-ATPase (22). As mentioned above, $F_0$ is the membrane-spanning unit of the ATPase motor. It remains embedded in the mitochondrial or cellular membrane. In 1978, it was discovered that a chemical potential gradient for protons is formed across the inner mitochondrial membrane or the proton-motive force (8). This force is utilized by the ATPase enzyme to produce ATP. The structure of $F_0$-ATPase is not as well known as its $F_1$ counterpart, which has been fully resolved (18, 23–28). The mechanochemical and quantitative models that explain how the ion-motive force is converted into the rotation of the $\gamma$-subunit were described in (15, 29–33).

The first hybrid nanoassembly structures powered by $F_1$-ATPase was proposed in (34). Nano-fabricated Ni posts, about 80 nm in diameter and 200 nm in height, each separated by about 2.5 $\mu$m were built. Upon these posts they attached specially produced recombinant biotinylated $F_1$-ATPases using histidine tags into their $\beta$-subunit coding sequences. A streptavidin molecule was bound to the $\gamma$-subunit, and finally Ni propellers of lengths 750 to 1400 nm were attached to them. In an action that is reverse of its ATP-producing cycle, the $F_1$-ATPase consumed externally provided ATP and produced anticlockwise rotation with a speed of about eight rotations per second. To date, this achievement remains a landmark in bionanotechnology.

## The Kinesin, Myosin, Dynein, and Flagella Molecular Motors

With modern microscopic tools, we view a cell as a set of many different moving components powered by molecular machines rather than a static environment. Molecular motors that move unidirectionally along protein polymers (actin or microtubules) drive the motions of muscles, as well as much smaller intracellular cargoes. In addition to the $F_0F_1$-ATPase motors inside the cell, there are linear transport motors present, tiny vehicles known as motor proteins, that transport molecular cargoes (35) and also require ATP for functioning. These minute cellular machines exist in three families: kinesins, myosins, and dyneins (36). The cargoes can be organelles, lipids, or proteins, etc. They play an important role in cell division and motility.

There are over 250 kinesin-like proteins, and they are involved in processes as diverse as the movement of chromosomes and the dynamics of cell membranes. The only part they have in common is the catalytic portion known as the motor domain. They have significant differences in their location within cells, their structural organization, and the movement they generate (37). Muscle myosin, whose study dates back to 1864, has served as a model system for understanding motility for decades. Kinesin, however was not discovered until 1985, using in vitro motility assays (38). Conventional kinesin is a highly processive motor that can take several hundred steps on a microtubule without detaching (39, 40), whereas muscle myosin executes a single stroke and then dissociates (41). Detailed analysis and modeling of these motors has been done (38, 42).

Kinesin and myosin make for an interesting comparison. Kinesin is microtubule based; it binds to and carries cargoes along microtubules, whereas myosin is actin based. The motor domain of kinesin weighs one third that of myosin and one tenth of that of dynein (43). Before the advent of modern microscopic and analytic techniques, it was believed that these two had little in common. However, the crystal structures available today indicate that they probably originated from a common ancestor (44).

THE MYOSIN LINEAR MOTOR Myosin is a diverse superfamily of motor proteins (45). Myosin-based molecular machines transport cargoes along actin filaments, the two-stranded helical polymers of the protein actin that are about 5–9 nm in diameter. They do this by hydrolyzing ATP and utilizing the released energy (46). In addition to transport, they are also involved in the process of force generation during muscle contraction, wherein thin actin filaments and thick myosin filaments slide past each other. Not all members of the myosin superfamily have been characterized. However, much is known about their structure and function. Myosin molecules were first seen (in the late 1950s) through electron microscope protruding out from thick filaments and interacting with the thin actin filaments (47–49). Since that time, ATP has been known to play a role in myosin-related muscle movement along actin (50); however, the exact mechanism was unknown, until it was explained in (51).

STRUCTURE: MYOSIN MOLECULAR MOTOR A myosin molecule binding to an actin polymer is shown in Figure 4*a* (see color insert) (52). A myosin molecule has a size of about 520 kDa, including two 220-kDa heavy chains and light chains of sizes between 15–22 kDa (53, 54). They can be visualized as two identical globular motor heads, also known as motor domains, each having a catalytic domain (actin, nucleotide, and light chain binding sites) and ~8 nm long lever arms. One of the heads, sometimes referred to as S1 regions (subfragment 1), is shown in green (only the active head is visible); the lever arms or the light chains, in red and yellow. Both heads are connected via a coiled coil made of two $\alpha$-helical coils (green) to the thick base filament. The light chains have considerable sequence similarity with the protein calmodulin and troponin C and are sometimes referred to as calmodulin-like chains. They act as links to the motor domains and do not play any role in their ATP binding activity (55) except for some exceptions (56, 57).

The motor domain in itself is sufficient for moving actin filaments (58). Three-dimensional structures of a myosin head revealed that it is a pear-shaped domain, about 19 nm long and 5 nm in maximum diameter (58, 59).

FUNCTION: MYOSIN MOLECULAR MOTOR A crossbridge-cycle model for the action of myosin on actin has been widely accepted since 1957 (47, 60, 61). Since the time the atomic structures of actin monomer (62, 63) and myosin (59) were resolved, this model has been refined into a lever-arm model which is now acceptable (64). Only one motor head is able to connect to the actin filament at a time, the other head remains passive. Initially, the catalytic domain in the head has ADP and Pi bound to it and, as a result, its binding with actin was weak. With the active motor head docking properly to the actin-binding site, the Pi has to be released. As soon as this happens, the lever arm swings counterclockwise (65) owing to a conformational change (49, 66–71), which pushes the actin filament down by about 10 nm along its longitudinal axis (38). The active motor head now releases its bound ADP, and another ATP molecule, by way of Brownian motion, quickly replaces it, making the binding of the head to the actin filament weak again. The myosin motor then dissociates from the actin filament, and a new cycle starts. However, nano-manipulation of single S1 molecules (motor domains) shows that myosin can take multiple steps per ATP molecule hydrolyzed, moving in 5.3 nm steps and resulting in displacements of 11 to 30 nm (72).

THE KINESIN LINEAR MOTOR The kinesin (43) and dynein families of proteins are involved in cellular cargo transport along microtubules, in contrast to myosin, which transports along actin (73). Microtubules are 25-nm diameter tubes made of protein tubulin and are present in the cells in an organized manner. Microtubules have polarity; one end being the plus (fast-growing) end while the other end is the minus (slow-growing) end (74). Kinesins move from the minus end to the plus end of the microtubule, whereas dyneins move from the plus end to the minus end. Microtubule arrangement varies in different cell systems. In nerve axons, they are arranged longitudinally such that their plus ends point away from the cell body and into the axon. In epithelial cells, their plus ends point toward the basement membrane. They extend radially out of the cell center in fibroblasts and macrophages with the plus end protruding outward (75). Similar to myosin, kinesin is also an ATP-driven motor. One unique characteristic of the kinesin family proteins is their processivity; they bind to microtubules and literally walk on it for many enzymatic cycles before detaching (76, 77). Also, each of the globular heads/motor domains of kinesin is made of a single polypeptide unlike myosin (heavy and light chains and dynein heavy, intermediate, and light chains).

STRUCTURE: KINESIN MOLECULAR MOTOR Much structural information about kinesin is now available through the crystal structures (44, 78, 79). The motor domain contains a folding motif similar to that of myosin and G proteins (36). The two heads or the motor domains of kinesin are linked via neck linkers to a long coiled coil, which extends up to the cargo (Figure 4*b*). These heads interact with the $\alpha$- and $\beta$-subunits of the tubulin hetrodimer along the microtubule protofilament. The heads contain nucleotide- and microtubule-binding domains.

FUNCTION: KINESIN MOLECULAR MOTOR Although kinesin is also a two-headed linear motor, its modus operandi is different from myosin in the sense that both of its heads work together in a coordinated manner in contrast to one being left out in the case of myosin. Figure 4*b* shows the kinesin walk. Each of the motor heads is near the microtubule in the initial state, with each motor head carrying an ADP molecule. When one of the heads loosely binds to the microtubule, it loses its ADP molecule to facilitate a stronger binding. Another ATP molecule replaces the ADP, which facilitates a conformational change such that the neck region of the bound head snaps forward and zips on to the head (37). In the process, it pulls the other ADP-carrying motor head forward by about 16 nm so that it can bind to the next microtubule-binding site. This results in the net movement of the cargo by about 8 nm (80). The second head now binds to the microtubule by losing its ADP, which is promptly replaced by another ATP molecule (Brownian motion). The first head, meanwhile hydrolyzes the ATP and loses the resulting Pi. It is then snapped forward by the second head while it carries its ADP forward. Hence coordinated hydrolysis of ATP in the two motor heads is the key to the kinesin processivity (81, 82). Kinesin is able to take about 100 steps before detaching from the microtubule (39, 76, 83), while moving at 1000 nm/s and exerting forces of the order of 5–6 pN at rest (84, 85).

THE DYNEIN MOTOR The dynein superfamily of proteins was discovered in 1965 (86). Dyneins exist in two isoforms: cytoplasmic and axonemal. Cytoplasmic dyneins are involved in cargo movement, whereas axonemal dyneins are involved in producing bending motions of cilia and flagella (87–97). Figure 5 shows a typical cytoplasmic dynein molecule.

STRUCTURE: DYNEIN MOLECULAR MOTOR The structure consists of two heavy chains in the form of globular heads, three intermediate chains, and four light intermediate chains (98, 99). Recent studies have exposed a linker domain connecting the stem region below the heads to the head itself (100). Also the microtubule-binding domains (the stalk region, not visible in the figure) protrude from the top of the heads (101). The ends of these stalks have smaller ATP-sensitive globular domains that bind to the microtubules. Cytoplasmic dynein is associated with a protein complex known as dynactin, which contains 10 subunits (102). Some are shown in the Figure 5 as p150, p135, actin-related protein 1 (Arp1), actin, dynamitin, capping protein, and p62 subunit. These play an important regulatory role in the binding ability of dynein to the microtubules. The heavy chains forming the two globular heads contain the ATPase and microtubule motor domains (103).

One striking difference between dynein and the kinesins and myosins is that dynein has AAA (ATPases associated with a variety of cellular activities) modules

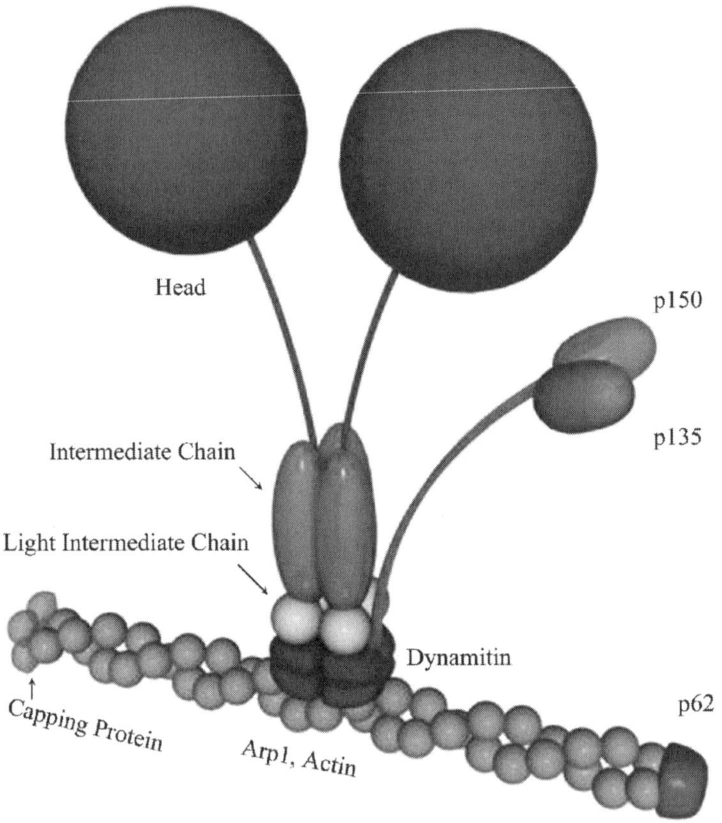


**Figure 5** A dynein molecule. Shown are the globular heads (heavy chains) connected to the intermediate chains and the light chains. Dynactin complex components p150, p135, dynamitin, p62, capping proteins, Arp1, and Actin are also shown.

(104–106), which indicate that its mode of working will be entirely different from kinesins and myosins. This puts dyneins into the AAA superfamily of mechanoenzymes. The dynein heavy chains contain six tandemly linked AAA modules (107, 108), with the head having a ring-like domain organization, which is typical of a AAA superfamily. Four of these are nucleotide-binding motifs, named P1–P4, but only P1 (AAA1) is able to hydrolyze ATP.

FUNCTION: DYNEIN MOLECULAR MOTOR Because dynein is a larger and more complex structure than other motor proteins, its mode of operation is not as well known. However, electron microscopy and image processing was used (100) to show the structure of a flagellar dynein at the start and end of its power stroke, which gives some insight into its possible mode of force generation. When the dynein contains bound ADP and $V_i$ (vandate), it is in the prepower stroke conformation.

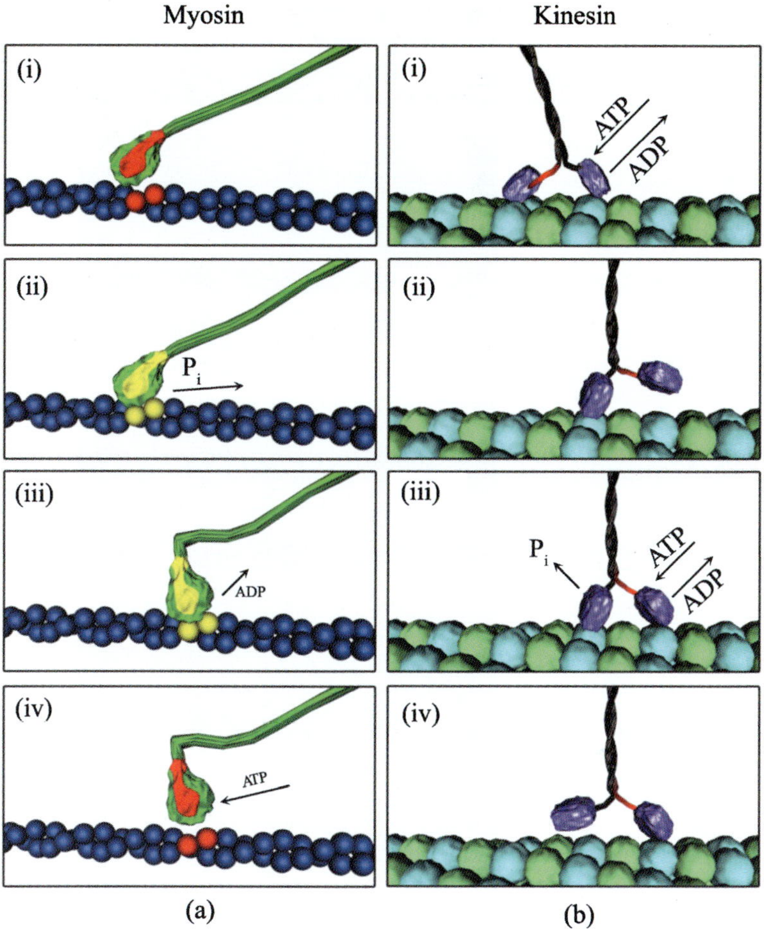


**Figure 4** The kinesin-myosin walks. (*a*) Myosin motor mechanism. (i) Motor head loosely docking to the actin-binding site; (ii) the binding becomes tighter along with the release of Pi; (iii) lever arm swings to the left with the release of ADP; and (iv) replacement of the lost ADP with a fresh ATP molecule results in dissociation of the head. (*b*) Kinesin heads working in conjunction. (i) Both ADP-carrying heads come near the microtubule and one (*black neck*) binds; (ii) loss of bound ADP and addition of fresh ATP in the bound head moves the other (*red neck*) to the right; (iii) the second head (*red*) binds to microtubule while losing its ADP, and replacing it with a new ATP molecule, whereas the first head hydrolyzes its ATP and loses Pi; (iv) the ADP-carrying black neck will now be snapped forward, and the cycle will be repeated.

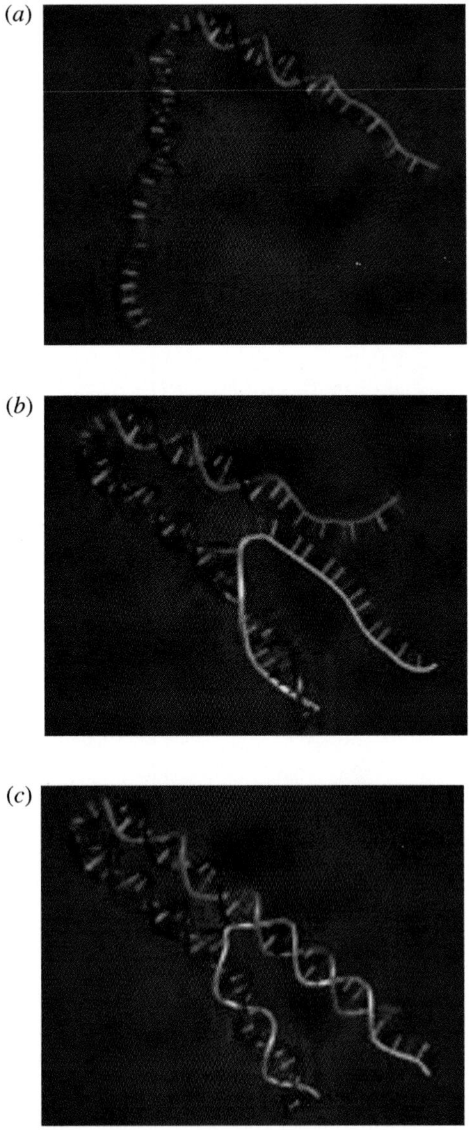


**Figure 7** The DNA tweezers. (*a*) The machine is in the open conformation with the central strand (*black*) partially hybridized to the two side strands (*red* and *green*); (*b*) a fuel strand (*white*) is introduced; and (*c*) the fuel strand hybridizes with the two free ends to bring the device into a closed conformation. With the addition of complement to the fuel strand, it can be removed to leave the system back to state (*a*). Figure reprinted with permission from Bernard Yurke, Lucent Technologies.

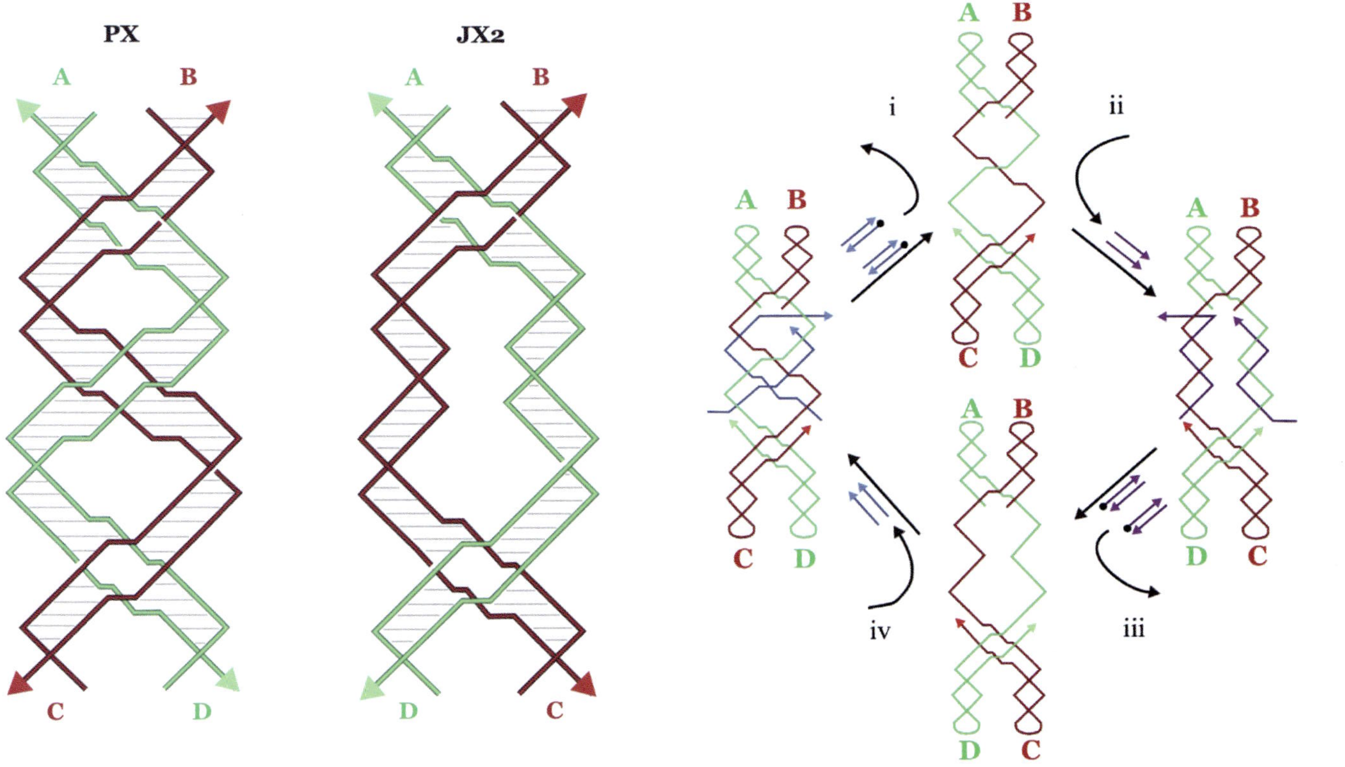


**Figure 8** (*a*) PX and $JX_2$ topological DNA motifs. The two lower double helices, C and D, are rotated by 180° during transition from PX to $JX_2$. (*b*) Working principle of the rotary DNA machine: (stage i) Type 1 strands (*blue*) are removable from PX motifs by the addition of their respective complementary strands (*black dots at ends*); (stage ii) the addition of Type 2 strands (*purple*) results in a rotation of C and D units; (stage iii) Type 2 strands can then be removed by adding their complementary strands; (stage iv) Type 1 strands added again to revert the motif back to PX state.

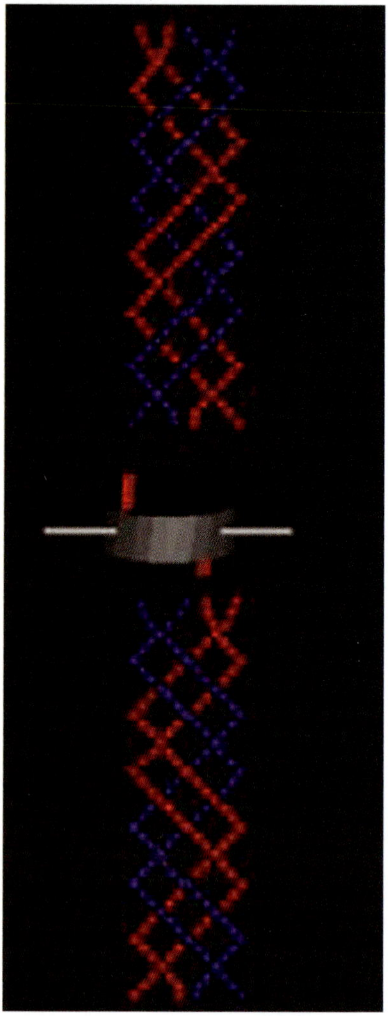

**Figure 9** A possible application of two DNA rotary machines to rotate a central disc by half a rotation at a time to achieve one full rotation. Red tags on the disc are stoppers that will allow linkage to the motifs.

The state when it has lost the two, known as the apo-state, is the more compact post-power stroke state. There is a distinct conformational change involving the stem, linker, head, and the stalk that produces about 15 nm of translation onto the microtubule bound to the stalk (100).

THE FLAGELLA MOTORS Unicellular organisms such as *E. coli* have an interesting mode of motility (see 109–111). They have a number of molecular motors, about 45 nm in diameter, that drive their feet or the flagella, which help the cell to swim. Motility is critical for cells, as they often have to travel from a less favorable to a more favorable environment. The flagella are helical filaments that extend out of the cell into the medium and perform a function analogous to what the oars perform to a boat. The flagella and the motor assembly are called a flagellum. The motor assembly imparts a rotary motion into the flagella (112, 113). In addition to a rotary mechanism, the flagellar machines consist of components such as rate meters, particle counters, and gearboxes (114). These are necessary to help the cell decide which way to go, depending on the change of concentration of nutrients in the surroundings. The rotary motion imparted to the flagella needs to be modulated to ensure the cell is moving in the proper direction, as well as to ensure that all flagella of the given cell are providing a concerted effort toward it (115). When the motors rotate the flagella in a counterclockwise direction, as viewed along the flagella filament from outside, the helical flagella create a wave away from the cell body. Adjacent flagella subsequently intertwine in a propulsive corkscrew manner and propel the bacteria. When the motors rotate clockwise, the flagella fly apart, causing the bacteria to tumble or change its direction (116). These reversals occur irregularly, giving the bacterium a random walk, unless, of course, there is a preferential direction of motility due to reasons mentioned earlier. The flagella motors allow the bacteria to move at speeds of as much as 25 $\mu$m/s, with directional reversals occurring approximately 1 per second (117). A number of bacterial species in addition to *E. coli* depend on flagella motors for motility: e.g., *Salmonella enterica* serovar, Typhimurium (*Salmonella*), *Streptococcus*, *Vibrio* spp., *Caulobacter*, *Leptospira*, *Aquaspirrilum serpens*, and *Bacillus*. The rotation of flagella motors is stimulated by a flow of ions through them, which is a result of a build-up of a transmembrane ion gradient. There is no direct ATP-involvement; however, the proton gradient needed for the functioning of flagella motors can be produced by ATPase.

STRUCTURE: THE FLAGELLA MOTORS A complete part list of the flagella motors is not yet available. Continued efforts dating back to early 1970s have, however, revealed much of their structure, composition, genetics, and function. Newer models of the motor function are still being proposed with an aim to explain observed experimental phenomena (118, 119) because we still do not fully understand the functioning of this motor (110). A typical flagella motor from *E. coli.* consists of ~20 different proteins (110), and many more are involved in its assembly and operation. There are 14 Flg-type proteins, FlgA–FlgN; 5 Flh-type proteins,

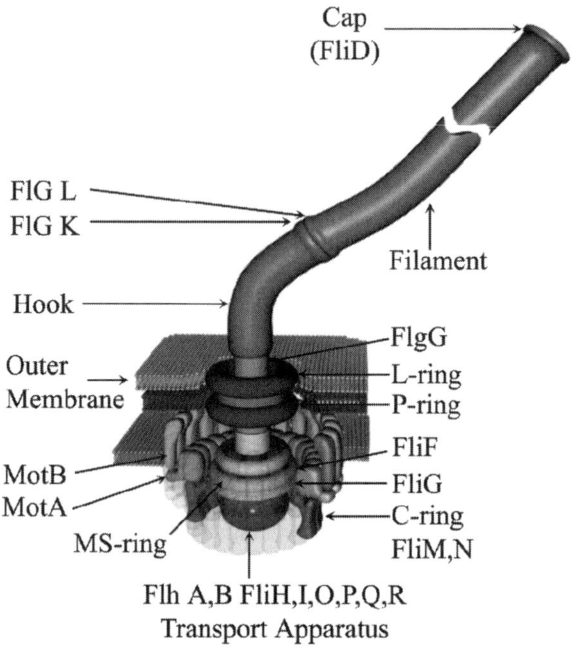


**Figure 6** A typical flagellum. A filament (FliC) is connected to the hook (FlgE), which connects to the transmembrane motor unit through a shaft. Hook-related proteins (FlgK, FlgL, and FliD) help in assembly and stability of the hook and filament. The L-ring is embedded in the outer cell membrane, the P-ring in the peptidoglycan layer, and the MS-ring (FliF) along with FliG (rotor) and parts of stator (MotA and MotB) are embedded in the inner cell membrane. The C-ring and the transport apparatus are located inside the cell.

FlhA–FlhE; 19 Fli-type proteins, FliA–FliT; with MotA and MotB making a total of 40 related proteins. The group names Flg, Flh, Fli, and Mot correspond to the related genes (120). Within the main structural proteins are other proteins: FliC or the filament; FliD (filament cap); FliF or the MS-ring; FliG, FliM, and FliN (C-ring); FlgB, FlgC, and FlgF (proximal rod); FlgG (distal rod); FlgH (L-ring); FlgI (P-ring); FlgK and FlgL (hook-filament junction); and MotA-MotB (torque-generating units) (see Figure 6). It was initially believed that the M and S were two separate rings (M, membrane; S, supramembranous) (121). However, they are now called the MS-ring because they were found to be two domains of the same protein, FliF (122, 123). The C-ring stands for cytoplasmic (124–126); the e names for the P and L-rings come from peptidoglycan and lipopolysaccharide, respectively, indicating their location as seen in Figure 6. FlhA, B, FliH, I, O, P, Q, and R constitute the transport apparatus.

The hook and filament part of the flagellum is located outside the cell body. The motor portion is embedded in the cell membrane, with the C-ring and the transport apparatus inside the inner membrane in the cytoplasmic region. MotA and MotB are arranged in a circular array embedded in the inner membrane, with the MS-ring at the center. Connected to the MS-ring is the proximal end of a shaft, to which the P-ring, embedded in the peptidoglycan layer, is attached. Moving further outward, is the L-ring, which is embedded in the outer cell membrane, followed by the distal shaft end that protrudes out of the cell. To this end there is an attachment of the hook and the filament, both of which are polymers of hook-protein and flagellin respectively.

*Function: the flagella motors* The flagellar motors in most cases are powered by protons flowing through the cell membrane (proton-motive force) barring exceptions such as certain marine bacteria, for example, the *Vibrio* spp., which are driven by $Na^+$ ions (127). There are about 1200 protons required to rotate the motor by one rotation (128). A complete explanation of how this proton flow is able to generate torque is not yet available. From what is known, the stator units of MotA and MotB play an important role in torque generation. They form a MotA/MotB complex that when oriented properly binds to the peptidoglycan and opens proton channels through which protons can flow (129). It is believed that there are eight such channels per motor (130). The proton-motive force is a result of the difference of pH between the outside and inside of the cell. The *E. coli* cells like to maintain an internal pH of 7.6–7.8, so depending on the pH of the surroundings, the proton-motive force will vary, and hence the speed of rotation of their motors. To test how the speed of rotation depends on the proton-motive force, the motors were powered by external voltage with attached markers acting as heavy loads (131). As expected, the rotation was found to depend directly on the proton-motive force. According to the most widely accepted model, MotA/MotB complex interacts with the rotor via binding sites. The passage of protons through a MotA/MotB complex (stator or torque generator) moves it so that the protons bind to the next available binding site on the rotor, thereby stretching their linkage. When the linkage recoils, the rotor assembly has to rotate by one step. Hence whichever complex receives protons from the flux will rotate the rotor and generate torque. The torque-speed dependence of the motor has been studied in detail (132, 133) and indicates the torque range of about 2700 to 4600 pN-nm.

## DNA-BASED MOLECULAR MOTORS/DEVICES

As mentioned above, nature chose DNA mainly as an information carrier. There was no mechanical work assigned to it. Energy conversion, trafficking, and sensing, for example, were the tasks assigned mainly to proteins. Probably for this reason, DNA turns out to be a simpler structure, with only four kinds of nucleotide bases, adenosine, thiamine, guanine, and cytosine (A, T, G, and C), attached in a linear fashion that takes a double-helical conformation when paired with a complementary strand. Such structural simplicity vis-à-vis proteins, made of some 20 amino acids with complex folding patterns, results in a simpler structure and predictable behavior. There are certain qualities that make DNA an attractive choice for the construction of artificial nanomachines. In recent years, DNA has found use not only in mechanochemical but also in nanoelectronic systems (134–137). A DNA double-helical molecule is about 2 nm in diameter and has 3.4–3.6-nm helical pitch no matter what its base composition is, a structural uniformity not achievable with protein structures if one changes their sequence. Furthermore, double-stranded DNA (ds-DNA) has a respectable persistence length of about 50 nm (138), which provides it enough rigidity to be a candidate component of molecular machinery. Single-stranded DNA (ss-DNA) is very flexible and cannot be used where rigidity is required; however, this flexibility allows its application in machine components such as hinges or nanoactuators (139). Its persistence length is about 1 nm, covering up to 3 base pairs (140) at 1M salt concentration.

Other than the above structural features, two important and exclusive properties make DNA suitable for molecular level constructions: molecular recognition and self-assembly. The nucleotide bases A and T on two different ss-DNA have affinity for each other, so do G and C. Effective and stable ds-DNA structures are formed only if the base orders of the individual strands are complementary. Hence, if two complementary single strands of DNA are in a solution, they will eventually recognize each other and hybridize, or zip-up, forming a ds-DNA. This property of molecular recognition and self-assembly has been exploited in a number of ways to build complex molecular structures (141–148). From a mechanical perspective, if the free energy released by hybridization of two complementary DNA strands is used to lift a hypothetical load, a force capacity of 15 pN can be achieved (F.C. Simmel & B.Yurke, unpublished data), comparable to that of other molecular machines such as kinesin (5 pN) (150).

The first artificial DNA-based structure in the form of a cube in 1991 was presented in (143, 151). More complex structures such as knots (152, 153) and Borromean rings (147) were also developed. In addition to these individual constructs, two-dimensional arrays (145, 154, 155) were made with the help of the double-crossover (DX) DNA molecule (156–158). This DX molecule gave the structural rigidity required to create a dynamic molecular device, the B-Z switch (159). DNA double helices can be of three types: A-, B-, or Z-DNA. The B-DNA is the natural, right-handed helical form of DNA, whereas the A-DNA is a shrunken, low-humidity form of the B-DNA. Z-DNA, obtained from certain CG base repeat sequences occurring in B-DNA, can take a left-handed double helical form (160). The CG-repeated base pair regions can be switched between the left and the right-handed conformations by changing ionic concentration (161). The switch was designed in such a way that it had three cyclic strands of DNA, two of them wrapped around a central strand that had the CG repeat region in the middle. On the two free ends of the side strands fluorescent dyes were attached in order to monitor the conformational change. With the change in ionic concentration the central CG repeat sequence could alternate between the B and the Z modes bidirectionally, which was observed through fluorescence resonance energy transfer (FRET) spectroscopy.

## The DNA Tweezers

An artificial DNA-based molecular machine that also accepted DNA as a fuel was recently developed (162). The machine, called DNA tweezers, consisted of three strands of DNA labeled A, B and C. Strands B and C are partially hybridized on to the central strand A with overhangs on both ends (Figure 7, see color insert). This conformation of the machine is the open conformation. When F, an auxiliary fuel strand designed to hybridize with both overhang regions, is introduced, the machine attains a closed conformation. The fuel strand is then removed from the system by the introduction of its exact complement, leaving the system to go back to its original open conformation. In this way a reversible motion is produced, which can be observed by attaching fluorescent tags to the two ends of the strand A. In this case the 5′ end was labeled with the dye TET (tetrachloro-fluorescein phosphoramidite), and the 3′ end was labeled with TAMRA (carboxy-tertamethylrhodamine). Aside from the creation of a completely new molecular machine, this showed a way of selective fueling of such machines. The fuel strands are sequence specific, so they will work on only those machines toward which they are directed and will not trigger other machines surrounding them.

This machine was later improved to form a three-state device (163), which had two robust states and one flexible intermediate state. A variation of the tweezers came about as the DNA-scissors (164).

## Rotary DNA Actuator Concept

Based on the principle of branch migration and targeted fueling as achieved in the DNA tweezers, a rotary machine element made of DX-DNA (double-crossover DNA) molecules was introduced. This element was based on the reversible transition between two states, the paranemic crossover (PX) (165) DNA, and its topoisomer, $JX_2$ (Figure 8*a*, see color insert).

The PX-DNA is known to play a role in recombination process. As seen in Figure 8*b*, the PX-DNA is formed by brown, green, and blue DNA strands. However, the top and bottom double-helical regions of the brown and green strands are connected to each other by a single-stranded region. These single-stranded regions are partially hybridized by blue strands with overhangs that will act as 'sticky ends' to adhere to incoming fuel strands. When exact complements of the blue strands are supplied (i), the blue strands are displaced from the PX motif and bind with their complements. This makes possible the addition of a different set of strands into the gap. In stage ii, when the purple strands are added into the gap, the PX molecule changes conformation to $JX_2$ state with the lower double helices C and D rotating by 180°. The purple strands can then be removed in a fashion similar to displacing the blue ones, and fresh blue strands can be added to the remaining intermediate, which will result in another rotation such that the C and D portions come back to their PX-positions. In a very smart complex molecular construction, the researchers attached half-hexagonal DNA structures formed by DX and ds-DNA onto one of the ds regions (brown or green, Figure 8) of PX motifs arranged in a linear array (166). Because of the larger size of the structures, they could be visualized using an atomic force microscope to prove that the rotary device indeed rotates. A possible application of two DNA rotary machines to rotate a central disc is shown in Figure 9 (see color insert).

## INORGANIC (CHEMICAL) MOLECULAR MACHINES

In the past two decades, chemists have been able to create, modify, and control numerous types of chemical molecular machines. Many of these machines carry a striking resemblance to our everyday macroscale machines such as gears, propellers, shuttles, etc. In addition, all of these molecular machines are easy to synthesize artificially and are generally more robust than the natural molecular machines. Most of these machines are organic compounds of carbon, nitrogen, and hydrogen, with the presence of a metal ion being required occasionally. Electrostatic interactions and covalent and hydrogen bonding play essential roles in the performance of these machines. Such artificial chemical machines can be controlled in various ways—chemically, electrochemically, and photochemically (through irradiation by light). Some are even controlled in several ways, rendering them more flexible, which enhances their utility. A scientist can have more freedom with respect to the design of chemical molecular machines depending on the performance requirements and conditions. Rotaxanes (167–169) and catenanes (170, 171) make the basis of many of the molecular machines described in this section. These are families of interlocked organic molecular compounds with a distinctive shape and properties that guide their performance and control.

### The Rotaxanes

Rotaxane family of molecular machines is characterized by two parts: a dumbbell-shaped compound with two heavy chemical groups at the ends and a light, cyclic component, called a macrocycle, interlocked between the heads (Figure 10).

A reversible switch can be made with a rotaxane setup (172). For this, one needs to have two chemically active recognition sites in the neck region of the dumbbell. In this particular example, the thread was made of polyether, marked by recognition sites of hydroquinol units and terminated at the ends by large triisoproplylsilyl groups. A tetracationic bead was designed and self-assembled into the system that interacts with the recognition sites. The macrocycle has a natural, low-energy state on the first recognition site, but can be switched reversibly between the two sites upon application of suitable stimuli. Depending on the type of rotaxane setup, the stimuli can be chemical, electrochemical, or photochemical (173, 174). The stereo-electronic properties of the recognition sites can be altered by protonation or deprotonation, or by oxidation or reduction, thereby changing the affinity of the sites toward the macrocycle. In a recent example, light-induced acceleration of rotaxane motion was achieved by photoisomerization (175). Similar controls through alternating current (oscillating electric fields) had previously been shown (176).

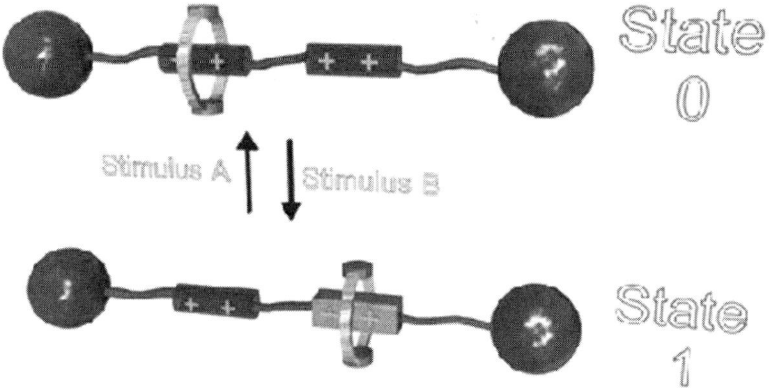


**Figure 10** A typical rotaxane shuttle setup. The macrocycle encircles the thread-like portion of the dumbbell with heavy groups at its ends. The thread has two recognition sites that can be altered reversibly so as to make the macrocycle shuttle between the two sites.

There are various ways for making rotaxanes by supramolecular synthesis (177). They can be self-assembled (178) using template-directed synthesis (179) methods such as threading, clipping, and slippage (180–182). In addition, various other rotaxane shuttles and means of controlling the switching motion have been described (183–192).

## The Catenanes

The catenanes are also a special type of interlocked structures that represent a growing family of molecular machines. They are synthesized by supramolecular assistance to molecular synthesis (177). The general structure of a catenane is that of two interlocked ring-like components that are noncovalently linked via a mechanical bond, i.e., they are held together without any valence forces. Both macrocyclic components have recognition sites composed of atoms or groups of atoms that are redox active or photochemically reactive. It is possible to have both rings with similar recognition sites. In such a scenario, one of the rings may rotate inside the other with the conformations stabilized by noncovalent interactions, but the two states of the inner ring, differing by 180°, will be undistinguishable (degenerate) (193). For better control and distinguishable molecular conformations, it is desirable to have different recognition sites within the macrocycles. Then they can be controlled independently through their own specific stimuli. The stereo-electronic property of a recognition site within a macrocycle can be varied such that at one point it has more affinity for the sites on the other ring. At this instant, the force balance will guide the rotating macrocycle for a stable conformation, which requires that particular site to be inside the other macrocycle. Similarly, with other stimuli, this affinity can be turned off, or even reversed, along with an

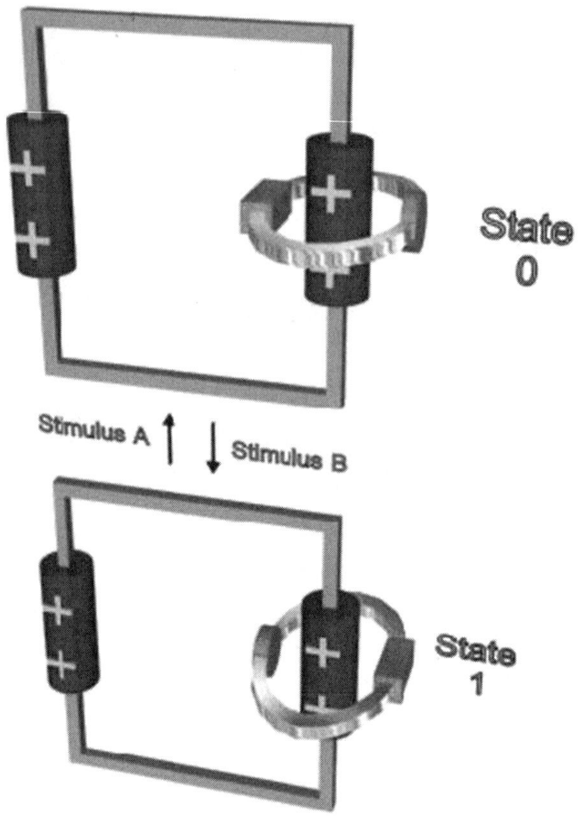


**Figure 11** A nondegenerate catenane. One of the rings (the moving ring) has two different recognition sites in it. Both sites can be turned off or on with different stimuli. When the trapezoidal-shaped site is activated, the force and energy balance results in the first conformation, whereas when the disc-shaped site is activated, the second conformation results. They can be called states 0 and 1, analogous to binary machine language.

increase of the affinity of the second recognition site on the rotating macrocycle toward those on the static one. There is a need for computational modeling, simulation, and analysis of such molecular machine motion (194). Catenanes can also be designed for chemical, photochemical, or electrochemical control (195–199). Figure 11 describes one such catenane molecular motor.

For both rotaxane- and catenane-based molecular machines, it is desirable to have recognition sites such that they can be easily controlled externally. Hence, it is preferable to build sites that are either redox active or photo active (173). Catenanes can also be self-assembled (200). An example of a catenane-assembled molecular motor is the electronically controllable bistable switch (201). An intuitive way of looking at catenanes is to think of them as molecular equivalents of ball and socket and universal joints (196, 202, 203).

Pseudorotaxanes are structures that contain a ring-like element and a thread-like element that can be threaded or dethreaded onto the ring upon application of various stimuli. Again, the stimuli can be chemical, photochemical, or electrochemical (204). These contain a promise of forming molecular machine components analogous to switches and nuts and bolts from the macroscopic world.

## Other Inorganic Molecular Machines

Many other molecular devices reported in the past four decades bear a striking resemblance to macroscopic machinery. Chemical compounds behaving as bevel gears and propellers that were reported in the late 1960s and early 1970s are still being studied today (205–208). A molecular propeller can be formed when two bulky rings such as the aryl rings (209) are connected to one central atom, often called the focal atom. Clockwise rotation of one such ring induces a counterclockwise rotation of the opposite ring about the bond connecting it to the central atom. It is possible to have a three-propeller system as well (210–212). Triptycyl and amide ring systems have been shown to observe a coordinated gear-like rotation (213–217). "Molecular turnstiles," which are rotating plates inside a macrocycle, have been created (218, 219). However, such rotations are not controllable. A rotation of a molecular ring about a bond could be controlled by chemical stimuli, as was shown for the case of a molecular brake (220). A propeller-like rotation of a 9-triptycyl ring system, which was used in gears, this time connected to a 2,2′-bipyridine unit, could be controlled by the addition and subsequent removal of a metal. Thus free rotations along single bonds can be stopped and released at will. Soon after demonstrating the brake, A similar structure, called the molecular ratchet, was also proposed (221, 222). Again, the polycyclic structure was allowed only one degree of rotational freedom about a single bond connecting triptycene and benzophenantherene (223). On similar lines and by the same group, a chemically powered unidirectional rotary machine was introduced (224–226). The demonstrations, as for most chemical machines, were done by $^1$H NMR techniques.

An additional type of molecular switch is the chiroptical molecular switch (227). Another large cyclic compound was found to be switchable between its two stable isomeric forms P and M′ (right- and left-handed) stimulated by light. Depending on the frequency of the bombarded light, the *cis* and *trans* conformations of the compound 4-[9′(2′-meth-oxythioxanthylidene)]-7-methyl-1,2,3,4-tetrahydrophenanthrene can be interconverted. Allowing a slight variation to this switch, a striking molecular motor driven by light and/or heat was introduced in (228). In contrast to the rotation around a single bond in the ratchet described above, this rotation was achieved around a carbon-carbon double bond in a helical alkene. Ultraviolet light or the change in temperature could trigger a rotation involving four isomerization steps in the compound (3R,3′R)-(P,P)-*trans*-1,1′,2,2′,3,3′,4,4′-octahydro-3,3′-dimethyl-4,4′,-biphenanthrylidene. A second-generation motor along with eight other motors from the same material is now operational (229). This redesigned motor has distinct upper and lower portions, and it operates at a higher speed. It also provides a good example of how controlled motion at the molecular level can be used to produce a macroscopic change in a system that is visible to the naked eye. The light-driven motors when inside liquid crystal (LC) films can produce a color change by inducing a reorganization of mesogenic molecules (230).

# OTHER PROTEIN-BASED MOTORS UNDER DEVELOPMENT

In this section we present two protein-based motors that are at initial developmental stages and yet possess some very original and interesting characteristics.

## Viral Protein Linear Motors

The idea of viral protein linear motors (231) stems from the fact that a family of retroviruses like the influenza virus (232) and HIV-1 (233) has a typical mechanism of infecting a human cell. When such a virus comes near the cell, it is believed that it experiences a drop in pH of its surroundings owing to the environment surrounding the cell. This is a sort of signal to the virus that its future host is near. The drop of pH changes the energetics of the outer (envelope glycoprotein) protein of the viral membrane in such a way that there is a distinct conformational change in a part of it (234, 235). A triple-stranded coiled coil domain of the membrane protein changes conformation from a loose random structure to a distinctive $\alpha$-helical conformation (236). It is proposed to isolate this domain from the virus and trigger the conformational change by variation of pH in vitro. Once this is realized, attachments can be added to the N or C (or both) terminals of the peptide, and a reversible linear motion can be achieved. Figure 12 shows a triple-stranded coiled coil structure at a pH of 7.0; the inverted hairpin-like coils shown in the front view in Figure 12*a* and top view shown in Figure 12*b* that change conformation into extended helical coils as seen in Figure 12*b*.

## Synthetic Contractile Polymers

In a recent development, large plant proteins that can change conformation when stimulated by positively charged ions were separated from their natural environment and shown to exert forces in orthogonal directions (237, 238). Proteins from sieve elements of higher plants that are a part of the microfluidics system of the plant were chosen to build a new protein molecular machine element. These elements change conformations in the presence of $Ca^{2+}$ ions and organize themselves inside the tubes to stop the fluid flow in case there is a rupture downstream. This is a natural defense mechanism seen in such plants. The change in conformation is akin to a balloon inflating and extending in its lateral as well as longitudinal directions. These elements, designated as forisomes, adhered to glass tubes, were shown to reversibly swell in the presence of $Ca^{2+}$ ions and shrink in their absence, hence performing a pulling/pushing action in both directions. Artificially prepared protein bodies such as the forisomes could be a useful molecular machine component in a future molecular assembly, producing forces of the order of micronewtons (237). Unlike the ATP-dependant motors discussed previously, these machine elements are more robust because they can perform well in the absence of their natural environment.

## CONCLUSIONS

The recent explosion of research in nanotechnology, combined with important discoveries in molecular biology, has created a new interest in biomolecular machines and robots. The main goal in the field of biomolecular machines is to use various biological elements—whose function at the cellular level creates a motion, force, or a signal—as machine components that perform the same function in response to the same biological stimuli but in an artificial setting. In this way, proteins and DNA could act as motors, mechanical joints, transmission elements, or sensors. If all these components were assembled together they could form nanodevices with

(*a*)

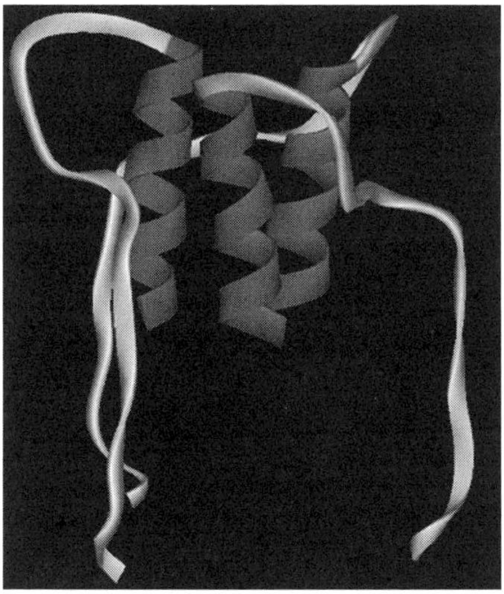

**Figure 12** (*a*) VPL motor at neutral pH. Front view of the partially $\alpha$-helical triple stranded coiled coil. VPL motor is in the closed conformation. (*b*) VPL Motor in the open conformation at acidic pH. The random coil regions are converted into well-defined helices and an extension occurs at lower pH.

(*b*)

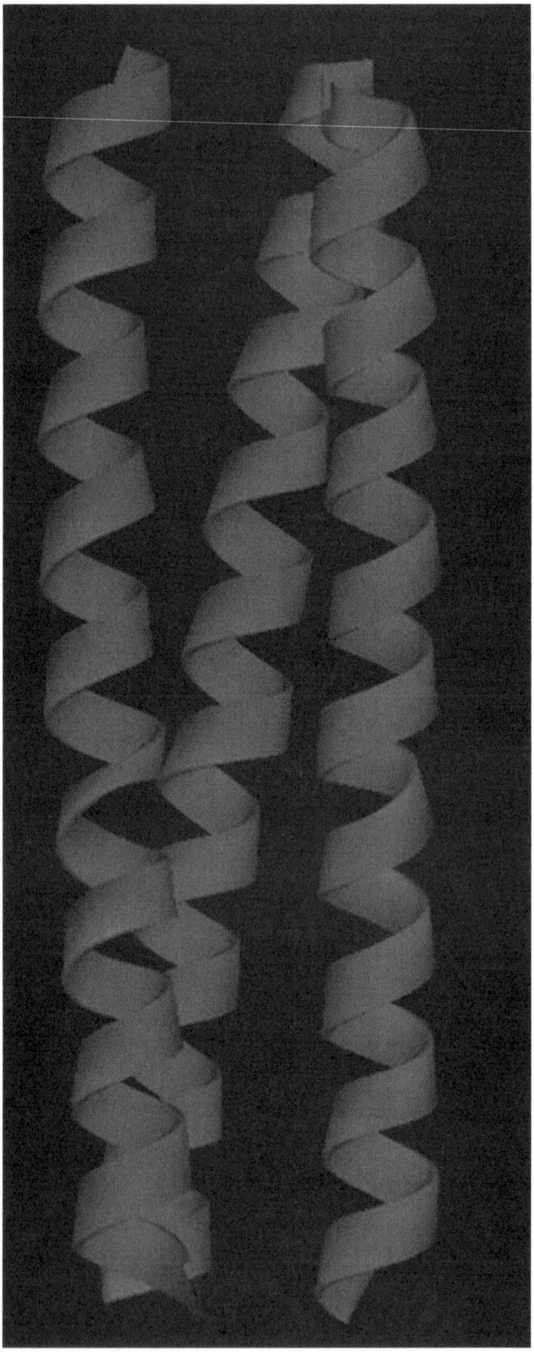

**Figure 12** (*Continued*)

multiple degrees of freedom, able to apply forces and manipulate objects in the nanoscale world, transfer information from the nano- to the macroscale world, and even travel in a nanoscale environment.

The future of molecular machinery is bright. We are at the dawn of a new era in which many disciplines will merge, including robotics, mechanical, chemical, and biomedical engineering, chemistry, biology, physics, and mathematics, so that fully functional systems will be developed. However, challenges toward such a goal abound. Developing a complete database of different biomolecular machine components and the ability to interface or assemble different machine components are some of the challenges to be faced in the near future. The problems involved in controlling and coordinating several biomolecular machines will come next.

## ACKNOWLEDGMENTS

This work was supported by the National Science Foundation (DMI-02,28103 and DMI-03,03950). Any opinions, findings, conclusions, or recommendations expressed in this publication are those of the authors and do not necessarily reflect the views of the National Science Foundation. The authors thank Kevin Nikitczuk of the Department of Biomedical Engineering at Rutgers University for providing assistance in the creation of the graphics for this paper.

**The *Annual Review of Biomedical Engineering* is online at http://bioeng.annualreviews.org**

## LITERATURE CITED

1. Oster G. 2003. How protein motors convert chemical energy into mechanical work. In *Molecular Motors*, ed. M Schliwa, pp. 207–28. New York: Wiley
2. Boyer PD. 1998. Energy, life, and ATP. *Biosci. Rep.* 18:97–117
3. Lipmann F. 1941. Metabolic generation and utilization of phosphate bond energy. *Adv. Enzymol.* 1:99
4. Yasuda R, Noji H, Kinosita K Jr, Yoshida M. 1998. F1-ATPase is a highly efficient molecular motor that rotates with discrete 120 degree steps. *Cell* 93:1117–24
5. Fernandez-Moran H. 1962. Molecular organization of cell membranes. *Circulation* 26:1039–65
6. Kagawa Y, Racker E. 1966. Partial resolution of the enzymes catalyzing oxidative phosphorylation. *J. Biol. Chem.* 241:2475–82
7. Oster G, Wang H. 1999. ATP synthase: two motors, two fuels. *Struct. Fold Des.* 7: R67–72
8. Mitchell P. 1979. Keilin's respiratory chain concept and its chemiosmotic consequences. *Science* 206:1148–59
9. Dimroth P. 1991. $Na^+$-coupled alternative to $H^+$-coupled primary transport systems in bacteria. *BioEssays* 13:463–68
10. Knowles AF, Penefsky HS. 1972. The subunit structure of beef heart mitochondrial adenosine triphosphatase. Physical and chemical properties of isolated subunits. *J. Biol. Chem.* 247:6624–30
11. Boyer PD, Cross RL, Momsen W. 1973. A new concept for energy coupling in oxidative phosphorylation based on a molecular explanation of the oxygen exchange reactions. *Proc. Natl. Acad. Sci. USA* 70: 2837–39

12. Walker JE. 1998. ATP Synthesis by rotary catalysis (Nobel Lecture). *Angew. Chem. Int. Ed.* 37:2308–19
13. Noji H, Yasuda R, Yoshida M, Kinosita K Jr. 1997. Direct observation of the rotation of F1-ATPase. *Nature* 386:299–302
14. Jones PC, Fillingame RH. 1998. Genetic fusions of subunit c in the $F_0$ sector of $H^+$-transporting ATP synthase. Functional dimers and trimers and determination of stoichiometry by cross-linking analysis. *J. Biol. Chem.* 273:29701–5
15. Dimroth P, Wang H, Grabe M, Oster G. 1999. Energy transduction in the sodium F-ATPase of *Propionigenium modestum*. *Proc. Natl. Acad. Sci. USA* 96:4924–29
16. Sambongi Y, Iko Y, Tanabe M, Omote H, Iwamoto-Kihara A, et al. 1999. Mechanical rotation of the c subunit oligomer in ATP synthase (F0F1): direct observation. *Science* 286:1722–24
17. Rastogi VK, Girvin ME. 1999. Structural changes linked to proton translocation by subunit c of the ATP synthase. *Nature* 402: 263–68
18. Stock D, Leslie AG, Walker JE. 1999. Molecular architecture of the rotary motor in ATP synthase. *Science* 286:1700–5
19. Seelert H, Poetsch A, Dencher NA, Engel A, Stahlberg H, Muller DJ. 2000. Structural biology. Proton-powered turbine of a plant motor. *Nature* 405:418–19
20. Stahlberg H, Muller DJ, Suda K, Fotiadis D, Engel A, et al. 2001. Bacterial $Na^+$-ATP synthase has an undecameric rotor. *EMBO Rep.* 2:229–33
21. Fillingame RH. 1990. Molecular mechanics of ATP synthesis in $F_1$ $F_0$-type $H^+$-transporting ATP synthases. *Bacteria* 12:345–91
22. Wang H, Oster G. 1998. Energy transduction in the $F_1$ motor of ATP synthase. *Nature* 396:279–82
23. Abrahams JP, Leslie AG, Lutter R, Walker JE. 1994. Structure at 2.8 Å resolution of F1-ATPase from bovine heart mitochondria. *Nature* 370:621–28
24. Shirakihara Y, Leslie AG, Abrahams JP, Walker JE, Ueda T, et al. 1997. The crystal structure of the nucleotide-free alpha 3 beta 3 subcomplex of F1-ATPase from the thermophilic Bacillus PS3 is a symmetric trimer. *Structure* 5:825–36
25. Bianchet MA, Hullihen J, Pedersen PL, Amzel LM. 1998. The 2.8-Å structure of rat liver F1-ATPase: configuration of a critical intermediate in ATP synthesis/hydrolysis. *Proc. Natl. Acad. Sci. USA* 95:11065–70
26. Menz RI, Walker JE, Leslie AG. 2001. Structure of bovine mitochondrial $F_1$-ATPase with nucleotide bound to all three catalytic sites: implications for the mechanism of rotary catalysis. *Cell* 106:331–41
27. Groth G. 2002. Structure of spinach chloroplast $F_1$-ATPase complexed with the phytopathogenic inhibitor tentoxin. *Proc. Natl. Acad. Sci. USA* 99:3464–68
28. Rodgers AJ, Wilce MC. 2000. Structure of the gamma-epsilon complex of ATP synthase. *Nat. Struct. Biol.* 7:1051–54
29. Dimroth P, Kaim G, Matthey U. 2000. Crucial role of the membrane potential for ATP synthesis by $F_1F_0$ ATP synthases. *J. Exp. Biol.* 203 Pt 1:51–59
30. Oster G, Wang H, Grabe M. 2000. How Fo-ATPase generates rotary torque. *Philos. Trans. R. Soc. London Ser. B.* 355: 523–28
31. Dimroth P. 2000. Operation of the $F_0$ motor of the ATP synthase. *Biochim. Biophys. Acta* 1458:374–86
32. Grabe M, Wang H, Oster G. 2000. The mechanochemistry of V-ATPase proton pumps. *Biophys. J.* 78:2798–813
33. Oster G, Wang H. 2000. Reverse engineering a protein: the mechanochemistry of ATP synthase. *Biochim. Biophys. Acta* 1458:482–510
34. Soong RK, Bachand GD, Neves HP, Olkhovets AG, Craighead HG, Montemagno CD. 2000. Powering an inorganic nanodevice with a biomolecular motor. *Science* 290:1555–58
35. Howard J. 1997. Molecular motors:

structural adaptations to cellular functions. *Nature* 389:561–67
36. Vale R. 1996. Switches, latches, and amplifiers: common themes of G proteins and molecular motors. *J. Cell Biol.* 135:291–302
37. Farrell CM, Mackey AT, Klumpp LM, Gilbert SP. 2002. The role of ATP hydrolysis for kinesin processivity. *J. Biol. Chem.* 277:17079–87
38. Vale RD, Milligan RA. 2000. The way things move: looking under the hood of molecular motor proteins. *Science* 288: 88–95
39. Block SM, Goldstein LS, Schnapp BJ. 1990. Bead movement by single kinesin molecules studied with optical tweezers. *Nature* 348:348–52
40. Howard J, Hudspeth AJ, Vale RD. 1989. Movement of microtubules by single kinesin molecules. *Nature* 342:154–58
41. Finer JT, Simmons RM, Spudich JA. 1994. Single myosin molecule mechanics: piconewton forces and nanometre steps. *Nature* 368:113–19
42. Hackney DD. 1996. The kinetic cycles of myosin, kinesin, and dynein. *Annu. Rev. Physiol.* 58:731–50
43. Block SM. 1998. Kinesin, what gives? *Cell* 93:5–8
44. Kull FJ, Sablin EP, Lau R, Fletterick RJ, Vale RD. 1996. Crystal structure of the kinesin motor domain reveals a structural similarity to myosin. *Nature* 380:550–55
45. Sellers JR. 2000. Myosins: a diverse superfamily. *Biochim. Biophys. Acta* 1496: 3–22
46. Howard J. 1994. Molecular motors. Clamping down on myosin. *Nature* 368: 98–99
47. Huxley HE. 1957. The double array of filaments in cross-striated muscle. *J. Biophys. Biochem. Cytol.* 3:631–48
48. Huxley HE. 1953. Electron microscope studies of the organisation of the filaments in striated muscle. *Biochim. Biophys. Acta* 12:387–94
49. Hanson J, Huxley HE. 1953. Structural basis of the cross-striations in muscle. *Nature* 153:530–32
50. Huxley HE. 1969. The mechanism of muscular contraction. *Science* 164:1356–65
51. Lymn RW, Taylor EW. 1971. Mechanism of adenosine triphosphate hydrolysis by actomyosin. *Biochemistry* 10:4617–24
52. For videos of myosin and kinesin movement visit http://sciencemag.org/feature/data/1049155.shl.
53. Lowey S, Slayter HS, Weeds AG, Baker H. 1969. Substructure of the myosin molecule. I. Subfragments of myosin by enzymic degradation. *J. Mol. Biol.* 42:1–29
54. Weeds AG, Lowey S. 1971. Substructure of the myosin molecule. II. The light chains of myosin. *J. Mol. Biol.* 61:701–25
55. Wagner PD, Giniger E. 1981. Hydrolysis of ATP and reversible binding to F-actin by myosin heavy chains free of all light chains. *Nature* 292:560–62
56. Citi S, Kendrick-Jones J. 1987. Regulation of non-muscle myosin structure and function. *BioEssays* 7:155–59
57. Sellers JR. 1991. Regulation of cytoplasmic and smooth muscle myosin. *Curr. Opin. Cell Biol.* 3:98–104
58. Schroder RR, Manstein DJ, Jahn W, Holden H, Rayment I, et al. 1993. Three-dimensional atomic model of F-actin decorated with *Dictyostelium* myosin S1. *Nature* 364:171–74
59. Rayment I, Rypniewski WR, Schmidt-Base K, Smith R, Tomchick DR, et al. 1993. Three-dimensional structure of myosin subfragment-1: a molecular motor. *Science* 261:50–58
60. Huxley AF. 2000. Cross-bridge action: present views, prospects, and unknowns. *J. Biomech.* 33:1189–95
61. Huxley AF, Simmons RM. 1971. Proposed mechanism of force generation in striated muscle. *Nature* 233:533–38
62. Kabsch W, Mannherz HG, Suck D, Pai EF, Holmes KC. 1990. Atomic structure of the

actin:DNase I complex. *Nature* 347:37–44

63. Holmes KC, Popp D, Gebhard W, Kabsch W. 1990. Atomic model of the actin filament. *Nature* 347:44–49
64. Spudich JA. 1994. How molecular motors work. *Nature* 372:515–18
65. Baker JE, Brust-Mascher I, Ramachandran S, LaConte LE, Thomas DD. 1998. A large and distinct rotation of the myosin light chain domain occurs upon muscle contraction. *Proc. Natl. Acad. Sci. USA* 95:2944–49
66. Houdusse A, Kalabokis VN, Himmel D, Szent-Gyorgyi AG, Cohen C. 1999. Atomic structure of scallop myosin subfragment S1 complexed with MgADP: a novel conformation of the myosin head. *Cell* 97:459–70
67. Jontes JD, Wilson-Kubalek EM, Milligan RA. 1995. A 32 degree tail swing in brush border myosin I on ADP release. *Nature* 378:751–53
68. Veigel C, Coluccio LM, Jontes JD, Sparrow JC, Milligan RA, Molloy JE. 1999. The motor protein myosin-I produces its working stroke in two steps. *Nature* 398:530–33
69. Corrie JE, Brandmeier BD, Ferguson RE, Trentham DR, Kendrick-Jones J, et al. 1999. Dynamic measurement of myosin light-chain-domain tilt and twist in muscle contraction. *Nature* 400:425–30
70. Irving M, St Claire Allen T, Sabido-David C, Craik JS, Brandmeier B, et al. 1995. Tilting of the light-chain region of myosin during step length changes and active force generation in skeletal muscle. *Nature* 375:688–91
71. Forkey JN, Quinlan ME, Shaw MA, Corrie JE, Goldman YE. 2003. Three-dimensional structural dynamics of myosin V by single-molecule fluorescence polarization. *Nature* 422:399–404
72. Kitamura K, Tokunaga M, Iwane AH, Yanagida T. 1999. A single myosin head moves along an actin filament with regular steps of ~5.3 nm. *Nature* 397:129–34
73. Howard J. 1996. The movement of kinesin along microtubules. *Annu. Rev. Physiol.* 58:703–29
74. Howard J, Hyman AA. 2003. Dynamics and mechanics of the microtubule plus end. *Nature* 422:753–58
75. Hirokawa N. 1998. Kinesin and dynein superfamily proteins and the mechanism of organelle transport. *Science* 279:519–26
76. Vale RD, Funatsu T, Pierce DW, Romberg L, Harada Y, Yanagida T. 1996. Direct observation of single kinesin molecules moving along microtubules. *Nature* 380:451–53
77. Berliner E, Young EC, Anderson K, Mahtani HK, Gelles J. 1995. Failure of a single-headed kinesin to track parallel to microtubule protofilaments. *Nature* 373:718–21
78. Sablin EP, Kull FJ, Cooke R, Vale RD, Fletterick RJ. 1996. Crystal structure of the motor domain of the kinesin-related motor ncd. *Nature* 380:555–59
79. Sack S, Muller J, Marx A, Thormahlen M, Mandelkow EM, et al. 1997. X-ray structure of motor and neck domains from rat brain kinesin. *Biochemistry* 36:16155–65
80. Schnitzer MJ, Block SM. 1997. Kinesin hydrolyses one ATP per 8-nm step. *Nature* 388:386–90
81. Peskin CS, Oster G. 1995. Coordinated hydrolysis explains the mechanical behavior of kinesin. *Biophys. J.* 68:202–11
82. Lohman TM, Thorn K, Vale RD. 1998. Staying on track: common features of DNA helicases and microtubule motors. *Cell* 93:9–12
83. Hackney DD. 1995. Highly processive microtubule-stimulated ATP hydrolysis by dimeric kinesin head domains. *Nature* 377:448–50
84. Hunt AJ, Gittes F, Howard J. 1994. The force exerted by a single kinesin molecule against a viscous load. *Biophys. J.* 67:766–81
85. Svoboda K, Block SM. 1994. Force

and velocity measured for single kinesin molecules. *Cell* 77:773–84
86. Gibbons IR, Rowe AJ. 1965. Dynein: a protein with adenosine triphosphate activity from cilia. *Science* 149:424–26
87. Schroer TA, Steuer ER, Sheetz MP. 1989. Cytoplasmic dynein is a minus end-directed motor for membranous organelles. *Cell* 56:937–46
88. Schnapp BJ, Reese TS. 1989. Dynein is the motor for retrograde axonal transport of organelles. *Proc. Natl. Acad. Sci. USA* 86:1548–52
89. Lye RJ, Porter ME, Scholey JM, McIntosh JR. 1987. Identification of a microtubule-based cytoplasmic motor in the nematode *C. elegans*. *Cell* 51:309–18
90. Paschal BM, Shpetner HS, Vallee RB. 1987. MAP 1C is a microtubule-activated ATPase which translocates microtubules in vitro and has dynein-like properties. *J. Cell Biol.* 105:1273–82
91. Hirokawa N, Sato-Yoshitake R, Yoshida T, Kawashima T. 1990. Brain dynein (MAP1C) localizes on both anterogradely and retrogradely transported membranous organelles in vivo. *J. Cell Biol.* 111:1027–37
92. Waterman-Storer CM, Karki SB, Kuznetsov SA, Tabb JS, Weiss DG, et al. 1997. The interaction between cytoplasmic dynein and dynactin is required for fast axonal transport. *Proc. Natl. Acad. Sci. USA* 94:12180–85
93. Lin SX, Collins CA. 1992. Immunolocalization of cytoplasmic dynein to lysosomes in cultured cells. *J. Cell Sci.* 101 (Pt 1):125–37
94. Corthesy-Theulaz I, Pauloin A, Rfeffer SR. 1992. Cytoplasmic dynein participates in the centrosomal localization of the Golgi complex. *J. Cell Biol.* 118: 1333–45
95. Aniento F, Emans N, Griffiths G, Gruenberg J. 1993. Cytoplasmic dynein-dependent vesicular transport from early to late endosomes. *J. Cell Biol.* 123:1373–87
96. Fath KR, Trimbur GM, Burgess DR. 1994. Molecular motors are differentially distributed on Golgi membranes from polarized epithelial cells. *J. Cell Biol.* 126:661–75
97. Blocker A, Severin FF, Burkhardt JK, Bingham JB, Yu H, et al. 1997. Molecular requirements for bi-directional movement of phagosomes along microtubules. *J. Cell Biol.* 137:113–29
98. King SJ, Bonilla M, Rodgers ME, Schroer TA. 2002. Subunit organization in cytoplasmic dynein subcomplexes. *Protein Sci.* 11:1239–50
99. King SM. 2000. The dynein microtubule motor. *Biochim. Biophys. Acta* 1496:60–75
100. Burgess S, Walker ML, Sakakibara H, Knight PJ, Oiwa K. 2003. Dynein structure and power stroke. *Nature* 421:715–18
101. Koonce MP. 1997. Identification of a microtubule-binding domain in a cytoplasmic dynein heavy chain. *J. Biol. Chem.* 272:19714–18
102. Gill S, Schroer T, Szilak I, Steuer E, Sheetz M, Cleveland D. 1991. Dynactin, a conserved, ubiquitously expressed component of an activator of vesicle motility mediated by cytoplasmic dynein. *J. Cell Biol.* 115:1639–50
103. Straube A, Enard W, Berner A, Wedlich-Soldner R, Kahmann R, Steinberg G. 2001. A split motor domain in a cytoplasmic dynein. *EMBO J.* 20:5091–100
104. Vale RD. 2000. AAA proteins: lords of the ring. *J. Cell Biol.* 150:13F–20
105. Neuwald AF, Aravind L, Spouge JL, Koonin EV. 1999. AAA+: a class of chaperone-like ATPases associated with the assembly, operation, and disassembly of protein complexes. *Genome Res.* 9:27–43
106. Confalonieri F, Duguet M. 1995. A 200-amino acid ATPase module in search of a basic function. *BioEssays* 17:639–50
107. King SM. 2000. AAA domains and organization of the dynein motor unit. *J. Cell Sci.* 113(Pt 14):2521–26

108. Asai DJ, Koonce MP. 2001. The dynein heavy chain: structure, mechanics and evolution. *Trends Cell Biol.* 11:196–202
109. Berry RM, Armitage JP. 1999. The bacterial flagella motor. *Adv. Microb. Physiol.* 41:291–337
110. Berg HC. 2003. The rotary motor of bacterial flagella. *Annu. Rev. Biochem.* 72:19–54
111. Blair DF. 1995. How bacteria sense and swim. *Annu. Rev. Microbiol.* 49:489–522
112. Berg HC, Anderson RA. 1973. Bacteria swim by rotating their flagellar filaments. *Nature* 245:380–82
113. Fahrner KA, Ryu WS, Berg HC. 2003. Biomechanics: bacterial flagellar switching under load. *Nature* 423:938
114. Berg HC. 2000. Motile behavior of bacteria. *Phys. Today* 53:24–29
115. Scharf BE, Fahrner KA, Turner L, Berg HC. 1998. Control of direction of flagellar rotation in bacterial chemotaxis. *Proc. Natl. Acad. Sci. USA* 95:201–6
116. Macnab RM. 1977. Bacterial flagella rotating in bundles: a study in helical geometry. *Proc. Natl. Acad. Sci. USA* 74:221–25
117. Elston TC, Oster G. 1997. Protein turbines. I: the bacterial flagellar motor. *Biophys. J.* 73:703–21
118. Walz D, Caplan SR. 2000. An electrostatic mechanism closely reproducing observed behavior in the bacterial flagellar motor. *Biophys. J.* 78:626–51
119. Schmitt R. 2003. Helix rotation model of the flagellar rotary motor. *Biophys. J.* 85:843–52
120. Iino T, Komeda Y, Kutsukake K, Macnab RM, Matsumura P, et al. 1988. New unified nomenclature for the flagellar genes of *Escherichia coli* and *Salmonella typhimurium*. *Microbiol. Rev.* 52:533–35
121. Berg HC. 1974. Dynamic properties of bacterial flagellar motors. *Nature* 249:77–79
122. Ueno T, Oosawa K, Aizawa S. 1992. M ring, S ring and proximal rod of the flagellar basal body of *Salmonella typhimurium* are composed of subunits of a single protein, FliF. *J. Mol. Biol.* 227:672–77
123. Ueno T, Oosawa K, Aizawa S. 1994. Domain structures of the MS ring component protein (FliF) of the flagellar basal body of *Salmonella typhimurium*. *J. Mol. Biol.* 236:546–55
124. Driks A, DeRosier DJ. 1990. Additional structures associated with bacterial flagellar basal body. *J. Mol. Biol.* 211:669–72
125. Khan IH, Reese TS, Khan S. 1992. The cytoplasmic component of the bacterial flagellar motor. *Proc. Natl. Acad. Sci. USA* 89:5956–60
126. Francis NR, Sosinsky GE, Thomas D, DeRosier DJ. 1994. Isolation, characterization and structure of bacterial flagellar motors containing the switch complex. *J. Mol. Biol.* 235:1261–70
127. Yorimitsu T, Homma M. 2001. $Na^+$-driven flagellar motor of *Vibrio*. *Biochim. Biophys. Acta* 1505:82–93
128. Meister M, Lowe G, Berg HC. 1987. The proton flux through the bacterial flagellar motor. *Cell* 49:643–50
129. Van Way SM, Hosking ER, Braun TF, Manson MD. 2000. Mot protein assembly into the bacterial flagellum: a model based on mutational analysis of the motB gene. *J. Mol. Biol.* 297:7–24
130. Blair DF, Berg HC. 1988. Restoration of torque in defective flagellar motors. *Science* 242:1678–81
131. Fung DC, Berg HC. 1995. Powering the flagellar motor of *Escherichia coli* with an external voltage source. *Nature* 375:809–12
132. Berg H, Turner L. 1993. Torque generated by the flagellar motor of *Escherichia coli*. *Biophys. J.* 65:2201–16
133. Chen X, Berg HC. 2000. Torque-speed relationship of the flagellar rotary motor of *Escherichia coli*. *Biophys. J.* 78:1036–41
134. Seeman NC. 2003. DNA in a material world. *Nature* 421:427–31
135. Dekker C, Ratner M. 2001. Electronic properties of DNA. *Phys. World* August: 29–33

136. Robinson BH, Seeman NC. 1987. The design of a biochip: a self-assembling molecular-scale memory device. *Protein Eng.* 1:295–300
137. Seeman NC, Belcher AM. 2002. Emulating biology: building nanostructures from the bottom up. *Proc. Natl. Acad. Sci. USA* 99:6451–55
138. Smith SB, Cui Y, Bustamante C. 1996. Overstretching B-DNA: the elastic response of individual double-stranded and single-stranded DNA molecules. *Science* 271:795–99
139. Simmel FC, Yurke B. 2001. Using DNA to construct and power a nanoactuator. *Phys. Rev. E.* 63:041913
140. Tinland B, Pluen A, Sturm J, Weill G. 1997. Persistence length of single-stranded DNA. *Macromolecules* 30: 5763–65
141. Seeman NC. 1997. DNA components for molecular architecture. *Acc. Chem. Res.* 30:347–91
142. Niemeyer CM. 1999. Progress in "engineering up" nanotechnology devices utilizing DNA as a construction material. *Appl.Phys. A* 68:119–24
143. Chen JH, Seeman NC. 1991. Synthesis from DNA of a molecule with the connectivity of a cube. *Nature* 350:631–33
144. Zhang Y, Seeman NC. 1994. Construction of a DNA-truncated octahedron. *J. Am. Chem. Soc.* 116:1661–69
145. Winfree E, Liu F, Wenzler LA, Seeman NC. 1998. Design and self-assembly of two-dimensional DNA crystals. *Nature* 394:539–44
146. Yan H, Zhang X, Shen Z, Seeman NC. 2002. A robust DNA mechanical device controlled by hybridization topology. *Nature* 415:62–65
147. Mao C, Sun W, Seeman NC. 1997. Assembly of Borromean rings from DNA. *Nature* 386:137–38
148. Mao C, LaBean TH, Relf JH, Seeman NC. 2000. Logical computation using algorithmic self-assembly of DNA triple-crossover molecules. *Nature* 407:493–96
149. Deleted in proof
150. Coppin CM, Pierce DW, Hsu L, Vale RD. 1997. The load dependence of kinesin's mechanical cycle. *Proc. Natl. Acad. Sci. USA* 94:8539–44
151. Seeman NC. 1991. Construction of three-dimensional stick figures from branched DNA. *DNA Cell Biol.* 10:475–86
152. Wang H, Du SM, Seeman NC. 1993. Tight single-stranded DNA knots. *J. Biomol. Struct. Dyn.* 10:853–63
153. Seeman NC. 1998. Nucleic acid nanostructures and topology. *Angew. Chem. Int. Ed.* 37:3220–38
154. Mao C, Sun W, Seeman NC. 1999. Designed two-dimensional DNA Holliday junction arrays visualized by atomic force microscopy. *J. Am. Chem. Soc.* 121:5437–43
155. LaBean TH, Yan H, Kopatsch J, Liu F, Winfree E, et al. 2000. Construction, analysis, ligation, and self-assembly of DNA triple crossover complexes. *J. Am. Chem. Soc.* 122:1848–60
156. Fu TJ, Seeman NC. 1993. DNA double-crossover molecules. *Biochemistry* 32: 3211–20
157. Zhang S, Fu TJ, Seeman NC. 1993. Symmetric immobile DNA branched junctions. *Biochemistry* 32:8062–67
158. Li X, Yang X, Jing Q, Seeman NC. 1996. Antiparallel DNA double crossover molecules as components for nanoconstruction. *J. Am. Chem. Soc.* 118:6131–40
159. Mao C, Sun W, Shen Z, Seeman NC. 1999. A nanomechanical device based on the B-Z transition of DNA. *Nature* 397:144–46
160. Rich A, Nordheim A, Wang AHJ. 1984. The chemistry and biology of left-handed Z-DNA. *Annu. Rev. Biochem.* 53:791–846
161. Pohl FM, Jovin TM. 1972. Salt-induced co-operative conformational change of a synthetic DNA: equilibrium and kinetic studies with poly (dG-dC). *J. Mol. Biol.* 67:375–96
162. Yurke B, Turberfield AJ, Mills AP, Simmel FC, Neumann JL. 2000. A

DNA-fuelled molecular machine made of DNA. *Nature* 415:62–65
163. Simmel FC, Yurke B. 2002. A DNA-based molecular device switchable between three distinct mechanical states. *Appl. Phys. Lett.* 80:883–85
164. Mitchell JC, Yurke B. 2002. DNA scissors. In *DNA Computing. Proc. 7th Int. Meet. DNA-Based Computers*, ed. SN Jonoska, N Seeman. Univ. So. FL, Tampa. Heidelberg: Springer Verlag
165. Seeman NC. 2001. DNA nicks and nodes and nanotechnology. *Nano Lett.* 1:22–26
166. Yang X, Wenzler LA, Qi J, Li X, Seeman NC. 1998. Ligation of DNA triangles containing double crossover molecules. *J. Am. Chem. Soc.* 120:9779–86
167. Schill G. 1971. *Catenanes, Rotaxanes and Knots*. New York: Academic
168. Ashton PR, Ballardini R, Balzani V, Belohradsky M, Gandolfi MT, et al. 1996. Self-assembly, spectroscopic, and electrochemical properties of [n]rotaxanes. *J. Am. Chem. Soc.* 118:4931–51
169. Amabilino DB, Asakawa M, Ashton PR, Ballardini R, Balzani V, et al. 1998. Aggregation of self-assembling branched [n]rotaxanes. *N. J. Chem.* 9:959–72
170. Sauvage J-P, Dietrich-Buchecker C, eds. 1999. *Molecular Catenanes, Rotaxanes and Knots*. Weinheim: Wiley-VCH
171. Harada A. 2001. Cyclodextrin-based molecular machines. *Acc. Chem. Res.* 34: 456–64
172. Anelli P-L, Spencer N, Stoddart JF. 1991. A molecular shuttle. *J. Am. Chem. Soc.* 113:5131–33
173. Balzani VV, Credi A, Raymo FM, Stoddart JF. 2000. Artificial molecular machines. *Angew. Chem. Int. Ed. Engl.* 39: 3348–91
174. Schalley CA, Beizai K, Vogtle F. 2001. On the Way to rotaxane-based molecular motors: studies in molecular mobility and topological chirality. *Acc. Chem. Res.* 34:465–76
175. Gatti FG, Leon S, Wong JKY, Bottari G, Altieri A, et al. 2003. Photoisomerization of a rotaxane hydrogen bonding template: light-induced acceleration of a large amplitude rotational motion. *Proc. Natl. Acad. Sci. USA* 100:10–14
176. Bermudez VV, Capron N, Gase T, Gatti FG, Kajzar F, et al. 2000. Influencing intramolecular motion with an alternating electric field. *Nature* 406:608–11
177. Fyfe MCT, Stoddart JF. 1997. Synthetic supramolecular chemistry. *Acc. Chem. Res.* 30:393–401
178. Whitesides GM, Mathias JP, Seto CT. 1991. Molecular self-assembly and nanochemistry: a chemical strategy for the synthesis of nanostructures. *Science* 254:1312–19
179. Gaviña P, Sauvage JP. 1997. Transition-metal template synthesis of a rotaxane incorporating two different coordinating units in its thread. *Tetrahedron Lett.* 38:3521–24
180. Raymo FM, Houk KM, Stoddart JF. 1998. The mechanism of the slippage approach to rotaxanes. Origin of the "all-or-nothing" substituent effect. *J. Am. Chem. Soc.* 120:9318–22
181. Whitesides GM, Simanek EE, Mathias JP, Seto CT, Chin DN, et al. 1995. Noncovalent synthesis: using physical-organic chemistry to make aggregates. *Acc. Chem. Res.* 28:37–44
182. Asakawa M, Ashton PR, Ballardini R, Balzani V, Belohradsky M, et al. 1997. The slipping approach to self-assembling [n]rotaxanes. *J. Am. Chem. Soc.* 119:302–10
183. Brouwer AM, Frochot C, Gatti FG, Leigh DA, Mottier L, et al. 2001. Photoinduction of fast, reversible translational motion in a hydrogen-bonded molecular shuttle. *Science* 291:2124–28
184. Bissell RA, Córdova E, Kaifer AE, Stoddart JF. 1994. A chemically and electrochemically switchable molecular shuttle. *Nature* 369:133–37
185. Martínez-Díaz M-V, Spencer N, Stoddart JF. 1997. The self-assembly of a

switchable [2]rotaxane. *Angew. Chem. Int. Ed. Engl.* 36:1904–7
186. Ashton PR, Ballardini R, Balzani V, Baxter I, Credi A, Fyfe MCT, et al. 1998. Acid-base controllable molecular shuttles. *J. Am. Chem. Soc.* 120:11932–42
187. Armaroli N, Balzani V, Collin JP, Gaviña P, Sauvage JP, Ventura B. 1999. Rotaxanes incorporating two different coordinating units in their thread: synthesis and electrochemically and photochemically induced molecular motions. *J. Am. Chem. Soc.* 121:4397–408
188. Benniston AC, Harriman A, Lynch VM. 1995. Photoactive [2]rotaxanes: structure and photophysical properties of anthracene- and ferrocene-stoppered [2]rotaxanes. *J. Am. Chem. Soc.* 117: 5275–91
189. Benniston AC, Harriman A. 1993. A light-induced molecular shuttle based on a [2]rotaxane-derived triad. *Angew. Chem. Int. Ed. Engl.* 32:1459–61
190. Benniston AC, Harriman A, Lynch VM. 1994. Photoactive [2]rotaxanes formed by multiple-stacking. *Tetrahedron Lett.* 35:1473–76
191. Murakami H, Kawabuchi A, Kotoo K, Kunitake M, Nakashima N. 1997. A light-driven molecular shuttle based on a rotaxane. *J. Am. Chem. Soc.* 119:7605–6
192. Kaufmann C, Müller WM, Vögtle F, Weinman S, Abramson S, Fuchs B. 1999. Rotaxanes with chiral stoppers and photoresponsive central unit. *Synthesis* 5: 849–53
193. Ashton PR, Goodnow TT, Kaifer AW, Reddington MV, Slawin AMZ, et al. 1989. A [2]catenane made to order. *Angew. Chem. Int. Ed. Engl.* 28:1396–99
194. Deleuze MS. 2000. Can benzylic amide [2]catenane rings rotate on graphite? *J. Am. Chem. Soc.* 122:1130–43
195. Raymo FM, Houk KN, Stoddart JF. 1998. Origins of selectivity in molecular and supramolecular entities: solvent and electrostatic control of the translational isomerism in [2]catenanes. *J. Org. Chem.* 63:6523–28
196. Sauvage J-P. 1998. Transition metal containing rotaxanes and catenanes in motion: toward molecular machines and motors. *Acc. Chem. Res.* 31:611–19
197. Cambron J-C, Sauvage J-P. 1998. Functional rotaxanes: from controlled molecular motions to electron transfer between chemically nonconnected chromophores. *Chem. Eur. J.* 4:1362–66
198. Blanco MJ, Jimenez MC, Chambron J-C, Heitz V, Linke M, Sauvage J-P. 1999. Rotaxanes as new architectures for photoinduced electron transfer and molecular motions. *Chem. Soc. Rev.* 28:293–305
199. Leigh DA, Murphy A, Smart JP, Deleuze MS, Zerbetto F. 1998. Controlling the frequency of macrocyclic ring rotation in benzylic amide [2]catenanes. *J. Am. Chem. Soc.* 120:6458–67
200. Fujita M. 1999. Self-assembly of [2]catenanes containing metals in their backbones. *Acc. Chem. Res.* 32:53–61
201. Collier CP, Mattersteig G, Wong EW, Luo Y, Beverly K, et al. 2000. A [2]catenane-based solid state electronically reconfigurable switch. *Science* 289:1172–75
202. Balzani VV, Gomez-Lopez M, Stoddart JF. 1998. Molecular machines. *Acc. Chem. Res.* 31:405–14
203. Johnston MR, Gunter MJ, Warrener RN. 1998. Templated formation of multiporphyrin assemblies resembling a molecular universal joint. *Chem. Commun.* 28:2739–40
204. Amabilino DB, Anelli P-L, Ashton PR, Brown GR, Cordova E, et al. 1995. Molecular meccano. 3. Constitutional and translational isomerism in [2]catenanes and [n]pseudorotaxanes. *J. Am. Chem. Soc.* 117:11142–70
205. Vacek J, Michl J. 1997. A molecular "Tinkertoy" construction kit: computer simulation of molecular propellers. *N. J. Chem.* 21:1259–68
206. Michl J, Magnera TF. 2002. Supramolecular chemistry and self-assembly special

feature: two-dimensional supramolecular chemistry with molecular Tinkertoys. *Proc. Natl. Acad. Sci. USA* 99:4788–92
207. Vacek J, Michl J. 2001. Molecular dynamics of a grid-mounted molecular dipolar rotor in a rotating electric field. *Proc. Natl. Acad. Sci. USA* 98:5481–86
208. Gimzewski JK, Joachim C, Schlittler RR, Langlais V, Tang H, Johannsen I. 1998. Rotation of a single molecule within a supramolecular bearing. *Science* 281:531–33
209. Gust D, Mislow K. 1973. Analysis of isomerization in compounds displaying restricted rotation of aryl groups. *J. Am. Chem. Soc.* 95:1535–47
210. Finocchiaro P, Gust D, Mislow K. 1974. Correlated rotation in complex triarylmethanes. I. $^{32}$-isomer system and residual diastereoisomerism. *J. Am. Chem. Soc.* 96:3198–205
211. Finocchiaro P, Gust D, Mislow K. 1974. Correlated rotation in complex triarylmethanes. II. $^{16}$- and $^{8}$-isomer systems and residual diastereotopicity. *J. Am. Chem. Soc.* 96:3205–13
212. Mislow K. 1976. Stereochemical consequences of correlated rotation in molecular propellers. *Acc. Chem. Res.* 9:26–33
213. Clayden J, Pink JH. 1998. Concerted rotation in a tertiary aromatic amide: towards a simple molecular gear. *Angew. Chem. Int. Ed. Engl.* 37:1937–39
214. Hounshell WD, Johnson CA, Guenzi A, Cozzi F, Mislow K. 1980. Stereochemical consequences of dynamic gearing in substituted bis (9-triptycyl) methanes and related molecules. *Proc. Natl. Acad. Sci. USA* 77:6961–64
215. Cozzi F, Guenzi A, Johnson CA, Mislow K, Hounshell WD, Blount JF. 1981. Stereoisomerism and correlated rotation in molecular gear systems. Residual diastereomers of bis(2,3-dimethyl-9-triptycyl)methane. *J. Am. Chem. Soc.* 103:957–58
216. Kawada YIH. 1981. Bis(4-chloro-1-triptycyl) ether. Separation of a pair of phase isomers of labeled bevel gears. *J. Am. Chem. Soc.* 103:958–60
217. Johnson CA, Guenzi A, Mislow K. 1981. Restricted gearing and residual stereoisomerism in bis(1,4-dimethyl-9-triptycyl)methane. *J. Am. Chem. Soc.* 103:6240–42
218. Bedard TC, Moore JS. 1995. Design and synthesis of a "molecular turnstile." *J. Am. Chem. Soc.* 117:10662–71
219. Ugi I, Marquarding D, Klusacek H, Gillespie P, Ramirez F. 1971. Berry pseudorotation and turnstile rotation. *Acc. Chem. Res.* 4:288–96
220. Kelly TR, Bowyer MC, Bhaskar KV, Bebbington D, Garcia A, et al. 1994. A molecular brake. *J. Am. Chem. Soc.* 116:3657–58
221. Kelly TR, Tellitu I, Sestelo JP. 1997. In search of molecular ratchets. *Angew. Chem. Int. Ed. Engl.* 36:1866–68
222. Kelly TR, Sestelo JP, Tellitu I. 1998. New molecular devices: in search of a molecular ratchet. *J. Org. Chem.* 63:3655–65
223. Davis AP. 1998. Tilting at windmills? The second law survives. *Angew. Chem. Int. Ed. Engl.* 37:909–10
224. Kelly TR, De Silva H, Silva RA. 1999. Unidirectional rotary motion in a molecular system. *Nature* 401:150–52
225. Davis AP. 1999. Synthetic molecular motors. *Nature* 401:120–21
226. Kelly TR, Silva RA, De Silva H, Jasmin S, Zhao Y. 2000. A rationally designed prototype of a molecular motor. *J. Am. Chem. Soc.* 122:6935–49
227. Feringa BL, Jager WF, De Lange B, Meijer EW. 1991. Chiroptical molecular switch. *J. Am. Chem. Soc.* 113:5468–70
228. Koumura N, Zijlstra RW, van Delden RA, Harada N, Feringa BL. 1999. Light-driven monodirectional molecular rotor. *Nature* 401:152–55
229. Koumura N, Geertsema EM, van Gelder MB, Meetsma A, Feringa BL. 2002. Second generation light-driven molecular motors. Unidirectional rotation controlled by a single stereogenic center with

near-perfect photoequilibria and acceleration of the speed of rotation by structural modification. *J. Am. Chem. Soc.* 124: 5037–51

230. van Delden RA, Koumura N, Harada N, Feringa BL. 2002. Unidirectional rotary motion in a liquid crystalline environment: color tuning by a molecular motor. *Proc. Natl. Acad. Sci. USA* 99:4945–49
231. Dubey A, Thornton A, Nikitczuk KP, Mavroidis C, Yarmush ML. 2003. Viral protein linear (VPL) nano-actuators. Presented at *Proc. 2003 3rd IEEE Conf. Nanotechnology, San Francisco*
232. Wilson IA, Skehel JJ, Wiley DC. 1981. Structure of the haemagglutinin membrane glycoprotein of influenza virus at 3 Å resolution. *Nature* 289:366–73
233. Chan DC, Fass D, Berger JM, Kim PS. 1997. Core structure of gp41 from the HIV envelope glycoprotein. *Cell* 89:263–73
234. Bentz J. 2000. Minimal aggregate size and minimal fusion unit for the first fusion pore of influenza hemagglutinin-mediated membrane fusion. *Biophys. J.* 78:227–45
235. Bentz J. 2000. Membrane fusion mediated by coiled coils: a hypothesis. *Biophys. J.* 78:886–900
236. Carr CM, Kim PS. 1993. A spring-loaded mechanism for the conformational change of influenza hemagglutinin. *Cell* 73:823–32
237. Knoblauch M, Noll GA, Muller T, Prufer D, Schneider-Huther I, et al. 2003. ATP-independent contractile proteins from plants. *Nat. Mater.* 2:600–3
238. Mavroidis C, Dubey A. 2003. Biomimetics: from pulses to motors. *Nat. Mater.* 2:573–74

Annu. Rev. Biomed. Eng. 2004. 6:397–426
doi: 10.1146/annurev.bioeng.6.040803.140203

First published online as a Review in Advance on April 8, 2004

# ENGINEERING SYNTHETIC VECTORS FOR IMPROVED DNA DELIVERY: Insights from Intracellular Pathways

Charles M. Roth[1,2] and Sumati Sundaram[1]

*[1]Department of Chemical and Biochemical Engineering and [2]Department of Biomedical Engineering, Rutgers University, Piscataway, New Jersey 08854; email: cmroth@rci.Rutgers.edu*

**Key Words** intracellular trafficking, targeted delivery, antisense oligonucleotides, nonviral gene delivery, rational design

■ **Abstract** Significant progress has been made in the area of nonviral gene delivery to date. Yet, synthetic vectors remain less efficient by orders of magnitude than their viral counterparts. Research continues toward unraveling and overcoming various barriers to the efficient delivery of DNA, whether in plasmid form encoding a gene or as an oligonucleotide for the selective inhibition of target gene expression. Novel components for overcoming these hurdles are continually being incorporated into the design of synthetic vectors, leading to increasingly more virus-like particles. Despite these advances, general principles defining the design of synthetic vectors are yet to be developed fully. A more quantitative analysis of the cellular uptake and intracellular processing of these vectors is required for the rational manipulation of vector design. Mathematical frameworks with a more conceptual basis will help obtain an integrated perspective on these complex systems. In this review, we critically examine the progress made toward the improved design of synthetic vectors by the strategic exploitation of intracellular mechanisms and explore newer possibilities to overcome obstacles in the practical realization of this field.

CONTENTS

## INTRODUCTION—SCOPE OF REVIEW

The concept of gene therapy was originally developed nearly three decades ago (1). The idea rapidly emerged as a field with immense potential and has been reviewed extensively since then. In addition to the ability to introduce genes into cells to replace those that are defective or missing, revolutionary advances in molecular biology have provided us with many tools to modulate gene expression. Several well-developed methodologies are available today, each with its own strategy of where and how the flow of genetic information is perturbed (2–4). These can be classified as either antigene based [e.g., DNA repair oligonucleotides (ONs), triple helix-forming ONs, and DNA decoys] or anti-mRNA based (e.g., RNA decoys, antisense DNA and RNA, DNAzymes and ribozymes, and short interfering RNAs). Because double-stranded plasmid DNA for gene therapy and single-stranded ONs (of varying chemistries) for antisense technology are by far the most widely studied and have already demonstrated their versatility in clinic and laboratory research, we mainly focus on these two forms of nucleic acids. Nonetheless, lessons learned in developing delivery strategies for these molecules will serve as a starting point for delivering other forms of nucleic acids.

Basic research studies and promising results from several proof-of-principle studies in vitro and in animal models have led to high expectations for the practical implementation of these technologies in the clinic. To date, more than 600 clinical trials have been initiated, comprising 3500 patients worldwide. Several products are in Phase II and Phase III stages (2, 4), and there already exists one commercial antisense product, Vitravene, a phosphorothioate oligodeoxynucleotide (PS ODN) for the treatment of an inflammatory viral infection of the eye caused by cytomegalovirus (5). Technologies based on addition, repair, or inhibition of genes are being developed and commercialized not only for therapeutic purposes but also as tools in cellular and molecular bioengineering (6). With the promise of specificity and low toxicity, it is anticipated that such technologies will have a lasting impact on medicine and biotechnology.

Despite a growing body of knowledge regarding the chemistry, biology, and pharmacology of genes and ONs, the widespread application of DNA-based therapeutics remains a daunting challenge. Practical implementation has been more difficult than originally expected. Efficient delivery of nucleic acids to specific sites of action remains the major obstacle in the further advancement of this field. Direct injection of naked DNA has been shown to induce transgene expression. However, plasmid DNA is rapidly eliminated from the bloodstream owing to extensive uptake by the liver and kidney (7), exhibits poor cellular uptake owing to the large size and highly anionic nature of DNA, and generally results in quite low levels of transduced gene expression (8). The natural ability of viruses to deliver genetic material has been exploited for the delivery of therapeutic transgenes (9). However, they are constrained with respect to the amount of genetic material they can carry. More important concerns include the stimulation of strong immune responses and the potential for oncogenic transformations. As a consequence, nonviral delivery vectors are being explored as potential alternatives to viruses for DNA delivery. Synthetic vectors, utilizing carriers such as polymers or lipids, are attractive owing to flexibility in design, ability to be chemically or biochemically functionalized, and tunable toxicity properties. However, synthetic vectors are still very inefficient in comparison with viral vectors.

In the past decade, numerous papers have been published describing the barriers to effective DNA delivery. More recently, this topic has been the subject of abundant review (10–14). These barriers include (*a*) physical and biochemical degradation in the extracellular space, (*b*) the extracellular matrix and cell surface interactions, (*c*) internalization, (*d*) trafficking from endosomes to lysosomes and subsequent degradation, (*e*) escape from endosomes into the cytoplasm, (*f*) dissociation of DNA from its carrier, (*g*) transfer into the nucleus, and (*h*) transcription (for gene transfer) or hybridization (for antisense inhibition). For in vivo applications, physicochemical properties of vectors that affect stability as well as interactions with extracellular systemic components and the immune system will also be of significant importance. It would be desirable to identify a single step as the rate-limiting barrier. However, any or all of these processes may pose significant hindrance to effectiveness in a given application.

Nonetheless, each of these steps provides opportunities for improving vector design. Attempts are being made to improve the efficiency of the vectors, primarily by structural modifications of the carrier. This process is evolving toward the development of multifunctional vectors, which mimic properties of viruses. However, it is still unclear how multiple synthetic components can be assembled into a functional virus-like particle. The process is quite empirical, and there are no defining principles to make vectors that are effective and specific for a particular target cell type. Attempts to improve the efficiency of one of these steps by an appropriate vector modification may modify the intracellular itinerary of the delivered DNA. It would therefore be of great utility to have a systems framework that can integrate multiple attributes of vectors in a cohesive manner. Quantitative experimentation and mathematical modeling will be critical tools enabling further progress in this area.

The purpose of this review is to investigate the intracellular barriers to DNA delivery and their relation to nonviral vector design properties. We highlight new opportunities for design, identify some of the challenges that remain, and discuss newer strategies for solving these problems. Because we are restricted by the size of the chapter, we do not provide a comprehensive review of various types of synthetic vectors, but instead refer the reader at appropriate points to several excellent reviews that already exist.

# BACKGROUND

Transfer of exogenous DNA into the cell is greatly impeded by the size and charge of the DNA. Furthermore, DNA must evade biochemical degradation and several cellular barriers before it can have the desired effect in the cell. Accomplishing this task calls for the use of a carrier molecule, and the resulting package—DNA plus carrier(s)—is termed a vector. In general, an ideal vector should be able to compact the DNA, enhance its entry into the specific target cell, assist in overcoming several intracellular barriers, confer resistance to nuclease attack, and display minimum toxicity. Engineering multiple functionalities with often conflicting demands into the vector is a considerable challenge.

## Design Properties of Vectors—Lessons from Viral Vectors

Despite intensive research during the past decade, nonviral vectors for gene delivery still do not compare with viral vectors in terms of efficiency. Thus, the development of nonviral vectors borrows from viruses many of their design features and properties. Viruses used for gene transfer are self-assembled biological particles on the order of 100 nm in diameter and composed of lipids, proteins, and nucleic acids that include the gene of interest (15). For retroviruses, lipids form a bilayer and separate the viral contents from the environment. In contrast, this function is accomplished in adenovirus by a set of tightly assembled coat proteins. Several types of proteins exist in viruses, including capsid proteins, which condense the nucleic acids; envelope proteins, which bind to receptors on cellular membranes; and enzymes, which aid in unpackaging and integration of the genetic material in the host cell. The genetic material may be either DNA or RNA. In the latter case, a reverse transcriptase is part of the viral vector to generate DNA inside the target cell.

Owing to their multiple components and evolutionarily optimized properties, viruses are able to achieve the multipronged task of infection. Despite the negative charge existing on both viruses and cell membranes, viruses are able to adsorb to cells, even without envelope protein binding to cellular receptors (16). Envelope-receptor interactions appear to prevent detachment and to anchor the virus to the cell membrane. Fusion with the cell membrane then occurs, for some viruses mediated by environmentally sensitive, amphipathic peptides. The nucleic acid is released into the cell, reverse transcribed if necessary, then enters into the nucleus where it is integrated into the genome. Retroviruses do not enter the nucleus until its host cell enters mitosis, thus restricting the application of retroviruses to dividing cells. Other viruses, such as adenovirus, are able to transduce nondividing cells through the presence of nuclear localization sequences (NLS) on capsid proteins, which mediate extrusion of the nucleic acids via the nuclear pore complex (NPC) (17).

Thus, viruses provide a set of design features that are mimicked in the development of nonviral vectors. Their capabilities include condensation of DNA into nanoparticles, protection from nuclease degradation, adsorption to cells, delivery into the cytoplasm and (for nondividing cells) the nucleus, and unpackaging to release the nucleic acids. By nature, viruses are inherently biocompatible as they are composed of wholly biological entities. However, biocompatibility is a consideration for nonviral vectors. The problems encountered in viral gene delivery, such as immunogenicity and the possibility of oncogenesis, also serve as lessons for the design and development of nonviral vectors.

## Components of Vectors

Currently, most synthetic vectors are based on polymers or lipids, which on interaction with DNA form polymer/DNA complexes called polyplexes and lipid/DNA complexes called lipoplexes (18). A number of peptides are also utilized as delivery agents. There are several reviews that describe these vectors in great detail (4, 19, 20). Commonly used components of nonviral vectors are summarized in Table 1.

A range of synthetic and natural polymers has been incorporated into vectors for DNA delivery. Synthetic polymers differ in their chemical composition, number of repeating units, and degree of branching. Polycations such as poly-L-lysine (linear), polyamines such as polyethyleneimine (PEI) (linear and branched), and polyamidoamine (PAMAM) dendrimers are examples of relatively well-studied polymeric delivery systems (4, 21, 22). Also under current investigation is a variety of block and graft copolymers, which broaden the repertoire of DNA complexation and in vivo pharmacokinetic and cell interaction properties (23, 24). Naturally occurring proteins, such as histones and albumin, and polysaccharides, such as chitosan, have also been incorporated into vectors for DNA delivery (24–26). Although efforts toward improving the efficiency of such polymeric systems by

**TABLE 1** Components of a nonviral vector

| Component | Rationale | Examples |
|---|---|---|
| Carrier molecule | DNA compaction, charge reduction, protection from nucleases | PLL (22), PEI (78, 81), PAMAM (79, 147), chitosan (25), lipids (28, 75, 148) |
| Hydrophilic moiety | Steric stabilization, reduction of nonspecific interactions | PEG (149), HPMA polymers (150, 151) |
| Targeting ligand | Enhanced targeted receptor-mediated cellular uptake | See Table 2—asialoglycoprotein, folate, EGF |
| Endosome disruptive agent | Escape from endosomes—unpackaging | pH-sensitive peptides (129, 152), protonable amine structures (80) |
| Nuclear localization signal (NLS) | Nuclear targeting | SV40 T-antigen (105, 153), hnRNP A1 protein M9 (100), (HIV-1) Rev, and Tat protein (154) |

the incorporation of various auxiliary molecules and backbone modifications are under way, several are already available commercially.

Liposomes represent a large class of DNA delivery agents. Cationic lipids possess a hydrophobic moiety; a positively charged headgroup; and a linker functional group, such as ester, amide, or carbamate, to bind these molecules together covalently. Lipids with monocationic head groups [e.g., N-[1-(2,3-dioleyloxy)propyl]-N,N,N-trimethylammonium chloride (DOTMA), N-[1-(2,3-dioleoyloxy)-propyl]-N,N,N-trimethylammonium methylsulfate (DOTAP), 3-$\beta$ [N-(N′,N′-dimethylami noethane)-carbamoyl] cholesterol (DC-Chol)] and those with polycationic head groups [e.g., 2,3-dioleyloxy-N-[2(sperminecarboxamido)ethyl]-N,N-dimethyl-1-propane ammonium trifluoroacetate (DOSPA) and dioctadecylamidoglycyl spermine (DOGS)] have been utilized as DNA delivery agents (27, 28). Various helper lipids, such as dioleoyl-phosphatidylethanolamine (DOPE), and neutral lipids, such as cholesterol and its derivatives, are used in many formulations for improving efficiencies (29). DNA has been successfully delivered to cells with cationic, neutral and anionic lipids, and mixtures thereof. More recently, vector systems consisting of nucleic acid condensed prior to complex formation with cationic liposomes are gaining popularity due to their higher transfection efficiencies (30, 31).

In addition to polymers and lipids, delivery systems that incorporate proteins, peptides, and other biological molecules to penetrate cellular membranes are being explored. Peptides are also widely used as targeting moieties or as auxiliary molecules attached to the polymer/DNA complex for a specific purpose. Many peptides and other biological ligands have been used as cell-targeting carrier molecules, including glycoproteins, mannose, insulin, antibodies, lectins, and folic acid (32–34). The pH sensitivity of fusogenic peptides is also being exploited to penetrate cellular membranes and deliver a cargo of DNA (35, 36).

## Structure and Characterization of Vectors

Formation of synthetic vectors relies on effective DNA packaging. Spontaneous electrostatic interactions between polycations and DNA have lead to the condensation of DNA into discrete particles and the formation of complexes of various morphologies, such as toroids, rods, and spheres (23, 37, 38). Although the major factor governing the compaction of DNA is charge neutralization, several other molecules (e.g., polyamines, alcohols, and neutral or anionic polymers with monovalent salts) are also found to aid in DNA compaction. Lipid/DNA complexes are also self-assembling systems. Mixing cationic liposomes with supercoiled plasmid DNA causes electrostatic interactions, leading to extensive reorganization, followed by DNA-induced aggregation of the cationic liposomes, vesicle rupture and fusion, and ultimately leading to the formation of lipoplexes of various structures (39, 40). In general, negatively charged complexes are found to have DNA extending from the surface of the particles, whereas those possessing excess positive charge are multilamellar aggregates with DNA effectively condensed between lipid bilayers (41).

Practical exploitation of self-assembly for the development of stable, monodisperse carrier/DNA formulations for in vitro and in vivo use is not trivial. Formation of complexes has been found to depend on a large number of factors, such as the chemistry and structure of both DNA and carrier, reaction conditions (e.g., buffer composition and ionic strength), rate of mixing, and the order in which components are mixed (42, 43). Most formulations are comprised of a heterogeneous population of particles with varying shapes and sizes, depending on the process conditions. Particles frequently aggregate to form larger particles, with more than tenfold increase in diameter when introduced in physiological media due to the increased ionic strength that reduces the charge repulsion between particles (44). Several strategies to create newer formulations with improved stability are being developed (45).

A range of physicochemical methods is utilized to characterize vector formulations. Initial characterization of self-assembly is typically achieved using a gel-shift electrophoretic assay, which distinguishes free and associated DNA based on size. The DNA is commonly detected by fluorescence, either via a label incorporated before complex formation or using a DNA-binding dye whose exclusion indicates that the DNA is bound and protected (46, 47). Techniques such as single- and dual-color fluorescent fluctuation spectroscopy (48, 49) and fluorescence resonance transfer (FRET) (41) have recently found applications in the more detailed analysis of polymer-DNA interactions. Size and surface charge are generally evaluated by photon correlation spectroscopy (PCS) and zeta potential measurements, respectively. Morphological investigation and evaluation of size polydispersity are achieved using techniques such as atomic force microscopy (AFM) (50, 51), transmission electron microscopy (TEM) (52, 53), or X-ray scattering (54, 55). Among these, AFM permits analysis in conditions closer to physiological as compared to others that require prior sample preparation.

# INTRACELLULAR PROCESSING OF SYNTHETIC VECTORS

DNA is generally maintained in the nuclei of cells, which do not have mechanisms for importing DNA from their surroundings. Efforts to do so artificially must overcome a set of cellular barriers present as part of the cell's internal organization and protection from its environment. Thus, a detailed understanding of the interactions of nonviral vectors with the components of cellular uptake and intracellular processing pathways is necessary for improving the design of vectors (see Figure 1).

## Internalization

In the absence of a carrier molecule, the highly anionic nature of DNA hinders its passive diffusion through the hydrophobic cell membrane. Even small ODNs, including natural ODNs, phosphorothioates, and uncharged methylphosphonates,

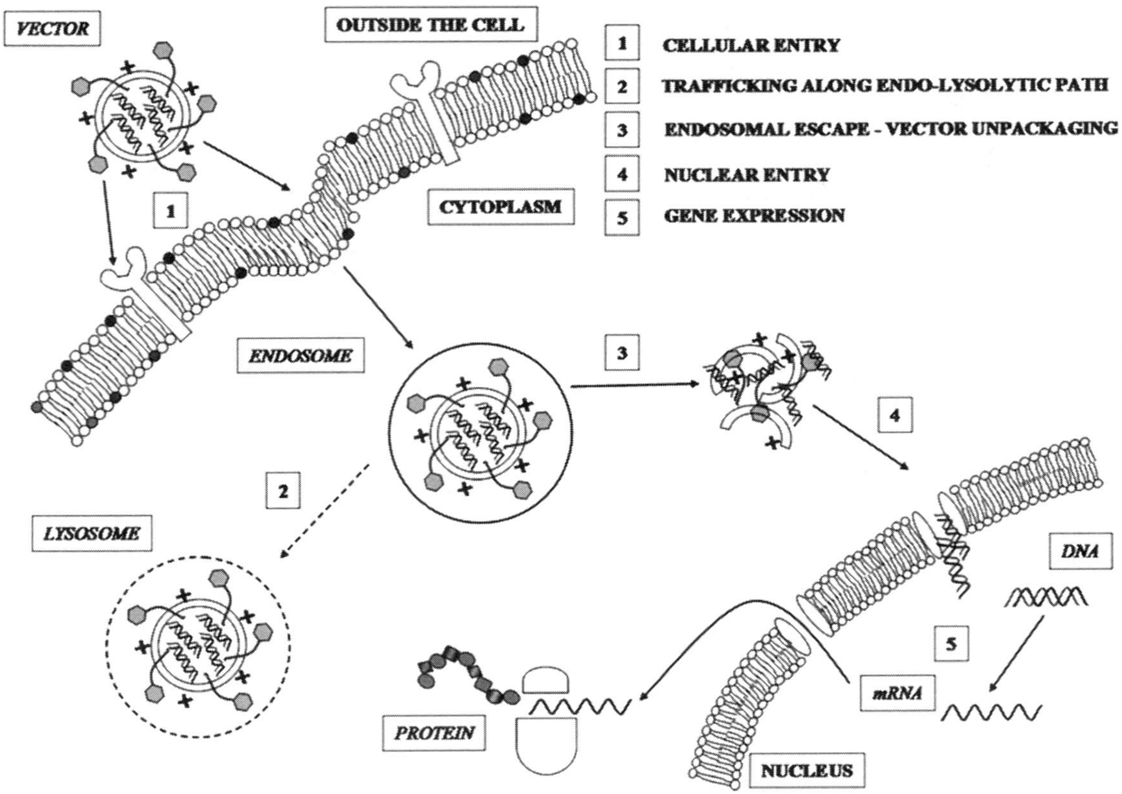


**Figure 1** Schematic of intracellular vector trafficking indicating various barriers to gene delivery. Vectors must bind to and traverse the cell membrane, in most cases avoid lysosomal degradation and achieve escape from endosomes, unpackage the complexed DNA, enter the nucleus, and be transcribed into mRNA from which the encoded protein is made.

cannot generally pass through in sufficient quantities to demonstrate activity (56). Association of DNA with a cationic polymer or other delivery agent greatly reduces the negative charge and aids in increased cellular uptake.

Carrier/DNA complexes associate with the negatively charged cell membrane, mainly due to nonspecific charge interactions, and are subsequently internalized by the cell. Electrostatic interactions with cell surface glycosaminoglycans (GAGs) have multiple implications for DNA delivery depending on the particular type of carrier molecule and GAG involved. For instance, DNA may be released from the complex or intracellular trafficking of carrier/DNA complexes may be altered (57, 58). In most cases, association with GAGs drastically reduces transfection efficiencies (59).

Most nonviral vectors exploit the endocytic pathway for uptake and subsequent processing within the cell. Light and electron microscopic studies show that clathrin-mediated endocytosis is the primary pathway (60, 61). Other pathways that may be involved in vector uptake include caveolae mediated, clathrin independent, macropinocytosis, and phagocytosis. Colloidal properties of carrier/DNA complexes, such as size and charge, and biochemical interactions of vectors with cellular interfaces determine the uptake mechanisms involved. Particles up to 200 nm can be internalized through clathrin-dependent processes, and larger particles (up to 500 nm) enter by clathrin-independent endocytosis mechanisms, for example, by recruiting caveolae (62). Even for lipid/DNA complexes, although some studies suggest cellular entry via fusion with the plasma membrane, internalization is considered to be largely via endocytosis (63, 64). As an alternative to such conventional uptake mechanisms, Kueltzo & Middaugh (65) recently proposed the involvement of nonclassical transport mechanisms in which vectors are transported through charge interactions with a cellular network of polyanions. However, the hypothesis still requires experimental verification. It seems plausible that vectors are internalized by multiple mechanisms, but it is difficult to assess the relative contribution of various uptake pathways in an experimental setting. Uptake of vectors is highly dependent on cell type. In various cell types, one or more of these mechanisms may be more active than others (66).

In particular, receptor-mediated endocytic pathways have been exploited to improve both the efficiency and selectivity of DNA and vector uptake. Targeting molecules that are attached to carrier/DNA complexes are designed to direct them to only those cells that express the corresponding receptor(s). A number of ligands (4, 67) targeting receptors that confer specificity for a cell type (e.g., asialoglycoprotein receptor for hepatocytes) or selectivity for a target cell subpopulation (e.g., tumor cells overexpressing epidermal growth factor receptor) have been used to increase efficiency in vitro and in vivo. Table 2 provides examples of ligands that are used to target specific receptors on various cell types.

The initial delivery of DNA, or any solute, via receptor-mediated endocytosis will be modulated by the finite number of receptors available on the cell surface for binding and internalization. It has been shown that in steady state, with all receptors

**TABLE 2** Ligands used for receptor-mediated targeting of synthetic vectors

| Receptor | Ligand | Target cell | Carrier (Reference) |
|---|---|---|---|
| Asialoglycoprotein | Asialoglycoprotein | Hepatocytes | PLL (37, 155), liposomes (156) |
| Receptor | Lactose | Hepatocytes | PLL (61), liposomes (157) |
| | Galactose | Hepatocytes | PLL (158), PEI (159, 160), liposomes (161, 162), chitosan (163) |
| | Mannose | Macrophages | PLL (164), PEI (165), liposomes (166) |
| LDL receptor | LDL | Smooth muscle cell | PLL (167, 168) |
| Transferrin receptor | Transferrin | Various | PLL (169, 170), PEI (171), liposomes (24, 152, 172), chitosan (22) |
| Folate receptor | Folate | Various | PLL (173, 174), PEI (175), copolymers (31, 176), lipopolyplex (28), liposomes (177) |
| EGF receptor | EGF | Various | PLL (70), PEI (178) |
| Various | Antibodies | Various | PLL (179), PEI (180), liposomes (181) |

recycling to the surface after dissociation from the ligand in the endosome, the uptake rate, $U$, of a delivered moiety can be expressed as

$$U = \frac{R_T}{\dfrac{1}{k_{on}[L]} + \dfrac{1}{k_i} + \dfrac{1}{k_r}}, \tag{1}$$

where $R_T$ is the total number of receptors; $[L]$ is the concentration of ligand; and $k_{on}$, $k_i$, and $k_r$ are rate constants for ligand binding, complex internalization, and receptor recycling, respectively. For example, K562 cells possess approximately 150,000 transferrin receptors per cell, with a 4–5 min receptor recycle time (68), leading to a hypothetical throughput of ~30,000 vectors/min in the presence of excess ligand. However, the interaction of a targeted vector with the receptor and endocytic machinery may be different than that for natural ligand. In particular, the binding affinity of the ligand to the receptor has been found to be dependent on the particular chemistry used to link the ligand to the carrier molecule (69, 70). An additional consideration is that targeted vectors are multivalent, and very high ligand density may cause a greater extent of receptor downregulation per internalized vector.

## Subcellular Trafficking on the Endocytic Pathway

The intracellular fates of internalized complexes appear to be related to the specifics of vector and internalization pathways. Nonetheless, some common features are expected irrespective of the uptake mechanism.

Upon internalization, endosomal compartments undergo continuous acidification from the initial cell surface pH (~7), ultimately to that found in lysosomes (~4), through the action of ATP-dependent proton pumps acting in conjunction with other ion transporters found in the membranes. Vectors initially appear in early endosomes that are characterized by their closeness to the cell surface and slightly acidic pH. These are further divided into sorting endosomes and recycling endosomes. Movement along the pathway from early endosomes to lysosomes is highly regulated and involves the microtubule network (71, 72). For hepatocytes, fluid phase and receptor-mediated endocytic pathways employ different early endosomes, but the pathways converge in prelysosomal compartments, such as the late endosome (73).

Whether and how compartmentalization of vectors into specific endosomes is influenced by vector properties is still not very clear. Microscopic investigations of subcellular distributions of gene carriers in various studies report fluorescence in the cell in punctate (speckled) patterns, which are generally described to be endosomes or lysosomes. In addition, antisense oligodeoxynucleotides (AS ODNs) bind to other cellular structures, such as intermediate filaments, the Golgi complex, and the endoplasmic reticulum (74, 75). Using a fluorescent technique, it is possible to determine the proportion of DNA taken into cells by endocytosis and the amount released into the cytoplasm (28). For effective delivery, the DNA must exit the pathway before it is degraded in the lysosomes.

Numerous studies have focused on elucidating the mechanism of escape of vectors from the endosomal pathway. Early observations of the interaction of cationic and anionic bilayers supported the flip-flop model in which lipid mixing between endosomal and cationic lipid membranes eventually leads to membrane disruption and release of DNA into the cytoplasm (76). Recently, correlations have been drawn between the structure of the lipids and transfection efficiency. Hexagonal lipoplexes are found to fuse more readily with the anionic lipidic vesicles, leading to easier release of DNA. Incorporation of lipids, such as DOPE and cholesterol, into the lipid formulations generally increases the release of DNA, leading to increased transgene expression. Such interactions of lipid with membranes leading to the release of DNA occur at the endosomal rather than at the cellular membrane, further highlighting the importance of lipid composition (76, 77).

Unlike liposomal vectors, most polymeric vectors do not fuse with lipid membranes. Polymer/DNA complexes have been detected in the cytoplasm as well as in the nucleus, suggesting that not free DNA but carrier-associated DNA is probably released from the endocytic pathway (78). For polycations, such as poly-L-lysine, although the mechanism of release has not been fully elucidated, some evidence favors physical disruption of the endosomal membrane caused by the cationic charge of the polymer (79). The higher transfection efficiencies generally observed with polyamines, such as PEI, have been attributed to its buffering capacity within the physiological pH range. This can be explained by an effect called the proton sponge hypothesis in which protonation of ionizable amine groups leads to chloride ion accumulation, with consequent osmotic endosome swelling causing rupture and enhanced escape of the polyplex (80). Although there have been suspicions about its validity (78, 81), experimental evidence based on chemical structure-function as well as direct measurements of acidification, chloride accumulation, and endosomal swelling has emerged to support the proton sponge effect (80, 82, 83).

Based on our current understanding of these mechanisms, several chemical and biochemical agents have been suggested for overcoming the endosomal barrier to DNA delivery. A number of lysomotropic agents (e.g., ammonium chloride, chloroquine, monensin, polyvinylpyrolidone, and sucrose) inhibit DNA degradation by dissipating the acidic pH of the endolysosomes, and they provide some increase in transfection efficiency in vitro (84). However, in some experimental settings, these agents do not improve delivery (25), and their use (at least as a chemical additive) is impractical for in vivo applications. Several synthetic peptides displaying pH-dependent fusogenic properties (e.g., GALA and KALA) have been shown to mediate acid-dependent increased vesicular escape and higher transfection efficiencies (36, 85). Compounds such as nocodazole or taxol, which regulate the polymerization states of microtubules, thus disrupting the typical transport from endosomes to lysosomes, enhance transfection efficiencies (72).

## DNA Release—Subsequent Fates of Carrier and DNA in the Intracellular Milieu

Exit from the endo-lysolytic pathway does not always result in high transfection efficiency. For the delivered DNA to be effective, the carrier/DNA complex should dissociate, causing release of DNA intracellularly, preferably close to the site of action. Literature suggests that vector unpackaging may pose a barrier to effective DNA delivery (64, 86). There needs to be an optimum degree of association between the DNA and carrier, as accelerated dissociation of the complex will lead to degradation of DNA by nucleases, whereas tightly bound rigid complexes may hinder the transport and functionality of DNA (i.e., transcription or hybridization). Vector design properties, influencing the kinetics and intracellular location of complex dissociation, will be of prime importance in determining the effectiveness of the delivery vector.

It is not very clear where and how carrier/DNA complexes release DNA inside the cell. Polyplex dissociation rates appear to vary dramatically depending on the chemistry of the polymer, as some studies have suggested very rapid dissociation (87), whereas others have observed intact polyplexes in the nucleus (64, 78, 86) as long as 48 h after transfection. In contrast to polyplexes, lipoplexes do not appear to undergo spontaneous dissociation. Instead, DNA release from the lipoplex seems to be synonymous with the exit from the endo-lysolytic pathway (77), as per the proposed flip-flop model (88). Ionic molecules present at high concentrations in the nucleus—such as ATP, polypeptides, RNA, spermidine, histones, as well as genomic DNA—have proven incapable of displacing DNA from the lipid/DNA complex (89). This is in agreement with the observation that liposomes microinjected directly into the nucleus are unable to release the complexed DNA (64).

Once DNA is released into the cytoplasm, it must still reach the site of action, which in most cases is the nucleus. Particularly for nonlipid carriers, it is not known whether the DNA is partially associated with the vector or is completely free. Transport of free DNA from the cytoplasm to the perinuclear region is proposed to be by diffusion. However, active transport along the cytoskeletal network has also been suggested for carrier/DNA complexes (90). Diffusion of large DNA molecules in the cytoplasm is lowered many fold compared to that in water. This phenomenon may be due to solvent viscosity effects or more likely due to the high protein concentrations and presence of organelles that impose an intense molecular crowding. The diffusion of DNA in the cytoplasm is hindered in a size-dependent manner. For example, the ratio of diffusion coefficients of DNA fragments in cytoplasm to that in water decreased from 0.19 for a 100-bp fragment to 0.06 for a 250-bp fragment and was $<0.01$ for $>2000$ bp (91). Because microinjected ODNs are uniformly distributed through the cytoplasm (92), the size, more than interactions with cytosolic proteins, is thought to be responsible for the poor diffusional characteristics of plasmid DNA in the cytoplasm.

DNA molecules, especially ODNs, in the cellular milieu are highly susceptible to nuclease attack, although those having secondary structures, such as loops or snail-like structures, have been found to be more nuclease resistant than linear ODNs (93). Delivery using vectors greatly reduces the possibility of DNA degradation due to nucleases. For example, when complexed with SuperFect™, the half-life of a linear ODN in HeLa cell lysate increases from less than 30 min to over 16 h (93). The relative importance of DNA stability (94) in the cytoplasm will depend on the vector dissociation mechanism. DNA that remains associated with the vector even after exit from the endocytic pathway will be less susceptible to nuclease activity during its transport from the cytoplasm to the nucleus. However, the possibility also exists of DNA damage signals and increased susceptibility of DNA to nuclease attack occurring as part of the unpackaging process (95).

Some efforts have been made to optimize the vector design properties that influence the kinetics and intracellular location of complex dissociation. In general, length of the polymer significantly influences dissociation rates. The dissociation rates of vectors using polylysine are inversely related to polymer chain length (86, 96). Strategies involving polymers with cleavable disulfide bonds for triggered DNA release in the reducing intracellular medium (45, 97, 98) are gaining importance. To improve the functionality of lipidic vectors, helper lipids capable of destabilizing the endosomal membranes are incorporated. Newer formulations that involve cationic lipids capable of forming pores in phospholipids bilayers might also prove useful for endosomal release of DNA (99). It is probable that functionalized polymer-based vectors might be utilized more effectively, as they present an opportunity to fine-tune intracellular DNA release properties, as opposed to lipid-based systems that seem to inherently function by lipid mixing and membrane fusion.

## Delivery to and Entry into the Nucleus

There is considerable evidence suggesting that the nuclear membrane presents a barrier to the entry of free or carrier-associated DNA from the cytoplasm (64, 87, 100, 101). In several studies, less than 0.1% of cytosolically injected plasmid DNA was found to be transcribed (87, 101). Even in the presence of lipofectin, less than 1% of cells stained positive for nuclear plasmid, although significant amounts of cytoplasmic plasmid were detected in nearly 80% of lipofected nondividing cells (103). In general, there are two paths to nuclear entry—one through the NPC and the other via nuclear disassembly that occurs during cell division.

Entry through the NPC may be passive or active. Passive diffusion through the NPC is determined mainly by the size of the molecule, with rates of diffusion found to be inversely related to the mass. As a general rule, molecules smaller than ~40 kD are found to diffuse through the NPC passively. DNA molecules up to 300 bp diffuse passively through the NPC (102), whereas larger plasmid molecules cannot. Consequently, for ODNs used in antisense experiments, nuclear entry does not usually present a hurdle (92). In contrast, for plasmid DNA size is a limitation, and carrier molecules may be used to aid DNA transport into the nucleus. Quantitative studies on the structural requirements for nuclear pore transport have demonstrated effective transport of intact polymer/DNA condensates through the NPC, with a particle size threshold of 25 nm, which is comparable to the diameter of the nuclear pore (103).

Active transport of proteins bearing NLS through the NPC occurs in an extremely regulated, energy-dependent manner at very high rates, up to 100 transport events per second. Therefore, signal-mediated active transport has been exploited for plasmids and other macromolecules larger than 60 kD that cannot traverse the NPC passively. Active transport of a macromolecule through the NPC requires attachment of NLS, a short amino acid sequence that behaves as a specific targeting signal, to the plasmid and/or carrier/DNA complex. A commonly used sequence is the SV40 Tag NLS, which has been found to provide an increase in transfection efficiencies, whereas nonclassical motifs, such as hnRNP A1 protein M9 NLS (100) and the (HIV-1) Rev protein are also currently being studied. More than 100 NLS sequences have been identified (104), but the relative effectiveness of these sequences has yet to be established. Design criteria for effective DNA nuclear delivery using NLS sequences have yet to be established. Conventional approaches of conjugating the NLS to DNA include electrostatic complexation of cationic NLS with DNA or covalent conjugation (102). The method of attachment must be such that the carrier or DNA does not interfere with the functionality of the NLS.

Other methods have been explored for trafficking plasmid to the nucleus. In some cases, use of plasmids containing specific DNA sequences, such as the SV40 enhancer region, which is known to bind to a variety of transcription factors, has been found to enhance nuclear delivery. This approach has also been utilized to increase nuclear uptake in a tissue-specific manner by using sequences specific to certain cell types (105). Novel approaches to providing functional NLS include the use of PNAs (peptide nucleic acids) to link molecules to DNA, which combine features of sequence-specific conjugation of the NLS and retention of NLS activity (106, 107).

The higher transfection rates of dividing cells compared to quiescent ones seem to suggest that DNA entry into the nucleus also takes place when the nuclear membrane disassembles. Evidence in favor of this mechanism comes from blocking the cell cycle in G1 phase by compounds such as aphidicolin or by releasing synchronized cells in G1 phase to progress through the cell cycle (108). The highest transfection efficiencies have been recorded for cells in the G2/M phase with a nearly 30–500-fold increase as compared to G1 cells for lipoplex- and polyplex-based transfections (108, 109). Nuclear delivery of AS ODNs is improved to a similar extent (110, 111). Such findings have significant implications for the utility of carrier systems in transfections involving nonproliferating cells, thus underlining the importance of introducing nuclear-targeting moieties, especially for in vivo applications. Furthermore, the often-observed variations in transfection efficiencies may be attributed to heterogeneity in different cell populations with regard to cell cycle.

## Genetic Integration or Hybridization—Limitations?

Entry into the nucleus, the proposed site of action, is generally reported as the final barrier to efficient nonviral DNA delivery (112). However, it has been noticed in several studies that the levels of DNA transfer into the nucleus and those of gene expression do not correlate (64, 86, 87, 95). This suggests the existence of additional factors that influence the efficiency of DNA transfer. It is likely that there exist barriers related to transgene expression (in the case of gene transfection) or hybridization of ODN to the specific target (in the case of antisense activity), which occur after DNA enters the nucleus.

Various groups have found limited gene expression in spite of substantial nuclear delivery of intact plasmids (64, 86, 87). One effect is simply saturation of gene expression, which has been observed when excess amounts of plasmids are delivered (113). Another explanation for the lack of correlation between gene expression and nuclear delivery of plasmids could be the methylation of plasmid DNA, which inhibits its expression in a sequence-dependent manner (114).

Furthermore, polymer carriers can impact the functionality of delivered DNA. Cellular transcription is known to be regulated by natural polycations, including histones and polyamines. Transcriptional regulation by synthetic polycations has also been observed in cell-free systems (115, 116). Thus, one would expect similar regulatory activity by synthetic carrier systems in cells. Indeed, the presence of carrier molecules in the nucleus has been observed in many cases, but it is not yet clear how the carrier molecule affects gene expression (78, 86). Existing studies of model polyplexes in the nucleus show very rapid disassembly (87, 103), but it remains to be seen if this tendency is general to new carrier molecules.

Although delivery of ODNs to the nucleus has been emphasized in many reports, the nucleus may not be the site of antisense activity (110, 117). Because antisense ODNs bind to a target mRNA, they could do so either in the nucleus as the mRNA is being formed and processed or in the cytoplasm when the mRNA is mature. Although previous studies have demonstrated AS ODN activity in the nucleus (118), others have shown a negative correlation between nuclear uptake and AS ODN activity (110). In any event, oligonucleotide hybridization to the target mRNA can be a significant barrier, as the association rate of ODN-mRNA binding varies over several orders of magnitude (119). ODN sequences can be designed for more rapid association and higher activity through molecular thermodynamic modeling (120, 121), but this rate may be affected by the carrier. Researchers have noted increased stability of hybrids with cationicity of associated polyamines (115) and following covalent conjugation to cationic peptides (121). Thus, nucleic acid hybridization can be enhanced by association with polymers, although it is not clear whether this actually occurs in the case of vector-mediated delivery.

The properties of nucleic acids may be altered by subtle changes in their chemistry. Phosphorothioate modification of ODNs is generally incorporated for increased resistance to nucleases, but this modification imparts deleterious effects on the stability of hybrids and increased nonspecific binding to cellular proteins. It has been reported that PS ODNs induce formation of PS bodies in the nucleus (123). Although DNA transported into the nucleus appears to be immobilized due to binding to proteins such as histones (91), PS ODNs have been found to continuously shuttle between the nucleus and cytoplasm (124). Such properties describing the interaction or influence of the particular carrier/DNA chemistry modification are significant in understanding unresolved effects that are observed in many systems.

## RATIONAL DESIGN OF SYNTHETIC VECTORS

Early approaches toward synthetic vector design involved the synthesis of carrier molecules with elegant chemistries, which provided for efficient condensation and protection of DNA. More recently, efforts have been directed toward incorporation of the existing mechanistic understanding of vector-cell interactions into vector design. With the identification of several barriers to effective DNA delivery, the properties of carriers can be altered by strategic structural modifications to overcome one or more of these individual barriers (82, 125). Despite the progress made so far, the field of synthetic vector development is still faced with two very important challenges: First, the best synthetic vectors available today still remain many orders of magnitude less efficient than the corresponding viral vectors; second, cell-type differences are significant. In light of these challenges, it is likely that vectors will have to be optimized for each application.

Detailed investigations of the intracellular processing of vectors have revealed the complexity and multitude of events that are associated with nonviral DNA delivery. Each of the steps detailed in Intracellular Processing of Synthetic Vectors, above, has been shown to be a limiting barrier to transfection under some circumstances. Furthermore, vector design variables may affect different steps to varying extents. A vector that is rationally designed to overcome one barrier may alter the cellular processing of the carrier, dramatically increasing the importance of other barriers. Therefore, systematic variation of one physical or chemical property is not likely to lead directly to a completely optimized vector, although it is evident that the efficiency of the DNA delivery process can be modulated by the properties of the delivery system. A more integrative approach that accounts for the interdependence of individual intracellular barriers and the effects of vector properties on the barriers seems essential. This will accelerate the process of optimization of various vector design variables for a range of cell types.

## Structure-Activity Relationships

In the quest for elucidating rational design principles, several researchers have attempted to draw structure-activity relationships for various vector systems. These studies generally involve determination of several biophysical properties of the carrier/DNA complexes such as size, shape, zeta-potential, and DNA condensation, as well as biological properties such as transfection efficiency and cytotoxicity. A correlation between these properties is proposed to serve as a basis for the future design of vectors.

Studies with series of structurally related polymers generally do not reveal significant correlations between the physical parameters and the biological activity (21, 35); however, strong correlations have been observed between the structure of the polymers and the physicochemical properties of their complexes with DNA (126, 127). Small sizes of the order of 100 nm are often required for entry through the endocytic pathway. However, larger aggregates of up to 500 nm sediment onto cells, especially in vitro, thereby providing high transfection efficiencies. In the case of cationic liposome/micelle-based systems, lipoplex size is a major determinant of lipofection efficiency in vitro, with larger lipoplex particles showing higher efficiency than smaller ones (128).

Alternatively, researchers have varied functional attributes of the carrier to affect various steps in the intracellular processing of vectors and have obtained interesting relationships. For example, balancing the relative contribution of cationic groups and endosomal escape moieties (pH-sensitive groups) resulted in lower cytotoxicity (125), and modifying the protonatible nitrogens in PEI highlighted the importance of amines in endosomal escape (82). Even a polymer such as PLL, which is notorious for its high cytotoxicity, has been found to exhibit much higher transfection efficiency when side chains of lower pKa, such as histidine, are attached to it (129). In the case of liposomes, studies have found transfection efficiency to be dependent on the membrane fluidity of the lipoplex membrane (29, 130). Combinatorial approaches to screen hundreds of structurally related polymers or lipids may prove useful in the identification of chemical structures that have enhanced DNA delivery properties (130). Such chemical structure-activity relationships provide additional insight into functionality that can then be engineered into vectors for higher efficiencies.

The utility of such structure-activity relationships will be judged by the success of their application to the rational design of future vectors. The fact that no useful correlations have been observed between the physical parameters and the biological activity of the complexes seems to suggest that such an approach oversimplifies the complexity of DNA delivery. One issue is the heterogeneity of the vectors, with the resulting concern that only a small fraction of the population may display the desired effect (132, 133). Nonetheless, attempting to optimize the biological functionality of the complex via one-dimensional structure-activity relationships may not be sufficient.

## Mathematical Modeling

How is one to interpret the accumulated set of structure-activity relationships derived for disparate conditions? Mathematical modeling of the DNA delivery pathway can provide a framework for quantifying the interplay among various design variables, consequently reducing the amount of experimentation required for optimizing vectors for various cell types. In addition, combined with quantitative experimentation, it can provide insight into the molecular mechanisms and rate-limiting steps for effective delivery.

Relatively few mathematical models exist for the analysis of nonviral DNA delivery, and to date there are essentially none characterizing the antisense ODN delivery pathway. Mathematical representations of plasmid delivery have been based on a compartmental model (134, 135), with mass action kinetics representing the various steps involved in the DNA delivery process (136). Data from previous experimental literature is generally used to obtain parameter values. Model outputs can be utilized to identify rate-limiting barriers and to make testable predictions. The values of some parameters, such as ligand-receptor binding and trafficking rates (for targeted delivery), may be known quite accurately, whereas others, such as rates of intracellular trafficking and degradation, are likely to be known to a much lesser degree of accuracy. Parameter-sensitivity analysis provides useful insights into the importance of model parameters in determining the gene delivery efficiency. Vectors with hypothetical (rationally designed) attributes could then be tested for their effectiveness by measuring several key parameters and relating the resulting model predictions to experimental observables.

Complete characterization of a mathematical model would require quantitative experimental data to be obtained under a consistent set of conditions (e.g., cell type, cell density, plasmid type, duration of exposure to vector). Commonly observed differences in cell type and heterogeneity in experimental conditions make predictions more difficult to assess. There is a clear need to develop assays for the accurate, quantitative determination of absolute numbers as well as the state of the DNA and carrier molecules in various subcellular compartments. Recent advances in fluorescent technology have led to the development of several analytical methods for the characterization and quantitation of various vector-cell interactions (137). By a combination of subcellular fractionation and flow cytometry, it is possible to obtain quantitative estimates of fluorescently labeled plasmids in various cellular compartments (138). However, care must be taken to ensure that measured levels represent intact DNA rather than degradation products. Techniques such as real-time PCR and Southern analysis, as well as in vitro transcription assays that do not require DNA labeling, might prove to be useful complements (100, 113, 136). Such quantitative evaluations are more challenging for systems involving ODNs, as many of the techniques applied to plasmids are not applicable to ODNs (139).

## Can We Create Virus-Like Multifunctional Vectors?

Integrating design solutions to the often-conflicting demands of DNA delivery necessitates the development of multifunctional vectors. As viruses are naturally occurring biological systems that have evolved to achieve high efficiency of transduction (see Structure and Characterization of Vectors, above), attempts to create virus-like particles for DNA delivery applications have been pursued for over a decade (140). Artificial viruses have been proposed to be mononuclear, stoichiometric, of viral size ($<$100 nm), and capable of transfection (141, 142). The aim of producing artificial viruses is to incorporate in a modular fashion several viral or virus-mimetic components to provide efficient cellular delivery characteristics, including DNA condensation, cell attachment, and release from the endosome.

Viral peptides, such as influenza virus hemagglutinin (HA), or synthetic peptides, such as GALA, have been utilized to impart endosomal disruptive functions to a polymer/DNA complex (140, 143). A major challenge in the incorporation of peptides into delivery vectors has been the display of the peptides in an ordered manner to optimally mimic viral functioning. Approaches to self-assembly of complete viral-mimetic particles have been based on the mixing of lipids bearing various functional head groups and DNA, leading to spontaneous compaction of DNA into lipid-coated particles, leaving surface molecular signals sticking out (144, 145). Supercoiled plasmid DNA is able to transform lipopolyamine micelles into a supramolecular organization characterized by ordered lamellar domains (146). Newer approaches involving size-controlled glycocluster nanoparticles (nonamine/noncationic/nonpolymeric) are being explored (141).

Identification and incorporation of viral functionalities (e.g., endosomal escape or nuclear targeting) into synthetic vectors has already resulted in some increase in efficiency. Yet, other properties of viruses have been explored and mimicked to a much lesser extent. For example, the ability of viruses to unpackage their nucleic acid cargo aids in its ability to traverse the nuclear membrane and be expressed within the nucleus. A major challenge remains in the incorporation of multiple types of biomolecules into a vector, each still maintaining its critical functionality for the artificial virus.

## SUMMARY

Cells present a variety of barriers that hinder the delivery of exogenous DNA. The magnitudes of these barriers vary significantly from one cell type to another. It is therefore difficult to extrapolate results from one system to another, and vector systems will have to be optimized for specific applications. It remains to be seen to what extent information obtained from gene delivery systems can be transferred to those for oligonucleotides, as the size and form of DNA may result in substantial differences in self-assembly with carriers. The trend in the field of nonviral DNA delivery is toward making virus-like particles. However, nature's design principles for self-assembling viruses are not yet well enough understood to be applied to the synthesis of fully self-assembling vectors. As a result, there remains considerable work to be done in the areas of multifunctional vector synthesis and comprehensive biological evaluation. A more integrated approach involving mathematical models and truly quantitative experiments may open new avenues to vector design and application. When these directives are accomplished, DNA-based therapies may yet fulfill their promise.

### ACKNOWLEDGMENTS

This work was supported in part by NIH Grant 1 R01 GM65913-01.

**The *Annual Review of Biomedical Engineering* is online at http://bioeng.annualreviews.org**

### LITERATURE CITED

1. Friedmann T, Roblin R. 1972. Gene therapy for human genetic disease? *Science* 175:949–55
2. Opalinska JB, Gewirtz AMA. 2002. Nucleic-acid therapeutics: basic principles and recent applications. *Nat. Rev. Drug Discov.* 1:503–14
3. Gewirtz AM, Sokol DL, Ratajczak MZA. 1998. Nucleic acid therapeutics: state of the art and future prospects. *Blood* 92:712–36
4. Merdan T, Kopecek J, Kissel TA. 2002. Prospects for cationic polymers in gene and oligonucleotide therapy against cancer. *Adv. Drug Deliv. Rev.* 54:715–58
5. Anderson KP, Fox MC, Brown-Driver V, Martin MJ, Azad RF. 1996. Inhibition of human cytomegalovirus immediate-early gene expression by an antisense oligonucleotide complementary to immediate-early RNA. *Antimicrob. Agents Chemother.* 40:2004–11
6. Lee LK, Roth CM. 2003. Antisense technology in molecular and cellular bioengineering. *Curr. Opin. Biotechnol.* 14:505–11

7. Crooke ST, Bennett CF. 1996. Progress in antisense oligonucleotide therapeutics. *Annu. Rev. Pharmacol. Toxicol.* 36:107–29
8. Wolff JA, Malone RW, Williams P, Chong W, Acsadi G, et al. 1990. Direct gene transfer into mouse muscle in vivo. *Science* 247:1465–68
9. Palsson B, Andreadis S. 1997. The physico-chemical factors that govern retrovirus-mediated gene transfer. *Exp. Hematol.* 25:94–102
10. Nishikawa M, Huang L. 2001. Nonviral vectors in the new millennium: delivery barriers in gene transfer. *Hum. Gene Ther.* 12:861–70
11. Lechardeur D, Lukacs GL. 2002. Intracellular barriers to non-viral gene transfer. *Curr. Gene Ther.* 2:183–94
12. Godbey WT, Mikos AG. 2001. Recent progress in gene delivery using non-viral transfer complexes. *J. Control Release* 72:115–25
13. Varga CM, Wickham TJ, Lauffenburger DA. 2000. Receptor-mediated targeting of gene delivery vectors: insights from molecular mechanisms for improved vehicle design. *Biotechnol. Bioeng.* 70:593–605
14. Davis ME. 2002. Non-viral gene delivery systems. *Curr. Opin. Biotechnol.* 13:128–31
15. Andreadis ST, Roth CM, Le Doux JM, Morgan JR, Yarmush ML. 1999. Large-scale processing of recombinant retroviruses for gene therapy. *Biotechnol. Prog.* 15:1–11
16. Davis HE, Morgan JR, Yarmush ML. 2002. Polybrene increases retrovirus gene transfer efficiency by enhancing receptor-independent virus adsorption on target cell membranes. *Biophys. Chem.* 97:159–72
17. Escriou V, Carriere M, Scherman D, Wils P. 2003. NLS bioconjugates for targeting therapeutic genes to the nucleus. *Adv. Drug Deliv. Rev.* 55:295–306
18. Felgner PL, Barenholz Y, Behr JP, Cheng SH, Cullis P, et al. 1997. Nomenclature for synthetic gene delivery systems. *Hum. Gene Ther.* 8:511–12
19. Niidome T, Huang L. 2002. Gene therapy progress and prospects: nonviral vectors. *Gene Ther.* 9:1647–52
20. Chirila TV, Rakoczy PE, Garrett KL, Lou X, Constable IJ. 2002. The use of synthetic polymers for delivery of therapeutic antisense oligodeoxynucleotides. *Biomaterials* 23:321–42
21. Gebhart CL, Kabanov AV. 2001. Evaluation of polyplexes as gene transfer agents. *J. Control Release* 73:401–16
22. De Smedt SC, Demeester J, Hennink WE. 2000. Cationic polymer based gene delivery systems. *Pharm. Res.* 17:113–26
23. Petersen H, Fechner PM, Martin AL, Kunath K, Stolnik S, et al. 2002. Polyethylenimine-graft-poly(ethylene glycol) copolymers: influence of copolymer block structure on DNA complexation and biological activities as gene delivery system. *Bioconjug. Chem.* 13:845–54
24. Read ML, Dash PR, Clark A, Howard KA, Oupicky D, et al. 2000. Physicochemical and biological characterisation of an antisense oligonucleotide targeted against the bcl-2 mRNA complexed with cationic-hydrophilic copolymers. *Eur. J. Pharm. Sci.* 10:169–77
25. Mao HQ, Roy K, Troung-Le VL, Janes KA, Lin KY, et al. 2001. Chitosan-DNA nanoparticles as gene carriers: synthesis, characterization and transfection efficiency. *J. Control Release* 70:399–421
26. Balicki D, Reisfeld RA, Pertl U, Beutler E, Lode HN. 2000. Histone H2A-mediated transient cytokine gene delivery induces efficient antitumor responses in murine neuroblastoma. *Proc. Natl. Acad. Sci. USA* 97:11500–4
27. de Lima MC, Simoes S, Pires P, Gaspar R, Slepushkin V, Duzgunes N. 1999. Gene delivery mediated by cationic liposomes: from biophysical aspects to enhancement of transfection. *Mol. Membr. Biol.* 16:103–9

28. Hope MJ, Mui B, Ansell S, Ahkong QF. 1998. Cationic lipids, phosphatidylethanolamine and the intracellular delivery of polymeric, nucleic acid-based drugs (review). *Mol. Membr. Biol.* 15:1–14
29. Ferrari ME, Rusalov D, Enas J, Wheeler CJ. 2002. Synergy between cationic lipid and co-lipid determines the macroscopic structure and transfection activity of lipoplexes. *Nucleic Acids Res.* 30:1808–16
30. Lee CH, Ni YH, Chen CC, Chou C, Chang FH. 2003. Synergistic effect of polyethylenimine and cationic liposomes in nucleic acid delivery to human cancer cells. *Biochim. Biophys. Acta* 1611:55–62
31. Gosselin MA, Guo W, Lee RJ. 2002. Incorporation of reversibly cross-linked polyplexes into LPDII vectors for gene delivery. *Bioconjug. Chem.* 13:1044–53
32. Roth CM, Reiken SR, Le Doux JM, Rajur SB, Lu X-M, et al. 1997. Targeted antisense modulation of inflammatory cytokine receptors. *Biotechnol. Bioeng.* 55:72–81
33. Lee LK, Siapati EK, Jenkins RG, McAnulty RJ, Hart SL, Shamlou PA. 2003. Biophysical characterization of an integrin-targeted non-viral vector. *Med. Sci. Monit.* 9:BR54–61
34. Stella B, Arpicco S, Peracchia MT, Desmaele D, Hoebeke J, et al. 2000. Design of folic acid-conjugated nanoparticles for drug targeting. *J. Pharm. Sci.* 89:1452–64
35. Wyman TB, Nicol F, Zelphati O, Scaria PV, Plank C, Szoka FC Jr. 1997. Design, synthesis, and characterization of a cationic peptide that binds to nucleic acids and permeabilizes bilayers. *Biochemistry* 36:3008–17
36. Lee H, Jeong JH, Park TG. 2001. A new gene delivery formulation of polyethylenimine/DNA complexes coated with PEG conjugated fusogenic peptide. *J. Control Release* 76:183–92
37. Bunnell BA, Askari FK, Wilson JM. 1992. Targeted delivery of antisense oligonucleotides by molecular conjugates. *Somat. Cell. Mol. Genet.* 18:559–69
38. Mannisto M, Vanderkerken S, Toncheva V, Elomaa M, Ruponen M, et al. 2002. Structure-activity relationships of poly (L-lysines): effects of pegylation and molecular shape on physicochemical and biological properties in gene delivery. *J. Control Release* 83:169–82
39. Xu YH, Hui SW, Frederik P, Szoka FC. 1999. Physicochemical characterization and purification of cationic lipoplexes. *Biophys. J.* 77:341–53
40. Oberle V, Bakowsky U, Zuhorn IS, Hoekstra D. 2000. Lipoplex formation under equilibrium conditions reveals a three-step mechanism. *Biophys. J.* 79:1447–54
41. Wiethoff CM, Gill ML, Koe GS, Koe JG, Middaugh CR. 2002. The structural organization of cationic lipid-DNA complexes. *J. Biol. Chem.* 277:44980–87
42. Zelphati O, Nguyen C, Ferrari M, Felgner J, Tsai Y, Felgner PL. 1998. Stable and monodisperse lipoplex formulations for gene delivery. *Gene Therapy* 5:1272–82
43. Mount CN, Lee LK, Yasin A, Scott A, Fearn T, Shamlou PA. 2003. The influence of physico-chemical and process conditions on the physical stability of plasmid DNA complexes using response surface methodology. *Biotechnol. Appl. Biochem.* 37:225–34
44. Lee LK, Mount CN, Shamlou PA. 2001. Characterisation of the physical stability of colloidal polycation-DNA complexes for gene therapy and DNA vaccines. *Chem. Eng. Sci.* 56:3163–72
45. Oupicky D, Carlisle RC, Seymour LW. 2001. Triggered intracellular activation of disulfide crosslinked polyelectrolyte gene delivery complexes with extended systemic circulation in vivo. *Gene Ther.* 8:713–24
46. Ferrari ME, Nguyen CM, Zelphati O, Tsai Y, Felgner PL. 1998. Analytical methods

for the characterization of cationic lipid-nucleic acid complexes. *Hum. Gene Ther.* 9:341–51
47. Parker AL, Oupicky D, Dash PR, Seymour LW. 2002. Methodologies for monitoring nanoparticle formation by self-assembly of DNA with poly(L-lysine). *Anal. Biochem.* 302:75–80
48. Van Rompaey E, Chen Y, Muller JD, Gratton E, Van Craenenbroeck E, et al. 2001. Fluorescence fluctuation analysis for the study of interactions between oligonucleotides and polycationic polymers. *Biol. Chem.* 382:379–86
49. Lucas B, Van Rompaey E, De Smedt SC, Demeester J, Van Oostveldt P. 2002. Dual-color fluorescence fluctuation spectroscopy to study the complexation between poly-L-lysine and oligonucleotides. *Macromolecules* 35:8152–60
50. Martin AL, Davies MC, Rackstraw BJ, Roberts CJ, Stolnik S, et al. 2000. Observation of DNA-polymer condensate formation in real time at a molecular level. *FEBS Lett.* 480:106–12
51. Wolfert MA, Seymour LW. 1996. Atomic force microscopic analysis of the influence of the molecular weight of poly(L)lysine on the size of polyelectrolyte complexes formed with DNA. *Gene. Ther.* 3:269–73
52. Liu G, Molas M, Grossmann GA, Pasumarthy M, Perales JC, et al. 2001. Biological properties of poly-L-lysine-DNA complexes generated by cooperative binding of the polycation. *J. Biol. Chem.* 276:34379–87
53. Labat-Moleur F, Steffan AM, Brisson C, Perron H, Feugeas O, et al. 1996. An electron microscopy study into the mechanism of gene transfer with lipopolyamines. *Gene Ther.* 3:1010–17
54. Koltover I, Salditt T, Safinya CR. 1999. Phase diagram, stability, and overcharging of lamellar cationic lipid-DNA self-assembled complexes. *Biophys. J.* 77:915–24
55. Lasic DD. 1997. Colloid chemistry. Liposomes within liposomes. *Nature* 387:26–27
56. Shoji Y, Akhtar S, Periasamy A, Herman B, Juliano RL. 1991. Mechanism of cellular uptake of modified oligodeoxynucleotides containing methylphosphonate linkages. *Nucleic Acids Res.* 19:5543–50
57. Ruponen M, Ronkko S, Honkakoski P, Pelkonen J, Tammi M, Urtti A. 2001. Extracellular glycosaminoglycans modify cellular trafficking of lipoplexes and polyplexes. *J. Biol. Chem.* 276:33875–80
58. Wiethoff CM, Smith JG, Koe GS, Middaugh CR. 2001. The potential role of proteoglycans in cationic lipid-mediated gene delivery. Studies of the interaction of cationic lipid-DNA complexes with model glycosaminoglycans. *J. Biol. Chem.* 276:32806–13
59. Ruponen M, Honkakoski P, Ronkko S, Pelkonen J, Tammi M, Urtti A. 2003. Extracellular and intracellular barriers in non-viral gene delivery. *J. Control Release* 93:213–17
60. Colin M, Maurice M, Trugnan G, Kornprobst M, Harbottle RP, et al. 2000. Cell delivery, intracellular trafficking and expression of an integrin-mediated gene transfer vector in tracheal epithelial cells. *Gene Ther.* 7:139–52
61. Klink D, Yu QC, Glick MC, Scanlin T. 2003. Lactosylated poly-L-lysine targets a potential lactose receptor in cystic fibrosis and non-cystic fibrosis airway epithelial cells. *Mol. Ther.* 7:73–80
62. Rejman J, Oberle V, Zuhorn IS, Hoekstra D. 2004. Size-dependent internalization of particles via the pathways of clathrin- and caveolae-mediated endocytosis. *Biochem. J.* 377:159–69
63. Friend DS, Papahadjopoulos D, Debs RJ. 1996. Endocytosis and intracellular processing accompanying transfection mediated by cationic liposomes. *Biochim. Biophys. Acta.* 278:41–50
64. Zabner J, Fasbender AJ, Moninger T,

Poellinger KA, Welsh MJ. 1995. Cellular and molecular barriers to gene transfer by a cationic lipid. *J. Biol. Chem.* 270: 18997–9007
65. Kueltzo LA, Middaugh CR. 2003. Nonclassical transport proteins and peptides: an alternative to classical macromolecule delivery systems. *J. Pharm. Sci.* 92: 1754–72
66. Zuhorn IS, Kalicharan R, Hoekstra D. 2002. Lipoplex-mediated transfection of mammalian cells occurs through the cholesterol-dependent clathrin-mediated pathway of endocytosis. *J. Biol. Chem.* 277:18021–28
67. Schaffer DV, Lauffenburger DA. 2000. Targeted synthetic gene delivery vectors. *Curr. Opin. Mol. Ther.* 2:155–61
68. Wagner E, Curiel D, Cotten M. 1994. Delivery of drugs, proteins and genes into cells using transferrin as a ligand for receptor-mediated endocytosis. *Adv. Drug Deliv. Rev.* 14:113–35
69. Wagner E, Cotten M, Foisner R, Birnstiel ML. 1991. Transferrin-polycation-DNA complexes: the effect of polycations on the structure of the complex and DNA delivery to cells. *Proc. Natl. Acad. Sci. USA* 88:4255–59
70. Schaffer DV, Lauffenburger DA. 1998. Optimization of cell surface binding enhances efficiency and specificity of molecular conjugate gene delivery. *J. Biol. Chem.* 273:28004–9
71. Rogers SL, Gelfand VI. 2000. Membrane trafficking, organelle transport, and the cytoskeleton. *Curr. Opin. Cell. Biol.* 12:57–62
72. Hasegawa S, Hirashima N, Nakanishi M. 2001. Microtubule involvement in the intracellular dynamics for gene transfection mediated by cationic liposomes. *Gene Ther.* 8:1669–73
73. Synnes M, Prydz K, Lovdal T, Brech A, Berg T. 1999. Fluid phase endocytosis and galactosyl receptor-mediated endocytosis employ different early endosomes. *Biochim. Biophys. Acta* 1421:317–28
74. Shoeman RL, Hartig R, Huang Y, Grub S, Traub P. 1997. Fluorescence microscopic comparison of the binding of phosphodiester and phosphorothioate (antisense) oligodeoxyribonucleotides to subcellular structures, including intermediate filaments, the endoplasmic reticulum, and the nuclear interior. *Antisense Nucleic Acid Drug Dev.* 7:291–308
75. Islam A, Handley SL, Thompson KS, Akhtar S. 2000. Studies on uptake, subcellular trafficking and efflux of antisense oligodeoxynucleotides in glioma cells using self-assembling cationic lipoplexes as delivery systems. *J. Drug Target* 7:373–82
76. Zelphati O, Szoka FC. 1996. Mechanism of oligonucleotide release from cationic liposomes. *Proc. Natl. Acad. Sci. USA* 93:11493–98
77. Marcusson EG, Bhat B, Manoharan M, Bennett CF, Dean NM. 1998. Phosphorothioate oligodeoxyribonucleotides dissociate from cationic lipids before entering the nucleus. *Nucleic Acids Res.* 26:2016–23
78. Godbey WT, Wu KK, Mikos AG. 1999. Tracking the intracellular path of poly(ethylenimine)/DNA complexes for gene delivery. *Proc. Natl. Acad. Sci. USA* 96:5177–81
79. Zhang ZY, Smith BD. 2000. High-generation polycationic dendrimers are unusually effective at disrupting anionic vesicles: membrane bending model. *Bioconjug. Chem.* 11:805–14
80. Sonawane ND, Szoka FC Jr, Verkman AS. 2003. Chloride accumulation and swelling in endosomes enhances DNA transfer by polyamine-DNA polyplexes. *J. Biol. Chem.*
81. Bieber T, Meissner W, Kostin S, Niemann A, Elsasser HP. 2002. Intracellular route and transcriptional competence of polyethylenimine-DNA complexes. *J. Control Release* 82:441–54
82. Thomas M, Klibanov AM. 2002. Enhancing polyethylenimine's delivery of

plasmid DNA into mammalian cells. *Proc. Natl. Acad. Sci. USA* 99:14640–45
83. Merdan T, Kunath K, Fischer D, Kopecek J, Kissel T. 2002. Intracellular processing of poly(ethylene imine)/ribozyme complexes can be observed in living cells by using confocal laser scanning microscopy and inhibitor experiments. *Pharm. Res.* 19:140–46
84. Choi YH, Liu F, Park JS, Kim SW. 1998. Lactose-poly(ethylene glycol)-grafted poly-L-lysine as hepatoma cell-tapgeted gene carrier. *Bioconjug. Chem.* 9:708–18
85. Lim DW, Yeom YI, Park TG. 2000. Poly (DMAEMA-NVP)-b-PEG-galactose as gene delivery vector for hepatocytes. *Bioconjug. Chem.* 11:688–95
86. Schaffer DV, Fidelman NA, Dan N, Lauffenburger DA. 2000. Vector unpacking as a potential barrier for receptor-mediated polyplex gene delivery. *Biotechnol. Bioeng.* 67:598–606
87. Pollard H, Remy JS, Loussouarn G, Demolombe S, Behr JP, Escande D. 1998. Polyethylenimine but not cationic lipids promotes transgene delivery to the nucleus in mammalian cells. *J. Biol. Chem.* 273:7507–11
88. Szoka FC, Xu YH, Zelphati O. 1997. How are nucleic acids released in cells from cationic lipid-nucleic acid complexes? *Adv. Drug Deliv. Rev.* 24:291
89. Xu YH, Szoka FC. 1996. Mechanism of DNA release from cationic liposome/DNA complexes used in cell transfection. *Biochemistry* 35:5616–23
90. Suh J, Wirtz D, Hanes J. 2003. Efficient active transport of gene nanocarriers to the cell nucleus. *Proc. Natl. Acad. Sci. USA* 100:3878–82
91. Lukacs GL, Haggie P, Seksek O, Lechardeur D, Freedman N, Verkman AS. 2000. Size-dependent DNA mobility in cytoplasm and nucleus. *J. Biol. Chem.* 275:1625–29
92. Leonetti JP, Mechti N, Degols G, Gagnor C, Lebleu B. 1991. Intracellular distribution of microinjected antisense oligonucleotides. *Proc. Natl. Acad. Sci. USA* 88:2702–6
93. Maksimenko AV, Gottikh MB, Helin V, Shabarova ZA, Malvy C. 1999. Physicochemical and biological properties of antisense phosphodiester oligonucleotides with various secondary structures. *Nucleosides Nucleotides* 18:2071–91
94. Lechardeur D, Sohn KJ, Haardt M, Joshi PB, Monck M, et al. 1999. Metabolic instability of plasmid DNA in the cytosol: a potential barrier to gene transfer. *Gene Ther.* 6:482–97
95. Tanswell AK, Staub O, Iles R, Belcastro R, Cabacungan J, et al. 1998. Liposome-mediated transfection of fetal lung epithelial cells: DNA degradation and enhanced superoxide toxicity. *Am. J. Physiol. Lung Cell. Mol. Physiol.* 275:L452–60
96. Ziady AG, Ferkol T, Dawson DV, Perlmutter DH, Davis PB. 1999. Chain length of the polylysine in receptor-targeted gene transfer complexes affects duration of reporter gene expression both in vitro and in vivo. *J. Biol. Chem.* 274:4908–16
97. Read ML, Bremner KH, Oupicky D, Green NK, Searle PF, Seymour LW. 2003. Vectors based on reducible polycations facilitate intracellular release of nucleic acids. *J. Gene Med.* 5:232–45
98. Balakirev M, Schoehn G, Chroboczek J. 2000. Lipoic acid-derived amphiphiles for redox-controlled DNA delivery. *Chem. Biol.* 7:813–19
99. Chanturiya A, Yang J, Scaria P, Stanek J, Frei J, et al. 2003. New cationic lipids form channel-like pores in phospholipid bilayers. *Biophys. J.* 84:1750–55
100. Subramanian A, Ranganathan P, Diamond SL. 1999. Nuclear targeting peptide scaffolds for lipofection of nondividing mammalian cells. *Nat. Biotech.* 17:873–77
101. Dowty ME, Williams P, Zhang G, Hagstrom JE, Wolff JA. 1995. Plasmid DNA entry into postmitotic nuclei of primary rat myotubes. *Proc. Natl. Acad. Sci. USA* 92:4572–76

102. Ludtke JJ, Zhang G, Sebestyen MG, Wolff JA. 1999. A nuclear localization signal can enhance both the nuclear transport and expression of 1 kb DNA. *J. Cell. Sci.* 112(Pt. 12):2033–41
103. Liu G, Li D, Pasumarthy MK, Kowalczyk TH, Gedeon CR, et al. 2003. Nanoparticles of compacted DNA transfect postmitotic cells. *J. Biol. Chem.* 278:32578–86
104. Cokol M, Nair R, Rost B. 2000. Finding nuclear localization signals. *EMBO Rep.* 1:411–15
105. Dean DA, Dean BS, Muller S, Smith LC. 1999. Sequence requirements for plasmid nuclear import. *Exp. Cell. Res.* 253:713–22
106. Vaysse L, Harbottle R, Bigger B, Bergau A, Tolmachov O, Coutelle C. 2004. Development of a self-assembling nuclear targeting vector system based on the tetracycline repressor protein. *J. Biol. Chem.* 279:5555–64
107. Branden LJ, Mohamed AJ, Smith CI. 1999. A peptide nucleic acid-nuclear localization signal fusion that mediates nuclear transport of DNA. *Nat. Biotechnol.* 17:784–87
108. Mortimer I, Tam P, MacLachlan I, Graham RW, Saravolac EG, Joshi PB. 1999. Cationic lipid-mediated transfection of cells in culture requires mitotic activity. *Gene Ther.* 6:403–11
109. Brunner S, Sauer T, Carotta S, Cotten M, Saltik M, Wagner E. 2000. Cell cycle dependence of gene transfer by lipoplex polyplex and recombinant adenovirus. *Gene Ther.* 7:401–7
110. Wu-Pong S, Bard J, Huffman J, Jimerson J. 1997. Oligonucleotide biological activity: relationship to the cell cycle and nuclear transport. *Biol. Cell.* 89:257–61
111. Helin V, Gottikh M, Mishal Z, Subra F, Malvy C, Lavignon M. 1999. Cell cycle-dependent distribution and specific inhibitory effect of vectorized antisense oligonucleotides in cell culture. *Biochem. Pharmacol.* 58:95–107
112. Rolland A. 1999. *Advanced Gene Delivery: From Concepts to Pharmaceutical Products*, 314:xv. Amsterdam: Harwood Acad.
113. Tachibana R, Harashima H, Ide N, Ukitsu S, Ohta Y, et al. 2002. Quantitative analysis of correlation between number of nuclear plasmids and gene expression activity after transfection with cationic liposomes. *Pharm. Res.* 19:377–81
114. Hong K, Sherley J, Lauffenburger DA. 2001. Methylation of episomal plasmids as a barrier to transient gene expression via a synthetic delivery vector. *Biomol. Eng.* 18:185–92
115. Antony T, Thomas T, Shirahata A, Thomas TJ. 1999. Selectivity of polyamines on the stability of RNA-DNA hybrids containing phosphodiester and phosphorothioate oligodeoxyribonucleotides. *Biochemistry* 38:10775–84
116. Kim WJ, Ishihara T, Akaike T, Maruyama A. 2001. Comb-type cationic copolymer expedites DNA strand exchange while stabilizing DNA duplex. *Chemistry* 7:176–80
117. Tari AM, Andreeff M, Kleine HD, Lopez-Berestein G. 1996. Cellular uptake and localization of liposomal-methylphosphonate oligodeoxynucleotides. *J. Mol. Med.* 74:623–28
118. Moulds C, Lewis JG, Froehler BC, Grant D, Huang T, et al. 1995. Site and mechanism of antisense inhibition by C-5 propyne oligonucleotides. *Biochemistry* 34:5044–53
119. Walton SP, Stephanopoulos GN, Yarmush ML, Roth CM. 2002. Thermodynamic and kinetic characterization of antisense oligodeoxynucleotide binding to a structured mRNA. *Biophys. J.* 82:366–77
120. Walton SP, Stephanopoulos GN, Yarmush ML, Roth CM. 1999. Prediction of antisense oligonucleotide binding affinity to a structured RNA target. *Biotechnol. Bioeng.* 65:1–9
121. Jayaraman A, Walton SP, Yarmush ML, Roth CM. 2001. Rational selection and quantitative evaluation of antisense

oligonucleotides. *Biochim. Biophys. Acta* 1520:105–14

122. Harrison JG, Balasubramanian S. 1998. Synthesis and hybridization analysis of a small library of peptide-oligonucleotide conjugates. *Nucleic Acids Res.* 26:3136–45
123. Lorenz P, Baker BF, Bennett CF, Spector DL. 1998. Phosphorothioate antisense oligonucleotides induce the formation of nuclear bodies. *Mol. Biol. Cell* 9:1007–23
124. Lorenz P, Misteli T, Baker BF, Bennett CF, Spector DL. 2000. Nucleocytoplasmic shuttling: a novel in vivo property of antisense phosphorothioate oligodeoxynucleotides. *Nucleic Acids Res.* 28:582–92
125. Putnam D, Gentry CA, Pack DW, Langer R. 2001. Polymer-based gene delivery with low cytotoxicity by a unique balance of side-chain termini. *Proc. Natl. Acad. Sci. USA* 98:1200–5
126. Tang MX, Szoka FC. 1997. The influence of polymer structure on the interactions of cationic polymers with DNA and morphology of the resulting complexes. *Gene Ther.* 4:823–32
127. Jones NA, Hill IR, Stolnik S, Bignotti F, Davis SS, Garnett MC. 2000. Polymer chemical structure is a key determinant of physicochemical and colloidal properties of polymer-DNA complexes for gene delivery. *Biochim. Biophys. Acta* 1517:1–18
128. Almofti MR, Harashima H, Shinohara Y, Almofti A, Li W, Kiwada H. 2003. Lipoplex size determines lipofection efficiency with or without serum. *Mol. Membr. Biol.* 20:35–43
129. Benns JM, Choi JS, Mahato RI, Park JS, Kim SW. 2000. pH-sensitive cationic polymer gene delivery vehicle: N-Acpoly(L-histidine)-graft-poly(L-lysine) comb shaped polymer. *Bioconjug. Chem.* 11:637–45
130. Zhdanov RI, Podobed OV, Vlassov VV. 2002. Cationic lipid-DNA complexes-lipoplexes-for gene transfer and therapy. *Bioelectrochemistry* 58:53–64
131. Akinc A, Lynn DM, Anderson DG, Langer R. 2003. Parallel synthesis and biophysical characterization of a degradable polymer library for gene delivery. *J. Am. Chem. Soc.* 125:5316–23
132. Lobo BA, Vetro JA, Suich DM, Zuckermann RN, Middaugh CR. 2003. Structure/function analysis of peptoid/lipitoid:DNA complexes. *J. Pharm. Sci.* 92:1905–18
133. Woodle MC, Scaria P. 2001. Cationic liposomes and nucleic acids. *Curr. Opin. Colloid Interface Sci.* 6:78–84
134. Ledley TS, Ledley FD. 1994. Multicompartment, numerical-model of cellular events in the pharmacokinetics of gene therapies. *Hum. Gene Ther.* 5:679–91
135. Banks GA, Roselli RJ, Chen R, Giorgio TD. 2003. A model for the analysis of nonviral gene therapy. *Gene Ther.* 10: 1766–75
136. Varga CM, Hong K, Lauffenburger DA. 2001. Quantitative analysis of synthetic gene delivery vector design properties. *Mol. Ther.* 4:438–46
137. Leopold PL. 2000. Fluorescence methods reveal intracellular trafficking of gene transfer vectors: the light toward the end of the tunnel. *Mol. Ther.* 1:302–3
138. James MB, Giorgio TD. 2000. Nuclear-associated plasmid, but not cell-associated plasmid, is correlated with transgene expression in cultured mammalian cells. *Mol. Ther.* 1:339–46
139. Tewary HK, Iversen PL. 1997. Qualitative and quantitative measurements of oligonucleotides in gene therapy: part I. In vitro models. *J. Pharm. Biomed. Anal.* 15:857–73
140. Wagner E, Plank C, Zatloukal K, Cotten M, Birnstiel ML. 1992. Influenza virus hemagglutinin HA-2 N-terminal fusogenic peptides augment gene transfer by transferrin-polylysine-DNA complexes: toward a synthetic virus-like gene-transfer vehicle. *Proc. Natl. Acad. Sci. USA* 89:7934–38
141. Aoyama Y, Kanamori T, Nakai T, Sasaki T, Horiuchi S, et al. 2003. Artificial

viruses and their application to gene delivery. Size-controlled gene coating with glycocluster nanoparticles. *J. Am. Chem. Soc.* 125:3455–57
142. Zuber G, Dauty E, Nothisen M, Belguise P, Behr JP. 2001. Towards synthetic viruses. *Adv. Drug Deliv. Rev.* 52:245–53
143. Plank C, Oberhauser B, Mechtler K, Koch C, Wagner E. 1994. The influence of endosome-disruptive peptides on gene transfer using synthetic virus-like gene transfer systems. *J. Biol. Chem.* 269:12918–24
144. Xu L, Frederik P, Pirollo KF, Tang WH, Rait A, et al. 2002. Self-assembly of a virus-mimicking nanostructure system for efficient tumor-targeted gene delivery. *Hum. Gene. Ther.* 13:469–81
145. Remy JS, Kichler A, Mordvinov V, Schuber F, Behr JP. 1995. Targeted gene transfer into hepatoma cells with lipopolyamine-condensed DNA particles presenting galactose ligands: a stage toward artificial viruses. *Proc. Natl. Acad. Sci. USA* 92:1744–48
146. Pitard B, Aguerre O, Airiau M, Lachages AM, Boukhnikachvili T, et al. 1997. Virus-sized self-assembling lamellar complexes between plasmid DNA and cationic micelles promote gene transfer. *Proc. Natl. Acad. Sci. USA* 94:14412–17
147. Helin V, Gottikh M, Mishal Z, Subra F, Malvy C, Lavignon M. 1999. Uptake and intracellular distribution of oligonucleotides vectorized by a PAMAM dendrimer. *Nucleosides Nucleotides* 18:1721–22
148. Simoes S, Pires P, Duzgunes N, Pedrosa de Lima MC. 1999. Cationic liposomes as gene transfer vectors: barriers to successful application in gene therapy. *Curr. Opin. Mol. Ther.* 1:147–57
149. Ogris M, Brunner S, Schuller S, Kircheis R, Wagner E. 1999. PEGylated DNA/transferrin-PEI complexes: reduced interaction with blood components, extended circulation in blood and potential for systemic gene delivery. *Gene Ther.* 6:595–605
150. Oupicky D, Konak C, Dash PR, Seymour LW, Ulbrich K. 1999. Effect of albumin and polyanion on the structure of DNA complexes with polycation containing hydrophilic nonionic block. *Bioconjug. Chem.* 10:764–72
151. Oupicky D, Ogris M, Howard KA, Dash PR, Ulbrich K, Seymour LW. 2002. Importance of lateral and steric stabilization of polyelectrolyte gene delivery vectors for extended systemic circulation. *Mol. Ther.* 5:463–72
152. Simoes S, Slepushkin V, Pires P, Gaspar R, de Lima MP, Duzgunes N. 1999. Mechanisms of gene transfer mediated by lipoplexes associated with targeting ligands or pH-sensitive peptides. *Gene Ther.* 6:1798–807
153. Nakanishi M, Eguchi A, Akuta T, Nagoshi E, Fujita S, et al. 2003. Basic peptides as functional components of non-viral gene transfer vehicles. *Curr. Protein Pept. Sci.* 4:141–50
154. Henderson BR, Percipalle P. 1997. Interactions between HIV Rev and nuclear import and export factors: the Rev nuclear localisation signal mediates specific binding to human importin-beta. *J. Mol. Biol.* 274:693–707
155. Chowdhury NR, Hays RM, Bommineni VR, Franki N, Chowdhury JR, et al. 1996. Microtubular disruption prolongs the expression of human bilirubin-uridinediphosphoglucuronate-glucuronosyltransferase-1 gene transferred into Gunn rat livers. *J. Biol. Chem.* 271:2341–46
156. Singh M, Kisoon N, Ariatti M. 2001. Receptor-mediated gene delivery to HepG2 cells by ternary assemblies containing cationic liposomes and cationized asialoorosomucoid. *Drug Deliv.* 8:29–34
157. Perouzel E, Jorgensen MR, Keller M, Miller AD. 2003. Synthesis and formulation of neoglycolipids for the

functionalization of liposomes and lipoplexes. *Bioconjug. Chem.* 14:884–98
158. Han J, Lim M, Yeom YI. 1999. Receptor-mediated gene transfer to cells of hepatic origin by galactosylated albumin-polylysine complexes. *Biol. Pharm. Bull.* 22:836–40
159. Kunath K, von Harpe A, Fischer D, Kissel T. 2003. Galactose-PEI-DNA complexes for targeted gene delivery: degree of substitution affects complex size and transfection efficiency. *J. Control. Release* 88:159–72
160. Zanta MA, Boussif O, Adib A, Behr JP. 1997. In vitro gene delivery to hepatocytes with galactosylated polyethylenimine. *Bioconjug. Chem.* 8:839–44
161. Kawakami S, Yamashita F, Nishikawa M, Takakura Y, Hashida M. 1998. Asialoglycoprotein receptor-mediated gene transfer using novel galactosylated cationic liposomes. *Biochem. Biophys. Res. Commun.* 252:78–83
162. Koike K, Hara T, Aramaki Y, Takada S, Tsuchiya S. 1994. Receptor-mediated gene transfer into hepatic cells using asialoglycoprotein-labeled liposomes. *Ann. NY Acad. Sci.* 716:331–33
163. Park IK, Kim TH, Kim SI, Park YH, Kim WJ, et al. 2003. Visualization of transfection of hepatocytes by galactosylated chitosan-graft-poly(ethylene glycol)/DNA complexes by confocal laser scanning microscopy. *Int. J. Pharm.* 257:103–10
164. Nishikawa M, Takemura S, Yamashita F, Takakura Y, Meijer DK, et al. 2000. Pharmacokinetics and in vivo gene transfer of plasmid DNA complexed with mannosylated poly(L-lysine) in mice. *J. Drug Target.* 8:29–38
165. Diebold SS, Kursa M, Wagner E, Cotten M, Zenke M. 1999. Mannose polyethylenimine conjugates for targeted DNA delivery into dendritic cells. *J. Biol. Chem.* 274:19087–94
166. Opanasopit P, Hyoudou K, Nishikawa M, Yamashita F, Hashida M. 2002. Serum mannan binding protein inhibits mannosylated liposome-mediated transfection to macrophages. *Biochim. Biophys. Acta* 1570:203–9
167. Yu L, Nielsen M, Han SO, Wan Kim S. 2001. TerplexDNA gene carrier system targeting artery wall cells. *J. Control Release* 72:179–89
168. Kim JS, Kim BI, Maruyama A, Akaike T, Kim SW. 1998. A new non-viral DNA delivery vector: the terplex system. *J. Control Release* 53:175–82
169. Chan CK, Jans DA. 1999. Enhancement of polylysine-mediated transferrinfection by nuclear localization sequences: polylysine does not function as a nuclear localization sequence. *Hum. Gene Ther.* 10:1695–702
170. Uike H, Sakakibara R, Iwanaga K, Ide M, Ishiguro M. 1998. Efficiency of targeted gene delivery of ligand-poly-L-lysine hybrids with different crosslinks. *Biosci. Biotechnol. Biochem.* 62:1247–48
171. Wightman L, Patzelt E, Wagner E, Kircheis R. 1999. Development of transferrin-polycation/DNA based vectors for gene delivery to melanoma cells. *J. Drug Target.* 7:293–303
172. Cheng PW. 1996. Receptor ligand-facilitated gene transfer: enhancement of liposome-mediated gene transfer and expression by transferrin. *Hum. Gene Ther.* 7:275–82
173. Ward CM, Pechar M, Oupicky D, Ulbrich K, Seymour LW. 2002. Modification of pLL/DNA complexes with a multivalent hydrophilic polymer permits folate-mediated targeting in vitro and prolonged plasma circulation in vivo. *J. Gene Med.* 4:536–47
174. Mislick KA, Baldeschwieler JD, Kayyem JF, Meade TJ. 1995. Transfection of folate-polylysine DNA complexes: evidence for lysosomal delivery. *Bioconjug. Chem.* 6:512–15
175. Guo W, Lee RL. 1999. Receptor-targeted gene delivery via folate-conjugated polyethylenimine. *AAPS PharmSci.* 1:E19

176. Benns JM, Mahato RI, Kim SW. 2002. Optimization of factors influencing the transfection efficiency of folate-PEG-folate-graft-polyethylenimine. *J. Control Release* 79:255–69
177. Gosselin MA, Lee RJ. 2002. Folate receptor-targeted liposomes as vectors for therapeutic agents. *Biotechnol. Annu. Rev.* 8:103–31
178. Blessing T, Kursa M, Holzhauser R, Kircheis R, Wagner E. 2001. Different strategies for formation of pegylated EGF-conjugated PEI/DNA complexes for targeted gene delivery. *Bioconjug. Chem.* 12:529–37
179. Suh W, Chung JK, Park SH, Kim SW. 2001. Anti-JL1 antibody-conjugated poly (L-lysine) for targeted gene delivery to leukemia T cells. *J. Control Release* 72: 171–78
180. Merdan T, Callahan J, Petersen H, Kunath K, Bakowsky U, et al. 2003. PEGylated polyethylenimine-fab' antibody fragment conjugates for targeted gene delivery to human ovarian carcinoma cells. *Bioconjug. Chem.* 14:989–96
181. Yuh IS, Lee SY, Hong BJ. 2003. Growth control of mouse mammary epithelial cells by keratin antibody-targeted liposome containing oligonucleotides antisense to epidermal growth factor receptor. *Cell. Biol. Int.* 27:409–14

Annu. Rev. Biomed. Eng. 2004. 6:427–52
doi: 10.1146/annurev.bioeng.6.040803.140100

First published online as a Review in Advance on April 13, 2004

# FRACTAL ANALYSIS OF THE VASCULAR TREE IN THE HUMAN RETINA

Barry R. Masters
*Formerly, Gast Professor, Department of Ophthalmology, University of Bern, 3010 Bern, Switzerland; email: brmail2001@yahoo.com*

**Key Words** fractals, fractal structures, eye, bronchial tree, retinal circulation, retinal blood vessel patterns, Murray Principle, optimal vascular tree, human lung, human bronchial tree

■ **Abstract** The retinal circulation of the normal human retinal vasculature is statistically self-similar and fractal. Studies from several groups present strong evidence that the fractal dimension of the blood vessels in the normal human retina is approximately 1.7. This is the same fractal dimension that is found for a diffusion-limited growth process, and it may have implications for the embryological development of the retinal vascular system. The methods of determining the fractal dimension for branching trees are reviewed together with proposed models for the optimal formation (Murray Principle) of the branching vascular tree in the human retina and the branching pattern of the human bronchial tree. The limitations of fractal analysis of branching biological structures are evaluated. Understanding the design principles of branching vascular systems and the human bronchial tree may find applications in tissue and organ engineering, i.e., bioartificial organs for both liver and kidney.

CONTENTS

# INTRODUCTION

## Scope of the Review

This review presents a critical evaluation of the literature on the application of fractal measurements to the retinal circulation of the living normal human retina. The goals of this research are to determine the fractal dimension of the retinal vascular branching patterns and to infer the mechanism and optimization principles of its formation. Where it is appropriate, a discussion of the optimization principles consistent with the branching structure of the human bronchial tree and other organs is included.

The vascular system in the human retina has a unique property: It is easily observed in its natural living state in the human retina by the use of a retinal camera (1). The retinal circulation is an area of active research by numerous groups, and there is general experimental agreement on the analysis of the patterns of the retinal blood vessels in the normal human retina. However, studies of the vascular systems in the human lung and the human heart are made from resin corrosion casts because the patterns of the vessels in these organs are not directly observable in the living person. For these reasons, I have restricted the main portion of this review to the retinal circulation in the normal living human retina.

This review covers the following topics: the historical development of fractal analysis, the various methods to determine the fractal dimension of branching vascular trees, fractal growth processes, the experimental results on the fractal analysis of the normal human retinal circulation, the implications of this pattern for both vasculariogenesis and diagnostics, the limitations of the experimental analysis and interpretation of the results, and, finally, a discussion of the optimal organization of vascular trees and the human bronchial tree.

This review covers studies of large vessels, arteries, and veins that are observed with a red-free fundus camera in the normal human eye. It is important to note that the major vessels feed and drain the small capillaries, which are the sites of exchange between the components of the blood (gas exchange, nutrient exchange) and the surrounding tissue.

## The Role of Fractal Analysis in Biology and Medicine

A number of books serve as a good introduction to the topics of shape, pattern formation, scaling, and fractals in biology and medicine (2–6). The applications of fractal analysis in biology and medicine can be divided into two groups: (*a*) spatial analysis of shapes and branching patterns and (*b*) temporal analysis of time-varying signals. The applications of fractals to biology and medicine cover a wide range of scale: molecules, cells, tissues, and organs (7). The goal of this methodology, as applied to branching structures in tissues and organs, is to determine the fractal dimension of these objects and structures and then to use this number as a classifier to discriminate the class of normal structures from abnormal and pathological structures.

During the early application of fractal geometry to medical diagnostics, preliminary studies attempted to demonstrate the diagnostic value of fractals in the diagnosis of retinal disease (36, 37, 70, 72, 74). For a diagnostic method to have clinical efficacy it should provide an early discriminant from the normal condition (including biological variability) and show appropriate sensitivity and specificity. Fractal analysis has utility in the ability to characterize the shapes of cellular organelles, cells, tissues, and organs. These shape descriptors may be shown to have sufficient sensitivity and specificity in diagnostic tests to discriminate the pathological from the normal. This has not been the case for the early diagnostics of retinal pathology based on fractal analysis of the blood vessel patterns in the retinal circulation. In the presence of severe retinal disease there are alterations in the patterns of the blood vessels; however, these vascular changes are easily observed with a retinal camera. For example, fractal geometry can be used to quantify the progression of severe proliferative diabetic retinopathy (70). But these severe alterations from the normal vascular patterns are readily observed with a retinal camera, and therefore this technique is not an important diagnostic method.

Most retinal microvascular abnormalities occur early in the disease process and are located in the capillaries and result in alterations of permeability (59, 80). These early vascular alterations are not detected by fractal analysis. The fractal analysis of the blood vessels in the retinal circulation is a global measure of the pattern of the blood vessels; as such, it is not sensitive to small alterations of a small region of the total pattern.

Alternatively, the fractal dimension can be used as an index of growth or development. An example of this type of fractal classification is the fractal analysis of neurons in which different classes of neurons are associated with a different fractal dimension (8–11). In addition, during the growth and development of neurons, the measured fractal dimension changes in a systemic way, and thus it provides a mathematical characterization of the development of the neuron associated with its increased branching during growth and development (12).

Fractal analysis has also been applied to branching structures in the heart (5, 13). These studies have shown that a number of cardiopulmonary structures are fractal in their design. Examples of such self-similar structures are the arterial and venous branching trees, the branching of some cardiac muscle bundles, the branching of the bronchial tree, and the branching of the His-Purkinje network.

Fractal geometry has also been used for the description of texture in medical images (14). Texture can be defined as the spatial distribution of intensity values in an image. For example, fractal methodology has been used for the classification of benign and malignant tumors from chest radiographs (15). The power spectrum of regions in chest radiographs has been subjected to fractal analysis to differentiate between normal and nodular regions (16). Because the branching structure of the airways and the vessels of the lung show geometric self-similarity they can be modeled as a fractal (17, 18). An example of a diagnostic application is a study in which the fractal dimension has been used to discriminate normal lung from interstitial lung in computerized tomography (CT) images (18).

Another class of applications involves the study of branching biological structures and patterns. The bronchial tree and its branching design is the subject of several works (19–23).

An important topic for the application of fractal analysis is the branching trees of the vascular system in various tissues and organs. The following examples illustrate the diversity of biological branching vascular trees that have been analyzed as fractals: the morphometry of the small pulmonary arteries in man (24), the branching vascular system in the kidney (25), the branching vascular system in the heart (13), and the retinal circulation in the human retina (26–28). The goal of these studies is to determine the fractal dimension that characterizes the vascular systems of these organs. From a determination of the fractal dimension, inferences can be made on the mechanisms of their pattern formation. The fractal dimension may also provide evidence for a particular fractal growth process and its physiological correlates. For example, Tsonis & Tsonis (29) studied the fractal property of blood vessels in the developing embryo and proposed a diffusion-limited aggregation model.

A second class of fractal studies in physiology and medicine involves the temporal domain; for example, the one-dimensional time series of physiological signals and processes (30). Fractal signals are signals that have detail on all temporal scales; they are statistically self-similar. Applications of fractals in the time domain include the following: the analysis of normal and pathological brain activity from electroencephalogram data, studies of normal and abnormal cardiac electrical activity (31), and the application of fractals to ion channel kinetics (32).

## How is Fractal Analysis Useful to Study Vascular Systems?

Physiologists have studied the vascular system for many years. These studies cover the spatial scales from angiogenic molecules to the global pattern of the vascular systems. For example, at the molecular level, there are active investigations on the molecular signals and mechanisms of blood vessel formation and development and studies on compounds that can block angiogenesis in tumors (33–35). At the global level, investigations of corrosion casts of vascular systems within the heart, lungs, and kidneys aim to characterize the branching patterns of blood vessels within these organs (25).

Scientists who study the patterns of the vascular system may pose the following questions: How can we characterize the pattern of the blood vessels? What parameters need to be measured? And finally, is there a theoretical model or optimization principle that is consistent with both the pattern and the computer simulations that yield the observed pattern of blood vessels?

Typically, what is measured in a vascular system are the spatial properties and the blood flow velocities within subsets of the vascular system (24). Experimentally, this is a geometrical determination of the blood vessel diameters, lengths, and branching angles, together with physiological blood flow measurements. These parameters are determined on a scale from the major artery that provides the input down to the capillary bed and to the veins that drain the tissue. The measured parameters are then examined to determine goodness of fit with theoretical optimization models of blood flow, bifurcation angles, and branching lengths.

A new and different approach to the study of vascular systems is to use fractal analysis to characterize the blood vessel patterns in the normal human retinal circulation (36). The first step is to determine if the vascular pattern can be characterized as a fractal (methods and concepts are developed in subsequent sections) and then to measure the fractal dimension, which is a number that characterizes the distribution of the branching vascular system in two-dimensional space. Finally, it would be both interesting and useful to determine if the growth processes that are consistent with the fractal dimension of the vascular system can be derived from one or more of the global optimization principles for blood vessel branching systems. An understanding of the design principles of the human vascular system may have applications in the synthetic design of vascular systems in tissue and organ engineering, i.e., bioartificial organs for both liver and kidney.

This review is limited to the development of the normal retinal circulation; however, there is another aspect of the development of the vascular system following injury: neovascularization. A fractal model was used to simulate patterns of corneal neovascularization by inverted diffusion-limited aggregation (37).

## HISTORICAL DEVELOPMENT OF FRACTAL ANALYSIS

Anyone who marvels at a tree, a leaf, a river system, or a lightning bolt must wonder about these branching patterns and their formation. The underlying unity of patterns in nature can be mathematically analyzed in terms of their scaling relations. This methodology is a sequel to the work of D'Arcy Thompson on scaling relations and biological structure and function during the early 1900s (38).

Throughout history, thinkers have wondered about the relations between numbers and physical reality (39, 40). First, someone discovered a relationship between objects (biological and nonbiological) and numbers. Then, philosophers, mathematicians, and theologians offered their explanations. These activities, which began thousands of years ago, continue to occur in our time.

The Greeks were aware of the principle of similitude or scaling (41, 42). They developed a linear scaling relation they called the "golden section" or "golden mean." This scaling relation was used in Greek sculpture and architecture. Later, during the thirteenth century at Pisa, the golden mean was developed in terms of a sequence of numbers that were later termed Fibonacci numbers (43). How did this happen? In 1201, a man named Leonardo of Pisa, whose nickname was Fibonacci, discovered the sequence while he was breeding rabbits. Four centuries later, Kepler determined the recursion formula for the Fibonacci series. The golden mean was renamed by Kepler, who chose the term "divine proportion." The sequence can be generated by starting with the number 1 and each additional term in the sequence is composed of the sum of the two preceding terms. For example: 1, 1, 2, 3, 5, 8, 13, .... The ratio of each number to its immediate predecessor approached the golden mean as a limit (~1.618...). The Fibonacci sequence appears in such diverse applications as biological scaling relations and the keys of a piano.

Natural structures seem to have a similar appearance when viewed at different magnifications. When the basic pattern is magnified, one can observe repeating levels of detail; thus, each level looks like the whole. Rivers, coastlines, and mountains are familiar examples. Biological patterns can also obey scaling relations; however, these examples may be less familiar. For example, trees are self-similar objects. As the magnification is changed, each smaller portion looks like the entire tree. This example illustrates the concept of self-similar. A self-similar object has structure on all length scales and every part is the same as the whole. There are also examples of self-similar objects in art, notably the paintings "The Great Wave" by K. Hokusai and "The Deluge" by Leonardo Da Vinci.

It is important to distinguish between the terms similar and self-similar. A photograph of a face and its enlargement have the same shape and are called similar. However, a small portion of the photograph, e.g., the mouth, when magnified does not look like the original face in the photograph. The idea of similarity also exists in geometry. Two polygons are similar if there are areas of correspondence between the vertices such that the corresponding sides of the polygons are proportional and the corresponding angles are equal. Self-similar objects have similar shapes over a range of scales. As explained by Mandelbrot (45), self-similar objects are formed from subregions that resemble the shape of the whole object.

There is a 2500-year linkage from the Greek geometer Pythagoras, to Euclid, to D'Arcy Thompson, to Mandelbrot. Throughout this period, there was a strong unity between geometry, art, and nature. The developments of fractal geometry by Mandelbrot and others over the past 30 years illustrates the generality of patterns and demonstrates the myriad connections between geometry, art, and natural forms and patterns (44, 45).

It was Mandelbrot who pioneered the applications of fractal concepts to describe complex natural shapes, forms, and patterns (45). In 1961, Richardson published a work in which he described a scaling relation for the length of coastlines. This related the measured length to the size of the length scale used, which was raised to an exponent of 1-D. Richardson did not assign any special significance to the quantity D, which was not an integer. It was Mandelbrot who interpreted D as a dimension, even though it was not an integer, and named it the fractal dimension (44, 45). He was able to generalize the idea and introduced the concept of fractal geometry. Mandelbrot coined the word fractal from the Latin fractus to describe highly irregular patterns, shapes, and mathematical sets. The name comes from the fact that complex shapes can be described by a number, the fractal dimension, which is usually a fraction. This theory differs from our everyday concept of objects in Euclidean space, which have integer dimensions. In Euclidean space, a line has a dimension of 1, a planar object has a dimension of 2, and a volume has a dimension of 3. Fractal geometry is used to describe complex shapes, such as clouds or mountains, for which the fractal dimension can be a fraction between 2 and 3. These concepts are contained in the following quotation from Mandelbrot: "Clouds are not spheres, mountains are not cones, coastlines are not circles, and bark is not smooth, nor does lightning travel in a straight line (45)." It is the almost universal applicability of fractal concepts in describing objects from trees to coastlines to galaxies that demonstrates the elegance and power of these mathematical concepts. This review applies these fractal concepts to the branching pattern of the normal human retinal circulation and explores the implications for the mechanism of its development (46, 47).

## What are Fractals?

Before one can apply fractal analysis to biological objects it is necessary to understand the definition of a fractal (4, 48). In the previous sections, the concept of self-similarity was illustrated and defined. Fractals or fractal objects are self-similar structures or scale-invariant structures (45). Fractals are objects that show self-similarity at different magnifications. The fractal dimension is a measure of the roughness of a fractal structure. It can be understood as a form of symmetry. Round objects, such as circles or disks, are symmetric under the operation of rotation. Fractals are symmetric under changes of scale, which means that fractals are invariant under a change of length scale. In other words, fractals look the same under various degrees of magnification or scale. This definition is true for regular or deterministic fractals, such as those that may be generated on a computer by joining together similar shapes according to an algorithm.

The fractals that are found in nature are called random fractals, and their structure shows self-similarity only in a statistical sense. Random fractals are better described by the term invariance rather than self-similarity. Fractals found in nature show scale invariance only over a finite range of scale (usually between two and four decades): from their smallest to their largest dimension. Another important property found in all fractals is that their density decreases with the distance from any fixed point on them.

In addition to regular and random fractals, there are also self-affine, or anisotropic, fractals (49, 50). Examples of self-affine fractals are fractal surfaces. The self-similarity of the regular fractals, or the statistical self-similarity of the random fractals, is equivalent to an isotropic rescaling of the dimension of length. The geometric properties remain the same in this case. However, in self-affine fractals, the scale invariance holds only if the lengths are rescaled differently along specific directions. Examples of self-affine fractals include single-valued, nondifferentiable functions and the plot of the distance from the origin versus time for a particle undergoing one-dimensional Brownian motion. Another example of a self-affine fractal is the silhouette of a mountain range. For this type of image, the variation of the horizontal and the vertical coordinate scale differently. This behavior is very different from the self-similar boundary of a coastline in which the pattern scales the same in all directions.

An interesting class of fractals is called Laplacian fractals (51). The Laplace equation is the mathematical basis of their formation. The two components in the generation of a Laplacian fractal are the Laplace equation and randomness. Laplacian fractals are useful for modeling such diverse growth phenomena as snowflakes, lightning, and crystal growth and aggregation. The many diverse phenomena that form Laplacian fractals involve the Laplace equation with different physical fields. In dielectric breakdown, the field is the electrostatic potential. In the process of viscous fingering, the physical field is the pressure field, and in dendritic solidification, the diffusion of heat is involved (52).

How do fractal objects differ from ordinary Euclidean objects? For Euclidean objects the mass of the object (M) scales with a length raised to an integral power; for example, the power of three for a sphere, the power of two for a plane, and the power of one for a line. The mass of a solid sphere M(r) is proportional to the radius, r, of the sphere raised to the third power. Fractal objects also obey the mass-length scaling relation; however, the exponent (the fractal dimension, D) is not equal to the Euclidean dimension d. The exponent is, in general, nonintegral and less than the Euclidean dimension.

There are many patterns in nature that show ramified, open branching structures. These objects can be described by fractal geometry in the following manner. The random, scale-invariant objects have a volume V(r) or unit mass density, M, that is a function of the linear size or the radius, r, of the object. It is found empirically that

$$M(r) \approx r^{+D}, \tag{1}$$

where D equals the fractal dimension. Equation 1 applies to fractals when they are self-similar. In general, the fractal dimension $D < d$, where d equals the Euclidean dimension of the space in which the fractal is embedded. The value of D is usually a noninteger. For objects in the real world, there is an upper and a lower cutoff size for which the relation holds. The reader may wish to consult some of the books that are devoted to the mathematical analysis of fractals (48, 50).

## BASIC PRINCIPLES OF FRACTAL ANALYSIS

### Techniques to Determine the Fractal Dimension

The first step in the fractal analysis of an object or pattern is to determine its fractal dimension. There are several methods to determine the fractal dimension D of an object over several bounded length scales (49, 53). Real objects are typically defined as fractal if a scaling relation can be demonstrated over several decades of scale: the upper bound being the size of the object and the lower bound being dependent on the resolution of the technique. The methods to determine the fractal dimension of random fractals include (*a*) box counting, (*b*) the mass-radius relation, and (*c*) the two-point density-density or pair correlation function method.

The computer method to determine the box-counting dimension is outlined below (44, 45, 54). The binary image is covered with square boxes of side length (L). The number of boxes (N) of side length L are counted and denoted as N(L). The size of the box is then incremented and the process is repeated. N(L) is tabulated versus the size of the box (L). A log-log plot of N(L) versus (L) is plotted, and a linear least squares regression is made to determine the slope of the plot. The slope of the linear region of the plot is −D, where D is the box-counting dimension that corresponds to the fractal dimension.

A second method, which is based on the same concept, involves the mass radius relation (44). A set of concentric circles with increasing radii are drawn centered on the point of the object. The mass (M) at a given radius (r), M(r), is determined as a function of the size of the radius. A log-log plot of M(r) versus r is plotted, and the slope gives the fractal dimension D.

A third method useful for random fractals is based on the scaling relation of the two-point density-density correlation function (55). The definition of the normalized density-density, or two-point correlation function, is shown in Equation 2,

$$\mathrm{C(r)} = 1/\mathrm{N} \sum_{\mathrm{r}'} \rho(\mathrm{r}+\mathrm{r}')\rho(\mathrm{r}'). \tag{2}$$

Another interpretation of C(r) is the normalized autocorrelation function. This equation gives the expectation value or probability of finding a particle at the position r + r′, if there is a particle at position r. N is the number of particles in the cluster. In Equation 2, $\rho$(r) equals the local density, i.e., p(r) = 1 if the point belongs to the object; otherwise, it is zero. Usually, fractal objects are isotropic, which is equivalent to stating that the correlations are independent of direction; therefore, r is a scalar quantity. If the object is scale-invariant (the definition of a fractal), the correlation function is unchanged up to a constant by rescaling by an arbitrary factor f. This relation is shown in Equation 3,

$$\mathrm{C(fr)} = \mathrm{f}^{-\alpha}\mathrm{C(r)}, \tag{3}$$

where $\alpha$ is a noninteger greater than zero and less than d, the Euclidean dimension. This equation is satisfied by a power law decay of the local density in the fractal shown in Equation 4,

$$\mathrm{C(r)} = \mathrm{r}^{-\alpha}, \tag{4}$$

where the exponent $\alpha$ is equal to the embedding dimension minus the fractal dimension.

$$\alpha = \mathrm{d} - \mathrm{D} \tag{5}$$

The power law dependence shown in Equation 4 corresponds to the algebraic decay of the local density, as the density-density correlation function is proportional to the density distribution surrounding a given point. Because for real biological branching systems the density-density correlation function method requires the subjective determination of the straight portion of a curving function plot there is some error in the evaluation of the fraction dimension.

For real fractals, a plot of C(r) shows three regions. For small r, C(r) is small and rapidly increases. In the middle region, the cluster is scale-invariant, and C(r) decays with the slope of $\alpha$. However, as r approaches the size of the object, the correlations rapidly approach zero.

The mass-radius technique probes the mass within a given length scale, whereas the density-density correlation function is an average over the entire cluster. Therefore, in small-scale simulations or in random patterns with a limited range of length scales, these two methods give slightly different values for the fractal dimension D.

Different analytical methods used to determine the scaling properties of real objects yield different measures of the fractal dimension. If the objects are isotropic, self-similar, and continuous, then the different methods should yield the same fractal dimension. There are a number of other computerized methods to determine the fractal dimension that are of special interest (53).

In some experimental studies, it is the projection of the object, rather than the object, that is studied. For example, the fractal analysis of the retinal circulation of the normal human retina is based on two-dimensional retinal images taken with a fundus camera. The retinal circulation is on a curved surface of the eye, and it is the projection of this image onto the image plane that forms the acquired photograph. One could ask the question, is the fractal dimension of the projection of an object equivalent to the fractal dimension of the object? The answer is yes. The projection of a fractal embedded in three dimensions to a plane does not change D as long a $D < d$. (56). They are equivalent as long as the measured fractal dimension D is less than the dimension of the space d in which the object is embedded. For the normal human retinal circulation, this is the case as the fractal dimension is 1.7 and the dimension of the two-dimensional space is 2.

## Fractal Growth Processes

There are many growing, branching patterns that can be described by fractal geometry (39). These patterns are self-similar in a statistical manner. Another way of formulating this concept is that the volume of the object V(R) scales with the increasing size of R.

$$V(R) \sim R^{+D} \tag{6}$$

The fractal dimension D is usually a noninteger number, and $D < d$, where d is the Euclidean dimension of the space in which the fractal object is embedded.

There are several computer models to simulate fractal growth (52). However, only one model is described in detail because it produces branching fractal objects that are similar to the patterns observed in the retinal circulation of the human retina.

Many growing, branching objects can be simulated by computer simulations in which the spatial dependence of a field (temperature, concentration, electric field, etc.) satisfies the Laplace equation with moving boundary conditions. Diffusion-limited growth is a class of these models in which the concentration of diffusing particles satisfies the Laplace equation (51).

One such model is the diffusion-limited aggregation model (DLA) formulated in 1981 by Witten & Sander (46, 57). DLA is a far from equilibrium process. In other words, DLA is a nonequilibrium process. The simulation of a DLA yields branching patterns similar to the branching patterns seen in the human retina owing to the retinal circulation of arteries and veins. The fractal dimension of diffusion-limited aggregates is usually $D = 1.71$ for a fractal embedded in a two-dimensional space (58).

# THE RETINAL VASCULAR SYSTEM

## The Retinal Circulation

The retina has the highest oxygen requirement per unit weight of any tissue in the body, and any alteration in circulation may result in functional impairment and tissue damage. Diseases of the retinal circulation that can lead to blindness if untreated include diabetic retinopathy, retinopathy of prematurity, and hypertensive vascular disease (59).

The retina is supplied by two major blood vessel systems (60). The inner layer (nerve fiber layer) of nerves and glial cells are supplied by the retinal circulation. The retinal circulation performs the nutritive function for the inner two-thirds of the retina. In human beings, this circulation is supplied by the central retinal artery and has one main collecting trunk, the central retinal vein. The arteries of the retinal circulation lie in the nerve fiber layer or ganglion cell layer just below the internal limiting membrane. Following bifurcation at the optic disc, the retinal artery and vein form extended branching patterns throughout the retina. The veins and arteries do not cross themselves, but a vein and an artery can overlap, forming arteriovenous crossings. There are smaller branches of these major vessels: arterioles, venules, and the smallest vessels, the capillaries. The capillaries form a vast network throughout the retina and are suspended between the arterial and venous systems. The retinal blood vessels enter and leave the retina at the optic disc (the center of each retinal image in Figures 1–4), and to the right of the optic disc is the avascular foveal region. The branching patterns of the retinal circulation in the living normal human retina are the subject of this review.

The second circulatory system of the retina is the choroidal circulation, which supplies the outer layer of the cells of the neural retina (photoreceptors) and the retinal pigment epithelium (59). The choroidal arteries and veins do not run parallel as in most vascular systems. The choroidal circulation is both a nutritive and a

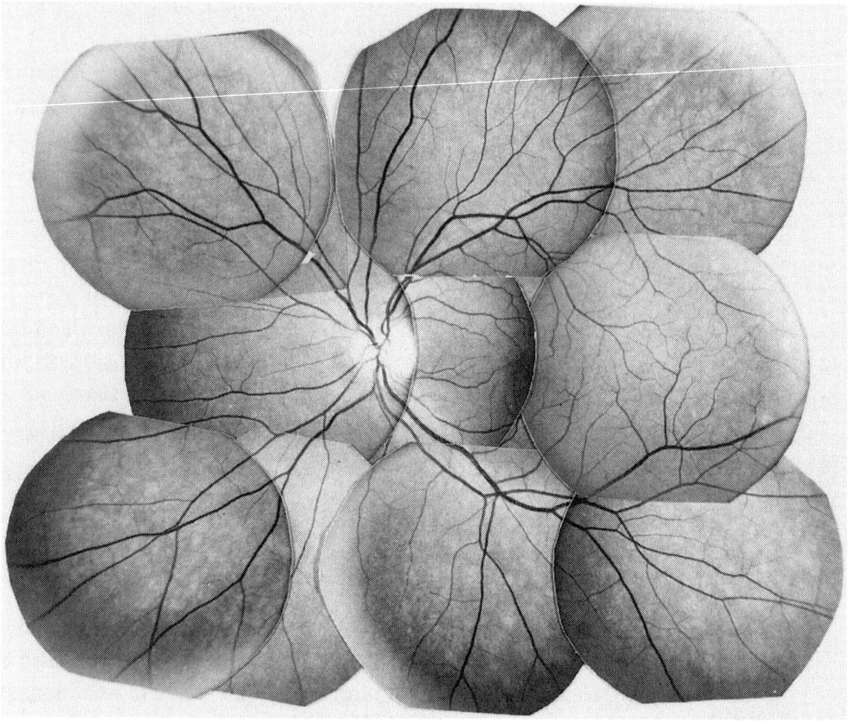

**Figure 1** Photomontage of retinal fields of normal human retina taken with a red-free (green filter) retinal camera. The bright region in the center of the photomontage from which the retina blood vessels appear is the optic nerve head. The major retinal arteries and veins appear black against a lighter background of the nerve fiber layer.

cooling system for the eye. The choroidal circulation system consists of three layers of choroidal vessels. The retinal circulation is visible clinically; however, the choroidal circulation is not visible except in pigmented areas of the retina. There are image-processing techniques, e.g., indocyanine green (ICG) choroidal angiography, to characterize choroidal blood flow (61, 62).

## Embryological Development of the Retinal Vascular System

In primates, the retinal vascularization proceeds via angiogenic sprouting from preexisting vessels in all regions and stages. Critical reviews of the cellular mechanisms in retinal vascular development have recently been published (63, 64).

The developing retinal vasculature may utilize novel sources of endothelial cells, such as recruitment of circulating stem cells and redeployment of mural cells from regressing vessel segments. Vascular growth occurs by two complementary mechanisms, vasculogenesis and angiogenesis. Controversy still exists over the mechanism of retinal vascular development (63). Vasculogenesis is the development of a vasculature by differentiation and organization of endothelial cell

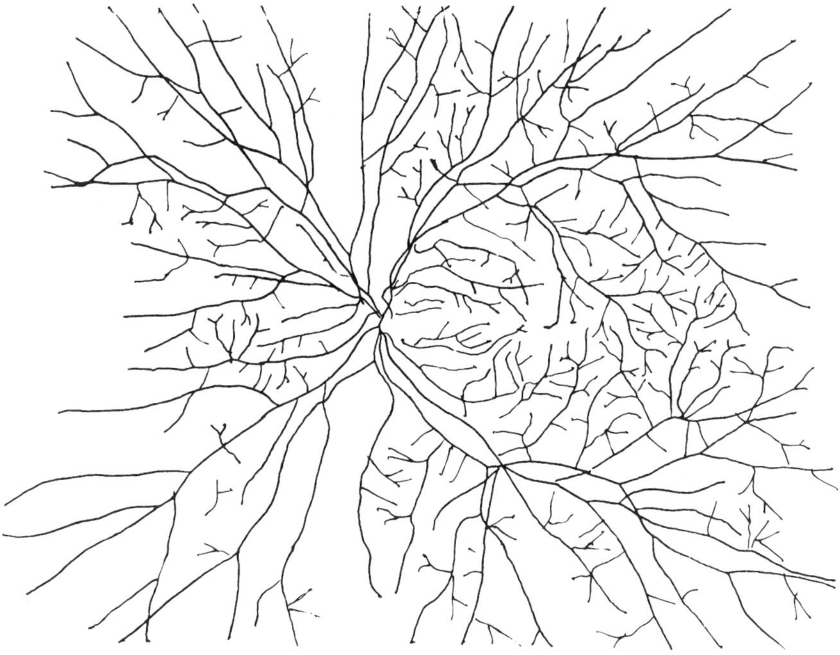

**Figure 2** Tracing of the retinal vessels from the photomontage shown in Figure 1.

precursors, angioblasts. Vasculogenesis is the process by which the initial vascular tree forms from an embryonic precursor cell. Angiogenesis is the formation of a blood vessel from an existing blood vessel by the migration and proliferation of endothelial cells. Angiogenesis is the process in which new vessels arise by sprouting of budlike and fine endothelial extensions from preexisting vessels. Angiogenesis changes the vascular tree created by vasculogenesis during embryogenesis and it results in the formation of pathologic vessels in tumors and other disease states, such as proliferative diabetic retinopathy (64).

In human beings, the retina remains avascular until the fourth month of fetal development (65). Up to this point of development, the hyaloid artery, which is the only intraocular blood vessel, has no retinal branches. At the end of the four-month period, the vascular mesenchymal cells enter the nerve fiber layer. The mesenchymal spindle cells spread out toward the periphery of the retina. Vascular growth occurs outward from the disc. The development of the mature vascular system probably involves a number of variables, including hemodynamic and metabolic factors and oxygen gradients.

Endothelial cells form a single layer that lines all blood vessels. Vessels develop from the walls of existing small vessels by the outgrowth of these endothelial cells. The endothelial cells are formed by the division of existing endothelial cells. New capillaries form by sprouting from existing small vessels and develop into new vessels. This process is called angiogenesis. The growth of the capillary network may be due to angiogenic factors released by the surrounding tissues.

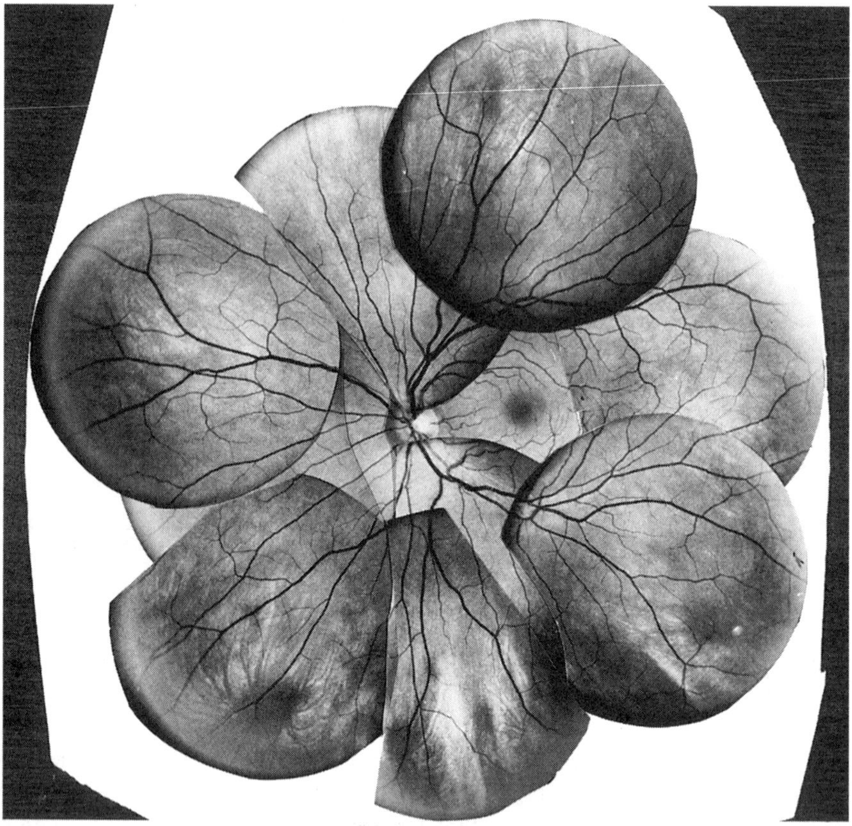

**Figure 3** Photomontage of retinal fields of normal human retina taken with a red-free (green filter) retinal camera. The retinal arteries and veins appear black against a lighter background of the nerve fiber layer.

A model for the development of the inner retinal circulation has been proposed by Kretzer and colleagues (66). Their hypothesis may be summarized as follows. There is a relation between inner retinal blood vessel development and maturation of the photoreceptors. In the course of development, the maturing photoreceptors consume progressively more oxygen, decreasing the oxygen available to support the respiratory needs of the inner retina. The migrating spindle cells in the avascular inner retina sense this diminished oxygen concentration and migrate toward the area of diminished oxygen concentration. The decrease in the transretinal flux of oxygen from the choroidal vasculature is compensated by a new vascular source on the inner retina. There is a putative relationship between inner retinal vascular development and the maturation of the photoreceptors. As the photoreceptors mature, they consume more oxygen; this is indicated by the increasing number and density of the mitochondria in their inner segments.

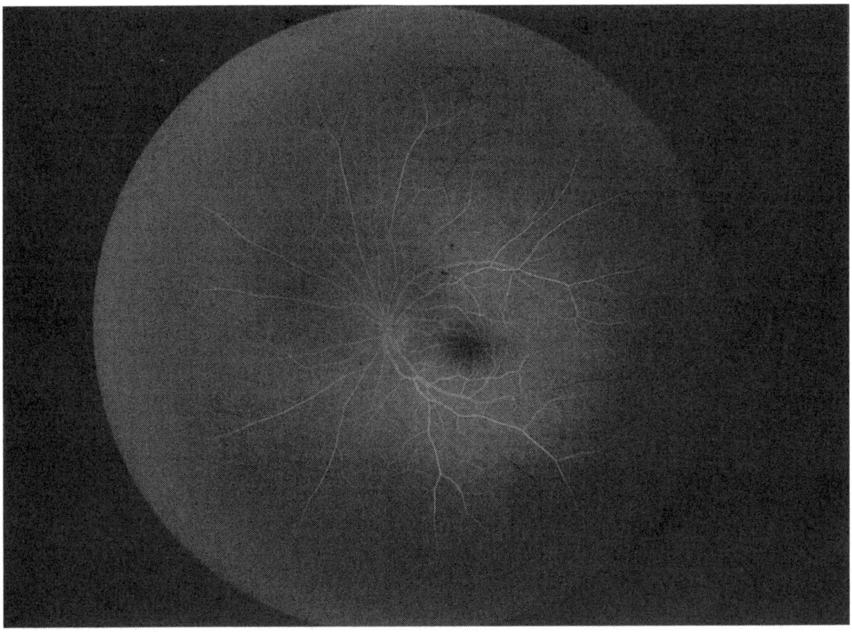

**Figure 4** An example of a fluorescein angiogram of the normal human retina from another subject. The image was taken with a 140° wide-field retinal camera. The retinal vessels appear white owing to the fluorescence of the fluorescein in the vessels.

In the case of pathology, i.e., retinopathy of prematurity, the spindle cells respond with the release of angiogenic factors (66). The angiogenic factors diffuse in the plane of the retina and stimulate the growth of new retinal blood vessels and the process of neovascularization. The diffusion of angiogenic factors is the physical process responsible for the new development of retinal vessel patterns.

Local oxygen tension has a large effect on the vasculature; it compensates vascular insufficiency through the induction of angiogenesis (67). This process is thought to be mediated by the hypoxia-inducible factor (HIF) complex, which is activated in hypoxic cells and increases transcription of a broad range of genes, including angiogenic growth factors such as VEGF. An important function for the vascular architecture is to bring the circulatory system into close contact with all cells. An important research question is how the vascular architecture develops and remodels in such a manner to insure that all areas of the tissue are adequately perfused.

## Fractal Analysis of the Human Retinal Circulation

The determination of the fractal dimension of the normal human retinal circulation is dependent on the quality and the type of retinal images. For a wide field of the retina to be imaged at high resolution, retinal photomontages are usually constructed from a series of images obtained with red-free retinal cameras; that is, the use of a green filter that causes the blood vessels in the retinal circulation to appear black. Examples of these photomontages are shown in Figures 1 and 3. The arteries and veins of the retinal circulation are seen as black vessels with a much lighter nerve fiber layer in the background. Alternatively, but not recommended, is the use of fluorescein angiograms of the retina. Masters has found that fractal analysis of retinal blood vessels based on the use of fluorescein angiograms shows great variability as compared to the use of red-free images taken with a retinal camera. An example is shown in Figure 4. These images show the veins and arteries of the retinal circulation as white lines owing to the bright fluorescence of the fluorescein that was injected into the circulatory system. The vessels of the retinal circulation that appear in the fluorescein angiograms depend on the time the image was acquired following the injection of the fluorescein. In addition, there is a bright background owing to leakage of the fluorescein. Therefore, there is great variability in detecting the vessels of the retinal circulation in these images. In most of the experimental work, the blood vessels are traced as shown in Figure 2, and one of the methods to determine the fractal dimension is used. It is important to note that the fractal analysis of the normal human retinal circulation may yield different results when applied to the diseased retina; however, the great variability of the results and analysis do not form the basis of a useful diagnostic tool at this time.

The application of fractals and fractal growth processes to the branching blood vessels of the normal human retinal circulation was introduced by Masters (68, 69) who worked in collaboration with Platt and Family (68, 69). A series of papers led to an estimate of the fractal dimension for the retinal vessels of $D = 1.7$, which is in good agreement with the dimension of a diffusion-limited aggregation cluster grown in two dimensions (68, 69). The early studies had difficulty in obtaining clinical fundus images of normal subjects and were also limited by lack of standardization in the acquisition of the fundus images and the methods of analysis to determine the fractal dimension. For example, this early investigation of six subjects only contained four normals and used various types of fundus cameras to acquire the images (30°, 60°, 140°). In addition, both the mass-radius and the two-point correlation function methods were used. This diversity of subjects, image acquisition, and fractal analysis methods results in a spread of the value of the fractal dimension. However, if the study is limited to the normal, human retina, and the mass-radius analysis method, then the measured fractal dimension is 1.72, which is consistent with a diffusion-limited growth process.

Several independent research groups have demonstrated that for the normal human retina over a range of ages, the patterns of the retinal vasculature are fractal. What is extremely interesting is that the patterns resemble a particular type of fractal-DLA cluster. The normal retinal vasculature and two-dimensional DLA models have fractal dimensions of approximately 1.7. As previously discussed, these are formed by a diffusion field that is governed by the Laplace diffusion equation. This fact may have implications on the mechanism of normal retinal vasculogenesis, which is the normal formation of blood vessels.

How does this study compare with our previous studies and with the results of others? Daxer (70) calculated the fractal dimension of normal human subjects with the density-density correlation function method. He reported that 14 normals had a fractal dimension of 1.708 $\pm$ 0.073 (mean $\pm$ standard deviation). This study used red-free retinal camera photographs as the source of data (70).

Two recent studies analyzed the retinal blood vessel patterns in fluorescein angiograms made with a 60° fundus camera. Landini et al. (71) determined the fractal dimension of the retinal blood vessels of 23 normal human subjects. The fractal dimension was determined with the box-counting method. The arterial and venous trees were manually traced separately and in combination. For retinal vessels in the size range 250–3200 $\mu$m, the following fractal dimensions were calculated: arteries 1.64, veins 1.66, and arteries and veins combined 1.76. These authors did not find differences with age (14–73 years) or sex (71). This study supports the view that a nonequilibrium Laplacian process could be involved in retinal angiogenesis. They also point out that small discrepancies in the estimation of the fractal dimension by various authors are related to image acquisition techniques rather than real differences in the fractal dimension.

In another study, Mainster (72) used the mass-radius method to analyze the fractal dimension of human subjects from their fluorescein angiograms. It is important to note that these are not normal human retinas; the subjects showed early background diabetic retinopathy. The retinal arteries had a fractal dimension of 1.63, and the veins had a fractal dimension of 1.71. Mainster is in agreement with the earlier suggestion of Masters (68) that a diffusion-limited growth process, based on the Laplace equation, may be involved in the development of the retinal blood vessel patterns (72).

One study of the fractal dimension of the normal human retinal circulation met all the criteria of standardized image acquisition, image tracing, and analysis (73, 74). The mean value and standard deviation of the fractal dimension (box-counting dimension) is 1.70 $\pm$ 0.02 (N = 10). All of the red-free images were obtained with a Zeiss fundus camera with a 30° field of view. A single ophthalmic photographer photographed all of the subjects. The subjects were previously examined by an ophthalmologist and were devoid of retinal pathology. The use of standard methods for both the data acquisition and the data analysis resulted in less variance in the data than was reported in our previous studies. In the limited sample, there were no differences between left and right eyes, nor with age in the range of 25–38 years (Table 1).

The blood vessel patterns of the retinal circulation of the normal human eye are self-similar structures with a fractal dimension (box counting dimension) of approximately 1.7. (74). This is the same fractal dimension that is found for a diffusion-limited growth process. The pattern is therefore consistent with the hypothesis that the development of human retinal blood vessels involves a diffusion process (75).

Two recent papers develop DLA from shear stress as a simple model of vasculogenesis (76). A model is proposed in which the formation of the vascular network

**TABLE 1** Fractal dimension (Bos-counting method) of the normal human retinal blood vessel patterns (74)

| Name[a] | Age | Eye[b] | Fractal dimension |
|---|---|---|---|
| AHS | 38 | OS | 1.70 |
| AHS | 38 | OD | 1.69 |
| BHS | 25 | OS | 1.68 |
| CHS | 28 | OD | 1.71 |
| DHS | 32 | OD | 1.72 |
| DHS | 32 | OS | 1.71 |
| EHS | 34 | OS | 1.71 |
| EHS | 34 | OD | 1.72 |
| FHS | 25 | OD | 1.68 |
| FHS | 25 | OS | 1.68 |

[a]Initials of each subject.
[b]OD, right eye; OS, left eye.

proceeds via a progressive penetration of the vessel ramification into a capillary mesh. The driving force is of hydrodynamic origin and results in a Laplacian growth mechanism. In their model, the growth of both arteries and veins follows the directions of high shear stress provoked by the blood flow on the endothelium wall of a preexisting capillary mesh. Their growth is driven by a field that satisfies the Laplace equation. This imposes a growth velocity on the tree surface that is proportional to the gradient of the field. The higher the flux, the higher the growth speed. Vasculogenesis occurs early in the growth process. There are two processes of vascular growth. The first is the transformation of cells into fibroblasts and endothelial cells. This results in the random formation of capillaries. The second is the proliferation and migration of endothelial cells found in the first vascular structure, which results in sprouting into previously avascular organs. The remodeling of the capillary network results in the formation of small vessels, which then enlarge in a process of maturation called pruning. The modeling of three-dimensional microvasculature by interlaced DLA includes a model of three-dimensional vascular formation, which is able to explain how the capillary system matures into two three-dimensional arborescent vasculatures, which interdigitate in the distal parts (77).

## LIMITATIONS OF FRACTAL ANALYSIS OF BRANCHING BIOLOGICAL STRUCTURES

It is important to understand the experimental and the theoretical limitations of the application of fractal analysis to the branching blood vessels of the normal human retinal circulation.

To achieve high precision and accuracy in the experimental determination of the fractal dimension of the branching patterns of the human retinal circulation, it is important to adhere to the following procedures. A single fundus photographer should acquire the retinal images of the normal subjects using the same retinal camera. The photomontages of the red-free fundus images should be made by the same person. The tracings of the branching vessels in the retinal circulation should be made by the same person. Comparison of the fractal dimension using the density-density correlation method does not always agree with the fractal dimension obtained from the same subjects using the box-counting or mass radius method owing to the subjective fit of the curve to a straight line, which introduces error. It was also observed that comparison of branching vessel patterns from red-free fundus photographs and their montages to obtain a wide field do not always agree with similar studies based on a fluorescein angiogram.

Some of these sources of error and discrepancies in the estimation of the fractal dimension have been previously discussed (78). Many of the variations in the experimental determination of the fractal dimension discussed in this paper can be attributed to the comparison of red-free retinal photographs with fluorescein angiograms in which the time of the image capture affects the visibility of the arteries and the veins in the retinal circulation, comparison of normal retinal with subjects showing disease states (e.g., 72), and comparison of computerized box-counting techniques with the more variable and subjective density-density correlation methods.

An alternative explanation for the different values of the fractal dimensions evaluated by different groups (79) is the crossover effect of several different fractal dimensions. However, the major differences discussed in the preceding paragraph were not addressed, i.e., use of subjects with retinal disease and use of subjective selection of a particular image from the set of angiograms.

The fractal dimension does not uniquely characterize the shape or form of the fractal object. It is a measure of how the fractal object fills up space. Nevertheless, there is some correspondence between the observed complexity or roughness of a pattern and its fractal dimension. As the complexity of how the object fills up space increases, the fractal dimension increases. In a plane, if the object is completely space filling, the fractal dimension is two. It is important to realize that there is not a unique relation between the shape of a pattern and its fractal dimension. Various patterns that fill space in the same way and show similar scaling relations have the same fractal dimension. Nevertheless, the single number may have important significance in characterizing the process that led to the formation of the pattern as a feature descriptor of the pattern.

What are the possible limitations of the preceding methodology? The mass-radius method assumes that the mass (the size of the object) is to be determined. The tracings convert a pattern comprised of vessels with a length and a width to a pattern comprised of lines. It is equivalent to having a vessel with an average width that does not vary with distance from the optic nerve head.

The geometry of the eye could also affect the experimental determination of the fractal dimension. A projection from a two-dimensional curved surface to a two-dimensional flat surface was used to produce a photograph of the retinal vessels. This projection involved the introduction of a fixed-length scale—the radius of curvature of the eye. Asymptotically, the measurement of the fractal dimension should not be sensitive to such an effect. In addition, the projection of a fractal embedded in three dimensions to a plane of two dimensions does not change D so long as the condition of $D < d$ holds. In the case of retinal blood vessels, D is approximately 1.7 and the Euclidean dimension is 2 for a plane. Therefore, the condition of $D < d$ is valid (56). Finally, it must be stated that the analysis was made over a limited range of length scales (approximately two decades) and therefore the conclusions are valid only in this regime.

Several studies attempt to use differences in the fractal dimension as a discriminant factor to detect and diagnose disease. The global analysis of the retinal circulation may miss the very early changes in the microvascular systems of the retinal circulation and, therefore, not be sensitive to the early manifestation of disease. Many disease processes show their first manifestations in the microvascular systems of the retina, and the studies covered in this review do not investigate the microvascular systems (80). Major alterations of the vessels in the retinal circulation would manifest themselves as alterations in the fractal dimension.

In addition to the fractal dimension, the property of lacunarity may be an additional useful discriminant in the study of branching blood vessels. Lacunarity is a measure of the size of gaps or holes within a structure and may complement the fractal dimension in the characterization of texture (81, 82).

Finally, however useful fractal analysis is to the study of the vascular system, it still suffers from the fundamental problem that it is not based on fundamental physical laws that can be expressed in mathematical form. Each branch of physics, from mechanics to thermodynamics, to electric and magnetic field theory, to quantum mechanics, to fluid flow, has fundamental physics laws that govern the phenomena. There is no fundamental equation that governs fractal geometry.

## OPTIMAL ORGANIZATION OF VASCULAR TREES AND THE HUMAN BRONCHIAL TREE

If we may assume that the design of branching biological trees, e.g., the human bronchial tree and the human retinal circulation, follows optimization principles, then a reasonable question to ask is what should be optimized? There are several general references that attempt to answer this question (19, 83–85).

There are many publications on the optimal organization of branching trees. Two early papers that developed the principles of optimal organization of branching trees were the work of Murray (86, 87). In 1926, Murray developed the principle of minimum work. He simultaneously minimized the energy-equivalent cost of blood flow and blood volume and concluded that the optimal economy of circulation can be realized if the flow is everywhere proportional to the third power of the vessel's diameter. This relationship is valid for the general flow in the entire vasculature; the flows in the individual vessels may differ owing to local conditions. A second paper by Murray applied the physiological principle of minimum work to the angle of branching arteries. The Murray Principle is based on Poisseuille's law for the flow of liquids in tubes. It was shown that the diameter, d, of a blood vessel is optimum when it is proportional to the cube root of the flow, q, in the vessel. Thus, the flow of blood past any section of artery shall be related to the cube of the radius of the vessel at that point.

The application of the Murray Principle to the normal human retinal circulation has been validated (88, 89). An advantage of study of the retinal vascular system is that in the retina, a large number of arterial bifurcations can be easily studied in vivo.

Horsfield (20) made a similar application of an optimization principle to the morphology of the bronchial tree in man. These authors used casts of the human bronchial tree and applied the principle of minimal work. This required that the airways of the human bronchial tree should have a maximum radius for minimal resistance to air flow. There is also a requirement that the airways should have a minimal volume for economy of space. The authors concluded that the morphology of the bronchial tree is appropriate to the function of airflow in the upper region of the tree and to molecular diffusion in the distal region, while maintaining a minimal volume compatible with these functions.

Another more recent application of the Murray Principle to optimal radii in microvascular networks makes the prediction that the flow is proportional to the cube of the vessel radius, and that at vessel junctions, the cube of the radius of the parent vessel equals the sum of the cubes of the daughter radii (90). This follows from the conservation of flow at vessel junctions. The authors studied the traverse arteriolar trees of the cat sartorius muscle and concluded that for entire trees with many junctions, the departure from the Murray Principle was small in energy terms.

Mayrovitz & Roy (91) tested the functional relationship between microvascular blood flow and arteriolar internal diameter. They studied paired blood velocity and arteriolar diameter in the cremaster muscle microvasculature of rats and concluded that for this vascular system, the flow is proportional to the cube of the diameter of the vessels (91).

In conclusion, design of the branching patterns of the human retinal circulation and the relation between vessel size and blood flow have been validated as first stated in the Murray Principle of 1926.

## CONCLUSIONS AND FUTURE DIRECTIONS

The biological mechanism for the formation of retinal vessel patterns in the developing human eye is unknown even though it is a question of importance. The current hypothesis is based on the existence of a variable oxygen gradient across the developing photoreceptors that stimulates the release of angiogenic factors, which diffuse in the plane of the retina and result in the growth of retinal vessels. This implies that the rate-limiting step in the formation of the vessel pattern is a diffusion process.

The branching patterns of the blood vessels in the normal human retinal circulation have a self-similar structure with a fractal dimension of approximately 1.7. This is the same fractal dimension found for a diffusion-limited growth process, and this is consistent with the hypothesis that the development of human retinal vessels involves a diffusion process. Furthermore, the experimental data supports the Murray Principle, i.e., the diameter of an artery is approximately proportional to the cube root of the flow that the artery is designed to convey (92).

Given that the normal human retinal circulation is a self-similar, fractal pattern, and that the Murray optimization principle is valid for the blood vessels in the normal human retinal circulation, it is exciting to pose the following question: What is the link, if any, between the observed fractal pattern and the theoretical formulation of the Murray principle? It is of interest to derive the fractal properties of the normal human retinal circulation from the Murray Principle.

The diagnostic potential of fractal analysis of the branching patterns of the blood vessels in the retinal circulation has not been demonstrated with high sensitivity and high specificity. This may be due to the fact that many retinal microvascular abnormalities occur early in the disease process, they are located in the capillaries, and result in alterations of permeability.

There is also the question of why fractals.

It has been suggested that fractal models have an appeal in that they are simple to encode genetically because the same branching mechanism is used repeatedly (93).

Fractal analysis of blood vessels may also find applications in the design and development of perfusion systems in artificial organs, e.g., kidney and liver, in which optimal exchange of metabolic components is desirable.

## ACKNOWLEDGMENTS

This work was supported by a grant from NIH, National Eye Institute, EY-06958. I thank Dr. Stephen Sinclair for providing the red-free montages of the human retinas.



## LITERATURE CITED

1. Wong D. 1991. The fundus camera. In *Duane's Clinical Ophthalmology*, eds. W Tasman, EA Jaeger, 61:1–14. Philadelphia, PA: J.B. Lippincott
2. Rashevsky N. 1960. *Mathematical Biophysics. Physico-Mathematical Foundations of Biology*. New York: Dover Publ. 3rd ed.

3. West BJ. 1990. *Fractal Physiology and Chaos in Medicine*. Singapore: World Sci.
4. Schroeder M. 1991. *Fractals, Chaos, Power Laws: Minutes from an Infinite Paradise*. San Francisco: W.H. Freeman. 429 pp.
5. Bassingthwaighte JB, Liebovitch LS, West BJ. 1994. *Fractal Physiology*. New York: Oxford Univ. Press
6. Iannaccone PM, Khokha M, eds. 1996. *Fractal Geometry in Biological Systems, An Analytical Approach*. Boca Raton, FL: CRC Press. 360 pp.
7. Stanley HE, Amaral LAN, Buldyrev SV, Goldberger AL, Havlin S, et al. 1996. Scaling and universality in living systems. *Fractals* 4:427–51
8. Smith TG Jr, Marks WB, Lange GD, Sheriff WH Jr, Neale EA. 1989. A fractal analysis of cell images. *J. Neurosci. Methods* 27:173–80
9. Caserta F, Stanley HE, Eldred WD, Daccord G, Hausman RE, Nittmann J. 1990. Physical mechanisms underlying neurite outgrowth: a quantitative analysis of neuronal shape. *Phys. Rev. Lett.* 64:95–98
10. Porter R, Ghosh S, Lange GD, Smith TG Jr. 1991. A fractal analysis of pyramidal neurons in mammalian motor cortex. *Neurosci. Lett.* 130:112–16
11. Reichenbach A, Siegel A, Senitz D, Smith TG Jr. 1992. A comparative fractal analysis of various mammalian astroglial cell types. *Neuroimage* 1:69–77
12. Smith TG Jr, Behar TN, Lange GD, Marks WB, Sheriff WH Jr. 1991. A fractal analysis of cultured rat optic nerve glial growth and differentiation. *Neuroscience* 41:159–66
13. Goldberger AL, Peng C-K, Hausdorff J, Mietus J, Havlin S, Stanley HE. 1996. Fractals and the heart. See Ref. 6, pp. 249–66
14. Einstein AJ, Wu H-S, Gil G. 1998. Self-affinity and lacunarity of chromatin texture in benign and malignant breast epithelial cell nuclei. *Phys. Rev. Lett.* 80:397–400
15. Peiss J, Verlande M, Ameling W, Gunther RW. 1996. Classification of lung tumors on chest radiographs by fractal texture analysis. *Invest. Radiol.* 31:625–29
16. Floyd CE Jr, Patz EF, Lo JY, Vittitoe NF, Stambaugh LW. 1996. Diffuse nodular lung disease on chest radiographs: a pilot study of characterization by fractal dimension. *Am. J. Radiol.* 167:1185–87
17. West BJ, Bhargava V, Goldberger AL. 1986. Beyond the principle of similitude: renormalization in the bronchial tree. *J Appl. Physiol.* 60:189–97
18. Uppaluri R, Hoffman EA, Sonka M, Hartley PG, Hunninghake GW, McLennan G. 1999. Computer recognition of regional lung disease patterns. *Am. J. Respir. Crit. Care Med.* 160:648–54
19. Weibel ER. 1963. *Morphometry of the Human Lung*. Berlin: Springer-Verlag
20. Horsfield K, Cumming G. 1967. Angles of branching and diameters of branches in the human bronchial tree. *Bull. Math. Biophys.* 29:245–59
21. Weibel ER. 1987. Scaling of structural and functional variables in the respiratory system. *Annu. Rev. Physiol.* 49:147–59
22. Horsfield K, Cumming G. 1968. Morphology of the bronchial tree in man. *J. Appl. Physiol.* 24:373–83
23. Horsfield K, Dart G, Olson DE, Filley GF, Cumming G. 1971. Models of the human bronchial tree. *J. Appl. Physiol.* 31:207–17
24. Horsfield K. 1978. Morphometry of the small pulmonary arteries in man. *Circ. Res.* 42:593–97
25. Sernetz M, Justen M, Jestczemski F. 1995. Dispersive fractal characterization of kidney arteries by three-dimensional mass-radius-analysis. *Fractals* 3:879–91
26. Masters BR, Family F, Platt DE. 1989. Fractal analysis of human retinal vessels. *Biophys. J.* 55:575a (Suppl.)
27. Masters BR. 1989. Fractal analysis of human retinal vessels. *SPIE Proc.* 1357:250–56
28. Masters BR. 1989. Fractal analysis of human retina blood vessel patterns: developmental aspects. *Int. Symp. Ocular Circ. Neovascularization, 2nd, Wilmer*

*Inst., Johns Hopkins Med. Inst.*, p. 45. Baltimore, MD
29. Tsonis AA, Tsonis PA. 1987. Fractals: a new look at biological shape and patterning. *Perspect. Biol. Med.* 30:355–60
30. Wornell GW. 1998. Fractal signals. In *The Digital Signal Processing Handbook*, ed. VK Madisetti, DB Smith, pp. 73-1–13. Boca Raton, FL: CRC Press
31. Goldberger AL, Bhargava V, West BJ, Mandell AJ. 1985. On a mechanism of cardiac electrical stability: the fractal hypothesis. *Biophys. J.* 48:525–28
32. Liebovitch LS. 1996. Ion channel kinetics. See Ref. 6, pp. 31–56
33. Folkman J. 1976. The vascularization of tumors. *Sci. Am.* 234:58–73
34. Folkman J, Haudenschild C. 1980. Angiogenesis in vitro. *Nature* 288:551–56
35. Yancopoulos GD, Klagsbrun M, Folkman J. 1998. Vasculogenesis, angiogenesis, and growth factors: ephrins enter the fray at the border. *Cell* 93:661–64
36. Masters BR. 1990. Fractal analysis of human retinal blood vessel patterns: developmental and diagnostic aspects. In *Noninvasive Diagnostic Techniques in Ophthalmology*, ed. BR Masters, pp. 515–27. New York: Springer Verlag
37. Landini G, Misson GP. 1993. Simulation of corneal neovascularization by inverted diffusion limited aggregation. *Invest. Ophthalmol. Vis. Sci.* 34:1872–76
38. Thompson DW. 1942. *On Growth and Form*. Cambridge: Cambridge Univ. Press
39. Stanley HE, Ostrowsky N, eds. 1986. *On Growth and Form*. Dordrecht: Martinus Nijhoff
40. West GB, Brown JH, Enquist BJ. 1997. A general model for the origin of allometric scaling laws in biology. *Science* 276:122–26
41. Cook TA. 1979. *The Curves of Life*. New York: Dover Publ.
42. Ball P. 1999. *The Self-Made Tapestry: Pattern Formation in Nature*. New York: Oxford Univ. Press
43. Livio M. 2002. *The Golden Ratio: The Story of Phi, The World's Most Astonishing Number.* New York: Random House
44. Mandelbrot BB. 1967. How long is the coast of Britain? Statistical self-similarity and fractional dimension. *Science* 156:636–38
45. Mandelbrot BB. 1982. *The Fractal Geometry of Nature*. San Francisco: WH Freeman. 460 pp.
46. Sander LM. 1987. Fractal Growth. *Sci. Am.* 256:94–100
47. Ben-Jacob E, Garik P. 1990. The formation of patterns in non-equilibrium growth. *Nature* 343:523–30
48. Peitgen H-O, Jürgens H, Saupe D. 1992. *Chaos and Fractals. New Frontiers of Science*. Berlin: Springer-Verlag. 984 pp.
49. Feder J. 1988. *Fractals*. New York: Plenum
50. Falconer K. 1997. *Techniques of Fractal Geometry*. New York: Wiley
51. Pietronero L, Erzan A, Evertsz C. 1988. Theory of Laplacian fractals: diffusion limited aggregation and dielectric breakdown model. *Physica A* 151:207–45
52. Vicsek T. 1992. *Fractal Growth Phenomena*. Singapore: World Sci. 488 pp. 2nd ed.
53. Landini G. 1996. Applications of fractal geometry in pathology. See Ref. 6, pp. 205–46
54. Bittner HR, Wlczek P, Sernetz M. 1989. Characterization of fractal biological objects by image analysis. *Acta Stereol.* 8:31–40
55. Bunde A, Havlin S, eds. 1991. *Fractals and Disordered Systems*. New York: Springer-Verlag
56. Weitz DA, Oliveria M. 1984. Fractal structures formed by kinetic aggregation of aqueous gold colloids. *Phys. Rev. Lett.* 52:1433–36
57. Witten TA, Sander LM. 1981. Diffusion-limited aggregation, a kinetic phenomena. *Phys. Rev. Lett.* 47:1400–3
58. Meakin P. 1986. A new model for biological pattern formation. *J. Theor. Biol.* 118:101–13
59. Ryan SJ. 1989. *Retina*. St. Louis: Mosby. Vols. 1, 2, 3

60. Hogan MJ, Alvarado JA, Weddel JE. 1971. *Histology of the Human Eye*. Philadelphia, PA: Saunders
61. Klein GJ, Baumgartner RH, Flower RW. 1990. An image processing approach to characterizing choroidal blood flow. *Invest. Ophthalmol.* 31:23–31
62. Lambrou GN. 1993. *Choroidal Plerometry: A Method for Evaluating the Choroidal Blood Supply in Clinical Practice*. The Hague: Kugler Publ.
63. Lutty GA, McLeod DS. 2003. Retinal vascular development and oxygen-induced retinopathy: a role for adenosine. *Prog. Retin. Eye Res.* 22:95–111
64. Gariano RF. 2002. Cellular mechanisms in retinal vascular development. *Prog. Retin. Eye Res.* 22:295–306
65. Ozanics V, Jakobiec FA. 1982. Prenatal development of the eye and its adnexa. In *Ocular Anatomy, Embryology and Teratology*, ed. FA Jakobiec, pp. 11–96. Philadelphia, PA: Harper Row
66. Kretzer FL, Hittner HM. 1988. Retinopathy of prematurity: clinical implications of retinal development. *Arch. Dis. Child.* 63:1151–67
67. Maxwell PH, Ratcliffe PJ. 2002. Oxygen sensors and angiogenesis. *Cell Develop. Biol.* 13:29–37
68. Masters BR, Platt DF. 1989. Development of human retinal vessels: a fractal analysis. *Invest. Ophthalmol. Vis. Sci.* 30:391 (Suppl.)
69. Family F, Masters BR, Platt DE. 1989. Fractal pattern formation in human retinal vessels. *Physica D* 38:98–103
70. Daxer A. 1993. Fractal analysis of new vessels in diabetic retinopathy. *Invest. Ophthalmol. Vis. Sci.* 34(Suppl.):718
71. Landini G, Misson GP, Murray P. 1993. Fractal analysis of the normal human retinal fluorescein angiogram. *Curr. Eye Res.* 12:23–27
72. Mainster MA. 1990. The fractal properties of retinal vessels: embryological and clinical implications. *Eye* 4:235–41
73. Masters BR, Sernetz M, Wlczek P. 1992. Image analysis of human retinal blood vessels and their characterization as fractals. *Acta Stereol.* 11(Suppl. 1):355–60
74. Masters BR. 1994. Fractal analysis of normal human retinal blood vessels. *Fractals* 2:103–10
75. Masters BR. 1991. Fractal patterns in the human retina and their physiological correlates. *Proc. SPIE* 1380:218–26
76. Fleury V, Schwartz L. 1999. Diffusion limited aggregation from shear stress as a simple model of vasculogenesis. *Fractals* 7:33–39
77. Fleury V, Schwartz L. 2000. Modelisation of 3-D microvasculature by interlaced diffusion limited aggregation. *Fractals* 8:255–59
78. Kyriacos S, Nekka F, Cartilier L, Vico P. 1997. Insights into the formation process of the retinal vasculature. *Fractals* 5:615–24
79. Sun T, Meakin P, Jossang T. 1995. Minimum energy dissipation and fractal structures of vascular systems. *Fractals* 3:123–53
80. Wong TY, Klein R, Klein BEK, Tielsch JM, Hubbard L, Nieto FJ. 2001. Retinal microvascular abnormalities and their relationship with hypertension, cardiovascular disease, and mortality. *Surv. Ophthalmol.* 46:59–80
81. Obert M. 1993. Numerical estimates of the fractal dimension D and the lacunarity L by the mass radius relation. *Fractals* 1:711–21
82. Landini G, Murray P, Misson GP. 1995. Local connected fractal dimensions and lacunarity analysis of 60° fluorescein angiograms. *Invest. Ophthalmol. Vis. Sci.* 36: 2749–55
83. Meinhardt H. 1982. *Models of Biological Pattern Formation*. London: Academic. 225 pp.
84. MacDonald N. 1983. *Trees and Networks in Biological Models*. New York: Wiley. 215 pp.
85. LaBarbera M. 1990. Principles of design of fluid transport systems in zoology. *Science* 249:992–1000

86. Murray CD. 1926. The physiological principle of minimum work. I. The vascular system and the cost of blood volume. *Proc. Natl. Acad. Sci.* USA. 12: 207–14
87. Murray CD. 1926. The physiological principle of minimum work applied to the angle of branching arteries. *J. Gen. Physiol.* 9: 835–41
88. Zamir M, Medeiros JS, Cunningham TK. 1979. Arterial bifurcations in the human retina. *J. Gen. Physiol.* 74:537–48
89. Zamir M. 2001. Fractal dimensions and multifractility in vascular branching. *J. Theor. Biol.* 212:183–90
90. Sherman TF, Popel AS, Koller A, Johnson PC. 1989. The cost of departure from optimal radii in microvascular networks. *J. Theor. Biol.* 136:245–65
91. Mayrovitz HN, Roy J. 1983. Microvascular blood flow: evidence indicating a cubic dependence on arteriolar diameter. *Am. J. Physiol. Heart Circ. Physiol.* 245(14):H1031–38
92. Zamir M, Medeiros JA, Cunningham TK. 1979. Arterial bifurcations in the human retina. *J. Gen. Physiol.* 74:537–48
93. Metzger RJ, Krasnow MA 1999. Genetic control of branching morphogenesis. *Science* 284:1635–39

Annu. Rev. Biomed. Eng. 2004. 6:453–95
doi: 10.1146/annurev.bioeng.5.040202.121601

First published online as a Review in Advance on April 2, 2004

# ADVANCES IN QUANTITATIVE ELECTROENCEPHALOGRAM ANALYSIS METHODS

Nitish V. Thakor and Shanbao Tong
*Biomedical Engineering Department, Johns Hopkins School of Medicine, Baltimore, MD 21205; email: nthakor@bme.jhu.edu, stong@bme.jhu.edu*

**Key Words** EEG analysis, signal processing, spectra, time-frequency analysis, entropy, complexity measure, information processing, fractal dimension applications

■ **Abstract** Quantitative electroencephalogram (qEEG) plays a significant role in EEG-based clinical diagnosis and studies of brain function. In past decades, various qEEG methods have been extensively studied. This article provides a detailed review of the advances in this field. qEEG methods are generally classified into linear and nonlinear approaches. The traditional qEEG approach is based on spectrum analysis, which hypothesizes that the EEG is a stationary process. EEG signals are nonstationary and nonlinear, especially in some pathological conditions. Various time-frequency representations and time-dependent measures have been proposed to address those transient and irregular events in EEG. With regard to the nonlinearity of EEG, higher order statistics and chaotic measures have been put forward. In characterizing the interactions across the cerebral cortex, an information theory-based measure such as mutual information is applied. To improve the spatial resolution, qEEG analysis has also been combined with medical imaging technology (e.g., CT, MR, and PET). With these advances, qEEG plays a very important role in basic research and clinical studies of brain injury, neurological disorders, epilepsy, sleep studies and consciousness, and brain function.

CONTENTS



1523-9829/04/0815-0453$14.00

## INTRODUCTION

Electroencephalogram (EEG) is a record of the electric activity from the scalp, obtained with the aid of an array of electrodes. After amplification, the signal is usually saved in graphic or digital format. EEG signals have been studied extensively since Dr. Hans Berger, a German neuro-psychiatrist, published the earliest research on human EEG in 1929 (1). It has been used as a clinical diagnostic and research tool ever since.

One of the most significant issues of EEG implementation is evaluating and quantifying the waves. The conventional clinical method of observing the waveform is thought to be subjective and laborious because the results depend on the technicians' experience and expertise. The development of quantitative EEG (qEEG) was motivated by the need for objective measures as well as some degree of automation. qEEG may also prove to be useful in understanding electrical brain activity and brain function. EEG analysis started from the long EEG recordings available since the end of the 1930s. Subsequent use of computers and digitization led to the evolution of qEEG methods. Before the 1980s, qEEG mainly consisted of frequency related analysis (2). Essentially, the signal was decomposed into its subband frequencies or the power spectrum was obtained. Since the 1990s, more novel techniques have been applied to EEG signal processing, including nonlinear and information theory-based methods (3–5). In this review, we outline the current methods in qEEG analysis and address the research issues.

Since its early use by Dr. Berger, EEG has been motivated by the need to study the mental (psychiatric) state and disease diagnosis. Before brain-imaging techniques became available, EEG was the main tool in this area. qEEG has been used in various applications:

1. Diagnosis of neural diseases: qEEG of various neural diseases, including Parkinson's (6), Alzheimer's (7–10), Wilson's (11–13), epilepsy (14–16), and brain tumors (17–21), have been studied to help diagnose and locate the focus of the seizures.
2. Neural functional and physiological evaluation: EEG has been accepted as a functional measure of the brain. qEEG helps to understand the electrophysiological and functional changes associated with mental and physiological states. qEEG analysis has been used to study different mental states, such as

relaxation/depression (22–25), attention (26, 27), anxiety (28), fatigue (29), and pain (30), and physiological states, such as sleep (31), arousal (32), and anesthesia (23–36).

3. Monitoring neurological injury: Detection and monitoring of brain injury is an important area of research. Nevertheless, there are currently no approved real-time approaches for detecting and monitoring such injury. qEEG analysis may provide a direct and noninvasive approach. EEG signals in the event of stroke (37–40), hypoxia-ischemia (41–43), trauma (44, 45), and coma (46) have been studied.
4. Combining EEG with brain imaging techniques: The EEG signal is limited by low spatial resolution, whereas the recent novel brain-imaging techniques, such as CT and MRI, can provide high spatial resolution. Thus, the combination of EEG and brain imaging techniques offers both high temporal and spatial resolutions (47–49).

# ELECTROENCEPHALOGRAM RECORDING AND PROPERTIES

## Physiological Basis of Electroencephalogram

EEG is the recording of the brain's electrical activity. Some of the activities recorded by scalp electrodes are generated by the action potentials of cortical neurons, but most are generated by excitatory postsynaptic potentials (50). Yet fine details about EEG generation are not fully understood. The EEG rhythms recorded on the scalp are the result of the summation effect of many excitatory and inhibitory postsynaptic potentials (EPSPs and IPSPs) produced in the pyramidal layer of the cerebral cortex. In humans, the thalamus is thought to be the main site of origin of EEG activities (Alpha and Beta bands) (2). Thalamic oscillations activate the firing of cortical neurons. The depolarization (mainly in layer IV) creates a dipole with negativity at layer IV and positivity at more superficial layers. The scalp electrodes will detect a small but perceptible far-field potential that represents the summed potential fluctuations (50). In clinical and experimental conditions, EEG is the recording of the potential difference between two electrodes (bipolar EEG) or one scalp electrode and the ear as the reference (unipolar EEG). Scalp electrodes cannot detect charges outside 6 $cm^2$ of the cortical surface area, and the effective recording depth is several millimeters.

The brain is an extremely complex system, constantly carrying out information transfer and processing. The neural system works through the interactions between large assemblies of neurons in the central nervous system (CNS) and the peripheral neural system. At the cellular level, neurons transfer and process the information via the action potentials and neural firing (also known as spikes). When this kind of electrical activity transfers to the surface of the cortex and to the surface of the scalp, we can record it as the EEG. One of the rationales for qEEG is that EEG signals originate in the brain and carry redundant physiological or pathological information inside the brain.

## Electroencephalogram Acquisition

To perform qEEG analysis, sensors, also known as electrodes, are positioned at standardized locations on the scalp. During the data acquisition phase of brain mapping, each electrode collects electrical signals from the CNS. The EEG recording system includes the (I) electrode and head stage, (II) preprocessing and quantitative EEG, and (III) data/results storage (Figure 1).

The early EEG recording systems were very large and cumbersome and could only be used in the EEG laboratory of a hospital. With the recent development of electronics and computer-aided instrumentation, there are more portable and powerful mini-systems for EEG recording and analysis.

1. Electrode: The EEG electrode is the electrical potential sensor. Electrodes are available in varied shapes and sizes depending on the task or experimental conditions, such as surface electrodes, needle electrodes, sphenoid electrodes, subdural strip electrodes, and depth electrodes. Currently, the

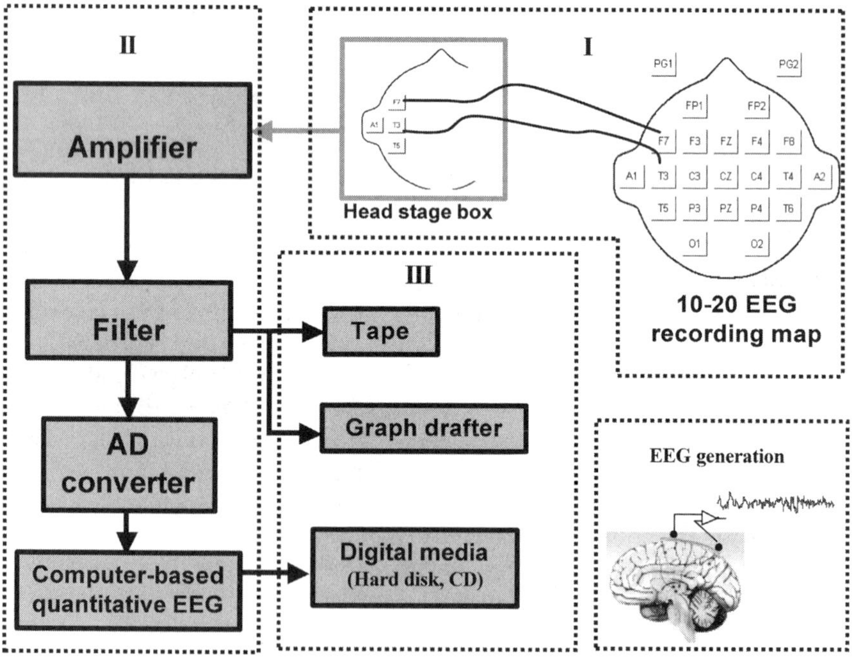


**Figure 1** Diagram of EEG recording and quantitative system: (I) Headstage and electrodes, (II) preprocessing and qEEG, and (III) data storage system. The right bottom box illustrates the principle of rhythmical scalp EEG activities.

most commonly used electrodes for routine clinical EEG are surface electrodes, which are affixed to the skin with gel. Various types of clinical and experimental EEG electrodes are shown in Reference 51.

2. Amplifier: The technique of EEG acquisition and amplification is very mature. The EEG signal bandwidth is 0.5–100 Hz in frequency (although the most interesting range components are below 30 Hz), and typical amplitudes are 10–300 $\mu$V. This requires an amplifier with specific features: good noise behavior, low leakage current, high CMRR (common mode rejection ratio), high input impedance, high PSRR (power supply rejection ratio), and high IMRR (isolation mode rejection ratio). For digitized EEG recording, the digital noise, sensitivity control, and filter cutoff frequency control should also be considered (52, 53).
3. Filtering: The routine EEG is usually sampled at a frequency of ~250 Hz, which theoretically covers the band of 0~125 Hz (in practice, the sampling rate may be quite a bit higher to obtain higher signal resolution). The EEG recording system may need a special filter to remove the power line artifacts (50 or 60 Hz). Because the EEG in different frequency bands [e.g., Delta (0.5–4 Hz), Theta (4–8 Hz), Alpha (8–12 Hz), Beta (12–30 Hz), and Gamma (>40 Hz)] is often of interest, then either analog or digital filters are provided by the EEG system. Many EEG recording systems provide the digital filter in their accompanying utility software.
4. Storage: Originally, the EEG was recorded with writing ink on a paper or saved on an analog tape. This type of storage has almost completely been taken over by computer-based data analysis, display, and storage. The analog EEG signal is converted to digital values by an analog-digital converter (ADC) device and saved in digital media, such as hard disks or compact discs. The digital storage is more convenient for computer-based qEEG analysis and subsequent archiving and retrieving.

## Electroencephalogram Properties

The properties of the EEG signal can be described as complex. The EEG complexity originates in the intricate neural system. Traditionally, the spontaneous EEG is characterized as a linear stochastic process with great similarities to noise. From the signal processing view, EEG has the following properties: (*a*) Noisy and pseudo-stochastic: The EEG is often between 10~300 $\mu$V, which is easily affected by various physiological and electrical noises. Meanwhile, artifacts from electrocardiogram (ECG), electrooculogram (EOG), electromyogram (EMG), and recording systems can also contaminate the signals. Even the EEG shows a high degree of randomness and nonstationarity. (*b*) Time-varying and nonstationary: EEG is not a stationary process; it varies with the physiological states. The waveforms may include a complex of regular sinusoidal waves, irregular spikes/polyspikes, or spindles/polyspindles. In most pathological conditions, such as epileptic seizures, the EEG may show evident singularity or nonstationarity. In practice, we regard

EEG as a stationary process over a relatively short period (~3.5 s for routine spontaneous EEG) (54). (*c*) High nonlinearity: Although the traditional linear models of EEG still play significant roles in EEG analysis and diagnosis, EEG is a nonlinear process (55). This kind of nonlinearity is also time-, state-, and site-dependent (56).

## Electroencephalogram Preprocessing

Because of experimental methods commonly adopted in laboratories, the raw data of the EEG signals are usually contaminated with various sources of noise and artifacts. The preprocessing of EEG deals mainly with these artifacts and interferences. The neural activity is at the level of 10 to 100 $\mu$V; thus, it is easily affected by various external and internal factors. The common artifacts include (*a*) movements from patients or animals during recording, such as blinking or jaw, tongue, or body/head movement; (*b*) the muscle artifacts; and (*c*) pulse wave or heart beat, usually appearing when wide interelectrode distance or the electrode pairs with the ear as the reference are used. Interferences include the power line (50/60 Hz), TV stations, radio pager, telephone ring, or cardiac pacemakers, which usually can be avoided by a notch filter and by properly grounding and shielding the recording system.

Most of the above artifacts are easy to recognize and can usually be removed by filtering. Nevertheless, some artifacts, such as EOG [in the rapid eye movement (REM) period of sleep study] and ECG, are present consistently and are difficult to reject. The removal of EOG and ECG artifacts is important because they overlap in amplitude and spectrum of EEG and sometimes interfere with qEEG analysis or diagnosis. In some pathological conditions, such as ischemia, when the EEG is weak, the ECG influence in EEG cannot be ignored. The normal ECG rhythm of a human is approximately 1~1.5 Hz oscillations; its second-order harmonics (2~3.0 Hz) are within the delta band. Therefore, for clinical EEG, the ECG artifact has little effect on the main spectrum of the EEG. In experimental studies with small animals, however, the heart rate is always much higher. The normal sinus rhythm of a rat is approximately 360 beats/min (~6 Hz). In addition, in small animals, the heart is close to the brain, and hence the ECG is more likely to affect the EEG. Our experiments on brain injury following cardiac arrest show evident ECG artifacts during the ischemia period and early recovery period. Either improved design and placement of the electrodes or some signal processing methods are needed to remove the ECG.

Recently, some novel methods have been proposed to remove the ECG or EOG/EMG artifact. We have applied the method of independent component analysis (ICA) to reject the ECG artifacts (57). The EEG contaminated with ECG artifacts is input to ICA, which separates the EEG and ECG components. Setting the ECG component to zero and multiplying the mixture matrix can remove the ECG artifacts. Figure 2 shows the EEG waveforms and spectrum before and after ICA.

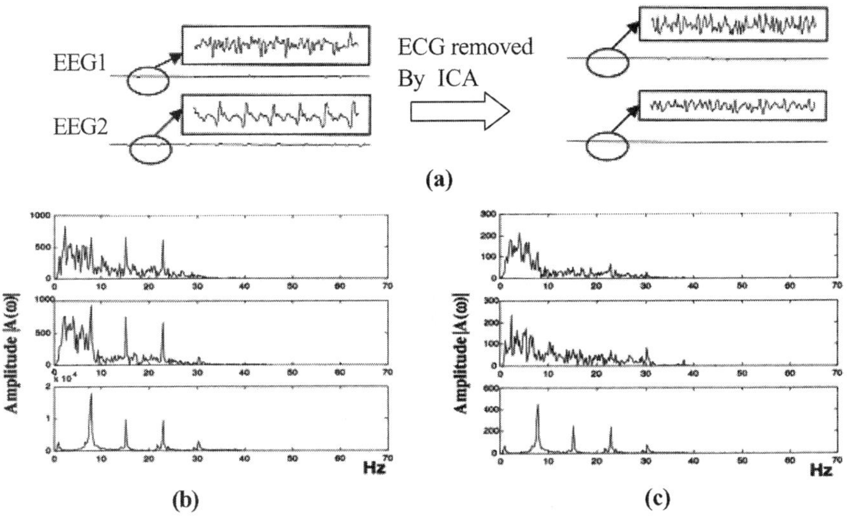


**Figure 2** Independent component analysis (ICA)–based ECG artifact removal from EEG signals. (*a*) Two segment EEG signals selected from the early recovery period of hypoxic-ischemic brain injury before and after ICA. (*b*) The EEG spectral traces before ICA and (*c*) after ICA. The bottom traces in (*b*) and (*c*) correspond to the ECG spectra. The interference of ECG is evident. After removal with ICA, the EEG is improved as seen clearly in the spectra (adapted from 57).

This method has also been applied to remove the EOG artifact (58) and other noise in the EEG (59).

After removing and depressing the artifacts and noise, the qEEG methods are further developed to analyze the signals. The traditional qEEG employs linear analysis methods. Recently, various nonlinear approaches have been introduced. And with the increased interest in brain imaging and function mapping, new areas of qEEG, such as information theoretic analysis, and combination of fMRI and qEEG have been developed (see Summary and Future Directions, below).

# LINEAR METHODS

## Time Domain Methods

Time domain methods usually try to model a time series of EEG signals with a specific mathematical expression. Two different EEG modeling methods have classically been used: parametric modeling and nonparameteric methods.

PARAMETRIC MODELING METHODS Parametric modeling preassumes that the EEG signals are created with equations, with unknown coefficients to be approximated, whereas the nonparametric methods study the features of EEG waveforms directly.

*Autoregressive model* The parametric modeling method fits the EEG with a mathematical model. The most popular one is the autoregressive (AR) model. Although the EEG signal is considered to be time varying and nonstationary, a short EEG segment can still be approximately considered as a stationary process, which can then be characterized by an AR model. The model parameters could be used to distinguish the EEG states. The method represents the EEG series with a $p$-order AR model:

$$x(n) = a_1 x(n-1) + a_2 x(n-2) + \cdots + a_p x(n-p) + w(n), \tag{1}$$

where $x(n)$ is the EEG signal, $\{a_i\}$ are AR parameters, $p$ is the order of the model, and $w(n)$ is white noise with a flat spectrum.

Two issues have to be determined before carrying out AR modeling: (*a*) The selection of the model order $p$. This is the central issue of AR modeling. A low $p$ value will result in oversmoothed spectra, but a high $p$ value may introduce false peaks in the spectrum (60). The criterion of $p$ is based on "goodness of fit." One popular criterion is the Akaike information criterion (AIC):

$$AIC(p) = N \log(Rp) + 2p \tag{2a}$$

$Rp$ is the error variance for model with order $p$. The optimal $p$ is the one that minimizes AIC($p$). Another criterion is by minimum description length (MDL), which is defined as

$$MDL(p) = N \log(Rp) + p \log(N). \tag{2b}$$

(*b*) The length of selected EEG: $N$. The choice of $x(n)$ length $N$ is optimized to minimize the error $Rp$. For the rat EEG, during normal baseline recording, the length of $x(n)$ is approximately 3.3 s (54, 61).

*Sinusoidal model* The sinusoidal model of EEG uses sinusoidal basis functions to represent the signal. The EEG signal is supposed to consist of a series of sinusoidal waves. The task of such modeling is to find the optimal coefficients of each sinusoidal function (Figure 3).

One of the classical sinusoidal model analyses is Fourier transform (FT), which represents the EEG with a series of harmonic waves:

$$\begin{cases} x(n) = \dfrac{1}{N} \displaystyle\sum_{k=1}^{N-1} (X_r(k)\sin(n\Omega_0 k) + jX_i(k)\cos(n\Omega_0 k)) \\ \Omega_0 = 2\pi/N \end{cases} . \tag{3}$$

The Fourier coefficients $X(k)$ indicate the strength of the signal at frequency. FT is the basis of spectral analysis, which is reviewed in the next section.

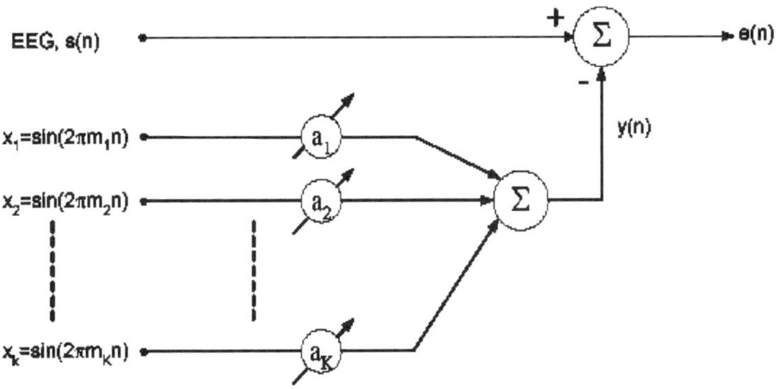


**Figure 3** Block diagram of the sinusoidal model of EEG. The EEG is supposed to be represented with a series of sinusoidal functions: $s(n) = \sum_{i=1}^{n} a_i \sin(2\pi m_i n)$. The coefficients may be adaptively obtained (adapted from 62).

Another sinusoidal model of EEG uses the Markov process proposed by Al-Nashash et al. (62), which simulates the stationary EEG with k-sinusoidal oscillations:

$$x(n) = \sum_{j=1}^{k} a_j(n) \sin(2\pi m_j n + \phi_j), \tag{4}$$

where $a_j(n)$ is the model amplitude, $m_j$ is the average $j^{th}$ frequency, $\phi_j$ is the initial phase, and $n$ is the time index. The $a_j(n)$ is estimated with a first-order Markov process:

$$a_j(n+1) = \gamma_j a_j(n) + \lambda_j(n)\xi_j(n). \tag{5}$$

The coefficients $\lambda_j(n)$ and $\xi_j(n)$ are estimated with the help of the least mean square (LMS) algorithm (62). This model can be used to simulate EEG in different conditions. Figure 4 illustrates a typical segment of EEG and its power spectral density (PSD), which matches well with the PSD of the EEG simulated by the sinusoidal model.

NONPARAMETRIC METHODS The nonparametric model independent methods study the waveforms directly. A coarse clinical evaluation is done by detecting amplitude change. The EEG is loosely described as low ($<20\ \mu$V), medium ($20\sim 50\ \mu$V), and high ($>50\ \mu$V) EEG. In some studies, the amplitude change is a significant feature. For example, in the study of animals with hypoxic-ischemic injury, the global amplitude changes with the different level of ischemia. As a result of the global injury, the EEG ceases. As the brain recovers, the amplitude also gradually returns to the normal level. In addition to the amplitude, another direct measure of the waveform is the energy change. By using a short time window, energy measurement can catch the strength change inside the signal. One of the

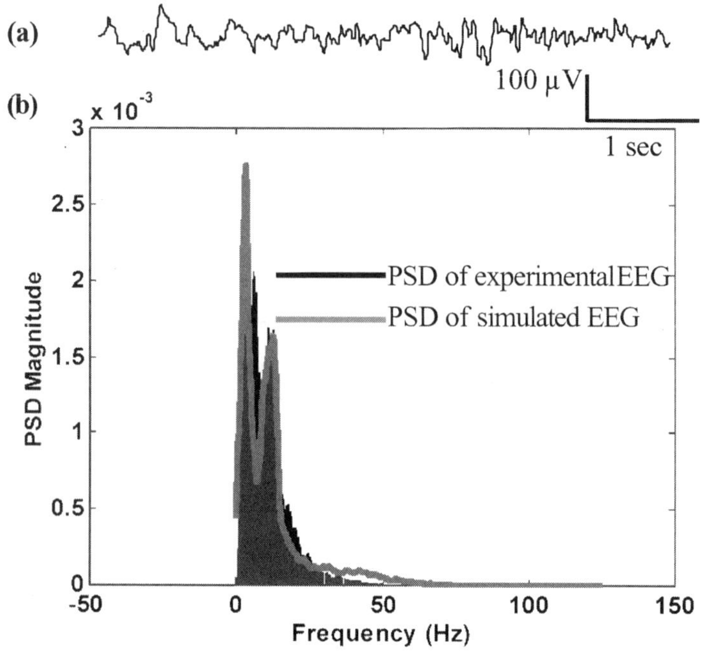


**Figure 4** (*a*) A typical baseline rat EEG segment, and (*b*) its power spectral density (PSD). The gray line corresponds to the PSD of the simulated EEG by the sinusoidal model, whereas the black line corresponds to the PSD of the experimental signal (adapted from 62).

energy measures, known as the teager energy operator (TEO) (63), has successfully described the abrupt energy change in the signals. The discrete-time TEO is defined as

$$\psi(n) = x^2(n) - x(n-1)x(n+1). \tag{6}$$

TEO is an approximation of the signal's energy, which depends on the frequency, and high frequencies are emphasized.

The amplitude of the routine EEG does not carry much information, however, because the amplitudes for different subjects may vary and may also be affected by the contact, location, or spacing of the electrodes. Another time approach is to evaluate the pattern complexity of the EEG waves. The Lempel-Ziv (L-Z) sequence complexity measure (64, 65) has been successfully applied to study the complexity of pattern in the EEG (66–68). The signal was first converted into a simple binary 0/1 sequence; a pattern-matching operation was then conducted to scan the sequence to find the new pattern. The number of different patterns is defined as the L-Z complexity. Zhang et al. (66, 67) have found that for different levels of anesthesia, the L-Z complexity is different. For example, under deep anesthesia, the EEG becomes simple (66, 67).

## Frequency Analysis

EEG frequency analysis usually means power spectral analysis, which was one of the first applications of qEEG analysis. The basic idea is to study the EEG in several classic nonoverlapping frequency bands: Delta wave (0.5∼4 Hz), Theta wave (4–8 Hz), Alpha wave (8–12 Hz), Beta1 (12∼18 Hz), and Beta2 (18∼30 Hz). Sometimes gamma bands (>30 Hz) are also studied in event-related and cognitive brain research (69, 70). The clinical technician interprets the EEG by the features or magnitudes of waves in each frequency band. Spectral analysis has been used for decades as the most important diagnostic tool. Even though the physicians do not calculate the spectrum, they usually focus on some specific wave rhythms (frequency components). The spectra can be estimated by the following methods.

MODEL FREE ESTIMATION The direct estimation of PSD is also called fast Fourier transform (FFT) and is the commonly used spectral estimation method (71). FFT is the fast algorithm of the discrete Fourier transform (DFT), which is defined as

$$X(k) = \frac{1}{N}\sum_{n=1}^{N} x(n)e^{-j2\pi nk/N}. \tag{7}$$

The power spectrum is obtained with

$$\|X(k)\|^2 = P(k). \tag{8}$$

FFT-based spectral estimation assumes that the signal is stationary and slowly varying. This kind of spectrum estimation has some drawbacks and limitations with respect to its resolution and leakage (or aliasing) effects (72). If the function to be transformed is not harmonically related to the sampling frequency, the response of an FFT looks like a *sinc* function (although the integrated power is still correct). Spectral leakage can be reduced by using a tapering function (such as gabor, hanning window, and others) or multitaper method (73, 74). Nevertheless, reduction of spectral leakage is at the expense of broadening the spectral response.

PARAMETRIC MODEL-BASED ESTIMATION The EEG series is represented with an AR model as in Equation 1, which can be rewritten as

$$w(n) = x(n) - a_1x(n-1) - a_2x(n-2) - \cdots - a_px(n-p). \tag{9}$$

Taking the $z$-transform yields

$$W(Z) = A(Z)X(Z). \tag{10}$$

Where $A(z) = 1 - \sum_{i=1}^{p} a_i z^{-i}$, then

$$X(Z) = A^{-1}(Z)W(Z). \tag{11}$$

If the $W$(Z) is a white noise input sequence, then its spectrum $W(\omega)$ will be flat. In practice, however, we can only approximately simulate white noise, so the

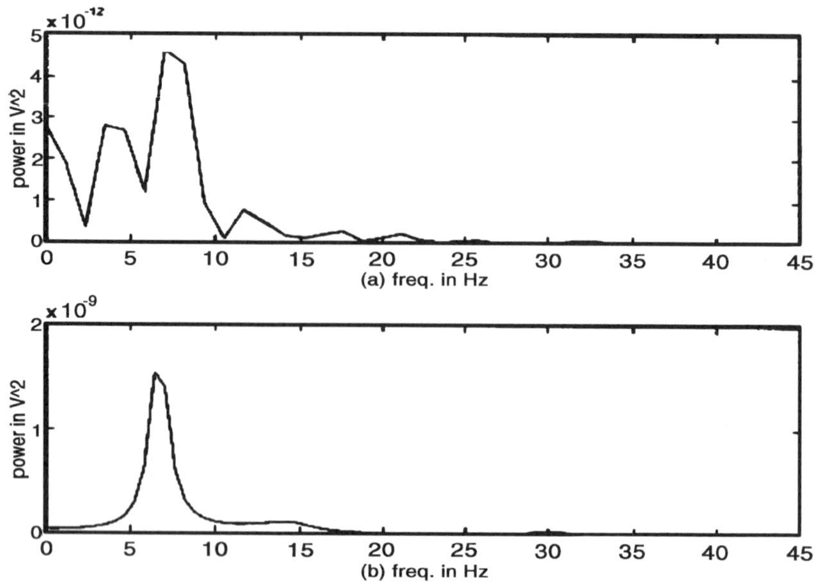


**Figure 5** Power spectra of a 150-point segment of baseline EEG waveform after filtering it with a low-frequency cutoff at 1 Hz and a high-frequency cutoff at 35 Hz: (*a*) spectrum using the FFT showing large components below 1 Hz owing to possible leakage effects; (*b*) spectrum using a tenth-order AR model (adapted from 72).

approximate estimation of spectrum $X(\omega)$ of $x(n)$ can be obtained by setting $z = e^{j\omega}$:

$$\bar{X}(\omega) = \frac{W(\omega)T}{\left|1 - \sum_{i=1}^{p} a_i e^{-j\omega T}\right|^2}, \tag{12}$$

where $T$ is the sampling frequency. The AR model-based methods include Burg's method, covariance method, modified covariance method, and Yule-Walker's method (60).

Compared to the periodogram method (FFT), AR-based estimation has a very significant improvement in frequency resolution (60). Figure 5 shows the power spectra of a segment of baseline rat EEG by FFT and AR modeling, which illustrates the advantages of AR model-based power spectrum in decreasing the leakage under 1 Hz.

SPECTRAL DISTANCE AND CEPSTRAL DISTANCE An important clinical problem is to determine the changes in EEG owing to injury or disease. For example, after ischemic brain injury, what is the quantitative change as compared with normal baseline? A series of AR model-based distance metrics can be defined to evaluate the EEG following injury or diseases. There are two distance measures, spectral distance (SD) and cepstral distance (CD), both of which have been applied to qEEG analysis.

AR-based SD measure (ARSD) is defined with the help of a spectrum obtained through Equation 12 by measuring the difference between two AR spectra, $X_t(\omega)$ and $X_r(\omega)$ (75):

$$ARSD(X_t, X_r) = \left\{ \frac{1}{L} \sum_{l=0}^{L-1} |X_t(j\Omega_l) - X_r(j\Omega_l)|^p \right\}^{1/p}, \tag{13}$$

where $\Omega_L = \pi l/L$ for $l = 0, 1, \ldots L - 1$.

CD is calculated from the first $p$ cepstral coefficients of the corresponding EEG and the reference EEG (usually the baseline EEG is chosen). The evaluation of CD is illustrated by the diagram in Figure 6.

CD calculates the difference of primary cepstral coefficients (first $p$-order) between a baseline and other states. In an experimental study of global ischemic brain injury in rodents, Geocadin et al. (61) found that the CD increases during the injury and correlates with the injury level. The CD of the EEG increases clearly during the injury period (Figure 7).

DOMINANT FREQUENCIES The peaks in the EEG spectrum, also called dominant frequencies, are usually of interest in qEEG analysis. The AR power spectrum can be written as

$$\bar{X}(\omega) = \frac{W(\omega)T}{\left| \prod_{k=1}^{p} \left(e^{-j\omega T} - P_k\right) \right|^2} \tag{14}$$

where $\{P_k\}$ are the complex poles of $\bar{X}(\omega)$. Therefore, at the frequencies satisfying $e^{-j\omega_k T} = P_k$, there are corresponding peaks in the spectrum. Therefore, the dominant frequencies can be obtained by

$$F_{dominant} = \frac{F_{sampling}}{2\pi} \cdot \omega_k. \tag{15}$$

The dominant frequency analysis extracts the power around the dominant frequency peaks $F_{dominant}$. Goel et al. (54) studied the power trend of the first three dominant frequencies of EEG after global ischemic brain injury (Figure 8). They found that the hypoxic-ischemic brain injury caused an increase of power in medium-high dominant frequency activity but a decrease in lower dominant frequency power over the course of hypoxia. These trends in dominant frequencies were shown to correlate with neurological deficits.

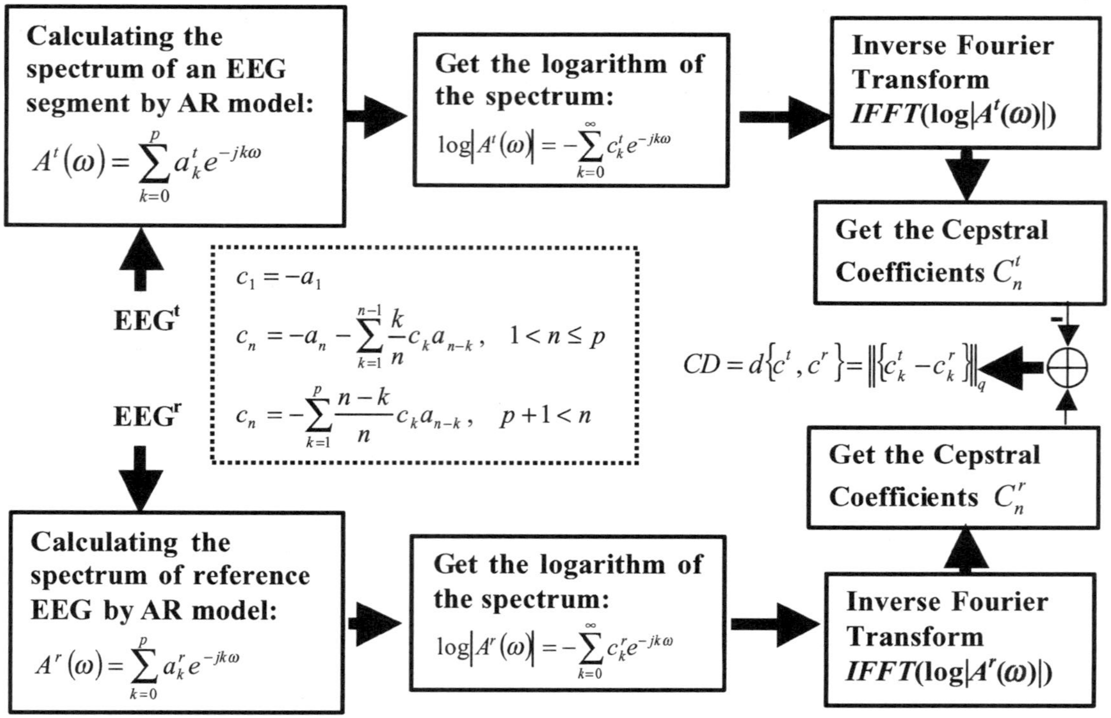


**Figure 6** Diagram of the cepstral distance (CD) evaluation. The cepstral coefficients of both EEG segments at time *t* (EEG$^t$) and baseline (EEG$^r$) are calculated. The CD is defined as the distance between their cepstral coefficients.

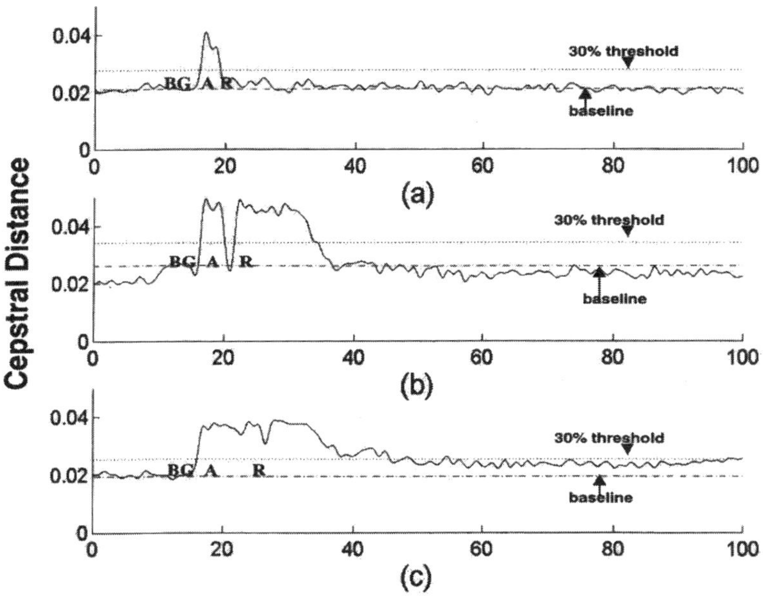


**Figure 7** Cepstral distance (CD) between reference EEG (baseline) and current EEG signals at various stages of the experiment. Wistar rats (n = 5/group) were anesthetized and subjected to global ischemia. Baseline recording of 10 min was followed by a 5-min washout to ensure the halothane did not have a significant effect on EEG. The durations of ischemia are indicated as (*a*) 1 min, (*b*) 5 min, and (*c*) 7 min. The different phases of the experiment are as follows: (*B*) baseline phase, (*G*) gas washout phase, (*A*) ischemic injury, and (*R*) start of resuscitation. The dashed line shows the 30% maximum CD value used as an ischemic injury indicator (adapted from 61).

## Time-Frequency Analysis

Time-domain analysis does not provide any frequency information. When signals such as EEG are time varying, the spectral analysis can provide the frequency details, but unfortunately, we do not know at what times the frequency changes occur. As described above, the EEG signal is dynamic, time varying, sometimes transient (spikes/bursts), mostly nonstationary, and usually corrupted by noise. In practice, we not only need to know the frequency components but we also want to know the time relation. Time-frequency analysis is especially suitable for addressing such problems (76). Time-frequency analysis has been successfully used to analyze the epileptic EEG (77) and electrocorticograms (ECoG) (78, 79) to locate the seizure source. The simplest method uses a short time FT (STFT) to increase the time resolution:

$$STFT(\omega, t) = \int_{-\infty}^{\infty} x(\tau)g(\tau - t)e^{-j\omega\tau}\,d\tau, \tag{16}$$

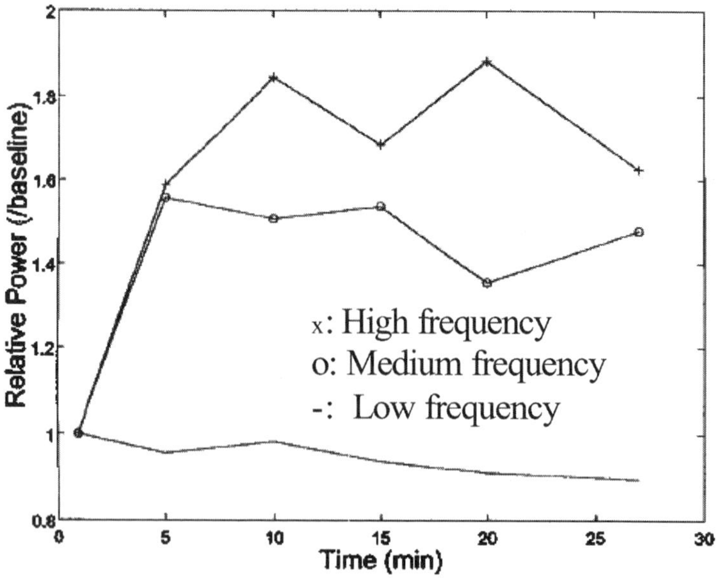


**Figure 8** Power trend of the three dominant frequency components during 30 min of hypoxia (10% oxygen) for a typical animal. The EEG was recorded from a neonatal piglet (adapted from 64).

where $g(t)$ is the window function. Equation 16 is also called Gabor transform. The FFT-based time-dependent spectrum is also called a spectrogram.

The spectrogram, however, has some pitfalls. STFT is based on FFT such that its time resolution cannot be high, and also there is bias at the boundaries. A high time and frequency resolution can be obtained through Wigner-Ville distribution (WVD):

$$Wx(\omega, t) = \int x\left(t + \frac{\tau}{2}\right)x^*\left(t - \frac{\tau}{2}\right)e^{-j\omega\tau}\,d\tau. \tag{17}$$

$Wx(\omega, t)$ is the FT of the autocorrelation function of signal $x(t)$ with respect to the delay variable. It can also be thought of as an STFT where the windowing function is a time-scaled, time-reversed copy of the original signal. In general, it has much better time and frequency resolution than does the STFT. Nevertheless, WVD has notable limitations: cross-term calculations may give rise to negative energy and the aliasing effect may distort the spectrum such that a high-frequency component may be misidentified as a low-frequency component.

The second pitfall of STFT is the fixed time and frequency resolutions. By the uncertainty principle, the product of the time uncertainty and frequency uncertainty is larger than a constant. In signal processing, we usually need more time accuracy in locating the transient waves (high frequency). For a slow waveform, we may be more interested in the frequency resolution. Such an analysis needs an

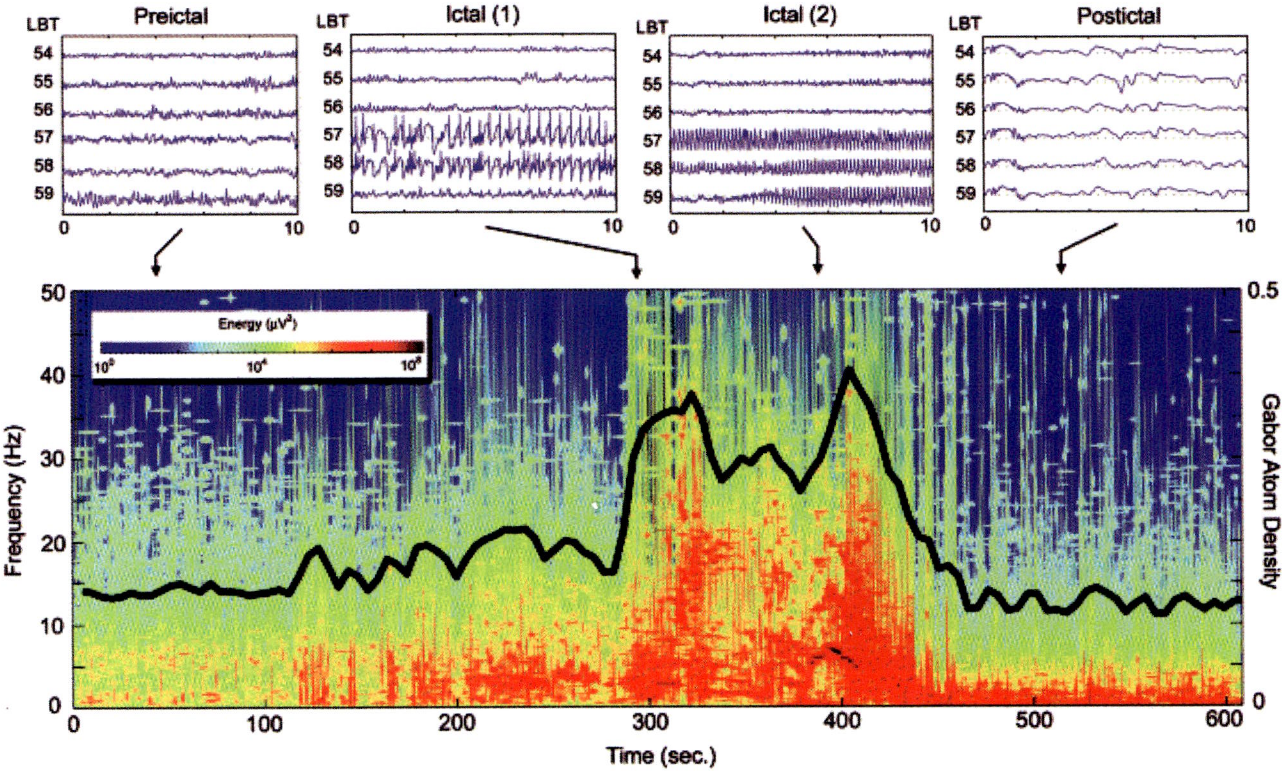


**Figure 10** Upper panels: EEG traces for four different periods (interictal, ictal 1 early in seizure, ictal 2 later in seizure, and postictal). Lower panel: color-coded time-frequency energy plot of the signal obtained by reconstruction of the atoms (*red*: high energy, *blue*: low energy). Energy scale is logarithmic. Superimposed over this plot is the corresponding Gabor atom density (GAD) (black trace) (adapted from 87).

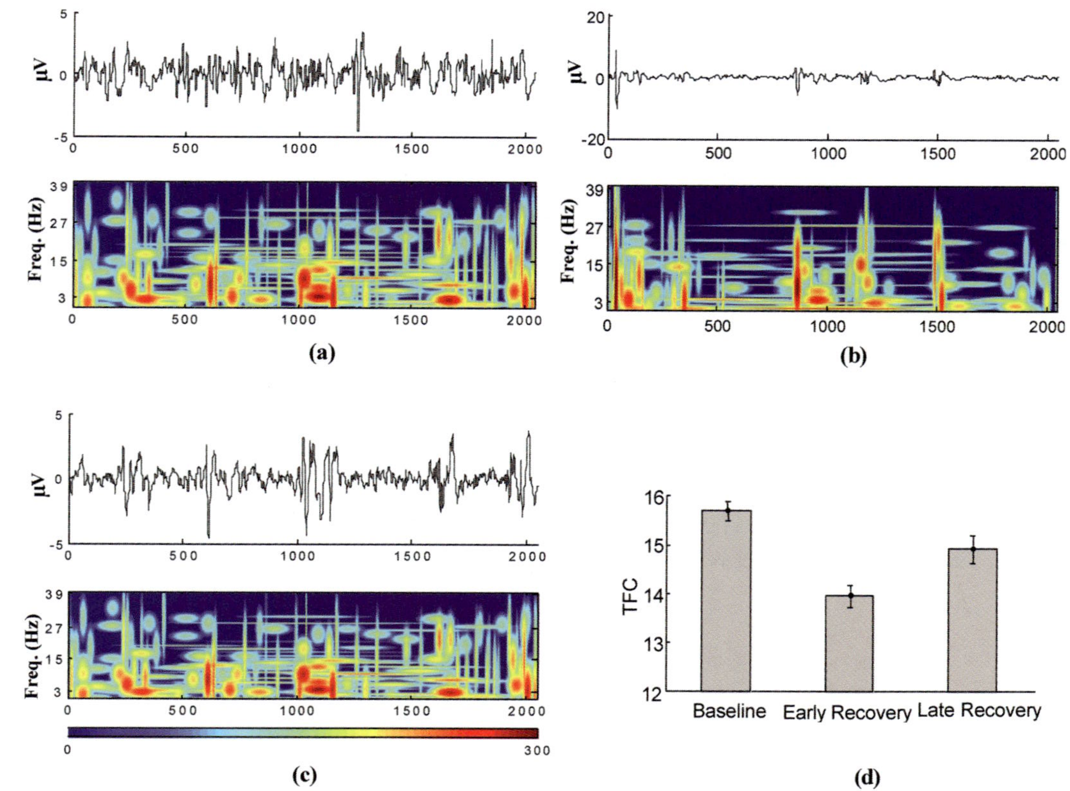


**Figure 15** Matching pursuits (MP)-based time-frequency representation (TFR) and time-frequency complexity (TFC) of EEG signals following 5 min of hypoxic-ischemic brain injury. (*a–c*): baseline, early recovery (30 min after CPR), and late recovery (2 h after CPR) EEG segments and its MP-based TFR; (*d*) TFC measures.

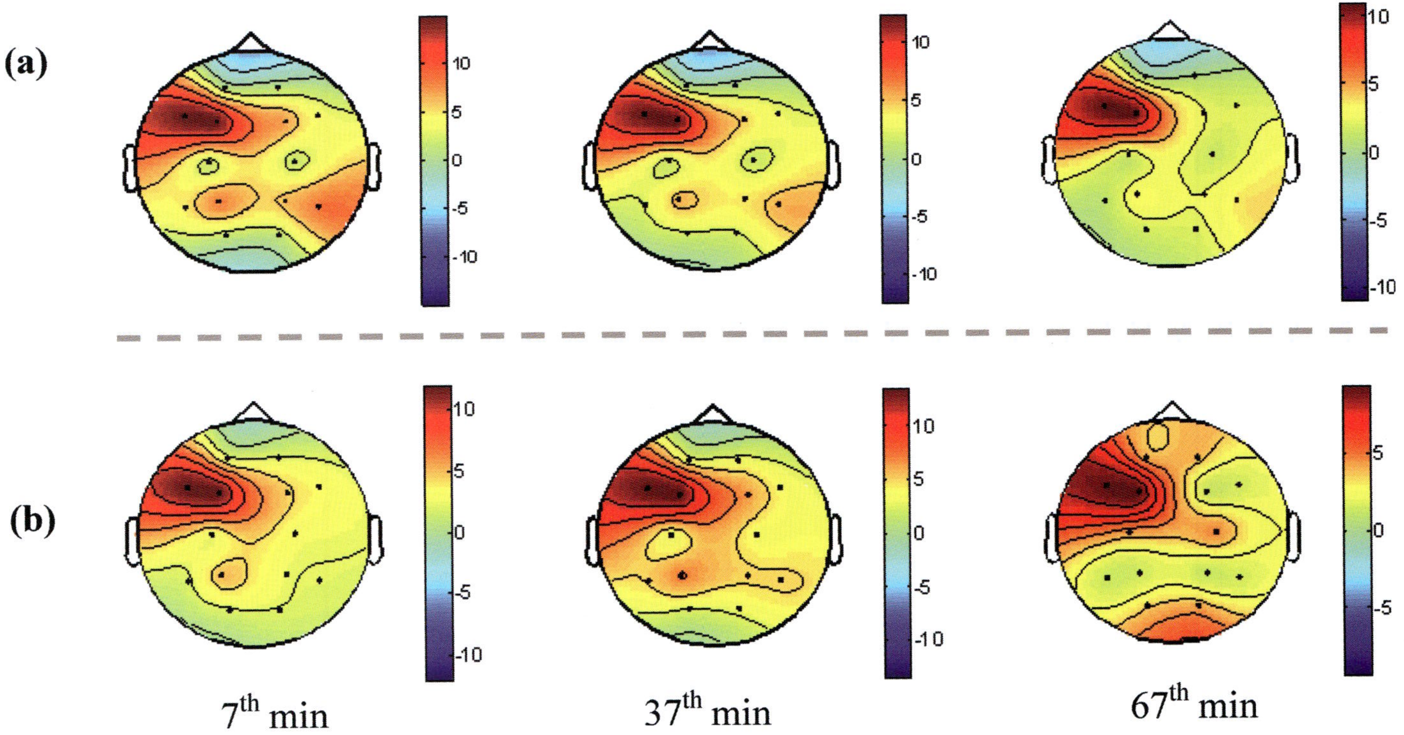


**Figure 16** Local flow of information (LFI) at different times after severe cardiac arrest. (*a*) 4-min cardiac arrest, 5-min CPR. (*b*) 20-min cardiac arrest, 30-min CPR. The start time for recording the EEG signals is 1 h after the cardiac arrest.

adaptive time-frequency analysis method. The wavelet transform (WT) is such a tool. By using a scalable function instead of the fixed-scale window function in Equation 16, the wavelet transform is defined as

$$Wx(a, b) = |a|^{-1/2} \int_{-\infty}^{\infty} x(t)\varphi\left(\frac{t-b}{a}\right)dt, \tag{18}$$

where $a$ and $b$ are the scaling and transiting parameters, respectively, and $\varphi$ is the mother wavelet function. For more methods of time-frequency distribution, refer to the software package available at http://crttsn.univ-nantes.fr/~auger/tftbtest.html (80).

Figure 9 is an illustration of the continuous WT (CWT)-based time-frequency analysis of the EEG signals recorded during the experimental studies of global

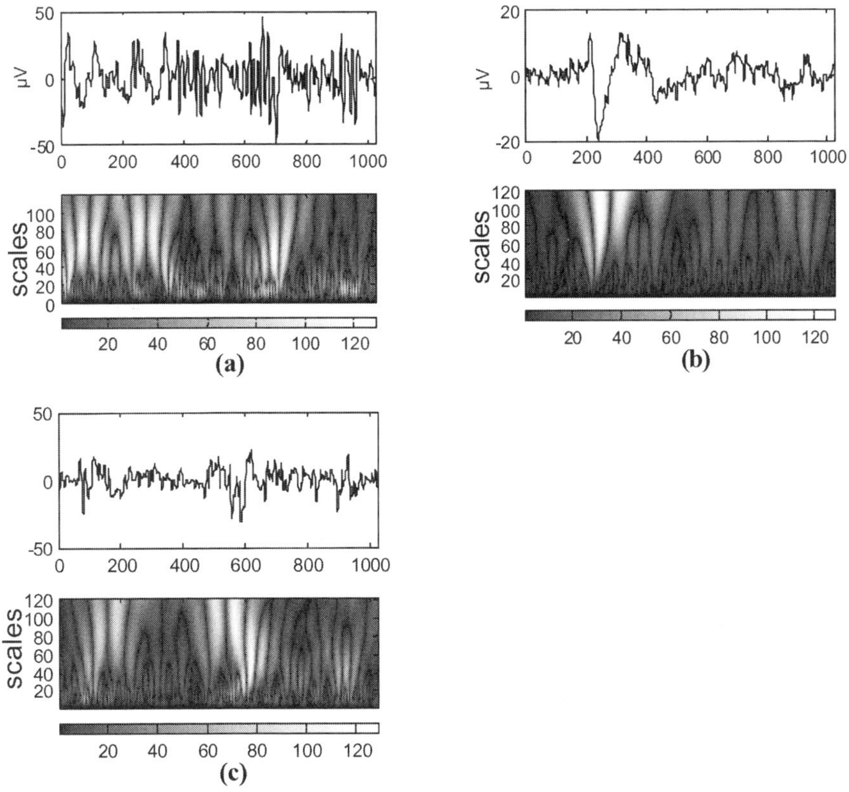


**Figure 9** Continuous wavelet transform (CWT)-based time-frequency representation of four-sec EEG signals at (*a*) baseline, (*b*) early hypoxic-ischemic injury recovery, and (*c*) later recovery. The CWT spectrum shows even spreading on the time-frequency plane for the baseline EEG, whereas there is highlighted area around the spikes during the postinjury recovery. The nonstationary time-frequency properties are clearly shown.

hypoxic-ischemic brain injury in rodents. The figures show the absolute values of the CWT coefficients for scale $a$ changing from 1 to 122. The fourth-order symlet wavelet is applied. The time-frequency map clearly indicates the changes caused by the spiking activities. The spiking activities correspond to larger coefficients in a broader frequency range (scale).

A new high-resolution time-frequency analysis based on matching pursuits (MPs) decomposition has recently been applied to analyze the EEG signals (81–84). MP was first proposed by Mallat & Zhang (85) to decompose a signal into a group of the atoms scaled, transmitted from a basis function. The idea of the MP algorithm is to use a redundant dictionary of atom functions for optimally matching the signal. The matching process involves the inner production between atom functions and the signal, so as to get the most coherent structure.

The basic procedure of the MP algorithm is as follows: First, a set of normalized functions (atom dictionary) is defined:

$$\begin{cases} D = \{g_1(t), g_2(t), \ldots, g_n\} \\ \|g_i\| = 1 \quad for \quad \forall g_i \in D \end{cases}. \tag{19}$$

Usually, the set $D$ is obtained by scaling, translating, and modulating a basis function $g(t)$ (as "mother wavelet" in wavelet decomposition):

$$g_i(t) = g_{\gamma_i}(t) = \frac{1}{\sqrt{s}} g\left(\frac{t-u}{s}\right) e^{i\xi t}, \tag{20}$$

where $\gamma_i = \{s_i, u_i, \xi_i\}$ corresponds to the parameters of scaling, translating, and modulating. $1/\sqrt{s}$ is used to normalize the atom. Each $\gamma_i$ determines one atom or structure pattern in $D$. The LastWave software offers approximately ten different types of atom windows (either blackman, hamming, hanning, gauss, spline0 (rectangular), spline1 (triangle), spline2, spline3, exponential, or FoF) (86). The MP's iterative decomposition is

$$\begin{cases} R^0 f = f \\ R^i f = \langle R^i f, g_{\gamma_i} \rangle g_{\gamma_i} + R^{i+1} f \\ g_{\gamma_i} = \arg\max_{g_{\gamma_i} \in D} |\langle R^i f, g_{\gamma_i} \rangle|, \end{cases} \tag{21}$$

where $\langle \bullet \rangle$ defines the inner product in Hilbert space $[\langle f, g \rangle = \int_{-\infty}^{+\infty} f(t)\bar{g}(t)dt]$. The iteration is convergent (85). For a signal with a simple structure, we need fewer atoms. Otherwise, for decomposing a complex structural signal, we need more atoms to reconstruct to the same level of energy. After $m$ iterations, the signal $f$ is decomposed into a linear expansion of $m$ atom functions with a residual error $R^m f$:

$$\begin{cases} f = \sum_{i=0}^{m-1} c_i g_{\gamma_i} + R^m f \\ c_i = \langle R^i f, g_{\gamma_i} \rangle \end{cases}. \tag{22}$$

We estimate the Wigner distribution of the approximate signal $f_{0.99}$ with linear atomic expansion in Equation 22. The basic cross Wigner distribution of two functions $f(t)$ and $g(t)$ is defined as

$$W[f_1, f_2](t, \omega) = \frac{1}{2\pi} \int_{-\infty}^{\infty} f_1(t + \tau/2) \bar{f}_2(t - \tau/2) e^{-j\omega\tau} d\tau. \tag{23}$$

By defining the $f_1(t) = f_2(t)$ and applying Equation 23 to Equation 22, we get the Wigner distribution of MP decomposition:

$$Wf(t, \omega) = \sum_{0}^{m_{0.99}-1} \|c_i\|^2 W g_{\gamma_i}(t, \omega) + \sum_{j=0}^{m_{0.99}-1} \sum_{k=0, k \neq j}^{m_{0.99}-1} c_j \cdot \bar{c}_k \cdot W[g_{\gamma_j} g_{\gamma_k}](t, \omega), \tag{24}$$

where $c_i$ is the coefficient shown in Equation 22. We throw away the second cross terms to get a clear picture of the time-frequency energy distribution of *f*:

$$Ef(t, \omega) \approx \sum_{0}^{m_{0.99}-1} \|c_i\|^2 W g_{\gamma_i}(t, \omega). \tag{25}$$

Jouny et al. (87) applied MP-based high-resolution time-frequency analysis to the detection of epileptic seizures (Figure 10, see color insert). The Gabor atom density (GAD) is extracted as a detector of seizure. During the preictal period, the GAD gradually increases and reaches the highest value with seizure bursts, and it returns to low level in the postictal phase.

GAD analyzes rapid, dynamically changing electroencephalographic manifestations of epileptic seizures. This method considers both temporal and spectral information of the signal. Compared with other methods, MP decomposition-based GAD gives a reliable signature of the intractable complex partial seizures (CPS).

# NONLINEAR METHODS

## Information Theory-Based Analysis

The distribution of the EEG signals is close to a random process. A series of statistical measures have been developed to evaluate the EEG signals in different domains, including time, frequency, or time-frequency. One measure calculates the information (entropy) of EEG signals in these three domains. Entropy is a method to quantify the order/disorder of a time series. It is calculated from the distribution $\{p_i\}$ of one of the signal parameters, such as amplitude, power, or time-frequency representation. Various formalisms of entropy have been defined: Shannon entropy (*SE*) (88), Renyi entropy (89), and nonextensive entropy (90).

By studying the mutual information between different regions on the cortex, we can understand the interdependence of different regions of the brain.

Recently, various entropy measures, such as time-dependent entropy, wavelet entropy, time-frequency complexity, and mutual information, have been applied to qEEG analysis.

TIME-DEPENDENT ENTROPY MEASURE The direct approach is to calculate the entropy from the time series of the EEG. The amplitudes of the EEG segment are partitioned into $M$ microstates; the raw sampled signal is denoted as $\{x(k): k = 1, \ldots, N\}$. The amplitude range $W$ is therefore divided into $M$ disjointed intervals $\{I_i : i = 1, \ldots, M\}$ such that

$$W = \bigcup_{i=1}^{M} I_i. \tag{26}$$

The probability distribution can be obtained by the ratio of the frequency of the samples $N_i$ falling into each bin ($I_i$) and the total sample number $N$:

$$p_i = N_i / N. \tag{27}$$

Then, the entropy can be defined with the amplitude distribution across the $M$ bins:

$$SE = -\sum_{i=1}^{M} p_i \ln(p_i). \tag{28}$$

This is the definition of the traditional $SE$ (88). $SE$ hypothesizes that the system is extensive or additive. We proposed the use of nonextensive time-dependent entropy (TDE) to analyze the EEG following brain injury. It is justifiable to take EEG as a nonextensive source (41, 42). The formalism of the nonextensive entropy was originally postulated in 1988 in a nonlogarithm format by Tsallis (90, 91), which is also called Tsallis entropy:

$$TE = \frac{1 - \sum_{i=1}^{M} p_i^q}{q - 1}. \tag{29}$$

The EEG is time-varying such that a time-dependent measure could be more effective in describing the temporal change. Therefore, we segment the EEG recordings into nonoverlapping windows: $W(n; w; \Delta) = \{x(i), i = 1 + n\Delta, \ldots, w + n\Delta\}$. Then, the entropy measure is applied to each window $W(n; w; \Delta)$. Correspondingly, the Shannon and Tsallis versions of TDE ($\mathrm{TDE_S}$ and $\mathrm{TDE_T}$, respectively) are defined as

$$TDE_S(n) = -\sum_{i=1}^{M} p_n(I_i) \ln(p_n(I_i)) \qquad \text{and} \tag{30}$$

$$TDE_T(n) = \frac{1 - \sum_{i=1}^{M} (p_n(I_i))^q}{q - 1}, \tag{31}$$

where $n$ is the window index and $q$ is the entropic index of Tsallis entropy, indicating the nonextensive degree. The probability that the signal $x(i) \in W(n; w; \Delta)$ falls into the interval $I_i$ is given by $p^n(I_i)$. There are three important issues regarding the estimation of the *TDE*.

***Partitioning number and partitioning methods*** There are two different approaches for partitioning the amplitude range: (*a*) fixed partitioning and (*b*) adaptive partitioning. Figure 11 illustrates these two different types of partitioning. The difference is that the adaptive partitioning can track the transient singularity changes in EEG but the fixed partitioning can track the energy change in the signal. Two segments of EEG with different variances are combined into one segment and the amplitudes are partitioned with fixed intervals (Figure 11*a*) and adaptive intervals (Figure 11*b*) for calculating TDE. Figure 11*c* shows that the TDE of the adaptive partitioning can be used to track the transient events, whereas the fixed partitioning can be used to track the amplitude change.

***Selection of entropic index q*** The entropic index $q$ in Equations 29 and 31 is related to the nonextensive degree of the system, which is usually determined by the system intrinsically. Reports in the literature describe the methods of obtaining the $q$ value in some specific physical systems (92–95). Currently, there are no methods to obtain the $q$ value of a time series. Some trials have been proposed to determine $q$ from the multifractal spectrum of the system (96). Usually, the choice of $q$ is empirical. $q$ has been proven sensitive to spiky/bursting activities in the EEG signals (97). A large $q$ value strengthens the bursts. The choice of $q$ should be different for different EEG signals. In the early recovery phase of hypoxic-ischemic brain injury, the typical EEG waveform feature is the presence of transient spiky signals. In Figure 12, the role of $q$ index is investigated. Higher $q$ emphasizes the spikes in the signals; however, higher $q$ suppresses spontaneous activities.

***Sliding step and window size*** The sliding step and window size decide the time resolution of TDE. Usually, if we focus on the local feature changes, the slide step is selected to be very small (e.g., sample by sample). If we are only interested in the general trend of the EEG, we can use nonoverlapping windows (slide step equal to the size of the window). To get a reliable and smooth probability density function (PDF), the window size should not be too small.

Figure 13 illustrates an application of the two types of TDE for the EEG following brain injury. Figure 13*a* shows a compact representation of a long experimental EEG, including a 15-min baseline (*I*), 5-min ischemia (*II*), immediate silent period (*III*), and 200 min of recovery (phases *IV* and *V*). Figure13*b* is the TDE for fixed

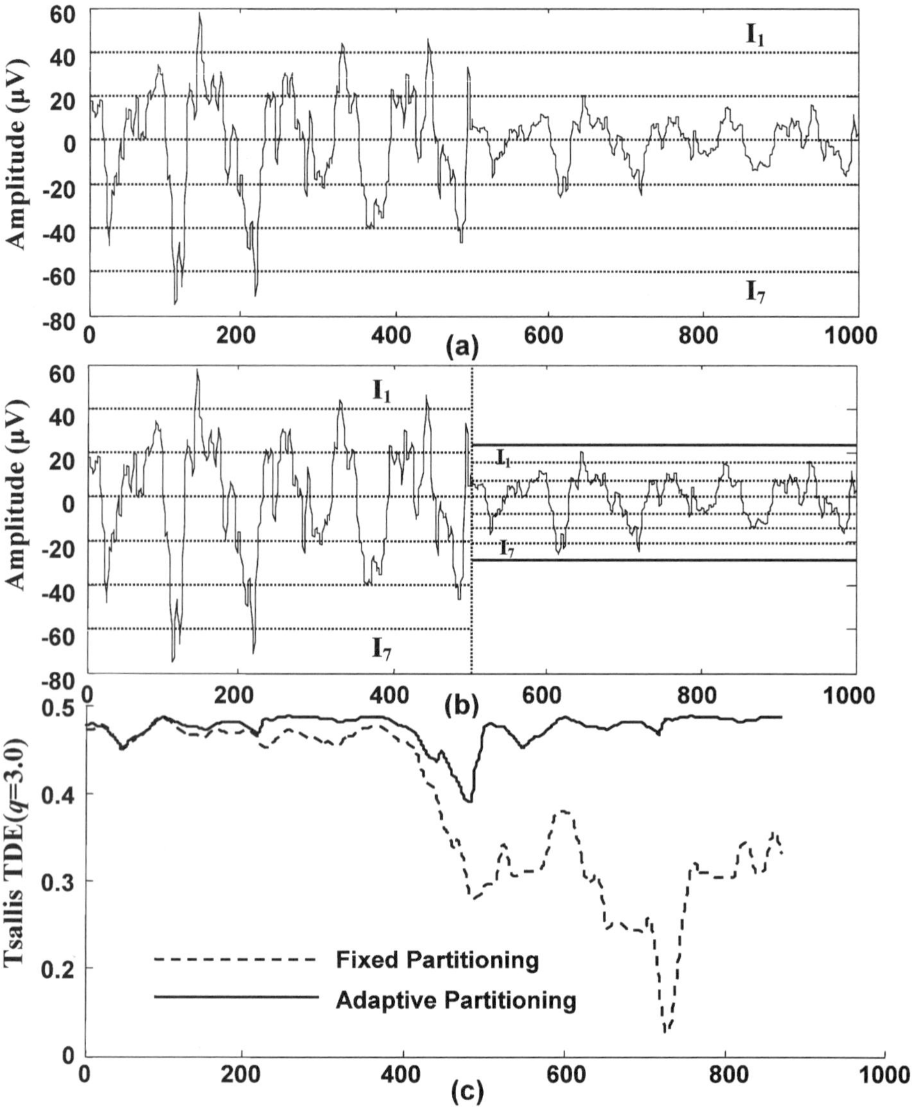


**Figure 11** Two different partitioning approaches in TDE analysis. The signal in both conditions consists of two segments of EEG with different variance. For calculating the TDE, the amplitudes are partitioned into a number of bins (M = 7). Two different partitioning approaches are applied: (*a*) fixed partitioning and (*b*) adaptive partitioning. (*c*) TDE results. Note that the TDE obtained by the adaptive partitioning is sensitive to the transient events, whereas the fixed partitioning can be used to track the amplitude change.

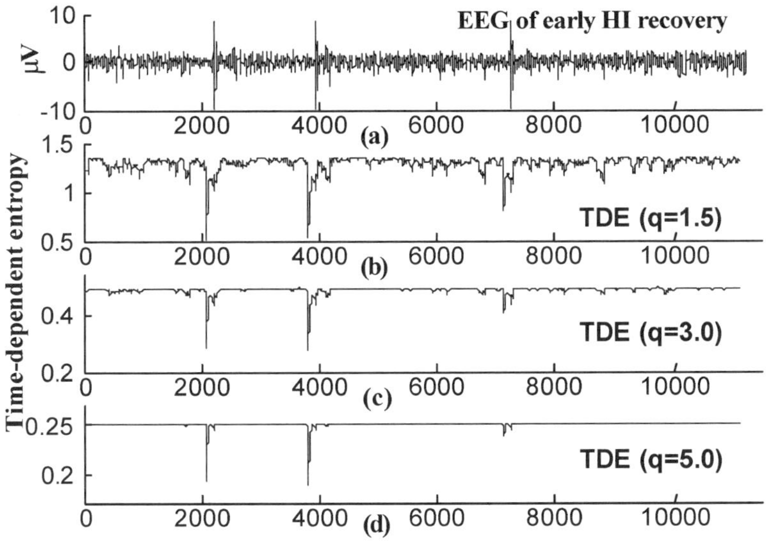


**Figure 12** The role of nonextensive parameter $q$ in TDE. (*a*) 40-s EEG segment selected from the recovery of brain ischemia, which includes three typical bursts in recovery phase. (*b–d*) are TDE plots for different nonextensive parameters ($q = 1.5$, 3.0, and 5.0, respectively). The size of sliding window is fixed at $w = 128$. The sliding step is one sample. Partition number $M = 10$ (adapted from 41).

partitioning, which shows the global trend of the brain activity mainly of spontaneous EEG. Figure 13*c* is the TDE for adaptive partitioning in which the spiking and bursting activities following CPR are clearly illustrated. There are two different rhythms in the EEG following hypoxic-ischemic brain injury: background spontaneous EEG and burst activities during the early recovery. Figure 13 indicates that TDE can exhibit these activities by different partitioning approaches.

WAVELET ENTROPY AND TIME-FREQUENCY COMPLEXITY TDE is useful for evaluating the complexity of EEG in the time domain. The EEG also shows complexity in the frequency domain. Rosso and colleagues proposed to use wavelet entropy to quantify the complexity of EEG in the time-frequency plane (77, 98, 99). The signal is represented with wavelets in different scale and time transit $\varphi_{j,k}(t)$ (Equation 32). The coefficients $\{c_{j,k}(t)\}$ provide a multiresolution analysis (MRA) of the signal:

$$f(t) = \sum_k \sum_j c_{j,k} \varphi_{j,k}(t). \tag{32}$$

The wavelet entropy evaluates the complexity of the energy distribution in a different frequency band (subbands). Wavelet entropy is defined using the Shannon

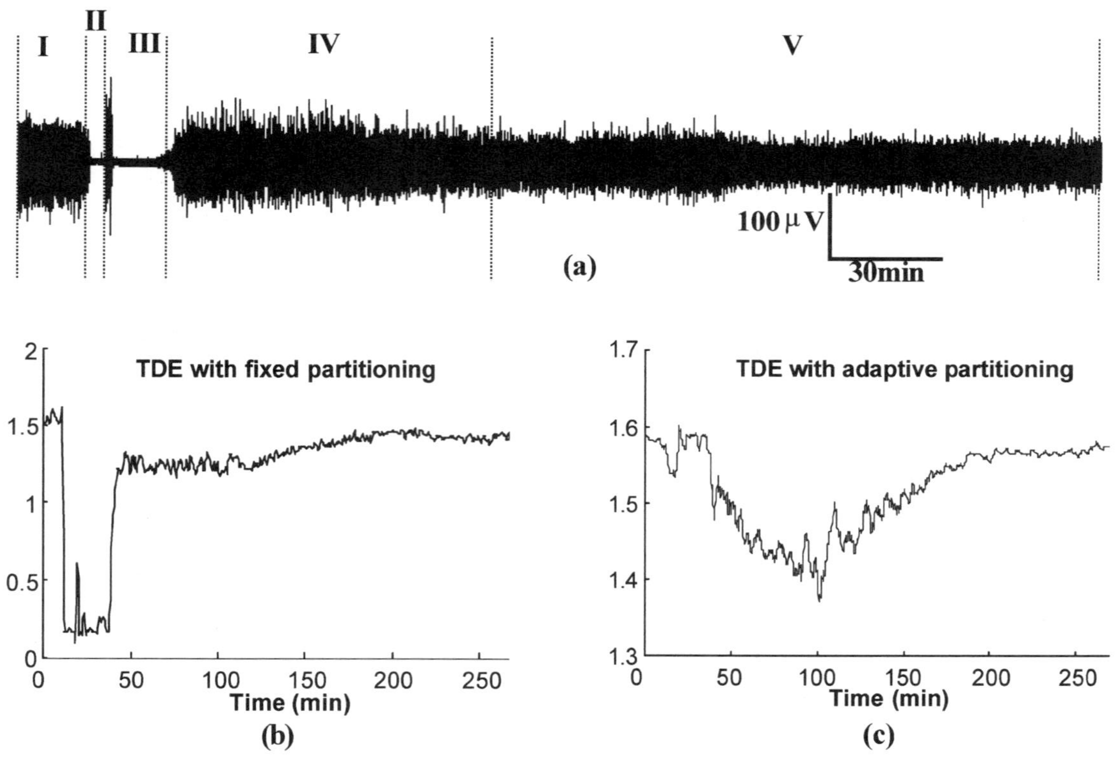


**Figure 13** Time-dependent entropy (TDE) analysis of the EEG of hypoxic-ischemic brain injury. (*a*) 4-h compressed trace of experimental hypoxic-ischemic EEG (15 min baseline, 5 min ischemia, 1 min CPR, and 250 min of recovery); (*b*) TDE with fixed partitioning; and (*c*) TDE with adaptive partitioning. To compensate between the specificity to detect the bursts (local) (it is better to use Tsallis entropy with high $q$) and the sensitivity to distinguish between different patterns of EEG (global) (it is better to use either Shannon or Tsallis entropy with low $q$), we selected Tsallis entropy with $q = 3$ in our previous analysis (41–43).

measure of entropy of the energy distribution:

$$\begin{cases} SWE = -\sum_i p_i \log(p_i) \\ p_j = \sum_k \|c_{j,k}\|^2 / \sum_j \sum_k \|c_{j,k}\|^2, \end{cases} \tag{33}$$

where $p_i$ actually is the ratio of the energy in $j^{th}$ scale and the total energy. Al-Nashash et al. (95) applied wavelet entropy to the specific frequency bands (Delta, Theta, Alpha, and Beta) of the EEG following hypoxic-ischemic injury, which is also called subband wavelet entropy (*SWE*). Wistar rats were given 3 min of global ischemia after 15 min of baseline recording; oxygen was then resupplied and the animals started to recover after resuscitation. Figure 14 shows the *SWE* before and after hypoxic-ischemic injury in Delta, Theta, Alpha, and Beta bands. Except in the Delta band, the *SWE* in other frequency bands shows strong correlations with the injury and its recovery.

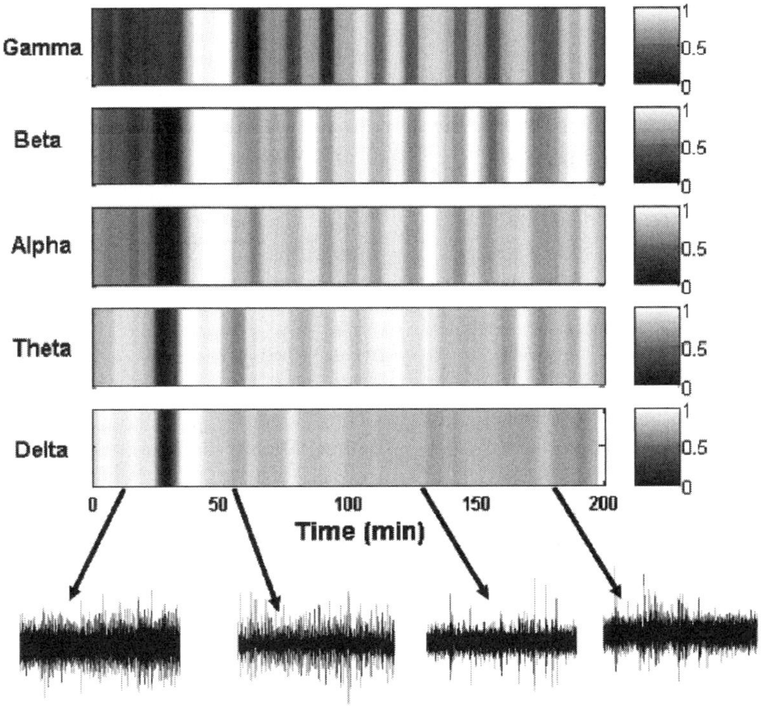


**Figure 14** Normalized gray level segments based on *SWE*. The animal received 3 min of asphyxic brain injury following 15 min of baseline recording. The weight given to each gray level is as shown in the respective gray level bars. The injury and silence periods are represented in black (adapted from 100).

As described above, wavelet entropy is estimated from the energy distribution in each scale. Therefore, it is actually measured in the frequency domain, thus containing little information in the time domain. For the time-varying characteristics of the EEG, a time-frequency complexity measure may provide more details of the signal. Andino et al. (101) proposed a Renyi entropy–based time-frequency measure on the time-frequency plane. The basic idea is to define the entropy in the two-dimensional (2-D) time-frequency plane:

1. Estimating the time-frequency representation (TFR) $C(t, \omega)$ [a free MATLAB toolbox for TFR is available from (81)]
2. Normalizing $C(t, \omega)$ as the time-frequency distribution function

$$\hat{C}(t, \omega) = \frac{C(t, \omega)}{\iint C(t, \omega) dt df} = \frac{C(t, \omega)}{\|s(t)\|^2}, \tag{34}$$

   where $\|s(t)\|^2$ is the total power of the EEG;
3. Estimating the entropy of the TFR:

$$RE = \frac{1}{1-\alpha} \log \iint (\hat{C}(t, \omega))^\alpha \tag{35}$$

Equation 35 is a format of Renyi entropy. We can also use Shannon or Tsallis entropy versions. One of the most important questions posed by this measure is which is the more suitable TFR to obtain the most accurate estimates of complexity for a given data set? To get a more accurate time-frequency complexity (TFC) measure, we describe the TFC with high-resolution time-frequency plane-based matching pursuits (102). TFC is defined as the *SE* of the distribution of time-frequency representation $Ef(t, \omega)$ of the signal $f(t)$:

$$TFC = -\iint_{t,\omega} p(t, \omega) \cdot \log(p(t, \omega)) dt d\omega, \tag{36}$$

where $p(t, \omega) = \frac{Ef(t,\omega)}{\iint_{t,\omega} Ef(t,\omega) dt d\omega}$ is the PDF of $Ef(t, \omega)$. $Ef(t, \omega)$ is the time-frequency energy distribution of signal $f(t)$ (see Equation 25 and Time-Frequency Methods, above).

By choosing a good time-frequency atom such as the Gabor function, this kind of MP-based TFC can be more useful in evaluating the complexity in the time-frequency domain.

Figure 15 (see color insert) illustrates the EEG before and after 5 min of global hypoxic-ischemic brain injury. Figure 15*a*–*c* are the MP-based TFRs of the baseline EEGs, early recovery, and late recovery. Figure 15*d* shows the corresponding TFC statistical results. TFC has the highest value in normal physiological conditions and is reduced considerably upon injury. As the brain recovers from the hypoxic-ischemic injury, TFC increases correspondingly. The evolution of EEG and its fine features can be seen more clearly by using these powerful segmentation procedures.

By highlighting these features, we hope to segment different phases of brain injury and assess the progress of recovery after injury.

MUTUAL INFORMATION The entropy measure in the time, frequency, or time-frequency domains can quantify the complexity of the EEG. But these measures do not consider interactions within the brain. In clinical neuroscience research, we not only want to monitor the activities of the brain but we also want to know more about the brain function through interactions between different regions. Mutual information (MI) is a useful measure for studying the dependence or relation between different regions of the brain. Mathematically, the MI between two cortical activity variables $X$ and $Y$ is defined with their joint probability density function, $p(x, y)$, and marginal probability density functions, $p(x)$ and $p(y)$. The MI($X$; $Y$) is the relative entropy between $p(x, y)$ and the product distribution $p(x)p(y)$ (103), i.e.,

$$MI(X,Y) = \sum_{x \in X} \sum_{y \in Y} p(x,y) \log \frac{p(x,y)}{p(x)p(y)}. \qquad (37)$$

MI is a general measure of the statistical dependencies between two time series. There are different parametric or nonparametric methods for MI estimation (104–107).

The entropy estimated with Equation 37 could achieve a contour map of MI between each pair of electrodes across the cerebral cortex. Sometimes we need to know how much a specific lobe contributes to the global information exchange and how active the cerebral cortex is at a specific point in time. We define two parameters, LFI (local flow of information) and GFI (global flow of information), as the total influx/efflux of information associated with a single electrode and the total flow of information associated with all electrodes across the cerebral cortex, respectively. By denoting the MI between two different electrodes, $E_i$, and $E_j$, as $\{MI(E_i, E_j) | E_i = Fp1, \ldots T6, E_j = Fp1, \ldots T6, \text{ and, } i \neq j\}$, LFI on electrode $E_i$ can be estimated by

$$LFI(E_i) = \sum_{\substack{j=1 \\ j \neq i}}^{L} MI(E_i, E_j), \qquad (38)$$

where $L$ is the total number of the electrodes. Then the GFI can be estimated from the summation of LFI directly:

$$GFI = \frac{1}{2} \sum_{i}^{L} \sum_{\substack{j=1 \\ j \neq i}}^{L} MI(E_i, E_j)$$

$$= \frac{1}{2} \sum_{i=1}^{L} LFI(E_i) \qquad (39)$$

The factor 1/2 is because $MI(E_i, E_j) = MI(E_j, E_i)$. GFI estimates the gross flow of information across the cortex.

MI calculated from an EEG and its delayed version [$MI(X(t), X(t+\tau))$, also called auto mutual information (AMI)] or other delayed channel [$MI(X(t), Y(t+\tau))$, also called cross mutual information (CMI)] can be used to measure the information propagation and interdependence between the channels (108). Na et al. (108) studied information transmission between different cortical areas in schizophrenics by estimating the average CMI (A-CMI), and they characterized the dynamic property of the cortical areas of schizophrenic patients from multichannel EEG by establishing the AMI. The schizophrenic patients had significantly higher interhemispheric and intrahemispheric A-CMI values than did the normal controls. In the study of Alzheimer's disease, Jeong (5) found that the local CMI in Alzheimer's disease subjects was lower than that in normal controls, especially over frontal and anterior-temporal regions. A prominent decrease in information transmission between distant electrodes in the right hemisphere and between corresponding interhemispheric electrodes was detected in the Alzheimer's disease patients. In addition, throughout the cerebrums of the Alzheimer's disease patients, AMI decreased significantly more over time than did the AMIs of normal controls. In our preliminary investigations of hypoxic-ischemic brain injury, we found that the frontal lobe and back lobes are more easily affected by hypoxic-ischemic brain injury in the LFI map (Figure 16, see color insert). These clinical studies are quite empirical and cannot reliably or fully explain these complex neurological disorders. Nevertheless, the tools of information and information flow can begin to help us understand complex interrelationships between different regions of the brain.

## High-Order Statistics

The power spectrum, also called first-order statistical analysis, provides the component contents in different frequencies. The power spectrum is only useful for studying the linear mechanisms governing the process because it suppresses phase relations between frequency components (109). The phase coupling (synchronization) between different frequency components plays an important role in the activities of the brain. EEG signals, especially during disorders such as epilepsy and burst suppression (109, 110), show complex oscillation frequencies and phase relationships. Higher-order statistical (HOS) analysis is a nonlinear method for describing the phase coupling. The most popular HOS index is bispectrum $B(\omega_1, \omega_2)$, which is the FT of the third-order cumulant. The highlighting advantages of HOS over the power spectra are (*a*) it can provide a measure of non-Gaussianity because the spectrum of the second and higher cumulants is zero if the signal is Gaussian, and (*b*) HOS is also suitable for multivariable analysis of measuring the extent of statistical dependence in the time series (111, 112). Mathematically, $B(\omega 1, \omega 2)$ of a time series is defined as

$$B(\omega_1, \omega_2) = E\{X(\omega_1)X(\omega_2)X^*(\omega_1 + \omega_2)\}, \tag{40}$$

where $X(\omega_i)$ is the complex Fourier coefficient spectrum of the EEG and $X^*$ is its complex conjugate. Two frequencies, $\omega_1$ and $\omega_2$, are said to be phase-coupled when a third component exists at a frequency of $\omega_1 + \omega_2$. To make different EEG comparable, the normalized bispectrum is extracted as bicoherence $bic(\omega_1, \omega_2)$:

$$bic(\omega_1, \omega_2) = \frac{|B(\omega_1, \omega_2)|}{\sqrt{P(\omega_1)P(\omega_2)P(\omega_1 + \omega_2)}}, \tag{41}$$

where $P(\omega_i) = \|X(\omega_i)\|^2$ is the power spectrum at frequency $\omega_i$ and $bic(\omega_1, \omega_2)$ varies between 0 to 1. When $P(\omega_1 + \omega_2)$ is not zero, $bic(\omega_1, \omega_2)$ shows the degree of the coupling between the frequencies $\omega_1$ and $\omega_2$. Muthuswamy et al. (109) studied the bispectrum of the burst patterns of EEGs following asphyxic arrest and during late recovery; it was found that the coupling within the Delta-Theta band of the EEG bursts was higher than found in baseline and late recovery waveforms (Figure 17).

In the EEG following asphyxic brain injury, the bicoherence indicates that the degree of phase coupling between two frequency components of a signal is significantly higher within the Delta and Theta bands of the EEG bursts than in the baseline or late recovery waveforms. The bispectral parameters show a more detectable trend than the power spectral parameters by taking advantage of the phase coupling among these frequencies during bursting and burst suppression events.

## Chaotic Measures

Nonlinear dynamics has been a rapidly developing area in physics since the late 1980s and has found extensive application in physiological signal processing (3, 4, 113, 114). The most commonly used descriptions are based on chaotic measures, such as dimension estimation (correlation dimension, information dimension, capacity dimension, and multifractal spectrum) (115), Lyapunov exponent spectrum (116), Poincare maps, Kolmogorov-Sinai entropy (3, 4), and approximate entropy (117). The motivation for nonlinear dynamics analysis of the EEG is the high complexity and limited predictability of the neurological signals, which may make them essentially stochastic. Theoretically, applying nonlinear dynamics theory to the nonlinear brain system may be helpful for understanding the underlying mechanisms. For example, in some studies, the EEG is considered a nonlinear and possibly even chaotic dynamic system (55, 115, 118, 119). Hence, various quantitative measures that help describe nonlinear and chaotic dynamics may be useful in characterizing EEG after trauma or neurological disorders.

### FRACTAL (CAPACITY, INFORMATION, AND CORRELATION) DIMENSION ESTIMATION

The fractal dimension is usually estimated through the measure of the signal in its embedded space.

***Reconstructing the phase space by time-delay embedding*** The fractal dimension is measured in the multidimensional space of the attractor of the system. For real

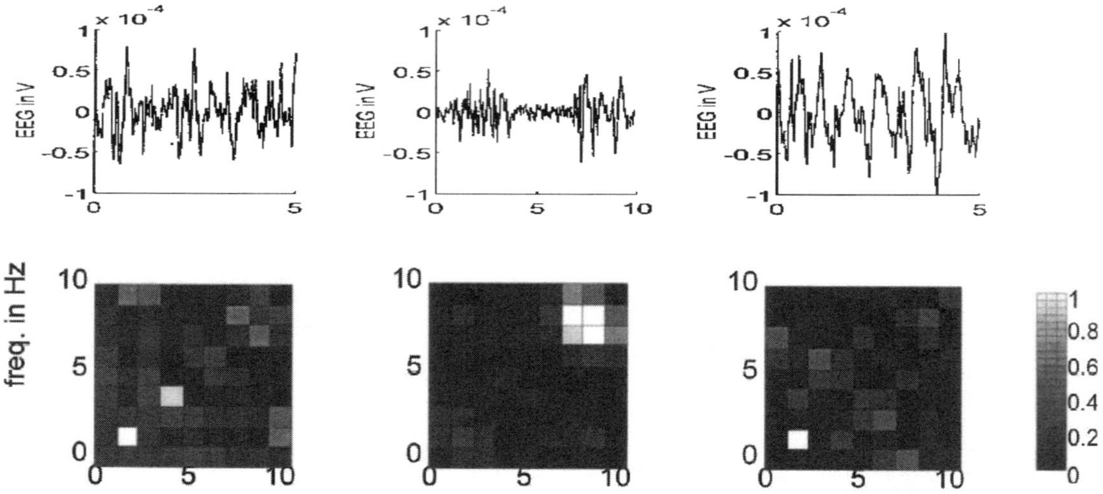


**(a)** **(b)** **(c)**

**Figure 17** The gray scale plots of the bicoherence indexes show only the region of interest, i.e., frequencies up to 10 Hz: (*a*) baseline, (*b*) burst suppression, and (*c*) recovery. These three plots correspond to the respective waveforms in the top. The bicoherence indexes were averaged along the diagonal up to a frequency of approximately 7 Hz. The significance level of the average bicoherence measure was later evaluated (adapted from 109).

experimental data, such as the EEG, however, we cannot record the multidimension signal. Takens (120) proposed a method to reconstruct the multidimension signal from the signal variable, digitalized, experimental time series generated by the undergoing nonlinear system. Suppose the recorded time series (EEG) is presented as $\{x(i)|i = 1, 2, \ldots, N\}$, then by Takens' embedding rule, the $m$-dimension phase space can be constructed by the samples with delayed and lagged selection from the raw signals:

$$\begin{cases} \vec{x}(1) = \{x(1), x(1+L), \cdots, x(1+(m-1)*L)\} \\ \vec{x}(2) = \{x(1+J), x(1+L+J), \cdots, x(1+(m-1)*L+J)\}\cdots, \\ \vec{x}(n) = \{x(1+(n-1)*J), x(1+L+(n-1)*J), \cdots, \\ \qquad x(n+(m-1)*L+(n-1)*J)\} \end{cases} \tag{42}$$

where $L$ is embedding lag, $J$ is the time jump, $m$ is the embedding dimension, and $\{\vec{x}(i)\}$ are the vectors in the $m$-dimensional phase space.

***Dimension estimation*** After constructing the $m$-dimension phase space by Takens' rule, the fractal dimension corresponding to this $m$-dimensional space can be estimated by the ratio of the logarithm of a measure [correlation integer $C(\varepsilon)$, capacity number $N(\varepsilon)$ occupying the space, or the information quantity $I(\varepsilon)$] and the logarithm of the resolution of the phase space $\varepsilon$. The correlation integer $C(\varepsilon)$ and the information quantity $I(\varepsilon)$ are defined as

$$C(\varepsilon) = \lim_{n\to\infty} \frac{1}{N^2} \sum_{\substack{i,j=1 \\ i\neq j}}^{N} H(\varepsilon - \|\vec{x}(i) - \vec{x}(j)\|) \qquad \text{and} \tag{43}$$

$$I(\varepsilon) = -\sum_{i=1}^{N} P_i(\varepsilon)\ln[P_i(\varepsilon)], \tag{44}$$

where $P_i(\varepsilon)$ is some nature measure or the probability that the $i^{th}$ element is populated. The capacity dimension ($D_{cap}$), information dimension ($D_{\inf}$), and correlation dimension ($D_{cor}$) are defined as follows, respectively:

$$\begin{cases} D_{cap} = -\dfrac{\log(N(\varepsilon))}{\log(\varepsilon)} \\ D_{\inf} = -\dfrac{\log(I(\varepsilon))}{\log(\varepsilon)} \\ D_{cor} = \dfrac{\log(C(\varepsilon))}{\log(\varepsilon)} \end{cases} . \tag{45}$$

Usually, $D_{cap} \leq D_{\inf} \leq D_{cor}$ is satisfied. This algorithm was originally proposed by Grassberg-Procassia (G-P algorithm) (121). Actually, $D_{cap}$, $D_{\inf}$, and $D_{cor}$ are the specific conditions of the multifractal spectrum:

$$D_q \equiv \frac{1}{q-1} \lim_{\varepsilon \to 0} \frac{\log(I(q,\varepsilon))}{\log(\varepsilon)}, \tag{46}$$

where $I(q,\varepsilon) = \sum_{i=1}^{N} [P_i(\varepsilon)]^q$. For $q = 0$, 1, and 2, $D_q$ is equal to $D_{cap}$, $D_{\inf}$, and $D_{cor}$, respectively.

Compared with the traditional spectrum analysis, nonlinear measures can provide additional details of the EEG mechanism. Figure 18*a*,*b* shows the power spectrum and the amplitude distributions of the EEG (F3-A1) of normal and schizophrenic patients. The EEG signals were recorded in an EEG lab; the experiments were performed in an acoustically and electrically shielded room where both the control subjects and the patients were seated comfortably in reclining chairs. Within the regular EEG frequency band (0~30 Hz) there is no evident difference between the control subjects and patients. By studying the correlation dimension (Figure 18*c*,*d*), an increase of EEG dimensional complexity in schizophrenia

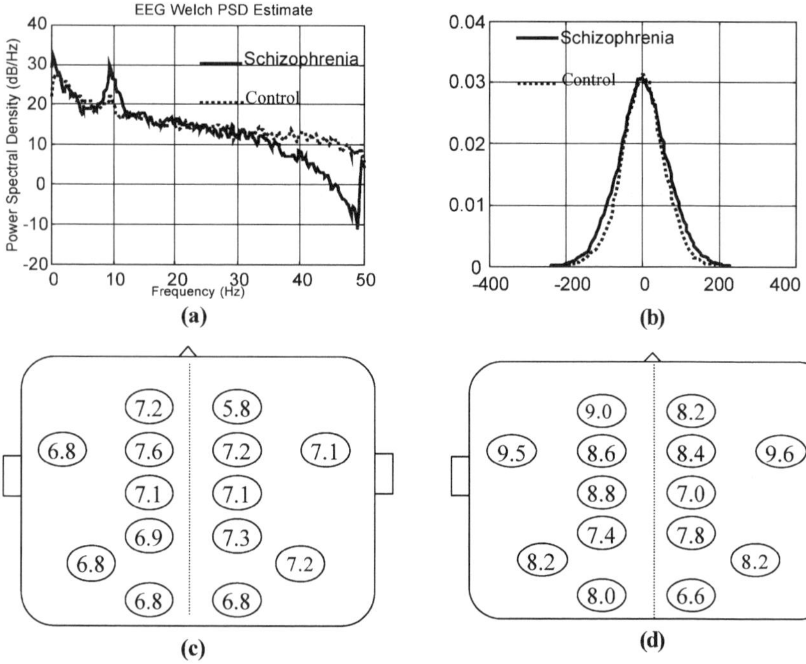


**Figure 18** Power spectrum and correlation dimension ($D_2$) of normal people and schizophrenics (n = 18 in each group). (*a*) Power spectrum from the channel F3-A1. (*b*) Amplitude distribution of the EEG from the channel F3-A1. The difference within the regular frequency band (0–30 Hz) is not clear. (*c*) $D_2$ of normal subject; (*d*) $D_2$ of schizophrenics. There is an apparent increase of $D_2$ in the schizophrenic group, especially in the left and front lobes (adapted from 118).

compared to controls with the measurement of $D_2$ was found. Moreover, by using a spatial embedding method, a relatively higher global correlation dimension was obtained in the left and frontal lobes of the schizophrenics (115, 118).

APPROXIMATE ENTROPY ESTIMATION Pincus (117) proposed approximate entropy (ApEn) to calculate complexity from the short data set, which is useful for real clinical and experimental studies. It is defined with the correlation integer at each point in the embedded space $C_i^m(r)$. The average logarithm of the correlation integer is obtained by

$$\Phi^m(r) = \frac{1}{N-m+1} \sum_{i=1}^{N-m+1} \log C_i^m(r). \tag{47}$$

Then, ApEn is

$$\mathrm{ApEn(m, r, N)(u)} = \Phi^{\mathrm{m}}(r) - \Phi^{m+1}(r), \mathrm{m} \geq 1. \tag{48}$$

Usually, $m$ is chosen as 1 or 2, and $r$ is selected as 0.1~0.2 standard deviation.

ApEn has been a useful tool in characterizing the irregularity and complexity of EEG (67, 122–124).

QUESTIONS ON CHAOTIC MEASURES The fractal dimensions can be interpreted as a measure of the degree of chaos in the underlying system. The difficulties in defining the chaotic measures of EEG signals lie in two issues. One is the G-P algorithm, which is currently the most widely used algorithm for estimating the correlation dimension (121, 125). Nevertheless, the analysis of biological signals by using such a method has encountered some problems. Many parameters have to be assigned arbitrarily, and improper assignment affects the value of $D_2$ and results in distortion and error. The G-P algorithm is unreliable for short data samples (126). In addition, there was a mimicked low-dimension component with the G-P algorithm (127, 128). Several modified methods have been found to make significant improvements on the G-P algorithm. Lee (118) proposed a spatial embedding method to reconstruct the $m$-dimensional phase space with the multichannel EEG.

The second issue originates in the EEG itself. The classic chaotic measures, such as fractal dimensions, hypothesize that the signal originates from a lower-dimensional nonlinear system. The recent literature reports, however, that the spontaneous EEG is ultrahigh dimensional (55). The usefulness of describing a high-dimensional nonlinear system with the measures better suited to describe a lower-dimensional system is still under question (55). Further, the EEG usually is a time-varying signal. In different physiological states, the attractors are always different; the complexity of the signals is also changing. In some pathological conditions, such as epileptic seizures, the EEG becomes relatively simpler and the chaotic measures have been confirmed to be effective in predicting the seizure by analyzing the preictal EEG (129, 130). Recently, the multifractal analysis has been recommended to analyze the ultracomplex EEG signals (131).

# BRAIN ACTIVITIES AND FUNCTIONAL IMAGING

In this section, we briefly review topics related to EEG signals, including EEG mapping, source localization, and combination with magnetic resonance imaging (MRI) techniques. This EEG-related research focuses on the visualization and structural analysis of the qEEG results.

## Multichannel Brain Activity Mapping

The EEG is a functional measure of brain activities. How to visualize the distribution of a specific functional measure on the scalp is the topic of brain mapping. The EEG-based brain mapping is also called BEAM (brain electric activity mapping), which requires multichannel EEG recordings. BEAM may use one index of EEG measures, such as amplitude (30, 132), phase synchronization (133), power spectrum (134), coherence (135, 136), or other measures (108), to show the distribution of this measure across the scalp.

One of the applications of BEAM is to localize the focal disease and explore the functional correlation. An important application of the multichannel EEG is to try to find the location of an epileptic focus (a small spot in the brain where the abnormal activity originates and then spreads to other parts of the brain) or a tumor, even when they are not visible in an X-ray or a computerized tomography (CT) scan of the head.

EEG brain mapping has proven to be a valuable method for diagnostic and therapeutic assessment in dementia trials (137–141), language studies (142), HIV/AIDS (143), brain hypoxia (144), and cerebral artery occlusion (145).

## Source Localization

EEG signals are the summated effect of large assemblies of neurons. Any spontaneous stimulation, cognition, or motion activity can give rise to a change in the EEG recordings. Source localization involves the recognition and localization of the neuronal signal generator inside the brain. The implementation of source localization includes neural dynamics and diagnosis of focal neural disease, such as epilepsy. Estimation of the electric field inside the brain with the EEG is usually also called the inverse problem. Source localization provides an interface between EEG and the electric field of the brain (146). The most crucial issue in source localization is the selection of head and source models.

SOURCE MODEL The simplest source model is a single dipole, which assumes that the electric field (where the EEG is recorded) is created by a point source of equivalent current dipole. Another model sometimes used is to divide the brain region into a large number of subregions. Each region is represented by a dipole, which is also called the multipole model (147, 148).

HEAD MODEL The most commonly used and simplest head model (134, 147) is a multilayer nested concentric sphere. The skull, scalp, cerebral cortex, etc. are modeled as different layers with different electrical conductivities (148). A more realistic model is an anisotropic, inhomogeneous, and nonspherical one. This type of accurate model uses anatomical information (obtained from CT or MRI).

Once the models are selected, the location of the source in the head model can be calculated by the inverse solution using numerical calculation of the Maxwell equations. The common method is the finite element method (FEM). Different source localization methods are compared in a study by Fernandez (149).

### Electroencephalogram and Functional Magnetic Resonance Imaging

MRI is a recent advanced technique for acquiring the anatomic image in a selected cross-section by activating (with brief radio frequency pulses) the inherent distribution of hydrogen atoms in the brain (150). The MRI has high spatial resolution, but low temporal resolution owing to the principle of the MRI technique. Compared with MRI, the EEG has very high temporal resolution, but low spatial resolution. Therefore, the combination of EEG and MRI techniques may provide both temporal and spatial resolutions (48).

Thatcher proposed the linkage between the MRI T2 relaxation time, the EEG coherence (151), and the EEG power spectrum (152). Dimitrov (153) made texturing three-dimensional (3-D) reconstructions of the brain with the EEG by using the data from an accompanying MRI scan. Bonmassar et al. (154) combined functional MRI (fMRI) and EEG data with the linear inverse estimation method to generate real-time spatiotemporal movies of brain activity. The spatial extent of the fMRI-constrained EEG localization is more focal than the results based on EEG measurements alone (154). Three distinct approaches have been used to combine EEG and fMRI images: converging evidence, direct data fusion, and computational neural modeling (47). By linking the EEG and fMRI, Baudewig et al. (49) successfully localized the epileptic activity.

## SUMMARY AND FUTURE DIRECTIONS

The task of qEEG is to provide an objective approach for experimental/clinical diagnostic studies and for understanding the brain's electrical function. qEEG methods have been developed from the traditional frequency analysis (decomposing into Delta, Theta, Alpha, and Beta bands) to various time, spectral, time-frequency, and nonlinear approaches. The characteristics of the EEG have been studied from different aspects. Although the new nonlinear methods can exploit more details from the stochastic time series, the traditional time and frequency analysis methods still serve as the most popular clinical tools. These linear methods can be applied when EEG waveform (or amplitudes) and rhythm (or frequencies) features designate the specific physiological status, e.g., in epilepsy diagnosis. But such spectrum-based methods take the EEG signal as a stationary process, which is a valid approximation for a short period. However, the EEG is expected to be nonstationary and time varying in experimental and clinical recordings. Therefore, time-frequency analysis and time-dependent parametric measures are recommended for tracking such signal components. For example, these can be the transient events in EEG, such as spikes and bursts. The nonlinear chaotic measures regard the source of the EEG as a dynamic system that provides a different quantitative view of EEG, such as any nonlinear, deterministic phenomena resulting from oscillations or coupling of different frequencies. When we study the interaction, correlation, causality, and neural pathway across the cortex or within the brain, the information theory-based methods can be useful. Thus, different qEEG methods provide different interpretations of the cortical rhythms. The selection of methods strongly depends on what kind of information we want to extract. A number of exciting new directions are emerging:

1. Methods for describing the interactions between different regions of the brain. The correlation, coherence, and mutual information measures can quantify the degree of interactions between different regions of the brain, but they cannot tell us the causality of such interactions or the direction of the information transferred. The directed transfer function (DTF) (155), directed mutual information (DMI) (156), and partial directed coherence (PDC) (157, 158) could be useful tools for describing directed interactions among the multichannel EEG recordings.
2. Time-varying and nonstationarity analysis. Most currently used qEEG methods approximate the EEG as a stationary process. Nevertheless, in most pathological conditions, the transient irregular components (such as seizures of epilepsy) are the most interesting waves. High-resolution time-frequency analysis and time-varying multifractal measures may help to extract more details inside the nonstationary EEG.
3. Combining with new imaging technologies. One of the features of EEG is high temporal but low spatial resolution. The imaging technologies, for example fast functional imaging methods such as CT, MRI, and positron emission tomography (PET) have higher spatial but lower temporal resolution. The combination of the EEG and imaging technology may provide good resolution in both the domains.

**The *Annual Review of Biomedical Engineering* is online at http://bioeng.annualreviews.org**

## LITERATURE CITED

1. Berger H. 1929. Über das Elektrenkephalogramm des Menschen (On the EEG in humans). *Arch. Psychiatr. Nervenkr.* 87:527–70
2. Hughes JR, John ER. 1999. Conventional and quantitative electroencephalography in psychiatry. *J. Neuropsychiatry Clin. Neurosci.* 11:190–208
3. Pritchard W, Duke D. 1992. Measuring chaos in the brain: a tutorial review of nonlinear dynamical EEG analysis. *Int. J. Neurosci.* 67:31–80

4. Pritchard W, Krieble K, Duke D. 1995. Measuring chaos in the brain—a tutorial review of EEG dimension estimation. *Brain Cogn.* 27:353–97
5. Jeong J, Gore JC, Peterson BS. 2001. Mutual information analysis of the EEG in patients with Alzheimer's disease. *Clin. Neurophysiol.* 112:827–35
6. Pezard L, Jech R, Ruzicka E. 2001. Investigation of non-linear properties of multichannel EEG in the early stages of Parkinson's disease. *Clin. Neurophysiol.* 112:38–45
7. Kowalski J, Gawel M, Pfeffer A, Barcikowska M. 2001. The diagnostic value of EEG in Alzheimer disease—correlation with the severity of mental impairment. *J. Clin. Neurophysiol.* 18:570–75
8. Jeong J. 2002. Nonlinear dynamics of EEG in Alzheimer's disease. *Drug Dev. Res.* 56:57–66
9. Bennys K, Rondouin G, Vergnes C, Touchon J. 2001. Diagnostic value of quantitative EEG in Alzheimer's disease. *Neurophysiol. Clin./Clin. Neurophysiol.* 31:153–60
10. Besthorn C, Forstl H, Geigerkabisch C, Sattel H, Gasser T, Schreitergasser U. 1994. EEG coherence in Alzheimer-disease. *Electronencephalgr. Clin. Neurophysiol.* 90:242–45
11. Nevsimalova S, Marecek Z, Roth B. 1986. An EEG study of Wilson's disease. Findings in patients and heterozygous relatives. *Electroencephalogr. Clin. Neurophysiol.* 64:191–98
12. Chu N-S, Chu C-C, Tu S-C, Huang C-C. 1991. EEG spectral analysis and topographic mapping in Wilson's disease. *J. Neurol. Sci.* 106:1–9
13. Giagheddu M, Tamburini G, Piga M, Tacconi P, Giagheddu A, et al. 2001. Comparison of MRI, EEG, EPs and ECD-SPECT in Wilson's disease. *Acta Neurol. Scand.* 103:71–81
14. Lehnertz K, Andrzejak R, Arnhold J, Kreuz T, Mormann F, et al. 2001. Nonlinear EEG analysis in epilepsy: its possible use for interictal focus localization, seizure anticipation, and prevention. *J. Clin. Neurophysiol.* 18:209–22
15. Van Cott A. 2002. Epilepsy and EEG in the elderly. *Epilepsia* 43:94–102
16. Benar C, Aghakhani Y, Wang Y, Izenberg A, Al-Asmi A, et al. 2003. Quality of EEG in simultaneous EEG-fMRI for epilepsy. *Clin. Neurophysiol.* 114:569–80
17. Van Leeuwen WS. 1950. EEG in metastatic brain tumour before, during and after radiation treatment. *Electroencephalogr. Clin. Neurophysiol.* 2:331–32
18. Silipo R, Deco G, Bartsch H. 1999. Brain tumor classification based on EEG hidden dynamics. *Intell. Data Anal.* 3:287–306
19. De Jongh A, De Munck JC, Baayen JC, Jonkman EJ, Heethaar RM, Van Dijk BW. 2001. The localization of spontaneous brain activity: first results in patients with cerebral tumors. *Clin. Neurophysiol.* 112:378–85
20. Dolisi C, Suisse G, Delpont E. 1990. Quantitative EEG abnormalities and asymmetries in patients with intracranial tumors. *Electroencephalogr. Clin. Neurophysiol.* 76:13–18
21. Decker DA, Knott JR. 1972. The EEG in intrinsic supratentorial brain tumors: a comparative evaluation. *Electroencephalogr. Clin. Neurophysiol.* 33:303–10
22. Armitage R, Roffwarg HP, Rush AJ, Calhoun JS, Purdy DG, Giles DE. 1992. Digital period analysis of sleep EEG in depression. *Biol. Psychiatry* 31:52–68
23. Armitage R, Husain M, Hoffmann R, Rush AJ. 2003. The effects of vagus nerve stimulation on sleep EEG in depression: a preliminary report. *J. Psychosom. Res.* 54:475–82
24. Knott V, Mahoney C, Kennedy S, Evans K. 2001. EEG power, frequency, asymmetry and coherence in male depression. *Psychiatry Res. Neuroimaging* 106:123–40
25. Knott V, Mahoney C, Kennedy S, Evans K. 2002. EEG correlates of acute and

chronic paroxetine treatment in depression. *J. Affect. Disord.* 69:241–49
26. Barry RJ, Clarke AR, Johnstone SJ. 2003. A review of electrophysiology in attention-deficit/hyperactivity disorder. I. Qualitative and quantitative electroencephalography. *Clin. Neurophysiol.* 114:171–83
27. Barry RJ, Johnstone SJ, Clarke AR. 2003. A review of electrophysiology in attention-deficit/hyperactivity disorder: II. Event-related potentials. *Clin. Neurophysiol.* 114:184–98
28. Papadimitriou GN, Kerkhofs M, Kempenaers C, Mendlewicz J. 1988. EEG sleep studies in patients with generalized anxiety disorder. *Psychiatry Res.* 26:183–90
29. Okogbaa OG, Shell RL, Filipusic D. 1994. On the investigation of the neurophysiological correlates of knowledge worker mental fatigue using the EEG signal. *Appl. Ergon.* 25:355–65
30. Chen ACN. 2002. Human brain measures of clinical pain—a review (1,2). Topographic mappings. *Pain* 54:115–44
31. Penzel T, Conradt R. 2000. Computer based sleep recording and analysis. *Sleep Med. Rev.* 4:131–48
32. Bonnet MH, Arand DL. 2001. Impact of activity and arousal upon spectral EEG parameters. *Physiol. Behav.* 74:291–98
33. Thomsen C, Prior P. 1996. Quantitative EEG in assessment of anaesthetic depth: comparative study of methodology. *Br. J. Anaesth.* 77:172–78
34. Koskinen M, Seppänen T, Tuukkanen J, Yli-Hankala A, Jäntti V. 2001. Propofol anesthesia induces phase synchronization changes in EEG. *Clin. Neurophysiol.* 112:386–92
35. Mi W, Sakai T, Kudo T, Kudo M, Matsuki A. 2003. The interaction between fentanyl and propofol during emergence from anesthesia: monitoring with the EEG-Bispectral Index™. *J. Clin. Anesth.* 15:103–7
36. Bo P, Soragna D, Specchia C, Chimento P, Favalli L. 2003. Quantified EEG analysis monitoring in a novel model of general anaesthesia in rats. *Brain Res. Protoc.* 11:155–61
37. Cohen BA, Bravo-Fernandez EJ, Anthony Sances J. 1976. Quantification of computer analyzed serial EEGs from stroke patients. *Electroencephalogr. Clin. Neurophysiol.* 41:379–86
38. Bassetti CL, Aldrich MS. 2001. Sleep electroencephalogram changes in acute hemispheric stroke. *Sleep Med.* 2:185–94
39. Murri L, Gori S, Massetani R, Bonanni E, Marcella F, Milani S. 1998. Evaluation of acute ischemic stroke using quantitative EEG: a comparison with conventional EEG and CT scan. *Neurophysiol. Clin./Clin. Neurophysiol.* 28:249–57
40. Nakajima Y, Homma S, Musha T, Okamoto Y, Ackerman RH, et al. 1990. Dipole-tracing of abnormal slow brain potentials after cerebral stroke—EEG, PET, MRI correlations. *Neurosci. Lett.* 112:59–64
41. Bezerianos A, Tong S, Thakor N. 2003. Tsallis entropy estimation of EEG rhythm changes following brain ischemia. *Ann. Biomed. Eng.* 31:221–32
42. Tong S, Bezerianos A, Paul J, Zhu Y, Thakor N. 2002. Nonextensive entropy measure of EEG following brain injury from cardiac arrest. *Physica A* 305:619–28
43. Tong S, Bezerianos A, Malhotra A, Zhu Y, Thakor N. 2003. Parameterized entropy analysis of EEG following hypoxic–ischemic brain injury. *Phys. Lett. A* 314: 354–61
44. Thatcher RW, Walker RA, Gerson I, Geisler FH. 1989. EEG discriminant analyses of mild head trauma. *Electroencephalogr. Clin. Neurophysiol.* 73:94–106
45. Legros B, Fournier P, Chiaroni P, Mercier C, Degiovanni E, et al. 1998. Emergency EEG and brain trauma. *Neurophysiol. Clin./Clin. Neurophysiol.* 28:111–20
46. Young G. 2000. The EEG in coma. *J. Clin. Neurophysiol.* 17:473–85
47. Horwitz B, Poeppel D. 2002. How can

EEG/MEG and fMRI/PET data be combined? *Hum. Brain Mapp.* 17:1–3
48. Alper J. 1993. EEG+MRI: a sum greater than the parts. *Science* 261:559
49. Baudewig J, Bittermann HJ, Paulus W, Frahm J. 2001. Simultaneous EEG and functional MRI of epileptic activity: a case report. *Clin. Electroencephalogr.* 112:1196–200
50. Misulis KE. 1997. *Essentials of Clinical Neurophysiology*. Boston: Butterworth-Heinemann
51. Spehimann R. 1981. *EEG Primer*. New York: Elsevier/North-Holland Biomed. Press
52. Webster JG. 1978. *Medical Instrumentation: Application and Design*. Boston: Houghton Mifflin
53. Yoo SK, Kim NH, Kim SH, Kim JL. 1995. The development of high precision EEG amplifier for the computerized EEG analysis. *Proc. IEEE Annu. Conf. Eng. Med. Biol. Soc., 17th*, 2:1651–52, Montreal, Quebec, Can.
54. Goel V, Brambrink AM, Baykal A, Koehler RC, Hanley DF, Thakor NV. 1996. Dominant frequency analysis of EEG reveals brain's response during injury and recovery. *IEEE Trans. Biomed. Eng.* 43:1083–92
55. Palus M. 1996. Nonlinear in normal human EEG: cycles, temporal asymmetry, nonstationarity and randomness, not chaos. *Biol. Cybern.* 75:389–96
56. Pijn J, Van Neerven J, Noest A, Lopes da Silva FH. 1991. Chaos or noise in EEG signals: dependence on state and brain site. *Electroencephalogr. Clin. Neurophysiol.* 79:371–81
57. Tong S, Bezerianos A, Paul J, Zhu Y, Thakor N. 2001. Removal of ECG interference from the EEG recordings in small animals using independent component analysis. *J. Neurosci. Methods* 108:11–17
58. Jung T, Makeig S, Westerfield M, Townsend J, Courchesne E, Sejnowski T. 2000. Removal of eye activity artifacts from visual event-related potentials in normal and clinical subjects. *Clin. Neurophysiol.* 111:1745–58
59. Jung T, Makeig S, Humphries C, Lee T, McKeown M, et al. 2000. Removing electroencephalographic artifacts by blind source separation. *Psychophysiology* 37: 163–78
60. Pardey J, Roberts S, Tarassenko L. 1996. A review of parametric modeling techniques for EEG analysis. *Med. Eng. Phys.* 18:2–11
61. Geocadin RG, Ghodadra R, Kimura T, Lei H, Sherman DL, et al. 2000. A novel quantitative EEG injury measure of global cerebral ischemia. *Clin. Neurophysiol.* 111:1779–87
62. Al-Nashash H, Al-Assaf Y, Paul JS, Thakor NV. 2004. EEG signal modeling using adaptive Markov process amplitude. *IEEE Trans. Biomed. Eng.* 51(5):744–51
63. Kaiser JF. 1990. On a simple algorithm to calculate the 'energy' of a signal. *Proc. Int. Conf. Acoustics, Speech, Signal Process., Albuquerque, NM*, pp. 381–84
64. Kaspar F, Schuster H. 1987. Easily calculable measure for the complexity of spatiotemporal patterns. *Phys. Rev. A* 36:842–48
65. Lempel A, Ziv J. 1976. Complexity of finite sequences. *IEEE Trans. Inf. Theory* 22:75–81
66. Zhang X, Roy R. 1999. Predicting movement during anaesthesia by complexity analysis of electroencephalograms. *Med. Biol. Eng. Comput.* 37:327–34
67. Zhang X, Roy R. 2001. Derived fuzzy knowledge model for estimating the depth of anesthesia. *IEEE Trans. Biomed. Eng.* 48:312–23
68. Xu J, Liu Z, Liu R, Yang QF. 1997. Information transmission in human cerebral cortex. *Physica D* 106:363–74
69. Crone N, Boatman D, Gordon B, Hao L. 2001. Induced electrocorticographic gamma activity during auditory perception. Brazier Award-winning article, 2001. *Clin. Neurophysiol.* 112:565–82

70. Crone N, Hao L, Hart JJ, Boatman D, Lesser R, et al. 2001. Electrocorticographic gamma activity during word production in spoken and sign language. *Neurology* 57:2045–53
71. Duhamel P, Vetterli M. 1990. Fast Fourier transforms: a tutorial review and a state of the art. *Signal Process.* 19:259–99
72. Muthuswamy J, Thakor NV. 1998. Spectral analysis methods for neurological signals. *J. Neurosci. Methods* 83:1–14
73. Thomson D. 1982. Spectrum estimation and harmonic-analysis. *Proc. IEEE* 70: 1055–96
74. Ghil M, Allen M, Dettinger M, Ide K, Kondrashov D, et al. 2002. Advanced spectral methods for climatic time series. *Rev. Geophys.* 40:1003
75. Kong X, Brambrink A, Hanley DF, Thakor NV. 1999. Quantification of injury-related EEG signal changes using distance measures. *IEEE Trans. Biomed. Eng.* 43:189–97
76. Thakor NV, Sherman DL. 1994. Biomedical problems in time-frequency-scale analysis—new challenges. *Proc. IEEE-SP Int. Symp. Time-Frequency Time-Scale Anal., Philadelphia*, pp. 536–39
77. Blanco S, Figliola A, Quiroga RQ, Rosso OA, Serrano E. 1998. Time–frequency analysis of electroencephalogram series (III): wavelet packets and information cost function. *Phys. Rev. E* 57:932–40
78. Williams WJ, Zaveri HP, Sackellares JC. 1995. Time-frequency analysis of electrophysiology signals in epilepsy. *IEEE Eng. Med. Biol. Mag.* 14:133–43
79. Zaveri HP, Williams WJ, Iasemidis LD, Sackellares JC. 1992. Time-frequency representation of electrocorticograms in temporal lobe epilepsy. *IEEE Trans. Biomed. Eng.* 39:502–9
80. Auger F. 1999. *Time-frequency distributions.* http://crttsn.univ-nantes.fr/~auger/tftbtest.html
81. Durka P, Blinowska K. 1995. Analysis of EEG transients by means of matching pursuit. *Ann. Biomed. Eng.* 23:608–11
82. Durka P, Blinowska K. 2001. A unified time-frequency parametrization of EEGs. *IEEE Eng. Med. Biol. Mag.* 20:47–53
83. Blinowska K, Durka P. 2001. Unbiased high resolution method of EEG analysis in time-frequency space. *Acta Neurobiol. Exp.* 61:157–74
84. Zygierewicz J, Blinowska KJ, Durka P, Szelenberger W, Niemcewicz S, Androsiuk W. 1999. High resolution study of sleep spindles. *Clin. Neurophysiol.* 110:2136–47
85. Mallat SG, Zhang Z. 1993. Matching pursuits with time-frequency dictionaries. *IEEE Trans. Signal Process.* 41:3397–415
86. Bacry E. 1997. *LastWave.* http://www.cmap.polytechnique.fr/~bacy/LastWave/
87. Jouny CC, Franaszczuk PJ, Bergey GK. 2003. Characterization of epileptic seizure dynamics using Gabor atom density. *Clin. Neurophysiol.* 114:426–37
88. Shannon CE. 1948. A mathematical theory of communication. *Bell Syst. Tech. J.* 27:379–423, 623–56
89. Renyi A. 1970. *Probability Theory.* Amsterdam: North-Holland
90. Tsallis C. 1988. Possible generalization of Boltzmann-Gibbs statistics. *J. Stat. Phys.* 52:479–87
91. Tsallis C. 1999. Nonextensive statistics: theoretical, experimental and computational evidences and connections. *Braz. J. Phys.* 29:1–35
92. Siekman WH. 2003. The entropic index of the planets of the solar-system. *Chaos Solitons Fractals* 16:119–24
93. Tatsuaki W, Takeshi S. 2001. When non-extensive entropy becomes extensive. *Physica A* 301:284–90
94. Tatsuaki W, Takeshi S. 2002. The additivity of the pseudo-additive conditional entropy for a proper Tsallis' entropic index. *Physica A* 305:186–89
95. Latora V, Baranger M, Rapisarda A, Tsallis C. 2000. The rate of entopy increase at the edge of chaos. *Phys. Lett. A* 273:97–103
96. De Moura FABF, Tirnakli U, Lyra ML.

2000. Convergence to the critical attractor of dissipative maps: log-periodic oscillations, fractality, and nonextensive. *Phys. Rev. E* 62:6361–65
97. Capurro A, Diambra L, Lorenzo D, Macadar O, Martin MT, et al. 1999. Human brain dynamics: the analysis of EEG signals with Tsallis information measure. *Physica A* 265:235–54
98. Yordanova J, Kolev V, Rosso OA, Schürmann M, Sakowitz OW, et al. 2002. Wavelet entropy analysis of event-related potentials indicates modality-independent theta dominance. *J. Neurosci. Methods* 117:99–109
99. Rosso OA, Blanco S, Yordanova J, Kolev V, Figliola A, et al. 2001. Wavelet entropy: a new tool for analysis of short duration brain electrical signals. *J. Neurosci. Methods* 105:65–75
100. Al-Nashash H, Paul J, Ziai W, Hanley D, Thakor N. 2003. Wavelet entropy for subband segmentation of EEG during injury and recovery. *Ann. Biomed. Eng.* 31:653–58
101. Andino SLG, Menendez RGD, Thut G, Spinelli L, Blanke O, et al. 2000. Measuring the complexity of time series: an application to neurophysiological signals. *Hum. Brain Mapp.* 11:46–57
102. Tong S, Thakor NV. 2003. Time-frequency complexity of EEG following hypoxic-ishemic brain injury. Presented at *25th IEEE-EMBS Conf., Cancun, Mex.*
103. Cover TM, Thomas JA. 1991. *Elements of Information Theory*. New York: Wiley
104. Darbellay GA, Vajda I. 1999. Estimation of the information by an adaptive partitioning of the observation space. *IEEE Trans. Inf. Theory* 45:1315–21
105. Darbellay GA. 1999. An estimator of the mutual information based on a criterion for independence. *Comput. Stat. Data Anal.* 32:1–17
106. Beirlant J, Dudewicz EJ, Gyorfi L, Meulen EC. 1997. Nonparametric entropy estimation: an overview. *Int. J. Math. Stat. Sci.* 6:17–39
107. Paninski L. 2003. Estimation of entropy and mutual information. *Neural Comput.* 15:1191–253
108. Na SH, Jin S-H, Kim SY, Ham B-J. 2002. EEG in schizophrenic patients: mutual information analysis. *Clin. Neurophysiol.* 113:1954–60
109. Muthuswamy J, Sherman DL, Thakor NV. 1999. Higher-order spectral analysis of burst patterns in EEG. *IEEE Trans. Biomed. Eng.* 46:92–99
110. Sherman DL, Brambrink AM, Walterspacher D, Dasika VK, Ichord R, Thakor NV. 1997. Detecting EEG bursts after hypoxic-ischemic injury using energy operators. *Proc. 19th Annu. Int. Conf. IEEE Eng. Med. Biol. Soc., Chicago*, 3:1188–90
111. Nikias CL, Mendel JM. 1993. Signal processing with higher-order spectra. *IEEE Signal Process. Mag.* 10:10–37
112. Akkarakaran S, Vaidyanathan PP. 2000. Bifrequency and bispectrum maps: a new look at multirate systems with stochastic inputs. *IEEE Trans. Signal Process.* 48:723–36
113. Kowalik ZJ, Elbert T. 1994. Changes of chaoticness in spontaneous EEG/MEG. *Integr. Physiol. Behav. Sci.* 29:270–82
114. Sarbadhikari S, Chakrabarty K. 2001. Chaos in the brain: a short review alluding to epilepsy, depression, exercise and lateralization. *Med. Eng. Phys.* 23:445–55
115. Lee YJ, Zhu YS, Xu YH, Shen MF, Zhang HX, Thakor NV. 2001. Detection of nonlinearity in the EEG of schizophrenic patients. *Clin. Neurophysiol.* 112:1288–94
116. Krystal A, Zaidman C, Greenside H, Weiner R, Coffey C. 1997. The largest Lyapunov exponent of the EEG during ECT seizures as a measure of ECT seizure adequacy. *Electroencephalogr. Clin. Neurophysiol.* 103:599–606
117. Pincus S. 1995. Approximate entropy (ApEn) as a complexity measure. *Chaos* 5:110–17
118. Lee YJ, Zhu YS, Xu YH, Shen MF, Tong SB, Thakor NV. 2001. The

nonlinear dynamical analysis of the EEG in schizophrenia with temporal and spatial embedding dimension. *J. Med. Eng. Technol.* 25:79–83

119. Stam C, Jelles B, Achtereekte H, Rombouts S, Staets J, Keunen R. 1995. Investigation of EEG non-linearity in dementia and Parkinson's disease. *Electroencephalogr. Clin. Neurophysiol.* 95: 309–20
120. Takens F. 1981. Detecting strange attractors in turbulenc. In *Dynamical Systems and Turbulence; Lecture Notes in Mathematics*, ed. D Rand, LS Young, 898:366–81. Berlin: Springer-Verlag
121. Grassberger P, Procaccia I. 1983. Measuring the strangeness of strange attractors. *Physica D* 9:189–208
122. Bruhn J, Ropcke H, Hoeft A. 2000. Approximate entropy as an electroencephalographic measure of anesthetic drug effect during desflurane anesthesia. *Anesthesiology* 92:715–26
123. Bhattacharya J. 2000. Complexity analysis of spontaneous EEG. *Acta Neurobiol. Exp.* 60:495–501
124. Gu FJ, Meng X, Shen EH, Cai ZJ. 2003. Can we measure consciousness with EEG complexities? *Int. J. Bifurc. Chaos* 13:733–42
125. Grassberger P, Procaccia I. 1983. Characterization of strange attractors. *Phys. Rev. Lett.* 50:346–49
126. Judd K. 1994. Estimating dimension from small samples. *Physica D* 71:421–29
127. Theiler J, Euband S, Longtin A, Galdrikian B, Farmer J. 1992. Testing for nonlinearity in time series: the method of surrogate data. *Physica D* 58:77–94
128. Rapp P, Albano A, Schmah T, Farwell L. 1993. Filtered noise can mimic low-dimensional chaotic attractors. *Phys. Rev. E* 47:2289–97
129. Le Van Quyen M, Martinerie J, Adam C, Varela F. 1999. Nonlinear analyses of interictal EEG map the brain interdependencies in human focal epilepsy. *Physica D* 127:250–66
130. Martinerie J, Adam C, Le Van Quyen M, Baulac M, Clemenceau S, et al. 1998. Epileptic seizures can be anticipated by non-linear analysis. *Nat. Med.* 4:1173–76
131. Ogo K. 1995. Chaos and fractal properties in EEG data. *Electron. Commun. Jpn. Pt. III* 78:27–36
132. Chen ACN. 2001. New perspectives in EEG/MEG brain mapping and PET/fMRI neuroimaging of human pain. *Int. J. Psychophysiol.* 42:147–59
133. Lachaux J-P, Rodriguez E, Martinerie J, Varela FJ. 1999. Measuring phase synchrony in brain signals. *Hum. Brain Mapp.* 8:194–208
134. Baillet S, Mosher JC, Leahy RM. 2001. Electromagnetic brain mapping. *IEEE Signal Process. Mag.* 18:14–30
135. Passynkova NR, Volf NV. 2001. Seasonal affective disorder: spatial organization of EEG power and coherence in the depressive state and in light-induced and summer remission. *Psychiatry Res. Neuroimaging* 108:169–85
136. Volf NV, Passynkova NR. 2002. EEG mapping in seasonal affective disorder. *J. Affect. Disord.* 72:61–69
137. Schellenberg R, Schwarz A, Knorr W, Haufe C. 1992. EEG-brain mapping. A method to optimize therapy in schizophrenics using absolute power and center frequency values. *Schizophr. Res.* 8:21–29
138. Galderisi S, Mucci A, Di Gregorio M, Bucci P, Maj M, Kemali D. 1990. C-EEG brain mapping in DSM-III schizophrenics after acute and chronic haloperidol treatment. *Eur. Neuropsychopharmacol.* 1:51–54
139. Galderisi S, Mucci A, Mignone M, Maj M, Kemali D. 1991. CEEG mapping in drug-free schizophrenics. Differences from healthy subjects and changes induced by haloperidol treatment. *Schizophr. Res.* 6:15–23
140. Kemali D, Galderisi S, Maj M, Mucci A, Di Gregorio M, Bucci P. 1992. Computerized EEG topography findings in

schizophrenic patients before and after haloperidol treatment. *Int. J. Psychophysiol.* 13:283–90

141. Saletu B, Kufferle B, Anderer P, Grunberger J, Steinberger K. 1990. EEG-brain mapping in schizophrenics with predominantly positive and negative symptoms. Comparative studies with remoxipride/haloperidol. *Eur. Neuropsychopharmacol.* 1:27–36
142. Angrilli A, Dobel C, Rockstroh B, Stegagno L, Elbert T. 2000. EEG brain mapping of phonological and semantic tasks in Italian and German languages. *Clin. Neurophysiol.* 111:706–16
143. Itil T, Ferracuti S, Freedman A, Sherer C, Mehta P, Itil K. 1990. Computer-analyzed EEG (CEEG) and dynamic brain mapping in AIDS and HIV related syndrome: a pilot study. *Clin. Electroencephalogr.* 21:140–44
144. Saletu B, Grunberger J, Linzmayer L, Anderer P. 1990. Brain protection of nicergoline against hypoxia: EEG brain mapping and psychometry. *J. Neural Transm. Parkinsons. Dis. Dement. Sect.* 2:305–25
145. Lu X-CM, Williams AJ, Tortella FC. 2001. Quantitative electroencephalography spectral analysis and topographic mapping in a rat model of middle cerebral artery occlusion. *Neuropathol. Appl. Neurobiol.* 27:481–95
146. Nunez PL. 1981. *Electric Fields of the Brain*. New York/Oxford: Oxford Univ. Press
147. Cuffin BN. 1998. EEG dipole source localization. *IEEE Eng. Med. Biol. Mag.* 17:118–22
148. Mosher JC, Leahy RM, Lewis PS. 1999. EEG and MEG: forward solutions for inverse methods. *IEEE Trans. Biomed. Eng.* 46:245–59
149. Fernandez DC, Menendez RGD, Andino SLG, Farras EO. 1995. Some limitations of spatio-temporal source models. *Brain Topogr.* 7:233–43
150. Gordon E. 1999. Brain imaging technologies: how, what, when and why? *Aust. NZ J. Psychiatry* 33:187–96
151. Thatcher RW, Biver C, McAlaster R, Salazar A. 1998. Biophysical linkage between MRI and EEG coherence in closed head inury. *Neuroimage* 8:307–26
152. Thatcher RW, Biver C, Gomez JF, North D, Curtin R, et al. 2001. Estimation of the EEG power spectrum using MRI T(2) relaxation time in traumatic brain injury. *Clin. Neurophysiol.* 112:1729–45
153. Dimitrov L. 1998. Texturing 3D-reconstructions of the human brain with EEG-activity maps. *Hum. Brain Mapp.* 6:189–202
154. Bonmassar G, Schwartz D, Liu A, Kwong K, Dale A, Belliveau J. 2001. Spatiotemporal brain imaging of visual-evoked activity using interleaved EEG and fMRI recordings. *Neuroimage* 13:1035–43
155. Korzeniewska A, Manczak M, Kaminski M, Blinowska K, Kasicki S. 2003. Determination of information flow direction among brain structures by a modified directed transfer function (dDTF) method. *J. Neurosci. Methods* 125:195–207
156. Liang H, Ding M, Bressler S. 2001. Temporal dynamics of information flow in the cerebral cortex. *Neurocomputing* 38:1429–35
157. Sameshima K, Baccala L. 1999. Using partial directed coherence to describe neuronal ensemble interactions. *J. Neurosci. Methods* 94:93–103
158. Baccala L, Sameshima K. 2001. Partial directed coherence: a new concept in neural structure determination. *Biol. Cybern.* 84:463–74

Annu. Rev. Biomed. Eng. 2004. 6:497–525
doi: 10.1146/annurev.bioeng.6.040803.140223

First published online as a Review in Advance on April 9, 2004

# ROBOTICS, MOTOR LEARNING, AND NEUROLOGIC RECOVERY

David J. Reinkensmeyer,[1,2] Jeremy L. Emken,[2] and Steven C. Cramer[3]
*[1]Department of Mechanical and Aerospace Engineering, [2]Department of Biomedical Engineering, and [3]Department of Neurology, University of California, Irvine, California 92697-3975; email: dreinken@uci.edu, jemken@uci.edu, scramer@uci.edu*

**Key Words** rehabilitation, neural systems, motor adaptation, neuroplasticity, neuromuscular control

■ **Abstract** Robotic devices are helping shed light on human motor control in health and injury. By using robots to apply novel force fields to the arm, investigators are gaining insight into how the nervous system models its external dynamic environment. The nervous system builds internal models gradually by experience and uses them in combination with impedance and feedback control strategies. Internal models are robust to environmental and neural noise, generalized across space, implemented in multiple brain regions, and developed in childhood. Robots are also being used to assist in repetitive movement practice following neurologic injury, providing insight into movement recovery. Robots can haptically assess sensorimotor performance, administer training, quantify amount of training, and improve motor recovery. In addition to providing insight into motor control, robotic paradigms may eventually enhance motor learning and rehabilitation beyond the levels possible with conventional training techniques.

CONTENTS

## INTRODUCTION

In the past decade, investigators increasingly have used robotic devices to manipulate and measure human movement, providing insight into how the nervous system learns to control movement. Here, we review knowledge generated by two new robotic paradigms: adaptation to robot-applied force fields and robot-assisted motor rehabilitation. We also provide examples of ways that robotic devices may ultimately enhance motor learning and recovery using these paradigms. Summaries of recent nonrobotic studies in motor learning (1–4) and motor rehabilitation (5–8) can be found elsewhere.

## MOTOR ADAPTATION TO ROBOT-APPLIED FORCE FIELDS

Moving requires interacting with dynamic environments. Gravity, water, the ground, clothes, tools, doors, bicycles, dance partners, and our limbs themselves have dynamics describable with nonlinear differential equations that dictate, along with muscle force, the trajectory of our limbs. Recently, investigators have used robots to create novel dynamic environments and investigate the human ability to adapt them.

The typical study design follows the one used by Shadmehr & Mussa-Ivaldi (9) (Figure 1). A two degrees-of-freedom (DOF) robotic device applied perturbing forces to the hands of unimpaired subjects who reached in a horizontal plane. The robot applied a force field for which force depended on hand velocity but pointed to it obliquely. The field initially curved the reaching path of the hand. With practice, however, the subjects adapted to the forces, straightening their hand

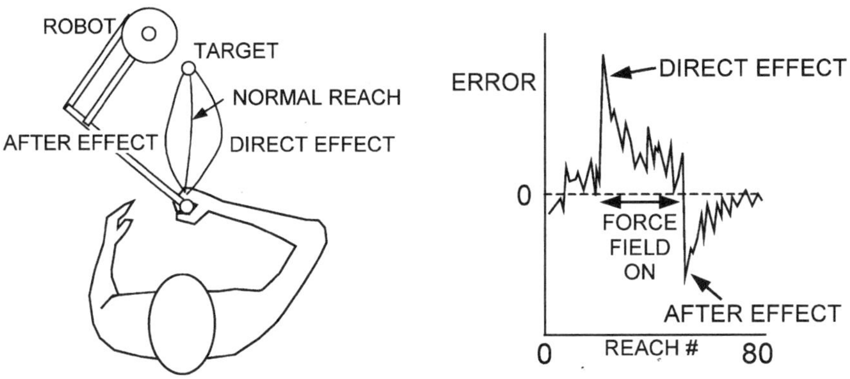


**Figure 1** Robotic force-field paradigm. A robot applies a force field to the subject's hand during reaching. The reach path is curved at first but straightens with time. When the force field is unexpectedly turned off, the subject exhibits an aftereffect that persists for tens of movements, which suggests that the nervous system formed an internal model of the force field. The graph (*right*) shows the reaching error (typically quantified as the maximum perpendicular distance or area between each reach and a normative reach) as the force field is applied then removed.

paths. When the forces were unexpectedly removed, the hand path was displaced in the direction opposite the force, along a roughly mirror-symmetric path to the one observed during initial exposure to the perturbation. The presence of this aftereffect proved that the nervous system generated a prediction of the expected perturbing forces using an internal model of the environment. Feedback or impedance control strategies would not generate aftereffects, provided the desired reach path remained constant throughout the experiment; they would cause the hand to move even straighter along the desired trajectory when the external, perturbing force field was removed.

The basic observation of aftereffects, and the inference of an internal model, is perhaps not surprising. If a person picks up a suitcase expecting that it is full when it is really empty, then he moves too fast and overshoots his intended endpoint. In other words, he exhibits an aftereffect because the internal model of the suitcase was incorrect. However, what the robotic force-field paradigm provides is the ability to create a wide range of force fields, to unexpectedly alter or revert them, and to precisely measure the forces and movements associated with them. In addition, the paradigm induces adaptation in a relatively short timescale—on the order of tens of movements, which makes it possible to perform motor-learning experiments quickly. As we review below, investigators have used these features in dozens of subsequent studies to elucidate the structure of neural control.

Subjects who participate in a force-field experiment often have several interesting impressions. First is the persistence of aftereffects following unexpected cessation of the applied field. The subject thinks an external force is still being applied for tens of movements, even though no force is being applied. Typically, the subject also decreasingly perceives the perturbation during adaptation, such that he is minimally aware that the force field is still on. Thus, conscious sense of effort appears to be heightened during periods of increased error rather than increased external force. That adaptation happens automatically, or subconsciously, for almost all subjects is also striking. Subjects who experience the force field even dozens of times still adapt to it. Put together, these observations suggest that a rather automatic or implicit process, linked to but separate from conscious control, guides internal model formation.

## Technical Requirements

The robotic force-field paradigm typically uses backdriveable robots, where "backdriveability" refers to low, intrinsic, endpoint impedance (10) or simply that the passive robot linkage moves easily when pushed. Backdriveable robots allow aftereffects to be measured and, more generally, a wide range of dynamic environments to be created. Most industrial robots are not backdriveable because they rely on highly geared motors to produce large forces. Backdriveability can be achieved easily for planar movement by mechanically grounding large motors that drive five bar linkages, a design often used in the robotic force-field paradigm (9, 11). Achieving high force with good backdriveability in three or more dimensions is more difficult. One commercial, haptic robot (PHANToM, Sensable Technologies, Inc.) used in force-field experiments (e.g., 12) uses cable and capstan transmission but generates only modest forces. Nonbackdriveable robots with high-bandwidth force control are another possibility for creating dynamic environments, but typically they are not as responsive as backdriveable robots and have not been widely used to study motor adaptation. Combining force control with a springy actuator provides good active backdriveability (13).

The robotic force-field paradigm also requires selecting an appropriate force field. Most experiments have used planar, velocity-dependent, or viscous force fields as the perturbing field. Typically the 2 by 2 damping gain matrix is chosen so that the force points obliquely, often perpendicularly, to the hand velocity (a viscous curl or conservative field). Investigators use a velocity-dependent field because it does not apply force when the subject is not moving, and thus it can be turned on or off unexpectedly between movements, allowing a kinematic glimpse of the consequences of the next feedforward command (i.e., the aftereffect). Inertial force fields could also be switched on unexpectedly, but acceleration signals are often more difficult to obtain or noisier than velocity signals. Inertial force fields have been created by adding weights to outriggers on a splint attached to the arm (14). Velocity-dependent force fields with a curl component are interesting because few external environments generate them, and thus they are ostensibly novel to most subjects. Velocity-dependent force fields have also been created with revolving rooms (15). Studies have begun to investigate force fields that represent nonrigid objects, such as a simulated mass and spring (16) or inverted pendulum (17), and suggest that internal model-based control is also used for such objects.

## State Dependence Versus Rote Memorization

Feedforward control could be achieved by simply memorizing and then replaying the time sequence of muscle forces required to cancel the novel dynamic environment or by forming a mapping (an internal model) between limb state and muscle forces. If learning were rote, then performance improvements would not generalize to a movement trajectory requiring a different time sequence of commands. However, the internal model formed during straight-line reaching movements generalized well to circular drawing movements (11). Subjects also adapted to a time-varying pattern of perturbing force by producing compensating forces that depended on the position and velocity of the arm and not on time (18). Subjects adapted to a force field that varied with movement sequence only if the sequence could be approximated with a state-dependent model (19). These observations suggest that the internal model computes muscle activations from limb states, rather than from memorized time sequences.

## Generalization

A motor control strategy is said to generalize or transfer if it can be used effectively in a situation different from the one in which it was learned. For example, the above experiments indicate that the internal model generalizes between different tasks (reaching and drawing circles) that share the same workspace, presumably because the model relies on a state-space representation of the field. Generalization of internal models across space, arms, directions, and speeds has also been observed.

Internal models generalize spatially, allowing subjects to compensate for a field in a region of the workspace different from the one in which they learned it. For example, subjects adapted to the field in a workspace on the right side of their bodies and then performed reaching movements in a workspace on the left side of their bodies (9). When the field was translated to the left workspace, subjects initially could not move straight. When the field orientation was rotated about the shoulder into the left workspace, however, subjects moved straight on their first reaches. Thus, the internal model learned in one part of the workspace transferred or generalized to another part of the workspace in a shoulder-centered coordinate frame. Other experiments have supported the concept that the internal model utilizes an intrinsic rather than extrinsic coordinate frame when generalizing to other regions of the workspace during same-limb reaching (20–22) or in a pole-balancing task in which the hand remained isometric (17). In contrast, learned dynamics appear to generalize from the dominant to the nondominant arm in extrinsic coordinates (23).

Instead of training in multiple directions in one workspace and then testing in other workspaces, investigators have also trained subjects in a single direction in one workspace and then tested generalization to other movement directions within the same workspace. In this situation, aftereffect magnitude decreased with increasing angle from the learned direction, which suggests that internal models are locally represented with respect to direction (20, 24). Predictive grasping forces used during bimanual manipulation also are learned locally with respect to direction (25).

Learning of a velocity-dependent force field for a reaching movement generalized to movements of the same orientation with increased velocity or amplitude (26). This generalization was best captured by a linear extrapolation of the force field represented in state space and may help people scale learned movements in time and space.

## Noise, Instability, and Impedance Control

In most force-field experiments, the force-field parameters (i.e., the gain matrix of the viscous field) were held constant throughout adaptation. In the real world, people often move in noisy dynamic environments. For example, a postal worker sorting boxes will experience a range of weights for a given size box. Trial-to-trial variability also arises from neural sources (27, 28) and is larger during childhood (29) or following an injury such as a stroke (30). When the gain of a viscous curl field was varied from reach to reach according to a normal distribution, the nervous system formed an internal model that estimated the mean gain of the field, although the estimate was low in some cases (12, 31). Children as young as age five can adapt to force fields even if additional external noise is superimposed using a force field on their already-noisy movement (29). Thus, the internal model formation algorithm appears robust to at least some degree of external and internal, trial-to-trial noise.

Robot experiments indicate that the nervous system uses impedance control along with internal models in noisy and unstable force fields. Subjects increased their arm impedance so that variations in the field strength produced less variation in trajectory error, and aftereffects were diminished following exposure to the noisy force field (12). Aftereffects were absent following adaptation to a destabilizing force field that amplified trajectory errors (an unstable spring in the direction perpendicular to movement) (32). Measurements of limb impedance during adaptation indicated that arm stiffness increased only in the direction necessary to stabilize the arm. These results suggest that directionally specific impedance control is combined with varying amounts of internal model–based control for noisy or unstable environments.

## Kinematic Versus Dynamic Optimization

That the nervous system optimizes movements by either a kinematic criterion, such as trajectory error or smoothness, or a dynamic criterion, such as force or effort, is an appealing idea. Scheidt et al. (33) applied a viscous force field perpendicular to the reaching direction to investigate this question, then monitored deadaptation when kinematic errors were either allowed to occur following removal of the field or prevented from occurring by imposing a virtual channel that restricted movement in the perpendicular direction. When kinematic errors were prevented from occurring, subjects persisted in generating corrective forces that were unnecessary to generate an accurate reach. However, the magnitude of these forces decayed slowly over time, with a time constant approximately 15 times longer than when kinematic errors were allowed. This experiment suggests that kinematic and dynamic criteria were optimized simultaneously but at different timescales. The nervous system responded quickly to correct trajectory errors but more slowly optimized muscle force given an acceptable level of trajectory error. Thus, the nervous system may do the same task the next time with less effort, provided it succeeds by a kinematic criterion in the previous attempt.

## Multiple Internal Models, Retention, and Interference

The nervous system presumably stores an internal model for each dynamic object with which it knows how to interact, switching between the models based on visual or other sensory clues (e.g., envision switching between a hammer, nail, and board). Several studies have investigated the development and switching of multiple internal models.

Brashers-Krug et al. (34) demonstrated that an internal model learned in the robotic force-field paradigm could be retained over time. When subjects learned to reach in a force field, then rested or even left the robot for a period, their next attempt at reaching in the field was straighter than their first attempt, although not as straight as their last attempt; this finding indicates partial retention of the learned model. Retention was observed after delays of up to five months (35). When subjects learned a second, conflicting field immediately after learning the first, retention of the first was decreased, a phenomenon called interference. The amount of interference depended on the temporal separation between the two conflicting force fields. A delay of five hours between two fields was sufficient for maximal retention, apparently owing to consolidation from short- to long-term memory.

The null field itself is an interfering field, as subjects who practiced reaching in the null field following adaptation to a force field showed little or no retention when experiencing the field a second time (29). However, as described above, subjects who walk away from the robot and move their arms in a null field at home (i.e., not attached to the robot) retain their robot model at a subsequent visit (34). These observations are consistent with the idea that the nervous system associates internal models with objects: We expect a tool (e.g., the robot arm) to behave as it did the last time we used it. When we are not using the tool, we apparently do not use the model associated with it to move our arm.

Several studies illustrate the difficulty in learning two different force fields presented in close opposition by one tool (i.e., the robot). Subjects were unable to predict two viscous force fields presented in alternating groups associated with colored lights or thumb posture (20). However, they predicted the fields with extended practice when the fields were associated with different handgrips. Thus, a single model may have been formed that predicted the different fields on the basis of the different arm/hand states, or two models may have been formed and switched between on the basis of the grip context. In either case, an intrinsic cue, related to joint posture, was apparently required to predict the two fields. This was somewhat surprising, given that we switch easily between internal models using visual cues in everyday life. Subjects could not predict two viscous force fields that were simply alternated reach-by-reach over four days, which suggests that temporal sequence was insufficient to learn and switch between two models (19).

However, Wada et al. (36) recently showed that subjects ultimately learned to predict randomly presented unstable and stable viscous force fields for a single DOF elbow movement, given days of practice and colors that signaled the field type. Thus, a conflicting force field presented in close temporal succession does not necessary cause catastrophic interference, and an intrinsic contextual clue is not necessarily needed for switching. Rather, the readiness with which multiple internal models are formed may depend on both the effectiveness of the contextual clues and the similarity of the force fields (36). For example, learning to switch between a robot-applied force field and a glass of water may be straightforward because of the different fields and contexts. Switching between two similar force fields on the robot, or between racquetball and tennis, may be more difficult because of the similarity of both the context and fields.

## Forward and Inverse Models

Forward models predict movement on the basis of a motor command, whereas inverse models predict the motor command needed to achieve a desired movement. Learning to cancel a force field ultimately requires an inverse dynamic computation of some form, whether implemented by an explicit inverse model, a neural network, or a feedback controller. Forward models, which are more difficult to isolate (37, 38), could be useful in motor learning for selecting inverse models and as state estimators for use in control. For example, the nervous system could use predictions from a forward model, compared to actual performance, to decide to switch between internal inverse models (39). Forward models could also be used to predict and cancel the sensory consequences of motor commands (40). A control architecture using both forward and inverse models best predicted reaching trajectories during force-field adaptation (41). Saccadic eye movements that track the hidden hand during reaching are controlled by a forward model that predicts the state of the arm about 200 ms in advance and takes into account the dynamics of the arm and its environment (42).

## Computational Models of Internal Model Formation

The evolution of movement error during application of a force field can be described with a simple finite difference equation (24, 31, 43):

$$e_i = a_1 e_{i-1} + b_0 B_i + b_1 B_{i-1}, \quad (1)$$

where $e_i$ is movement error on the $i^{th}$ trial, $B_i$ is field strength on the $i^{th}$ trial, and $a_1$, $b_0$, $b_1$ are regression coefficients.

This equation suggests that the nervous system updates its currently selected internal model on the basis of sensory information from only one previous trial and an internal state variable, performing a sort of moving average. If it is assumed that the measure of movement performance $x_i$ is related to a motor command $u_i$ and field strength $B_i$ by a static function that can be linearized as

$$x_i = f(B_i, u_i) = c_i B_i + d_i u_i, \quad (2)$$

where $u_i$ is motor command on the $i$th trial and $c_i$, $d_i$ are linearization coefficients, then the following simple, motor command update law produces Equation 1:

$$u_i = u_{i-1} + G e_{i-1}. \quad (3)$$

Thus, in this formulation, the nervous system calculates the next motor command by adjusting the previous command on the basis of the last error. In a related formulation, the desired trajectory for a feedback controller could be adjusted on a trial-by-trial basis using performance error, effectively producing the same sort of iterative, inverse computation but without an explicit internal model (44). By vectorizing such a finite difference equation to account for movement error in multiple directions, and by allowing an error in one direction to affect commands in other directions with a Gaussian weighting, error evolution for multi-target reaching can be more accurately modeled (24).

Another way to view the inverse model computation is as a function approximation problem, where the function that must be approximated is the applied force-field equation. Thoroughman & Shadmehr (24) suggested that the function may be approximated by a weighted sum of broadly overlapping Gaussians. In their paradigm, the Gaussian weights were incremented on the basis of force errors. Such a scheme predicted the curvature of reaches in a force field and poor compensation for a force field with high spatial frequency content. Other modeling studies of robotic force-field adaptation can be found in References 45 through 47.

## Relationship to Kinematic Models

The nervous system is also capable of forming an internal model of its kinematic environment, defining the relationship between perceived and actual motion. Krakauer et al. (48) suggested that internal models for kinematic and dynamic perturbations form independently because no interference occurred when subjects learned a dynamic perturbation (inertial load) shortly after a kinematic one (rotated spatial reference frame). However, when subjects first adapted to a position-dependent visuomotor rotation and then to a position-dependent rotary force field, the learning of visuomotor rotation was impaired, indicating interference (49). Thus, internal models of kinematic and dynamic perturbations are not independent when they rely on the same kinematic variable. The nervous system can combine and decompose kinematic and dynamic models. For example, reaching errors for the kinematic perturbations were smaller if subjects had first learned the combined transformation (50).

## Other Limb Systems

Investigators have applied velocity-dependent force fields to the leg during the swing phase of treadmill locomotion using a novel backdriveable robotic device (51, 52). Subjects adapted to the field and exhibited aftereffects, indicating formation of an internal model. Studies have also applied force fields to spinal transected rats stepping bipedally on a treadmill during the stance (53) and swing (54) phases of locomotion. The rats adapted to the force field by altering step timing and muscle activity, although with different timescales than in intact human adaptation with the arm and without clear evidence of aftereffects. Subjects exhibited aftereffects when robotic coupling of the hands was unexpectedly broken in a bimanual unloading task (55).

## Developmental Studies

Children ages 4 to 18 formed internal models of force fields produced by robotic devices (29, 56, 57). The accuracy of the model was comparable to that of adults, although the time required for adaptation or deadaptation was longer. Children also exhibited more trial-to-trial variability in their movements, both before and after adaptation (29). The youngest children, ages 5 to 7, more quickly reduced their variability with practice, giving the appearance of rapid learning even though their final variability levels were still higher than those in adults. Internal models formed in one workspace region transferred to an untrained region (56).

## Force-Field Adaptation after Neurologic Injury

Hemiparetic stroke patients with full reaching range of motion, but who were weakened by ~60%, still adapted to a mild perturbing force field by forming an internal model (58). However, more severely impaired stroke patients, with reduced reaching range of motion and weakness of more than 70%, showed no aftereffects and a continual reliance on feedback control to correct for the perturbation. This finding suggests that severe hemiparesis impairs either the ability to form or implement internal models. For example, destruction of brain areas responsible for internal model formation may impair feedforward control. Alternately, an inability to produce enough force, or perhaps force at a high-enough rate, may render feedforward control ineffective. Subjects with Parkinson's disease adapted to a force field but had decreased learning rates when adapting to a second, opposite curl field after learning the first (59).

## Neural Substrates

A number of studies have examined the brain structures in which activity changes in relation to motor learning during robot-applied force fields. Shadmehr & Holcomb (60) used positron emission tomography (PET) scanning to measure cerebral blood flow (CBF) at various phases of motor adaptation. Subjects learned to use their right arm to move a robotic arm in a viscous force field. Early during the learning process, motor output correlated with activation in bilateral sensorimotor cortices and the right striatum. This early learning, when compared to motor performance in an unlearnable random robotic force-field condition, was associated with relatively greater brain activation in areas such as the pulvinar nucleus and the right dorsolateral prefrontal cortex. When PET scans taken at the end of the learning phase were contrasted with scans taken 5.5 h later, however, the location of activation increases during motor task performance showed a relative shift to left posterior parietal cortex, left dorsal premotor cortex, and right cerebellum. This shift over time was not associated with a change in the quality of motor performance but may indicate the substrate underlying consolidation, or stabilization, of motor learning in this model. A later study by these authors (61) used a model of motor learning based on learning two different motor tasks separated either by a short time interval, making them compete for motor learning resources, or by a long time interval. This study suggested that the early phase of motor adaptation is associated with increased activity in the left putamen and bilateral dorsolateral prefrontal cortex. As motor performance reached a plateau, putaminal activation decreased.

Krebs et al. (62) studied various phases of motor learning by acquiring serial PET scans during adaptation to a force field imposed upon the right arm by a robot. Images taken early during the process of motor learning were contrasted with images taken during arm movement in the absence of a force field. The resulting images described brain activation during early motor learning, with increased activation in such areas as the right striatum (at a site more anteromedial than that in Reference 60), the left primary sensory cortex, and the bilateral parietal association areas. Images acquired as motor performance improved found that activation shifted to areas including the left motor and premotor cortices plus the right cerebellum. The role of the right striatum in motor learning, suggested in this study, is further supported by reports of poor motor learning in a patient with ischemic injury to this brain area (62).

Nezefat et al. (63) used PET to study CBF in cerebellum as subjects learned to use the right arm to control force-field changes introduced by a robot handle. In the right cerebellar hemisphere, posterior cortical activation increased during learning then declined as performance improved, whereas a reverse pattern was seen in the deep nuclei. Over the ensuing four weeks, during which motor performance remained stable, serial PET studies found a decrease in anterior cerebellar cortex activation. The results support a role for the cerebellum in the acquisition and retention of motor memories. Imamizu et al. (64) and Flament et al. (65), using fMRI, further supported changes in cerebellar activation in relation to motor adaptation. These findings are consistent with the observed motor learning deficiencies described in patients with cerebellar damage (63).

Donchin et al. (66) studied the influence of four pharmacological agents on acquisition and recall of new motor memories related to forces imposed by a robot arm. Lorazepam, a GABA-receptor agonist, and dextromethorphan, an NMDA-receptor antagonist, each impeded new motor learning, whereas lamotrigine, a sodium and calcium channel blocker, and scopolamine, a muscarinic-receptor antagonist, had no effect on learning. None of the four agents influenced motor memory recall. The findings support hypothesized relationships between synaptic plasticity and memory, and were novel in extending these relationships to memory in the motor system. Other models have found that lorazepam and dextromethorphan impair use-dependent plasticity in motor cortex (7). In addition, the results are important because they emphasize the presence of distinct neurobiological mechanisms for the processes of motor memory acquisition and recall.

Studies in primates agree with the above human brain mapping investigations. Gandolfo et al. (67) studied neuronal activity in primary motor cortex of two macaques as they learned to perform reaching movements in the presence of interfering external forces. A number of neuronal populations were described in relation to the arm movements. Activity in some cells was related to the direction of arm movement. Some of these cells changed their directional tuning during introduction of the force field, and a subset of these retained these changes. A large number of neurons changed directional tuning properties during adaptation to the force field. These changes in cell firing rate were not related to changes in muscle activity, which led the authors of this study to hypothesize that the neuronal changes were instead related to formation of an internal model within primary motor cortex. Li et al. (68) also found that some cells in primary motor cortex change their preferred direction of movement as a force field is learned.

Therefore, motor adaptation to force fields arises from brain areas that overlap incompletely with those areas related to motor skill acquisition. Early in motor adaptation, activation is increased relatively in cortico-striatal circuits, whereas later, performance is related to cortico-cerebellar circuits (4). Many of the substrates related to robot-mediated motor adaptation overlap with brain areas related to motor recovery after a CNS injury such as stroke (69, 70). This provides a theoretical framework for a possible clinical benefit of robot-related interventions in patients with stroke and other CNS insults. Note that the neurobiological substrate underlying motor adaptation may differ in several ways from that related to motor learning in other contexts such as motor sequence learning (4).

## Functional Relevance

Whether the knowledge gained from robotic force-field experiments can be expected to produce practical applications is an important question for biomedical engineering. For example, does the paradigm capture a fundamental-enough motor situation to provide general insight in a broad range of motor activities? Internal models are used pervasively throughout the day as we interact with tools and the environment, and indeed, every time we move our limbs, because our limbs themselves are dynamic objects. Internal models also may have several functional benefits. They allow movements to be made accurately in a more energy-efficient way, at least for predictable, stable environments. They may provide the mean for adjusting to morphological growth and tissue changes associated with development and aging, although the timescale of internal model formation seems much faster than what is necessary to keep up with such changes. They help us learn new tasks and tools and move in new environments, in a graceful, knowing way. We likely could get along without internal models, but our movements would be slower, less coordinated, less efficient, and more dependent on vision or feel. Therefore, the basic scientific knowledge gained with the robotic force-field paradigm most likely will lead to practical enhancements in motor learning, provided such enhancements are indeed possible.

For example, a thorough understanding of the error signals that drive adaptation may allow them to be amplified or filtered, thus accelerating learning. An understanding of the nature of generalization should facilitate the design of practice regimens for learning a new skill with the greatest generality and least amount of practice. Identifying factors that slow or interfere with learning, retention, or multiple model formation may suggest ways to minimize those factors. Finally, a thorough understanding of internal model formation, and the neural substrates for internal models, may lead to improved rehabilitation or neuroregeneration therapies for people with neurologic injuries. To define the relative role of, and optimal treatments for, different deficits of control, planning, sensing, and outflow pathways on the basis of the pattern of neurologic damage will be a key goal.

# ROBOT-ASSISTED MOTOR REHABILITATION

## Motivation for Robotic Therapy

Central nervous system diseases characterized by persistent motor deficits are common, a major source of disability, and expensive. Examples include stroke, multiple sclerosis, traumatic brain injury, Parkinson's disease, and spinal cord injury. For example, in patients with stroke a motor deficit is present in approximately 80% of patients early on, and in 50% at chronic time points, so that approximately two million stroke survivors in the United States have chronic arm impairment (71).

Two forces in rehabilitation medicine drove the development of robotic therapy devices, or rehabilitators (see Figure 2, see color insert), for patients with CNS diseases in the last decade. First, evidence increased that the injured motor system can reorganize in the setting of motor practice. However, the optimal training techniques for facilitating reorganization remained unclear, in part because of difficulties quantifying dose, type, and consistency of rehabilitation therapy. Robotic devices were seen as a possible way to precisely control and measure therapy.

Second, because of increasing pressure on the U.S. health care system, including the aging of baby boomers, patients began receiving less therapy following neurologic injuries such as stroke, even though studies suggested that more therapy was better. Robotic devices were seen as a possible way to automate labor-intensive training techniques, providing new tools for therapists and improved access to therapy for patients.

Four randomized, controlled studies of robotic therapy have been published: three for the upper extremity therapy after stroke (72–74) and one for gait training after stroke (75). Several robotic therapy studies have used chronic stroke or spinal cord–injured patients as their own baseline control (76–79). Other reviews of robotic therapy can be found in References 80 through 84.

## Robotic Therapy Algorithm Selection

Several modes of robot-assisted movement have been developed, including passive (72, 73, 75), active-constrained (73), counterpoise control (85), resistive (76), error-amplifying (86), and bimanual modes (73, 75, 87, 88). However, the primary therapy paradigm tested so far is active assistance (72–78), a clinical term that refers to exercises in which the patient attempts a movement (active) and in which a therapist manually helps complete the movement if the patient is unable (assistance). For example, a patient may try to reach to a target, and the therapist may guide the arm, if necessary. Such active assistance may improve recovery by enhancing proprioceptive input, reducing spasticity, restoring soft tissue suppleness, improving self-confidence, or by simply making exercise psychologically more tolerable, but it is labor intensive and has not been validated in controlled trials. It was a logical target when engineers and clinicians were presented with weak patients and force-generating robots.

Using devices to provide active assistance, however, is not new. For arm therapy, mobile arm supports, arm skateboards, and overhead slings are sometimes used in clinics to provide support against gravity, a passive form of active-assist exercise. For gait training, parallel bars, walkers, and overhead weight support systems are used to assist patients in standing and walking. Robotic devices, however, can provide programmable levels of assistance, do work against gravity, and automatically modify their output based on sensing.

## Robotic Therapy Devices for the Upper Extremity: First Results

The first robotic system to receive extensive clinical testing was MIT-MANUS, a two DOF backdriveable robot manipulator, similar to the one used by Shadmehr & Mussa-Ivaldi (9) in their original experiment. In a first report, 20 stroke patients received 4 to 5 1-h sessions a week for up to 9 weeks with MIT-MANUS, beginning on average 3 weeks after a single stroke (89). The device assisted planar pointing and drawing movements with an impedance controller. A control group received 1 h of sham therapy a week, in which they used the less-impaired limb

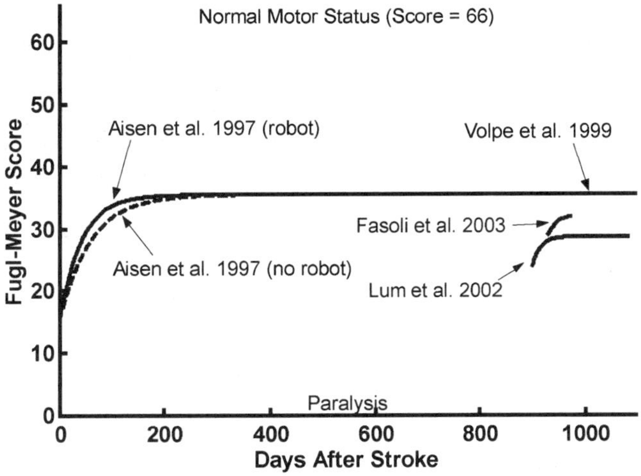


**Figure 3** Perspective on the magnitude of recovery of the upper extremity following stroke with robotic therapy. Plot summarizes data from four studies. The long solid curve (robot therapy) and dashed curve (no robot therapy) represent recovery reported in References 90 and 129. The two short curves represent data from References 76 (*upper curve*) and 73 (*lower curve*). All studies used the Fugl-Meyer upper extremity scale, which scores a series of movements 0, 1, or 2, then adds the individual movement scores to obtain the total score.

in the robot, or the robot interacted passively with the more-affected limb. When compared to the control group, the patients who received robotic therapy had reduced motor impairment of the shoulder and elbow according to the motor status score. The groups were still statistically different in terms of motor impairment at a three-year follow-up (90). These findings were confirmed with larger samples of 56 and 96 patients (72). Chronic stroke subjects who performed assistive and resistive exercises with MIT-MANUS also improved arm movement ability (76) (Figure 3).

This pioneering work suggests that supplemental robotic therapy can improve recovery in acute and now chronic stroke patients. However, these studies do not address whether robotic treatment offered unique advantages to conventional therapy or what the key components of the robotic therapy were (e.g., mechanical assistance by the robot versus an increased amount of sheer repetitive effort by the patient).

The MIME (mirror image movement enhancer) is a six-DOF, industrial robot manipulator (Puma 560) that applies forces to the paretic limb through a customized forearm splint. The robot can move the forearm through a large range of positions and orientations in three-dimensional space. A six-axis sensor measures the forces and torques between the robot and the paretic limb. Several modes of robot-assisted movement have been implemented with MIME, including passive, active-assisted, active-constrained, and bimanual modes, in which MIME copies the mirror image of the movement of a stroke subject's unimpaired limb, measured with a digitizing linkage.

The initial clinical testing of MIME compared the effectiveness of robotic therapy with an equally intensive program of conventional therapy (73). Twenty-seven chronic stroke subjects received 24 1-h sessions over 2 months. Subjects in the robot group practiced shoulder and elbow movements assisted by MIME in all four of its modes. Subjects in the control group received conventional treatment and five minutes of exposure to the robot in each session. The robot group had statistically larger improvements in the Fugl-Meyer score, a common clinical motor-impairment scale. The robot group also had larger gains in strength and reach extent. At the six-month follow-up, the groups were no longer different in terms of the Fugl-Meyer scale; however, the robot group had larger improvements in a scale that measured functional independence in activities of daily living (functional independence measure). These results suggest that robot-assisted therapy can be comparable, or perhaps even more effective, than conventional therapy.

A third device, the assisted rehabilitation and measurement (ARM) guide was designed to mechanically assist in reaching movements (91). Because reaching movements typically follow straight-line trajectories, the device uses a linear bearing to guide reaches by the subject. The linear bearing can be oriented at different yaw and pitch angles to allow subjects to reach to different workspace regions. Like MIT-MANUS and MIME, the device can assist or resist in movement and can measure hand movement and force generation. The device is statically counterbalanced so it does not gravitationally load the arm.

The goal of the initial clinical testing of the ARM guide was to identify the role of mechanical assistance in stimulating movement recovery, as opposed to unassisted, repetitive effort. Nineteen chronic stroke subjects received 24 therapy sessions over 2 months. Subjects in the robot group ($n = 10$) received mechanically assisted reaching exercise with the ARM guide. For this group, the subject initiated movement, and the ARM guide completed the movement along a smooth trajectory through the arm's full passive range if the subject was unable. Subjects in the free reaching group ($n = 9$) performed unassisted, repetitive reaching exercises, matched in the number of repetitions and target locations with the robot group. All subjects were evaluated using a set of clinical and biomechanical measures of arm movement. The subjects who received therapy with the ARM guide showed significant improvement in the time to complete functional tasks and in supported reaching range and velocity (92, 93). However, the amount of improvement in the free reaching group was not significantly different from the robot group and was, in fact, comparable in magnitude.

One interpretation of these results is that the action of repeatedly attempting to move, rather than the mechanical assistance provided by the ARM guide, was the primary stimulus to arm movement recovery for the subjects. This hypothesis is consistent with other repetitive-movement exercise paradigms that improve upper extremity movement ability following brain injury (e.g., 94–96). In addition, it is consistent with the observation that passive exercise engaged different brain areas and produced less motor learning when compared to active exercise in unimpaired subjects (97). Another possible explanation is that the particular movements (linear reaches) or form of robotic assistance provided by the ARM guide were suboptimal and that a higher DOF device with improved therapy algorithms may demonstrate a benefit over unassisted exercise.

Hesse et al. (77) developed a robotic device for the passive and active practice of bilateral forearm (supination/pronation) and wrist (flexion/extension) movements. Twelve chronic stroke subjects used the trainer for 15 min per day for 3 weeks. The subjects reported a reduction in spasticity, easier hand hygiene, and pain relief. A significant decrease in the modified ashworth score of wrist and finger spasticity was observed. No functional improvements were observed. Investigators have proposed or are developing other devices for arm and hand therapy (87, 88, 98–101), including vertical motion and wrist modules for MIT-MANUS (102, 103) and web-based teletherapy systems (104), but these devices have not undergone extensive clinical testing.

## Robotic Therapy Devices for Gait Training

Gait training with body weight support and manual assistance of the legs and pelvis is a promising new therapy technique that may manipulate spinal plasticity (8, 105–109), but it is labor intensive, requiring two to three therapists to assist the patient's legs and torso during each training session. In addition, the assistance provided, and thus the pattern of sensory input to the nervous system, can vary greatly between trainers and sessions. Recognizing this need, several research groups and a major U.S. healthcare provider (HealthSouth) are developing robotic devices for automating locomotor training in humans. The first device to undergo a controlled clinical trial was the mechanized gait trainer (MGT), a singly actuated mechanism that drives the feet through a gait-like trajectory using a doubled crank and rocker system (79).

The MGT was used in a crossover design to train subacute stroke patients to walk (75). A robot training group ($n = 15$) received two weeks of robotic gait training (A), followed by two weeks of human-assisted treadmill therapy (B), followed by two more weeks of robotic gait training (A). A control group ($n = 15$) received B-A-B. The patients were not significantly different before therapy in their overground walking ability but were after therapy, with the robot group performing better. Walking ability improved more rapidly for subjects in both groups during the robot-assisted training. Differences were not significant at a six-month follow-up. These results suggest that robot-assisted gait training can be as effective as conventional training, providing a significant reduction in manual labor.

Other devices for gait training are being developed, but they have not undergone extensive clinical testing yet. The Lokomat is a motorized exoskeleton worn by the patients during weight-supported stepping on a treadmill (78, 110). It drives hip and knee flexion/extension for each leg using precision ball screws connected to DC motors. The device was able to drive gait-like movement patterns in spinal cord–injured patients, reducing the labor burden on therapists who were assisting in step training. The Lokomat has been installed in dozens of research labs and clinics worldwide, and clinical testing results are forthcoming. ARTHuR (51) and PAM (111) are highly backdriveable robotic devices for measuring and manipulating stepping and pelvic motion, respectively. Small robots for training stepping by rats and mice have been developed to allow investigators to better study the neuromuscular plasticity that underlies step training (112). A new version of the MGT with more degrees of freedom is being developed (113).

## Robotic Assessment

Robotic devices provide a means to quantify sensory motor impairment, in addition to providing a means to implement and test specific forms of therapy. Backdriveable devices can act as motion capture devices and measure kinematic features of movements. Smoothness data from MIT-MANUS were used to develop the hypothesis that the nervous system has difficulty assembling movement primitives followings stroke (114). Directional error data gathered with a haptic robotic were used to support the hypothesis that increased variability in reaching after stroke is due to population coding, cosine tuning, neural firing rate noise, and cell death (115).

Nonbackdriveable robots can also quantify movement properties. For example, the pattern of forces reacted in high-impedance directions correlates with clinical measures of abnormal coordination (116, 117).

The active properties of robots can also be used to provide insight into sensorimotor impairment. Brisk stretches applied during reaching with the ARM guide illustrated that the presence of clinically observed spasticity does not necessarily mean an increase in arm stiffness during reaching (91, 118). Lateral forces applied during reaching can increase or decrease reaching range depending on their direction, which illustrates the coupled nature of directional force generation following stroke (58). Experiments have been performed with the Lokomat to identify the role of somatosensory input in gait generation following spinal cord injury (119). Asymptomatic carriers of the Huntington's disease gene had difficulty compensating for brief force pulses provided at the beginning of reaching movements, which suggests that feedback mechanisms are impaired by early damage to the basal ganglia and that robotic measures may provide a sensitive measure of disease onset (120). As reviewed in the previous section, investigators have noted an impaired ability to adapt to force fields after stroke (58) and Parkinson's disease (59).

## Functional Relevance

The first clinical studies of robotic therapy suggest that additional therapy provided by a robotic device can improve motor recovery and that robotic therapy is at least as effective as training with therapists alone in restoring arm function and gait after stroke. Investigators have not yet demonstrated conclusively that motorized therapy is superior to otherwise equivalent, nonmotorized therapy. The incremental improvements in clinical scales seen following intensive robotic therapy are statistically significant but small (Figure 3). They are arguably functionally insignificant from a third-party payer's point of view, although they are certainly meaningful to patients. The fate of robot therapy will be decided as the optimal components of therapy are defined. Robotic assessment techniques will play an important role in this process. In addition, there is a vast frontier that is virtually untouched in designing optimal rehabilitation therapies for specific patterns of neural damage, an important endeavor given the heterogeneity of stroke.

## ROBOT-ENHANCED MOTOR LEARNING AND RECOVERY

Could robotic devices enhance motor learning in health and injury beyond what is currently possible with conventional training techniques? Put another way, can the application of force to limbs in clever ways improve motor learning? To address this question, we first review a simple mathematical model of rehabilitation training that suggests conditions under which active assistance may be effective in promoting neurologic recovery. We then review experiments that suggest how three robotic training approaches may be more effective than unassisted, repetitive practice in promoting motor learning under certain conditions.

### A Mathematical Rationale for Active Assistance

Figure 4 shows a simple adaptive Markov model of sensory motor control that predicts the best movement recovery when an external trainer intervenes to correct errant movements on an as-needed basis, compared to no assistance or continual assistance (121). The basic assumptions of the model are, first, that the CNS probabilistically interprets somatosensory information in real time to generate motor output. To place this abstraction into a specific context, consider, for example, that changes in load-related afferent information during gait training cause functionally appropriate levels of limb extensor muscle activity to support the body (122). However, inherent variability exists in this response. Second, sensorimotor pathways become more reliable with repetitive activation in a sort of Hebbian learning. In other words, each time a sensorimotor transition is crossed, the probability associated with it is incremented, and competing pathways are decremented. Third, normal sensory input sometimes elicits abnormal motor output following neurologic injury owing to disrupted neural organization. Fourth, the external trainer generates a novel sensory state when it assists.

Given these assumptions, the model makes three intuitively appealing predictions (121). First, recovery can be enhanced by a trainer who actively assists abnormal movements, if the patient's sensorimotor impairment is not too severe. This

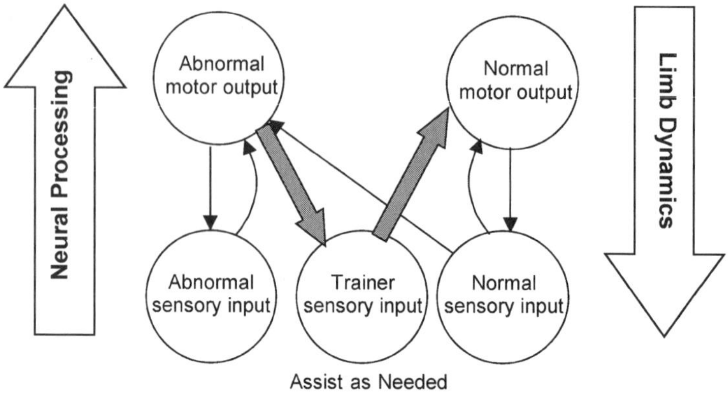


**Figure 4** Computational model of sensorimotor control. The model assumes that the nervous system interprets somatosensory information to create motor output and that motor output, in turn, creates sensory input. Motor and sensory states are abstracted into normal and abnormal states. The transitions between sensory and motor states are probabilistic, and the probabilities are modified with use in a Hebbian manner, resulting in an adaptive, Markov model. An external trainer (a therapist or robot) intervenes by recognizing abnormal motor output, assisting the limb and thereby creating a novel sensory state, which leads to a normal motor output (*large transition arrows*).

prediction corresponds well to the robotic studies reviewed above that have successfully used external mechanical assistance to retrain arm or locomotor ability after stroke.

Second, blindly assisting every movement of a patient is never beneficial compared to no assistance or assistance as needed, although it is equivalent in some situations. This prediction corresponds to the intuition that a therapist or robotic device that does not grade the level of assistance they provide will not be as effective as one that does.

Third, active assistance is unnecessary when sensory input is not directly coupled to motor output. Specifically, for a system in which abnormal sensory input does not always cause abnormal motor output, recovery does not require external assistance. This prediction suggests that there may be a fundamental difference in the optimal therapy approach for different sensorimotor systems. For example, attempts to retrain locomotion after spinal cord injury may benefit from active assistance because of the relatively tight coupling of somatosensory input and motor output in spinal-injured locomotion (123). In contrast, attempts to retrain arm movement after stroke may benefit less from active assistance because feedforward mechanisms appear largely sufficient for controlling arm movements, in the sense that sensory feedback is not required to trigger the next arm movement. Note, the model predicts that external assistance is not detrimental for uncoupled systems, but that its incorporation is simply unnecessary because unassisted, repetitive movement practice produces an equivalent result.

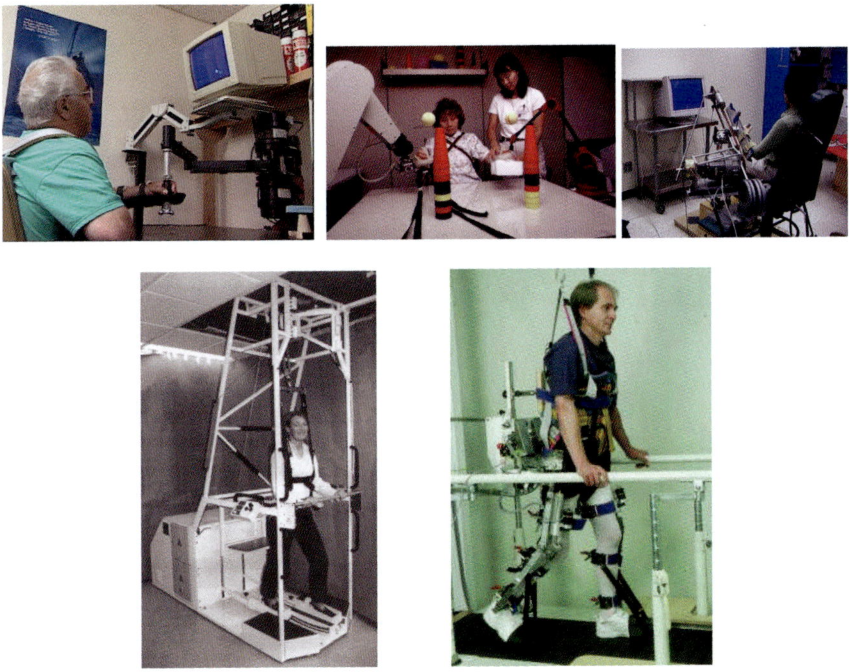

**Figure 2** Examples of robotic therapy devices (*clockwise from upper left*): MIT-MANUS allows horizontal planar motion of the arm using a two DOF robot (89); MIME uses a six DOF industrial robot arm to control arm motion and can be used in a bimanual mode in which the unimpaired arm of a stroke patient specifies the desired movement of the robot-controlled, impaired arm (73); the ARM Guide is a trombone-like, three DOF robot with one actuated DOF—the linear slide—which can be used to assist in reaching movements across the arm's workspace (91); the Lokomat drives hip and knee flexion and extension using ball-screw actuators attached to an exoskeleton (110); and the mechanized gait trainer uses a rock and cranker mechanism to drive the feet through a gait-like pattern (79). Figures reprinted with permission from the *Journal of Rehabilitation Research and Development*.

## Robot-Guided Training of Complex Trajectories

Feygin et al. (124) investigated the use of a robotic device to teach complex spatiotemporal trajectories to unimpaired subjects. Subjects learned the trajectory by holding a robot that moved along the trajectory (haptic learning), with or without vision, or by simply watching the robot move along the trajectory. Performance in replicating the trajectory was measured with and without vision and quantified using measures of spatial and temporal accuracy. Haptic learning with vision produced the best learning performance. Haptic learning without vision produced better learning of temporal features of the trajectory than vision alone. These results suggest that robotic devices may help therapists or coaches teach tasks of complex temporal patterning.

## Using Robot Force Fields to Teach Movement

Patton & Mussa-Ivaldi (125) are exploring the possibility of teaching desired movements using aftereffects from adaptation to robot-applied force fields. Different aftereffect trajectories were generated by shaping the force field, which demonstrates that movement kinematics can be sculpted by relying on implicit, subconscious motor adaptation. Determining how long the aftereffects persist, whether the aftereffect persists when the subject leaves the context of the robot, and whether learning a movement in this fashion is faster than learning it by simply being shown it and practicing are important questions for practical application.

Interesting preliminary data shows that stroke subjects can be taught to correct for systematic errors in directional control rather quickly using appropriately designed robotic force fields (86, 126). Specifically, if a force field is applied that amplifies a repeatable directional error (i.e., pushes the hand even further away from the target), then some subjects can adapt to the force field across tens of movements and return to their previous directional error levels. When the field is unexpectedly removed, the subject then moves more directly to the target (i.e., a beneficial aftereffect occurs that reduces the original directional error). The beneficial aftereffect may persist for some subjects. Thus, the neural processes associated with implicit motor adaptation may reshape sensorimotor mappings altered by stroke that cannot be altered simply by practicing movement.

## Guided Force Training

Recently, in comparing the results of the MIME and ARM guide studies of robotic therapy, Kahn et al. (127) observed a striking difference in a shared outcome measure (127). Despite similar therapy duration, therapy dosage, and subject characteristics, subjects who received therapy from the MIME device improved their active range of motion of free reaching by over 9 cm on average, whereas subjects who received therapy from the ARM guide device did not increase their active range of motion of free reaching. The control subjects from the studies who performed unassisted reaching therapy, or who received conventional therapy, also did not increase their active range of motion of free reaching.

MIME may have allowed a broader range of natural movements, perhaps enhancing functional retraining. Alternately, the bimanual training mode may have provided a unique stimulus for recovery of bilateral or ipsilesional neuromotor pathways. However, Kahn et al. (127) suggest that the MIME mode called active-constrained mode may be responsible. In active-constrained mode, the robot halted the subjects' movements when incorrect movement patterns were sensed, forcing subjects to learn how to generate the correct pattern at each troublesome workspace position. Active-constrained mode may thus be an effective way to functionally strengthen a weakened arm and to teach new muscle activation patterns necessary for coordinated movement.

## CONCLUSION

Robotic devices are helping us to understand the human motor controller and particularly the structure of feedforward control processes and their relationship to impedance and feedback control. Robotic devices are also helping us to understand how external force and movement practice influence motor recovery. New physical training modes, impossible with human teachers, are possible with robots. Elucidating how training can best manipulate physiology, and thus rationally defining the range of effective applications for robot trainers, is a key goal for future work. For example, clinical studies examining effectiveness of robotic training will need to devote increased attention to patient selection and the specific pattern of

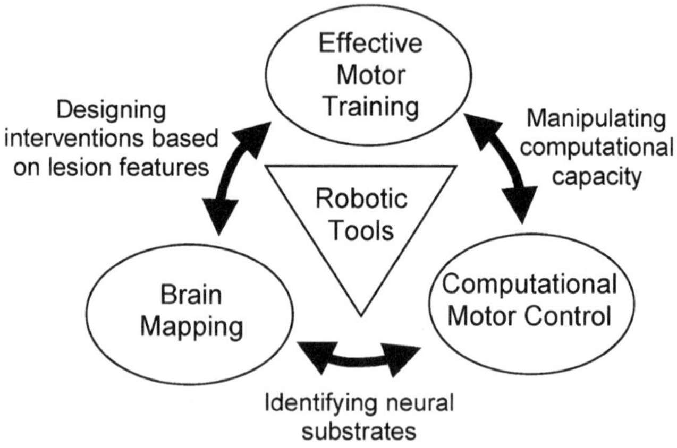


**Figure 5** Robots are facilitating an emerging synergy in which an improved understanding of the computational mechanisms and neural substrates of motor learning will drive improvements in motor rehabilitation.

neuropathology to be treated (128). We see the possibility of a new synergy facilitated by robotics, in which choice of patients and training techniques will arise logically from computational motor learning and brain mapping studies (Figure 5).

**The *Annual Review of Biomedical Engineering* is online at http://bioeng.annualreviews.org**

## LITERATURE CITED

1. Wolpert D, Ghahramani Z, Flanagan J. 2001. Perspectives and problems in motor learning. *Trends Cogn. Sci.* 5:487–94
2. Davidson P, Wolpert D. 2003. Motor learning and prediction in a variable environment. *Curr. Opin. Neurobiol.* 13:232–37
3. Sanes J. 2003. Neocortical mechanisms in motor learning. *Curr. Opin. Neurobiol.* 13:225–31
4. Doyon J, Penhune V, Ungerleider L. 2003. Distinct contribution of the cortico-striatal and cortico-cerebellar systems to motor skill learning. *Neuropsychologia* 41:252–62
5. Woldag H, Hummelsheim H. 2002. Evidence-based physiotherapeutic concepts for improving arm and hand function in stroke patients: a review. *J. Neurol.* 249:518–28
6. van der Lee J, Snels I, Beckerman H, Lankhorst G, Wagenaar R, Bouter L. 2001. Exercise therapy for arm function in stroke patients: a systematic review of randomized controlled trial. *Clin. Rehabil.* 15:20–31
7. Butefisch C, Davis B, Wise S, Sawaki L, Kopylev L, et al. 2000. Mechanisms of use-dependent plasticity in the human motor cortex. *Proc. Natl. Acad. Sci. USA* 97:3661–65
8. Hesse S, Werner C. 2003. Partial body weight supported treadmill training for gait recovery following stroke. *Adv. Neurol.* 92:423–28
9. Shadmehr R, Mussa-Ivaldi FA. 1994. Adaptive representation of dynamics during learning of a motor task. *J. Neurosci.* 14:3208–24
10. Krebs HI, Volpe BT, Aisen ML, Hogan N. 2000. Increasing productivity and quality of care: robot-aided neuro-rehabilitation. *J. Rehabil. Res. Dev.* 37:639–52
11. Conditt MA, Gandolfo F, Mussa-Ivaldi FA. 1997. The motor system does not learn the dynamics of the arm by rote memorization of past experience. *J. Neurophysiol.* 78:554–60
12. Takahashi C, Scheidt R, Reinkensmeyer D. 2001. Impedance control and internal model formation when reaching in a randomly varying dynamical environment. *J. Neurophysiol.* 86:1047–51
13. Robinson DW, Pratt JE, Paluska DJ, Pratt GA. 1999. Series elastic actuator development for a biomimetic walking robot. *1999 IEEE/ASME Int. Conf. Adv. Intell. Mechatronics*, pp. 561–68
14. Sainburg RL, Ghez C, Kalakanis D. 1999. Intersegmental dynamics are controlled by sequential anticipatory, error correction, and postural mechanisms. *J. Neurophysiol.* 81:1045–56
15. Lackner JR, Dizio P. 1998. Adaptation in a rotating artificial gravity environment. *Brain Res. Brain Res. Rev.* 28:194–202
16. Dingwell J, Mah C, Mussa-Ivaldi F. 2002. Manipulating objects with internal degrees of freedom: evidence for model-based control. *J. Neurophysiol.* 88:222–35
17. Mah C, Mussa-Ivaldi F. 2003. Evidence for a specific internal representation of motion-force relationships during object manipulation. *Biol. Cybern.* 88:60–72

18. Conditt MA, Mussa-Ivaldi FA. 1999. Central representation of time during motor learning. *Proc. Natl. Acad. Sci. USA* 96: 11625–30
19. Karniel A, Mussa-Ivaldi A. 2002. Does the motor control system use multiple models and context switching to cope with a variable environment? *Exp. Brain Res.* 143:520–24
20. Gandolfo F, Mussa-Ivaldi FA, Bizzi E. 1996. Motor learning by field approximation. *Proc. Natl. Acad. Sci. USA* 93:3843–46
21. Shadmehr R, Moussavi ZMK. 2000. Spatial generalization from learning dynamics of reaching movements. *J. Neurosci.* 20:7807–15
22. Malfait N, Shiller DM, Ostry DJ. 2002. Transfer of motor learning across arm configurations. *J. Neurosci.* 22:9656–60
23. Criscimagna-Hemminger SE, Donchin O, Gazzaniga MS, Shadmehr R. 2003. Learned dynamics of reaching movements generalize from dominant to nondominant arm. *J. Neurophysiol.* 89:168–76
24. Thoroughman KA, Shadmehr R. 2000. Learning of action through adaptive combination of motor primitives. *Nature* 407: 742–47
25. Witney AG, Wolpert DM. 2003. Spatial representation of predictive motor learning. *J. Neurophysiol.* 89:1837–43
26. Goodbody SJ, Wolpert DM. 1998. Temporal and amplitude generalization in motor learning. *J. Neurophysiol.* 79:1825–38
27. Lee D, Port NL, Kruse W, Georgopoulos AP. 1998. Variability and correlated noise in the discharge of neurons in motor and parietal areas of the primate cortex. *J. Neurosci.* 18:1161–70
28. Jones K, Hamilton A, Wolpert D. 2002. Sources of signal-dependent noise during isometric force production. *J. Neurophysiol.* 88:1533–44
29. Takahashi CD, Nemet D, Rose-Gottron CM, Larson JK, Cooper DM, Reinkensmeyer DJ. 2003. Neuromotor noise limits motor performance, but not motor adaptation, in children. *J. Neurophysiol.* 90:703–11
30. Kamper DG, McKenna AN, Kahn LE, Reinkensmeyer DJ. 2002. Alterations in reaching after stroke and their relationship to movement direction and impairment severity. *Arch. Phys. Med. Rehabil.* 83:702–7
31. Scheidt RA, Dingwell JB, Mussa-Ivaldi FA. 2001. Learning to move amid uncertainty. *J. Neurophysiol.* 86:971–85
32. Burdet E, Osu R, Franklin DW, Milner TE, Kawato M. 2001. The central nervous system stabilizes unstable dynamics by learning optimal impedance. *Nature* 414:446–49
33. Scheidt RA, Reinkensmeyer DJ, Conditt MA, Rymer WZ, Mussa-Ivaldi FA. 2000. Persistence of motor adaptation during constrained, multi-joint, arm movements. *J. Neurophysiol.* 84:853–62
34. Brashers-Krug T, Shadmehr R, Bizzi E. 1996. Consolidation in human motor memory. *Nature* 382:252–55
35. Shadmehr R, Brashers-Krug T. 1997. Functional stages in the formation of human long-term motor memory. *J. Neurosci.* 17:409–19
36. Wada Y, Kawabata Y, Kotosaka S, Yamamoto K, Kitazawa S, Kawato M. 2003. Acquisition and contextual switching of multiple internal models for different viscous force fields. *Neurosci. Res.* 46:319–31
37. Karniel A. 2002. Three creatures named 'forward model'. *Neural Netw.* 15:305–7
38. Mehta B, Schaal S. 2002. Forward models in visuomotor control. *J. Neurophysiol.* 88:942–53
39. Wolpert D, Kawato M. 1998. Multiple paired forward and inverse models for motor control. *Neural Netw.* 11:1317–29
40. Blakemore S, Wolpert D, Frith C. 2000. Why can't you tickle yourself? *Neuroreport* 11:R11–16
41. Bhushan N, Shadmehr R. 1999. Computational nature of human adaptive control

during learning of reaching movements in force fields. *Biol. Cybern.* 81:39–60

42. Ariff G, Donchin O, Nanayakkara T, Shadmehr R. 2002. A real-time state predictor in motor control: study of saccadic eye movements during unseen reaching movements. *J. Neurosci.* 22:7721–29
43. Takahashi CD, Nemet D, Rose-Gottron C, Larson JK, Cooper DM, Reinkensmeyer DJ. 2002. Computational motor adaptation—a kindergarten skill. *Proc. Second Joint EMBS/BMES Conf.* 3:2418–19
44. Gribble P, Ostry D. 2000. Compensation for loads during arm movements using equilibrium-point control. *Exp. Brain Res.* 135:474–82
45. Patton JL, Mussa-Ivaldi FA. 2002. Linear combinations of nonlinear models for predicting human-machine interface forces. *Biol. Cybern.* 86:73–87
46. Wang T, Dordevic GS, Shadmehr R. 2001. Learning the dynamics of reaching movements results in the modification of arm impedance and long-latency perturbation responses. *Biol. Cybern.* 85:437–48
47. Sanner RM, Kosha M. 1999. A mathematical model of the adaptive control of human arm motion. *Biol. Cybern.* 80:369–82
48. Krakauer JW, Ghilardi MF, Ghez C. 1999. Independent learning of internal models for kinematic and dynamic control of reaching. *Nat. Neurosci.* 2:1026–31
49. Tong C, Wolpert DM, Flanagan JR. 2002. Kinematics and dynamics are not represented independently in motor working memory: evidence from an interference study. *J. Neurosci.* 22:1108–13
50. Flanagan JR, Nakano E, Imamizu H, Osu R, Yoshioka T, Kawato M. 1999. Composition and decomposition of internal models in motor learning under altered kinematics and dynamics environments. *J. Neurosci.* 19(20):RC34
51. Reinkensmeyer D, Wynne J, Harkema S. 2002. A robotic tool for studying locomotor adaptation and rehabilitation. *Second Joint Meet. IEEE Eng. Med. Biol. Soc. Biomed. Eng. Soc.* pp. 2353–54
52. Emken JL, Reinkensmeyer DJ. 2003. *Evidence for an internal model dedicated to locomotor control.* Presented at 25th Annu. Int. IEEE EMBS, Cancun, Mexico
53. Timoszyk W, de Leon R, London N, Roy R, Edgerton V, Reinkensmeyer D. 2001. The lumbosacral spinal cord adapts to robotic loading during stance. *Soc. Neurosci. Abstr.* No. 297.20
54. Edgerton VR, de Leon RD, Harkema SJ, Hodgson JA, London N, et al. 2001. Retraining the injured spinal cord. *J. Physiol. (London)* 533:15–22
55. Lum PS, Reinkensmeyer DJ, Lehman SL, Li PY, Stark LW. 1992. Feedforward stabilization in a bimanual unloading task. *Exp. Brain Res.* 89:172–80
56. Jansen-Osmann P, Richter S, Konczak J, Kalveram KT. 2002. Force adaptation transfers to untrained workspace regions in children: evidence for developing inverse dynamic motor models. *Exp. Brain Res.* 143:212–20
57. Konczak J, Jansen-Osmann P, Kalveram K. 2003. Development of force adaptation during childhood. *J. Mot. Behav.* 35:41–52
58. Takahashi CD, Reinkensmeyer DJ. 2003. Hemiparetic stroke impairs anticipatory control of arm movement. *Exp. Brain Res.* 149:131–40
59. Krebs H, Hogan N, Hening W, Adamovich S, Poizner H. 2001. Procedural motor learning in Parkinson's disease. *Exp. Brain Res.* 141:425–37
60. Shadmehr R, Holcomb HH. 1997. Neural correlates of motor memory consolidation. *Science* 277:821–25
61. Shadmehr R, Holcomb HH. 1999. Inhibitory control of competing motor memories. *Exp. Brain Res.* 126:235–51
62. Krebs H, Brashers-Krug T, Rauch S, Savage C, Hogan N, et al. 1998. Robot-aided functional imaging: application to a motor learning study. *Hum. Brain Mapp.* 6:59–72

63. Nezafat R, Shadmehr R, Holcomb HH. 2001. Long-term adaptation to dynamics of reaching movements: a PET study. *Exp. Brain Res.* 140:66–76
64. Imamizu H, Miyauchi S, Tamada T, Sasaki Y, Takino R, et al. 2000. Human cerebellar activity reflecting an acquired internal model of a new tool. *Nature* 403:192–95
65. Flament D, Ellermann J, Kim S, Ugurbil K, Ebner T. 1996. Functional magnetic resonance imaging of cerebellar activation during the learning of a visuomotor dissociation task. *Hum. Brain Mapp.* 4:210–26
66. Donchin O, Sawaki L, Madupu G, Cohen LG, Shadmehr R. 2002. Mechanisms influencing acquisition and recall of motor memories. *J. Neurophysiol.* 88:2114–23
67. Gandolfo F, Li C, Benda BJ, Schioppa CP, Bizzi E. 2000. Cortical correlates of learning in monkeys adapting to a new dynamical environment. *Proc. Natl. Acad. Sci. USA* 97:2259–63
68. Li CS, Padoa-Schioppa C, Bizzi E. 2001. Neuronal correlates of motor performance and motor learning in the primary motor cortex of monkeys adapting to an external force field. *Neuron* 30:593–607
69. Rijntjes M, Weiller C. 2002. Recovery of motor and language abilities after stroke: the contribution of functional imaging. *Prog. Neurobiol.* 66:109–22
70. Cramer S. 2003. Functional magnetic resonance imaging in stroke recovery. *Phys. Med. Rehabil. Clin. N. Am.* 14:S47–55
71. Gresham G, Duncan P, Stason W, Adams H, Adelman A, et al. 1995. *Post-Stroke Rehabilitation.* Rockville, MD: Dep. Health Hum. Serv. Public Health Serv. Agency Health Care Policy Res.
72. Volpe B, Krebs H, Hogan N, Edelstein L, Diels C, Aisen M. 2000. A novel approach to stroke rehabilitation: robot-aided sensorimotor stimulation. *Neurology* 54:1938–44
73. Lum PS, Burgar CG, Shor PC, Majmundar M, Van der Loos M. 2002. Robot-assisted movement training compared with conventional therapy techniques for the rehabilitation of upper limb motor function following stroke. *Arch. Phys. Med. Rehabil.* 83:952–59
74. Kahn LE, Zygman M, Rymer WZ, Reinkensmeyer DJ. 2001. Effect of robot-assisted and unassisted exercise on functional reaching in chronic hemiparesis. *Proc. Annu. IEEE Eng. Med. Biol. Conf., 23rd, Istanbul,* October 25–28:39–44
75. Werner C, Von Frankenberg S, Treig T, Konrad M, Hesse S. 2002. Treadmill training with partial body weight support and an electromechanical gait trainer for restoration of gait in subacute stroke patients: a randomized crossover study. *Stroke* 33:2895–901
76. Fasoli S, Krebs H, Stein J, Frontera W, Hogan N. 2003. Effects of robotic therapy on motor impairment and recovery in chronic stroke. *Arch. Phys. Med. Rehabil.* 84:477–82
77. Hesse S, Schulte-Tigges G, Konrad M, Bardeleben A, Werner C. 2003. Robot-assisted arm trainer for the passive and active practice of bilateral forearm and wrist movements in hemiparetic subjects. *Arch. Phys. Med. Rehabil.* 84:915–20
78. Colombo G, Joerg M, Schreier R, Dietz V. 2000. Treadmill training of paraplegic patients with a robotic orthosis. *J. Rehabil. Res. Dev.* 37:693–700
79. Hesse S, Uhlenbrock D. 2000. A mechanized gait trainer for restoration of gait. *J. Rehabil. Res. Dev.* 37:701–8
80. Reinkensmeyer DJ, Hogan N, Krebs HI, Lehman SL, Lum PS. 2000. Rehabilitators, robots, and guides: new tools for neurological rehabilitation. In *Biomechanics and Neural Control of Posture and Movement,* ed. J Winters, P Crago, pp. 516–33. New York: Springer-Verlag
81. Volpe BT, Krebs HI, Hogan N. 2001. Is robot-aided sensorimotor training in stroke rehabilitation a realistic option? *Curr. Opin. Neurol.* 14:745–52

82. Reinkensmeyer D, Lum P, Winters J. 2002. Emerging technologies for improving access to movement therapy following neurologic injury. In *Emerging and Accessible Telecommunications, Information and Healthcare Technologies: Engineering Challenges in Enabling Universal Access*, ed. J Winters, C Robinson, R Simpson, G Vanderheiden, pp. 136–50. Arlington, VA: RESNA
83. Lum P, Reinkensmeyer D, Mahoney R, Rymer W. 2002. Robotic devices for movement therapy following stroke: current status and challenges to clinical acceptance. *Topics Stroke Rehabil.* 8:40–53
84. Reinkensmeyer D. 2003. Rehabilitators. In *Standard Handbook of Biomedical Engineering & Design*, ed. M Kutz, chapter 35. New York: McGraw-Hill
85. Reinkensmeyer DJ, Takahashi CD, Timoszyk WK, Reinkensmeyer AN, Kahn LE. 2000. Design of robot assistance for arm movement therapy following stroke. *Adv. Robotics* 14:625–37
86. Patton J, Mussa-Ivaldi F, Rymer W. 2001. Altering movement patterns in healthy and brain-injured subjects via custom designed robotic forces. *Proc. Annu. Int. Conf. IEEE Eng. Med. Biol. Soc., 23rd,* 2:1356–59
87. Lum PS, Lehman SL, Reinkensmeyer DJ. 1995. The bimanual lifting rehabilitator: a device for rehabilitating bimanual control in stroke patients. *IEEE Trans. Rehabil. Eng.* 3:166–74
88. Lum PS, Reinkensmeyer DJ, Lehman SL. 1993. Robotic assist devices for bimanual physical therapy: preliminary experiments. *IEEE Trans. Rehabil. Eng.* 1:185–91
89. Krebs HI, Hogan N, Aisen ML, Volpe BT. 1998. Robot-aided neurorehabilitation. *IEEE Trans. Rehabil. Eng.* 6:75–87
90. Volpe B, Krebs H, Hogan N, Edelsteinn L, Diels C, Aisen M. 1999. Robot training enhanced motor outcome in patients with stroke maintained over 3 years. *Neurology* 53:1874–76
91. Reinkensmeyer DJ, Kahn LE, Averbuch M, McKenna-Cole AN, Schmit BD, Rymer WZ. 2000. Understanding and treating arm movement impairment after chronic brain injury: progress with the ARM Guide. *J. Rehabil. Res. Dev.* 37: 653–62
92. Kahn LE, Averbuch M, Rymer WZ, Reinkensmeyer DJ. 2000. Comparison of robot-assisted reaching to free reaching in promoting recovery from chronic stroke. In *Integration of Assistive Technology in the Information Age*, ed. M Mokhtari, pp. 39–44. Amsterdam: IOS
93. Kahn L, Zygman M, Rymer W, Reinkensmeyer D. 2001. Effect of robot-assisted and unassisted exercise on functional reaching in chronic hemiparesis. *Proc. IEEE Eng. Med. Biol. Conf., Istanbul,* pp. 1344–47
94. Butefisch C, Hummelsheim H, Denzler P, Mauritz K. 1995. Repetitive training of isolated movement improves the outcome of motor rehabilitation of the centrally paretic hand. *J. Neurol. Sci.* 130:59–68
95. Liepert J, Bauder H, Miltner W, Taub E, Weiller C. 2000. Treatment-induced cortical reorganization after stroke in humans. *Stroke* 31:1210–16
96. Nudo RJ, Wise BM, SiFuentes F, Milliken GW. 1996. Neural substrates for the effects of rehabilitative training on motor recovery after ischemic infarct. *Science* 272:1791–94
97. Lotze M, Braun C, Birbaumer N, Anders S, Cohen L. 2003. Motor learning elicited by voluntary drive. *Brain* 126:866–72
98. Burdea G, Popescu V, Hentz V, Colbert K. 2000. Virtual reality-based orthopedic telerehabilitation. *IEEE Trans. Rehabil. Eng.* 8:430–32
99. Amirabdollahian F, Loureiro R, Driessen B, Harwin W. 2001. Error correction movement for machine assisted stroke rehabilitation. In *Integration of Assistive Technology in the Information Age*, ed. M Mokhtari, pp. 60–65. Amsterdam: IOS
100. Johnson MJ, Van der Loos HFM,

Burgar CG, Leifer L, Shor PC. 2000. Control strategies for a split-wheel car-steering simulator for upper limb stroke therapy. *Proc. Int. Conf. Robot. Autom., San Francisco*, pp. 1372–77
101. Merians A, Jack D, Boiau R, Tremaine M, Burdea G, et al. 2002. Virtual reality-augmented rehabilitation for patients following stroke. *Phys. Ther.* 82:898–915
102. Buerger SP, Krebs HI, Hogan N. 2001. Characterization and control of a screw-driven robot for neurorehabilitation. *Proc. 2001 IEEE Int. Conf. Control Appl.*, pp. 388–94
103. Williams DJ, Krebs HI, Hogan N. 2001. A robot for wrist rehabilitation. *Proc. Annu. Int. Conf. IEEE Eng. Med. Biol. Soc.* 23rd, 2:1336–39
104. Reinkensmeyer D, Pang C, Nessler J, Painter C. 2002. Web-based telerehabilitation for the upper-extremity after stroke. *IEEE Trans. Neural Sci. Rehabil. Eng.* 10: 1–7
105. Barbeau H, Norman K, Fung J, Visintin M, Ladouceur M. 2000. Does neurorehabilitation play a role in the recovery of walking in neurological populations? *Ann. NY Acad. Sci.* 860:377–92
106. Harkema SJ. 2001. Neural plasticity after human spinal cord injury: application of locomotor training to the rehabilitation of walking. *Neuroscientist* 7:455–68
107. Edgerton VR, Leon RD, Harkema SJ, Hodgson JA, London N, et al. 2001. Retraining the injured spinal cord. *J. Physiol.* 533:15–22
108. Dietz V, Wirz M, Colombo G, Curt A. 1998. Locomotor capacity and recovery of spinal cord function in paraplegic patients: a clinical and electrophysiological evaluation. *Electroencephalogr. Clin. Neurophys.* 109:140–53
109. Wernig A, Nanassy A, Muller S. 1999. Laufband (treadmill) therapy in incomplete paraplegia and tetraplegia. *J. Neurotrauma* 16:719–26
110. Colombo G, Wirz M, Dietz V. 2001. Driven gait orthosis for improvement of locomotor training in paraplegic patients. *Spinal Cord* 39:252–55
111. Ichinose W, Reinkensmeyer D, Aoyagi D, Lin J, Ngai K, et al. 2003. A robotic device for measuring and controlling pelvic motion during locomotor rehabilitation. *Proc. 2003 IEEE Eng. Med. Biol. Soc. Meet.*
112. Timoszyk WK, Merlo M, de Leon RD, Emken JL, Roy RR, et al. 2002. Second generation robotic systems for studying rodent locomotion following spinal cord injury. *Proc. Second Joint Meet. IEEE Eng. Med. Biol. Soc. Biomed. Eng. Soc., October 23–26, 2002, Houston, Texas*, pp. 2358–59
113. Schmidt H, Sorowka D, Hesse S, Bernhardt R. 2002. Robotic walking simulator for neurological gait rehabilitation. *Proc. Second Joint EMBS/BMES Conf.* 3:2356–57
114. Krebs HI, Aisen ML, Volpe BT, Hogan N. 1999. Quantization of continuous arm movements in humans with brain injury. *Proc. Nat. Acad. Sci USA* 96:4645–49
115. Reinkensmeyer D, Iobbi M, Kahn L, Kamper D, Takahashi C. 2003. Modeling reaching impairment after stroke using a population vector model of movement control that incorporates neural firing rate variability. *Neural Comput.* 11:In press
116. Lum PS, Burgar CG, Kenney DE, Van der Loos HF. 1999. Quantification of force abnormalities during passive and active-assisted upper-limb reaching movements in post-stroke hemiparesis. *IEEE Trans. Biomed. Eng.* 46:652–62
117. Reinkensmeyer DJ, Dewald JPA, Rymer WZ. 1999. Guidance-based quantification of arm impairment following brain injury: a pilot study. *IEEE Trans. Rehabil. Eng.* 7:1–11
118. Reinkensmeyer DJ, Schmit BD, Rymer WZ. 1999. Assessment of active and passive restraint during guided reaching after chronic brain injury. *Ann. Biomed. Eng.* 27:805–14
119. Dietz V, Mueller R, Colombo G. 2002.

Locomotor activity in spinal man: significance of afferent input from joint and load receptors. *Brain* 125:2626–34
120. Smith MA, Brandt J, Shadmehr R. 2000. Motor disorder in Huntington's disease begins as a dysfunction in error feedback control. *Nature* 403:544–49
121. Reinkensmeyer D. 2003. How to retrain movement after neurologic injury: a computational rationale for incorporating robot (or therapist) assistance. *Proceedings of the 2003 IEEE Eng. Med. Biol. Soc. Meet.*, Cancun, Mexico, pp. 1479–82
122. Harkema SJ, Hurley SL, Patel UK, Requejo PS, Dobkin BH, Edgerton VR. 1997. Human lumbosacral spinal cord interprets loading during stepping. *J. Neurophysiol.* 77:797–811
123. Lam T, Pearson KG. 2002. The role of proprioceptive feedback in the regulation and adaptation of locomotor activity. *Adv. Exp. Med. Biol.* 508:343–55
124. Feygin D, Keehner M, Tendick F. 2002. Haptic guidance: experimental evaluation of a haptic training method for a perceptual motor skill. *Proc. 10th Int. Symp. Haptic Interfaces Virtual Environ. Teleoperator Syst.* (*Haptics 2002*), *Orlando, Florida*, pp. 40–47
125. Patton J, Mussa-Ivaldi F. 2003. Robot-assisted adaptive training: custom force fields for teaching movement patterns. *IEEE Trans. Biomed. Eng.* 51:636–46
126. Raasch CC, Mussa-Ivaldi FA, Rymer WZ. 1997. Motor learning in reaching movements by hemiparetic subjects. *Soc. Neurosci. Abstr.* 23:2374
127. Kahn LE, Lum PS, Reinkensmeyer DJ. 2003. Selection of robotic therapy algorithms for the upper extremity in chronic stroke: Insights from MIME and ARM Guide results. *Proc. Int. Conf. Rehabil. Robot*, Daejeon, Korea pp. 208–10
128. STAIR II. 2001. Recommendations for clinical trial evaluation of acute stroke therapies. (Stroke Therapy Academic Industry Roundtable II). *Stroke* 32:1598–606
129. Aisen ML, Krebs HI, Hogan N, McDowell F, Volpe B. 1997. The effect of robot-assisted therapy and rehabilitative training on motor recovery following stroke. *Arch. Neurol.* 54:443–46

# Subject Index

## C

## I

## R

# Cumulative Indexes

## CONTRIBUTING AUTHORS, VOLUMES 1–6

# CHAPTER TITLES, VOLUMES 1–6

## Prefatory



## Imaging

## Biomechanical

## Biochemical